Frontiers in Anti-Infective Drug Discovery

Volume 2

Editor

Prof. Atta-ur-Rahman, *FRS*
Honorary Life Fellow
Kings College
University of Cambridge
UK

Co-Editor

Prof. M. Iqbal Choudhary
H.E.J. Research Institute of Chemistry
International Center for Chemical and Biological Sciences
University of Karachi
Pakistan

CONTENTS

CHAPTERS

PREFACE

Infections caused by viruses, bacteria, fungi and parasites are enduring threats to human well-being and survival. The discovery of antibiotics in 1928 had given the hope of controlling infectious diseases to human, livestocks and plants. However, wide spread and rapid emergence of multidrug resistance (MDR) in viruses and microorganisms, as well as their vectors, has posed a major challenge to the healthcare sector, creating a fear of return of the pre-antibiotic period. The emergence of MDR microorganisms and lack of effective antibiotics against them has direct impact on every sector of healthcare, including success of surgical interventions, post-surgical survival, neonatal and elderly care, *etc*. Unfortunately major pharmaceutical conglomerates have either closed down or downsized their anti-infectious drug discovery programs. Similarly, the number of academic researchers working on the anti-infectives agents has also reduced over he years. Ironically our understanding of infection in general, and spontaneous and acquired resistance in pathogens in particular at genetic and molecular levels, has improved substantially during the same period.

The volume entitled "*Frontiers in Anti-Infective Drug Discovery*" is our effort to highlight the continuous importance of research in this field. The volume contains five excellent articles by leading researchers in the field. These articles not only cover discoveries of anti-infective agents of natural and synthetic origins, but also review scientific work on the identification of molecular targets for new anti-infectious agents.

The article contributed by Novio *et al.* reviews the literature on antiviral properties of marine natural products, mainly from algal sources. The viruses targeted include HIV, herpes simplex, influenza and cytomegalovirus viruses.

Peptides have been known to possess a variety of biological activities, including antibacterial and cytotoxic properties. Hick and Clark have contributed a comprehensive review on the activity of synthetic peptides against the multidrug resistance bacteria and fungi, known to cause a variety of infections. Physicochemical properties concerning of peptide-cell wall lipid interactions of therapeutically important peptides, their mechanisms of action, as well as methods to overcome the problems associated with the therapeutic use natural and synthetic peptides (metabolic stability, lack of selectivity and stability, *etc*.) are also discussed.

Chopra *et al.* in their review focus on the diverse scaffolds of natural products and their anti-infective properties. These natural inhibitors provide excellent leads for further development. The advent of enabling technologies for the dereplication, isolation and structure determination of natural products, as well as the development of new biological screening methods, have further accelerated the process of discovery of new anti-infective agents from natural sources.

The understanding the multidrug resistance the mechanisms molecular level is the key to modern drug discovery and development against pathogenic agents. Salem and Zuel-Fakkar have reviewed the recent developments in the fields of molecular and structural biology and molecular genetics, related to intrinsic and acquired resistance in microorganisms, against available drugs. These complex molecular processes help us to understand the mechanisms of inhibition and to identify the targets for development of the next generations of antibiotics and MDR reversal agents.

Last but not least, Maderia and Phillips have reviewed the recent scientific work on the prevention and treatment of malaria through anti-malarial chemotherapies. Malaria being the major killer of human race, particularly in developing countries, remains a gigantic healthcare challenge for national governments and for pharmaceutical and biomedical R&D scientists. The development of new leads for malarial prevention and treatment is focused in this review.

We are confident that these contributions by experienced researchers will not only help the readers in developing a better understanding of the science behind anti-infection drug discovery and development, but most importantly will highlight the importance of systematic and sustainable efforts in this area. We are grateful to all the contributors for their diligent efforts in reviewing the recent literature on various aspects of the field in comprehensive and timely manner. We also acknowledge the efforts and hard work of the editorial team, particularly Mr. Mahmood Alam (Director Publication) and Miss. Hira Aftab (Assistant Manager) of Bentham Science Publishers.

Prof. Atta-ur-Rahman, *FRS*
Honorary Life Fellow
Kings College
University of Cambridge
UK

LIST OF CONTRIBUTORS

Sidharth Chopra
Central Drug Research Institute, Lucknow, UP, India

Ellen D. Beaulieu
SRI International, Biosciences Division, Menlo Park, CA, USA

Jeremiah P. Malerich
SRI International, Biosciences Division, Menlo Park, CA, USA

Silvia Novío
Department of Pharmacology, Lennart Levi Stress and Neuroimmunology Laboratory, School of Medicine, C/ San Francisco s/n, 15782 Santiago de Compostela, Spain

María Jesús Núñez
Department of Pharmacology, Lennart Levi Stress and Neuroimmunology Laboratory, School of Medicine, C/ San Francisco s/n, 15782 Santiago de Compostela, Spain

Manuel Freire-Garabal
Department of Pharmacology, Lennart Levi Stress and Neuroimmunology Laboratory, School of Medicine, C/ San Francisco s/n, 15782 Santiago de Compostela, Spain

Rickey P. Hicks
Department of Chemistry, East Carolina University, Greenville, NC 27858, USA

Tiffany D. Clark
Department of Chemistry, East Carolina University, Greenville, NC 27858, USA

Ana Maria Madeira M. Faísca Phillips
Department of Chemistry, Faculty of Sciences and Technology, Universidade Nova de Lisboa, Campus de Caparica, Quinta da Torre, 2829-516 Caparica, Portugal

Samar Abdallah M. Salem
Dermatology, Venereology and Anderology Department, Faculty of Medicine, Ain Shams University, Cairo, Egypt

Nehal M. Zuel-Fakkar
Dermatology, Venereology and Anderology Department, Faculty of Medicine, Ain Shams University, Cairo, Egypt

Send Orders for Reprints to reprints@benthamscience.net

Frontiers in Anti-Infective Drug Discovery, Vol. 2, 2014, 3-85

CHAPTER 1

Marine Red Algae as Source of Bioactive Therapeutic Molecules with Activity Against Viral Infection

Silvia Novío*, María Jesús Núñez and Manuel Freire-Garabal

Lennart Levi Stress and Neuroimmunology Laboratory, Department of Pharmacology, School of Medicine, C/ San Francisco s/n, 15782 Santiago de Compostela, Spain

Abstract: This chapter is an updated review of the literature published since 1980s about compounds with antiviral properties isolated from red seaweed (Rhodophyta). It integrates findings from molecular, experimental and cellular researches to show an overview of potential antiviral agents derived from Rhodophyta and their promising application in viral therapy. Extracts of and/or compounds isolated from red seaweed, mainly polysaccharides, play a protective role against different viruses such as human immunodeficiency virus, herpes simplex virus, influenza virus, cytomegalovirus, and others. The main target of the antiviral action of these algal compounds is the initial binding of pathogens to the host cells.

Keywords: Agars, antiviral activity, carrageenans, extracts, galactans, mannans, marine, natural, polysaccharides, rhodophyta, viruses.

INTRODUCTION

Viruses are ubiquitous, highly abundant and extraordinarily diverse [1]. They are the most abundant biological entities on the planet with the total number of virus particles exceeding the number of cells by at least an order of magnitude [2, 3]. Fig. **1** shows the classification of animal viruses according to their genomes and mode of propagation [4, 5].

***Address correspondence to Silvia Novío:** Lennart Levi Stress and Neuroimmunology Laboratory, Department of Pharmacology, School of Medicine, C/ San Francisco s/n, 15782 Santiago de Compostela, Spain; Tel: +34 981581744; Fax: +34 981573191; E-mail: snl@usc.es

Atta-ur-Rahman / M. Iqbal Choudhary (Eds.)

CLASS I (dsDNA)

Genome and transcription

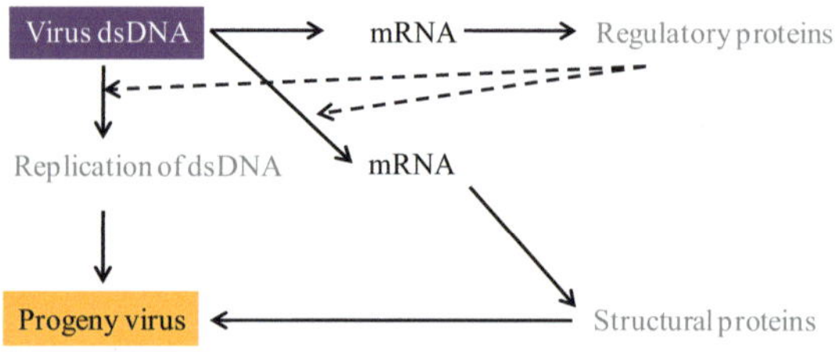

CLASS Ia (replication in the host-cell nucleus)

Examples of viruses

Adenovirus...

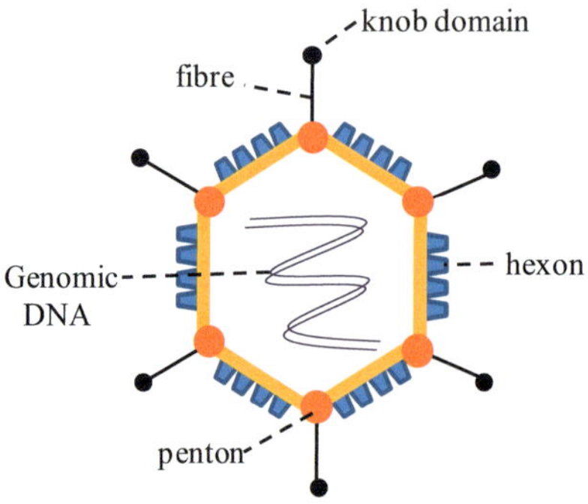

Characteristics [6]:

- Family: Adenoviridae
- Ubiquitous in human and animal populations
- More than 50 serotypes of adenovirus have been identified, which are further classified into subgroups: A-F
- The predominant serotypes differ among countries or regions and change over time
- It is isolated most commonly in infants and children
- It causes infections in the upper respiratory tract, gastroenteritis and conjunctivitis. Most infections are asymptomatic
- Treatment is controversial

Herpes simplex virus (HSV)...

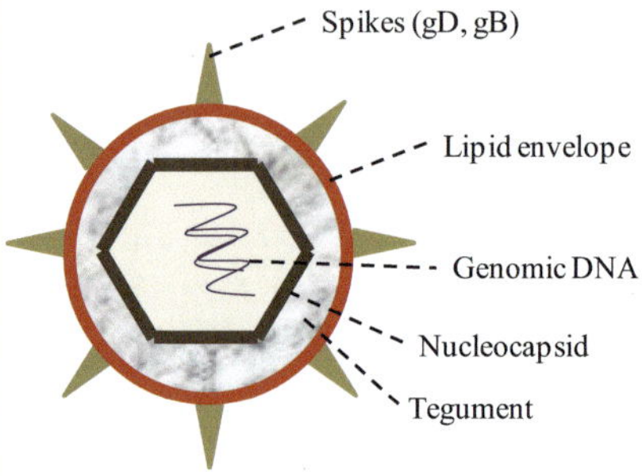

Characteristics [7]:

- Family: Herpesviridae
- 40-80% of people worldwide is infected by HSV
- HSV results in a lifelong infection
- Glycoproteins D (gD) and B (gB) play essential roles for HSV entry
- There are two types of HSV: type-1 (HSV-1) and type-2 (HSV-2)
- HSV is neurotropic. It can infect the nervous system and cause neurological diseases
- HSV-1 produces most cold sores and HSV-2 produces most genital herpes
- Acyclovir is the drug of choice

(Fig. 1) contd…..

Cytomegalovirus...

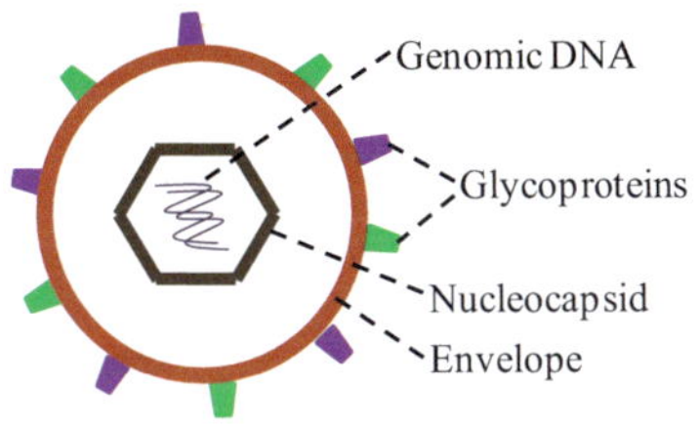

Characteristics [8]:

- Family: Herpesviridae
- It is one of the most successful human pathogens
- Infection is dependent on the functions of structural glycoproteins at multiple stages of the viral life cycle
- Transmission may occur *in utero,* perinatally or postnatally
- Most cytomegalovirus infections are asymptomatic; however, some people develop severe infections that can be life threatening

CLASS Ib (replication in the host-cell cytoplasm)

Examples of viruses

Variola virus...

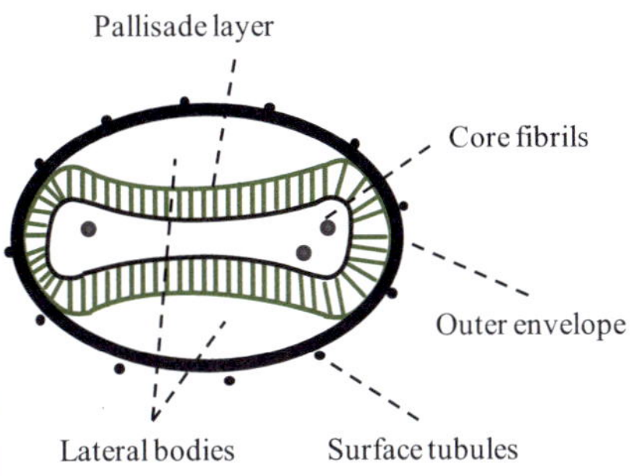

Characteristics [9]:

- Family: Poxviridae
- It is one of the most significant bioterrorist threat agents
- It is highly stable and retains its infectivity for long periods outside the host
- Virus transmission: face-to-face contact, direct contact with infected fluids and contaminated objects or through the air
- It causes smallpox (eradicated in 1979 through a worldwide vaccination campaign with Vaccinia virus)

CLASS II (ssDNA)

Genome and transcription

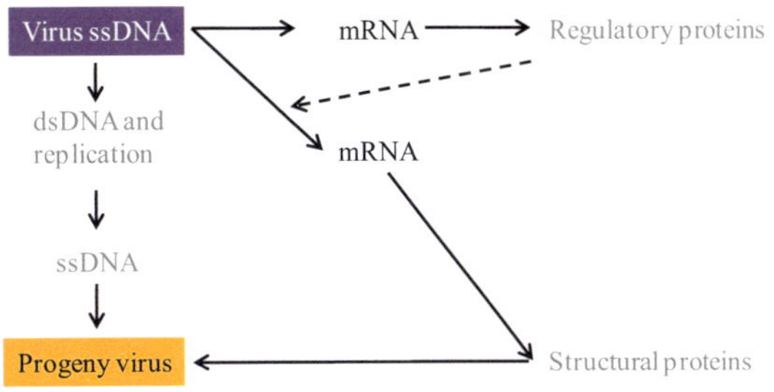

(Fig. 1) contd…..

Examples of viruses

Parvovirus…

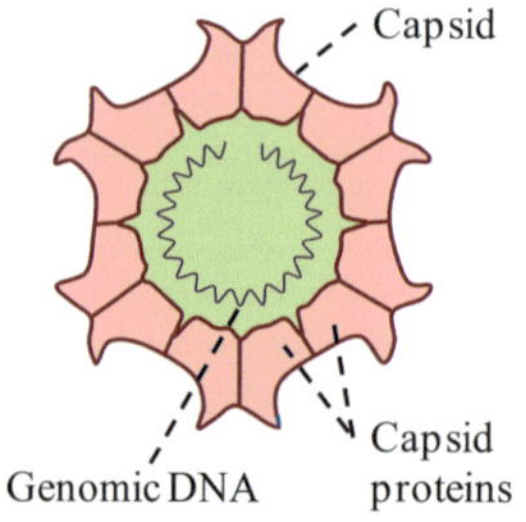

Characteristics [10]:

- Family: Parvoviridae
- Parvovirus B19 is the first (and until 2005 the only) known human virus in the family of parvoviruses
- It is primarily spread by infected respiratory droplets
- The only known host for B19 is humans
- Parvovirus B19 virus causes erythematous rash that affects the face, trunk and limbs of the body

CLASS III (dsRNA)

Genome and transcription

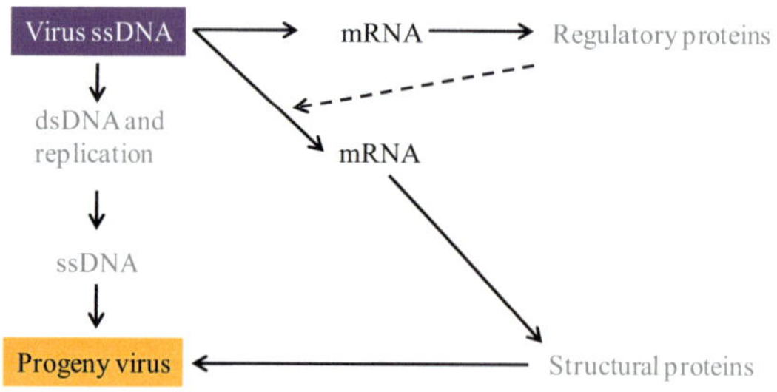

Examples of viruses

Orthoreovirus (reovirus)…

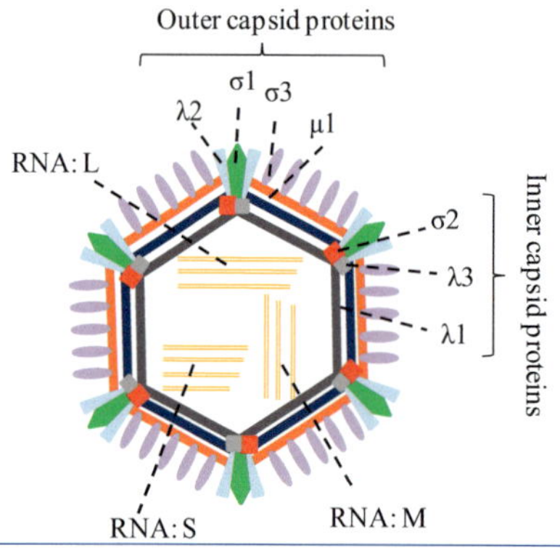

Characteristics [11]:

- Family: Reoviridae (the largest of the eight recognized dsRNA virus families)
- The orthoreovirus dsRNA genome contains 10 segments divided into three size classes: three large (L1, L2 and L3) segments, three medium segments (M1, M2 and M3), and four small segments (S1, S2, S3 and S4)
- It causes infections in the upper respiratory tract and gastrointestinal tract
- Reovirus is a wild-type oncolytic virus that is currently being investigated as a potential novel therapy for cancer

(Fig. 1) contd…..

Rotavirus…

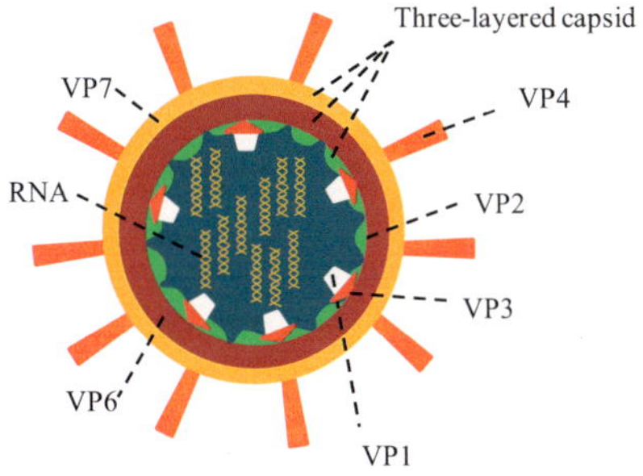

Characteristics [12]:

- Family: Reoviridae
- There are five species: A-E
- Structural proteins (VP1, VP2, VP3, VP4, VP6 and VP7) form the virus particle
- Nonstructural proteins (NSP1, NSP2, NSP3, NSP4, NSP5, NSP6) are only produced in cells infected by this virus
- It is transmitted by the faecal-oral route
- It is the most common cause of severe diarrheal illness in children
- Vaccination is now recommended by the World Health Organization for all children worldwide

CLASS IV ((+)ssRNA viruses)

Genome and transcription

Class IVa **Class IVb**

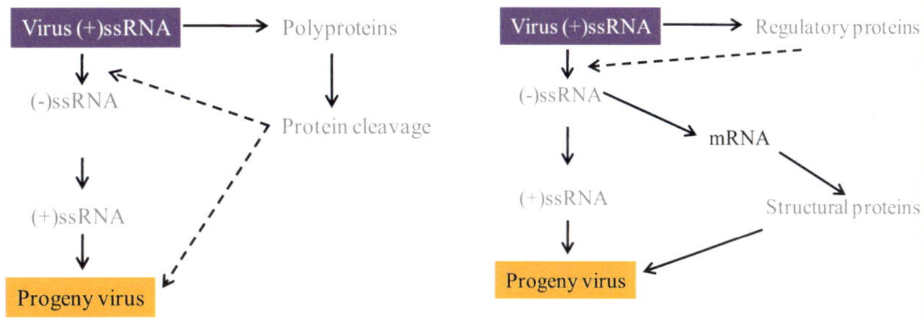

Examples of viruses

SARS coronavirus…

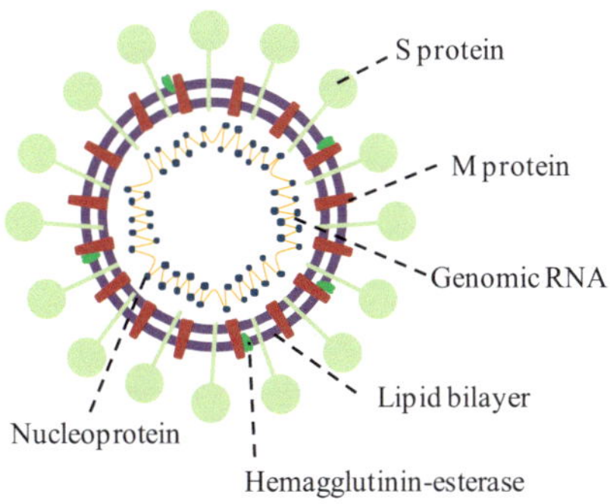

Characteristics [13]:

- Family: Coronaviridae
- It causes severe acute respiratory syndrome (SARS) that emerged in the human population in China in 2002
- The large spike protein (S) on the virion surface mediates both cell attachment and membrane fusion
- The coronavirus membrane protein (M) is the key player in the assembly of virions at intracellular membranes between endoplasmic-reticulum and Golgi-complex
- There is no agreed treatment for SARS other than management of symptoms. Drugs are under development and of particular interest are drugs that may block the protease (M(pro)) function

(Fig. 1) contd…..

Hepatitis A virus…

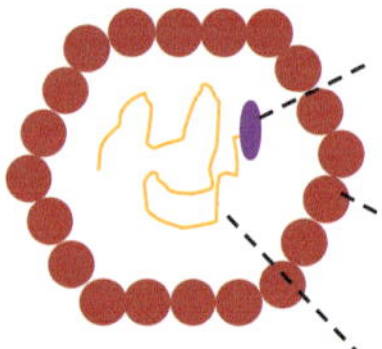

Characteristics [14]:

- Family: Picornaviridae
- Viral proteins genome-linked (VPgs) are involved in the replication of viral RNA and might serve as primers in the synthesis of viral RNA
- It is fecal-orally transmitted
- Hepatitis A is the most common infection of the liver worldwide
- Symptoms include fever, tiredness, loss of appetite, nausea, abdominal discomfort, dark urine, and jaundice
- There are two types of hepatitis A virus vaccine: inactivated and live attenuated, which confer significant protection for at least 2 and 5 years, respectively

Hepatitis C virus…

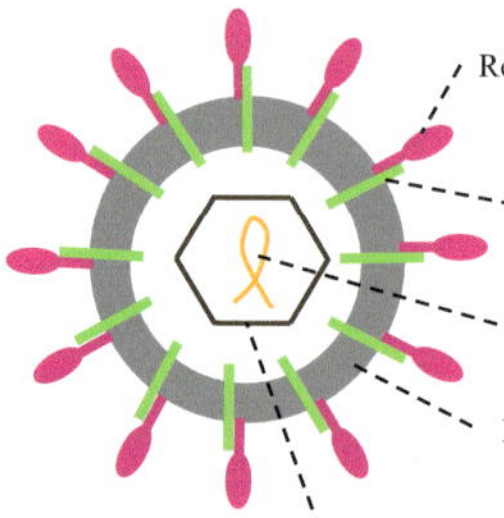

Characteristics [15]:

- Family: Flaviviridae
- Hepatitis C virus infection is the most common chronic bloodborne infection in the world
- HCV entry is a highly orchestrated process involving viral and host cell factors. These include the viral envelope glycoproteins E1 and E2, CD81, scavenger receptor BI, and tight junction proteins claudin-1 and occludin
- Hepatitis C virus infection can lead to cirrhosis, liver failure, and hepatocellular carcinoma
- Preventive modalities are absent and the current antiviral treatment is limited by resistance, toxicity, and very high costs

Alphavirus…

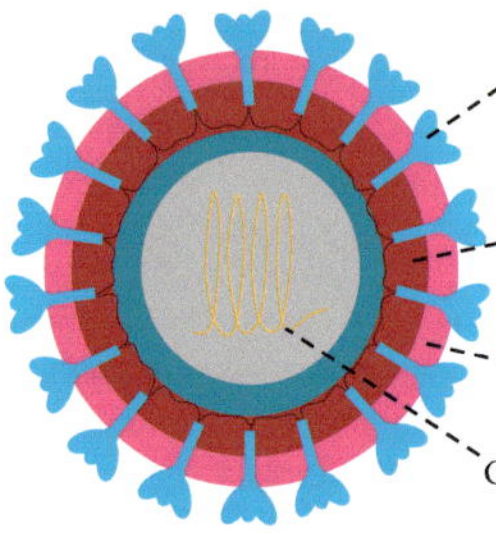

Characteristics [16]:

- Family: Togaviridae
- Alphavirus members include Semliki Forest virus, Sindbis virus, Western equine encephalitis virus…
- Trimers of E1/E2 heterodimers form the viral spikes complexes on the virion surface
- The viruses are transmitted by bloodsucking arthropods
- Alphaviruses can cause encephalitis and they have been associated with outbreaks of acute and persistent arthritis and arthralgia in humans
- Alphavirus vectors are very attractive for cancer treatment and vaccination

(Fig. 1) contd…..

Flavivirus (*e.g.* dengue virus)…

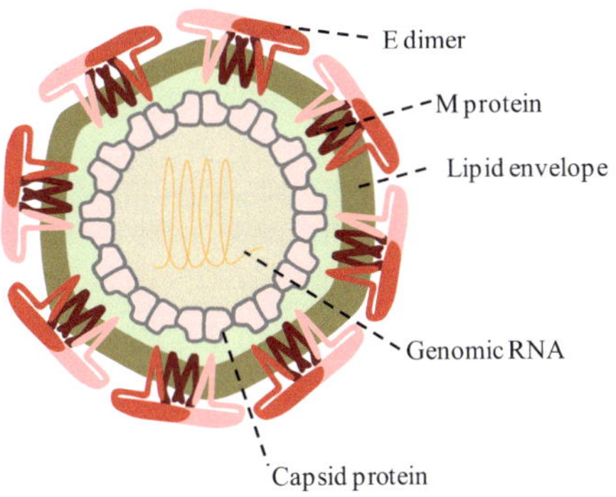

Characteristics [17]:

- Family: Flaviviridae
- Dengue virus is a major emerging arthopod-borne pathogen causing a significant burden of disease in tropical and subtropical areas of the world
- The envelope glycoprotein E and the membrane protein M are inserted in the lipid envelope. E protein is important in the initial attachment of the viral particle to the host cell, whereas M protein is implicated in the formation and maturation of the viral particle
- Dengue virus is the cause of dengue fever (muscle and joint pains, headache, fever, and skin rash that is similar to measles)

Enterovirus…

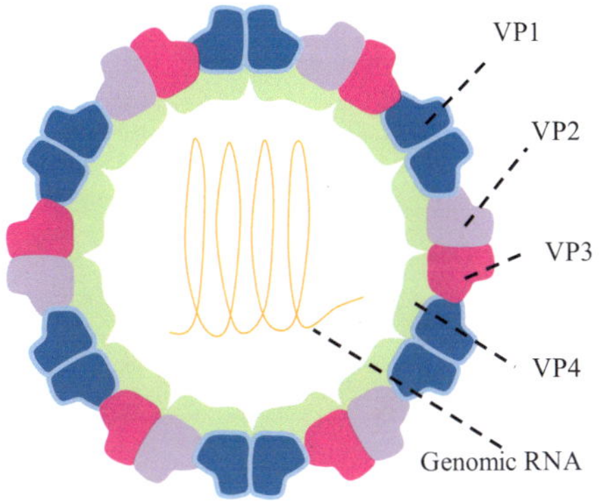

Characteristics [18, 19]:

- Family: Picornaviridae
- The viral capsid is composed of four proteins: VP1–4
- Enteroviruses include echoviruses, coxsackie A and B viruses, polioviruses…
- Enteroviruses are among the most common viruses causing disease in humans. A large proportion of enteroviral infections occur in neonates and infants
- Enterovirus infections range from benign short-lived febrile illnesses to life-threatening infections
- There are two types of coxsackie viruses namely type A and B. The first type causes muscle injury, paralysis and rarely death. The second one causes damage to internal organs although outcomes are less severe
- The coxsackie B viruses are the most common agent for myocarditis and dilated cardiomyopathy (50% of infections)
- Oral poliovirus vaccine is a highly effective tool although it has been associated to serious adverse effects

(Fig. 1) contd…..

CLASS V ((-)ssRNA viruses)

Genome and transcription

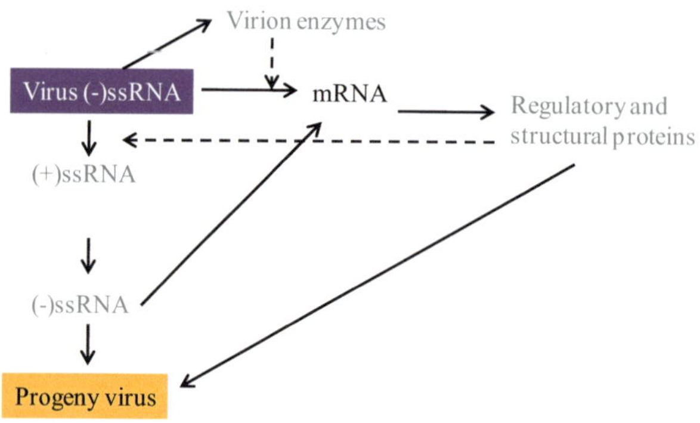

Vesicular stomatitis virus…

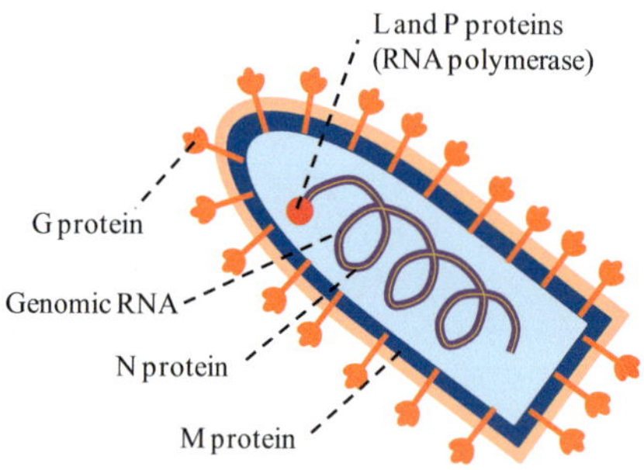

Characteristics [20]:

- Family: Rhabdoviridae
- Strand RNA is composed of 5 genes N, P, M, G, and L representing the nucleocapsid protein, phosphoprotein, matrix protein, glycoprotein (mediates viral attachment to the host cell), and the large protein, respectively
- Virus can be transmitted through direct contact with infected animals or by blood-feeding insects
- It causes vesicles, ulcers, erosions in the oral cavity and lesions at the mucocutaneous junctions of the lips

Influenza virus…

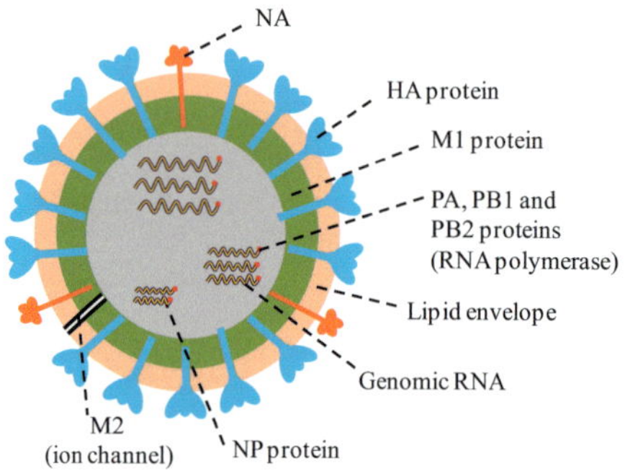

Characteristics [21, 22]:

- Family: Orthomyxoviridae
- RNA strands code for eleven proteins: HA (hemagglutinin), NA (neuraminidase), NP (nucleoprotein), NS1 and NEP (non-structural proteins), PA, PB1 and PB2 (RNA polymerase), PB1-F2 (induces apoptosis), M1 and M2 (matrix proteins)
- Influenza virus infections range from subclinical upper respiratory tract disease to fatal lower respiratory tract disease
- Immunization against influenza is considered an essential public health intervention to control both seasonal epidemic and pandemic influenza

(Fig. 1) contd…..

Respiratory syncytial virus (RSV)…

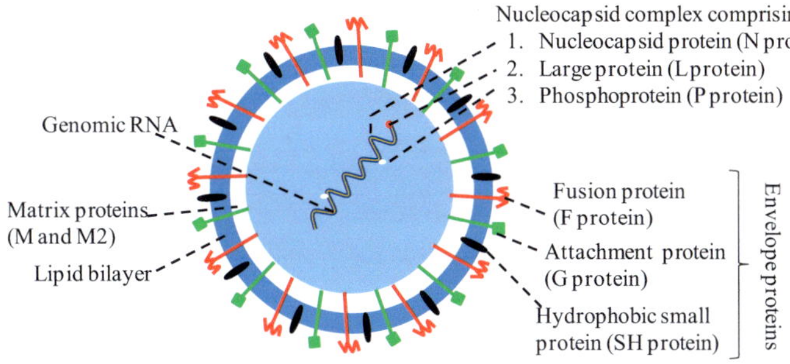

Characteristics [22]:

- Family: Paramyxoviridae
- By age 2, nearly all children have been infected with respiratory syncytial virus (RSV), with 1% to 3% hospitalized because of the infection
- The virus recruits immune cells to the lungs, triggering an inflammatory process that results in the production of a thick mucus that blocks alveoli in the bronchioles
- Successful treatment of RSV infection may require the use of an antiviral agent in combination with an anti-inflammatory agent

Parainfluenza virus (PIV)…

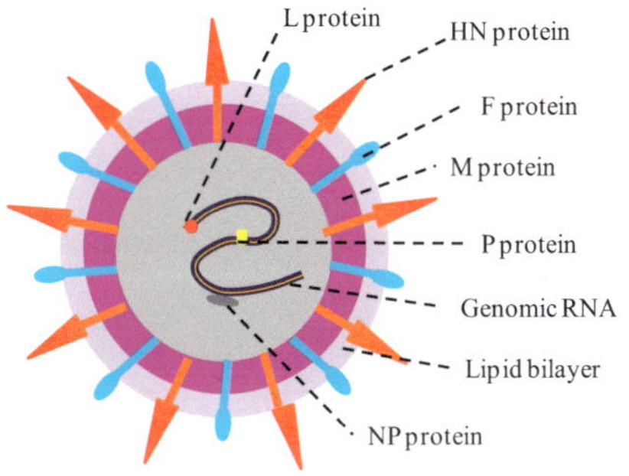

Characteristics [23]:

- Family: Paramyxoviridae
- Its genome encodes six key structural proteins: Hemagglutinin-neuraminidase (HN), fusion (F), matrix (M), nucleoprotein (NP), large (L) and phospho- (P) proteins
- PIV1 and PIV2 are best known to cause croup while PIV3 is a common cause of bronchiolitis and pneumonia
- There is no specific treatment/vaccine for the PIV infection

Arenavirus…

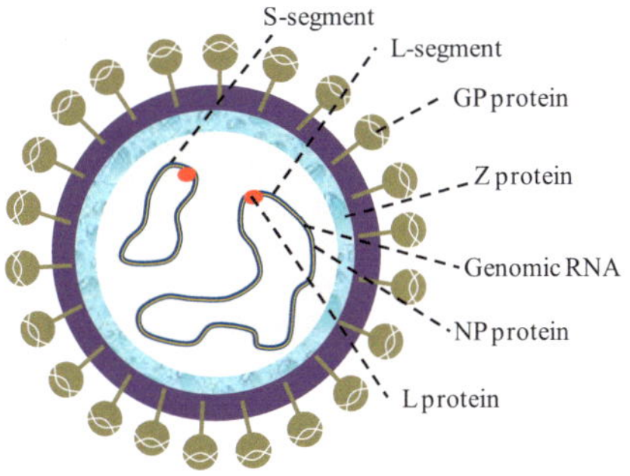

Characteristics [24]:

- Family: Arenaviridae
- Segmented RNA genome: The S-segment RNA encodes the viral nucleocapsid protein (NP) and glycoprotein (GP); the L-segment RNA encodes the viral RNA-dependent RNA-polymerase (L) and a small RING-domain containing protein (Z)
- Junin virus is the etiological agent of Argentine hemorrhagic fever
- Current treatment: early transfusion of immune plasma in standardized doses of neutralizing antibodies. Ribavirin has also shown some promise

(Fig. 1) contd…..

Measles virus…

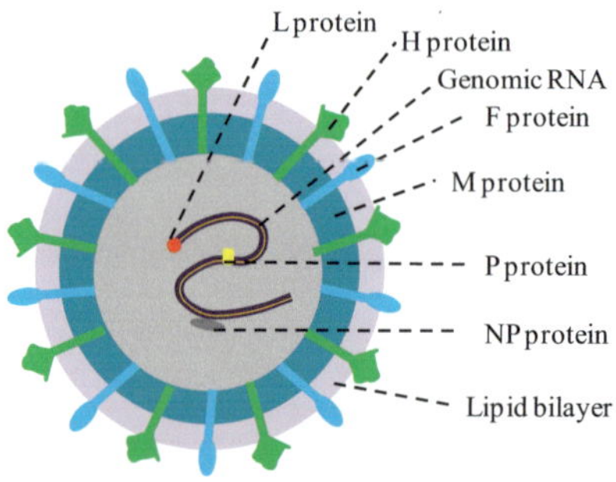

Characteristics [25]:

- Family: Paramyxoviridae
- The genome contains six genes that encode the nucleocapsid (NP), phospho- (P), matrix (M), fusion (F), haemagglutinin (H) and large (L) proteins
- The virus is transmitted *via* aerosol droplets
- It causes measles, one of the typical viral diseases of childhood
- Symptoms include fever, dry cough, runny nose, conjunctivitis, sore throat and a generalized maculopapular erythematous rash
- There is no specific treatment for measles

CLASS VI (ssRNA-RT)

Genome and transcription

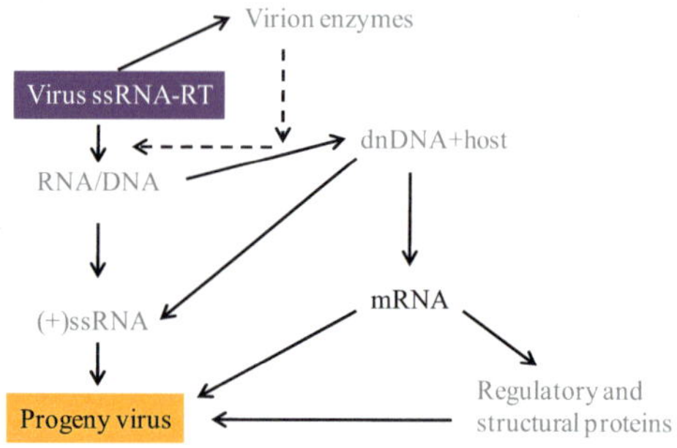

Examples of viruses

Human immunodeficiency virus (HIV)…

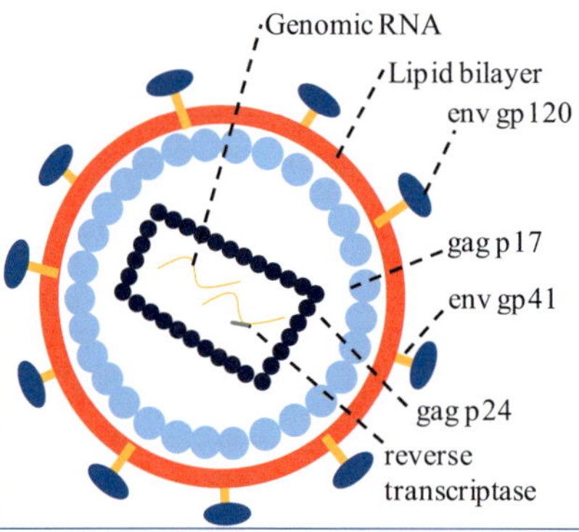

Characteristics [26]:

- Family: Retroviridae
- There are an estimated 39 million people living with HIV/AIDS worldwide, while about 25 million have died already
- Heterosexual transmission remains the dominant mode of transmission (85% of all HIV-1 infections)
- HIV causes acquired immunodeficiency syndrome (AIDS)
- Antiretroviral treatment is the best therapeutic option. However, current drugs do not eradicate HIV-1 infection and lifelong treatment might be needed

(Fig. 1) contd…..

CLASS VII (dsDNA-RT)

Genome and transcription

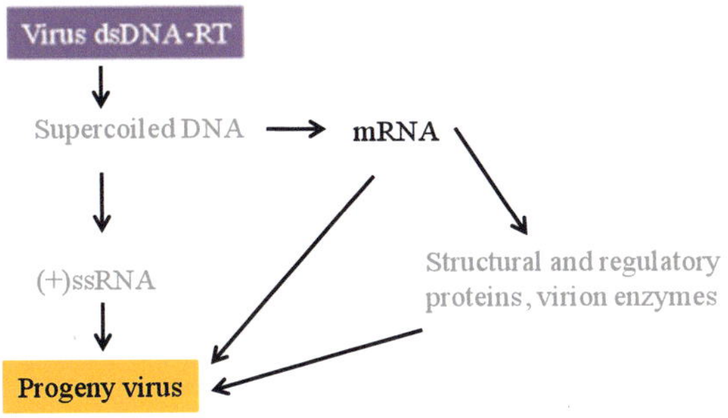

Examples of viruses

Hepatitis B virus (HBV)…

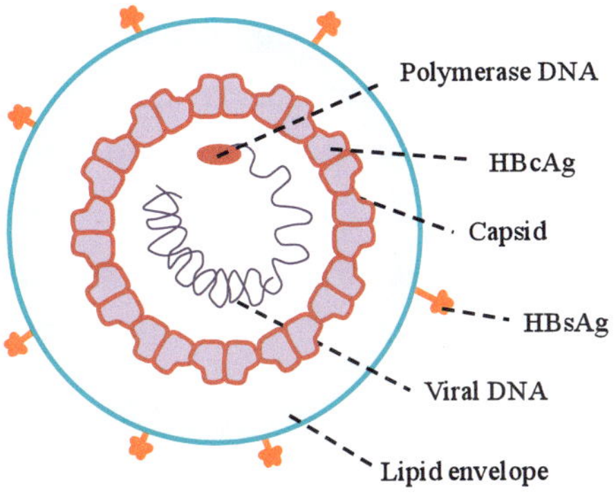

Characteristics [27]:

- Family: Hepadnaviridae
- HBsAg is made up of three glycoproteins (L, S, M) that are encoded by the same gene
- The main transmission routes include perinatal infection, the skin and mucous membrane infections caused by contaminated blood or body fluids, and sexual contacts
- Hepatitis B shows variable clinical manifestations ranging from asymptomatic HBV carriers to fulminant liver failure, and it becomes chronic, often progresses to chronic hepatitis, cirrhosis, and hepatocellular carcinoma
- Hepatitis B is a preventable disease; a safe and effective vaccine is available

Fig. (1). Classification of animal viruses according to their genomes and mode of propagation. Some of the most important viruses from a clinical point of view are indicated. Likewise, their structure as well as diseases that they cause more frequently are also detailed. Abbreviations: dsDNA: double-stranded DNA; dsRNA: double-stranded RNA; ssDNA: single-stranded DNA; ssRNA: single-stranded RNA; (+): positive strand; (-): negative strand.

Viral diseases have had a very important role throughout the mankind. In fact, they have been associated to huge tragedies. The “Spanish flu” pandemic of 1918 is a clear example. The 1918 flu pandemic killed more than 50 million people worldwide and it is thought to have contributed in the ending World War I. Nowadays, these diseases are still a leading cause of death in humans (*e.g.,* the SARS outbreak of early 2003 or the H1N1 flu pandemic that began in the Spring of 2009), particularly for immunocompromised individuals including: i) solid organ transplant recipients; ii) haematopoietic stem cell transplant recipients; iii) patients with primary immunodeficiency, and iv) HIV-infected patients [28, 29]. In this way, the control of viruses is a necessity of first order.

Numerous treatments have gained a notable success in reducing the severity of viral infections [30, 31], however no antiviral therapy could be considered perfect. It is said that an antiviral drug is effective if: its antiviral action is specific, it has a broad spectrum of activity and favourable pharmacodynamic properties, it irreversibly blocks viral synthesis in order to stop cell suicide due to the viral infection and restore normal cell synthesis, and it is not immunosuppressive [32]. However, one of the most important reasons for the lack of success in developing antiviral drugs is due to the nature of the infectious viral agents, which totally depend upon the cell they infect for their multiplication and survival, so that many compounds that may cause the death of viruses are also very likely to injure the host cell that harbor them [33]. Furthermore, these drugs are not always well-tolerated and viral mutans, which acquire resistance to drugs, have arisen during last decade. Thus, it would seem imperative search for new antiviral compounds [34-36].

Diverse strategies have been carried out to research on compounds which might be potential therapeutic agents targeting different steps in the viral replication cycle [37]. An understanding of the molecular mechanisms of viral invasion and replication are necessary to make the dream comes true. Since current antiviral therapies are insufficient for treating emerging, re-emerging and established viral diseases, screening of natural products derived from numerous species has afforded metabolites with interesting biological activities [36, 38-58]. They have been described as analgesic, anticancer, antidiabetic, anticoagulant, antiinflammatory and antimicrobial (antibacterial, antifungal or antiviral) agents, so they might find relevance in cosmetic/cosmeceutical and pharmaceutical applications [59-64]. This enormous body of knowledge however contrasts with the real potential that is thought these compounds have.

In this review, we will examine current progress in research of compounds with antiviral properties isolated from red seaweed. In the light of the evidence that will be mentioned later, the authors think that these natural products are a great promise as potentially effective new antiviral drugs. Besides offering major opportunities for finding novel structures that are active against a wide range of targets, they are generally molecules with drug-like properties (*i.e.,* they are capable of being absorbed and metabolized by the body), so costs of producing orally active medicines are likely to be much lower than that of biotechnological products or compounds produced from combinatorial chemistry.

Marine Environment

The marine environment represents approximately half of the global biodiversity. Algae are heterogeneous group of plants in the marine environment, which are grouped into two main classes: macroalgae (or seaweeds) and microalgae. Macroalgae are in the littoral zone and include green (division Chlorophyta), brown (division Phaeophyta) and red (division Rhodophyta) macroalgae. Microalgae occupy littoral and bentheic habitats and ocean waters as phytoplankton, this is diatoms (bacillariophyta), dinoflagellates (dinophyta), green and yellow-brown flagellates (chlorophyta, prasinophyta, prymnesiophyta, cryptophyta, chrysophyta and rhaphidiophyta) and blue-green algae (cyanophyta) [65]. Algae are an enormous resource for valuable natural compounds such as xanthophylls, vitamins, chlorophyll, carotenoids, terpenoids, amino acids, saturated and polyunsaturated fatty acids, acetogenins, antioxidants such as polyphenols, alkaloids, halogenated compounds and polysaccharides such as agars, carrageenans, proteoglycans, alginate, laminaran, rhamnan sulfate, galactosyl glycerol and fucoidan, besides others [66-90]. The resources of these compounds are potentially enormous, they can be extracted from various marine environments such as Mediterranean [91-93], Britain [94], India [95], Korea [96, 97], Japan [98], New Zealand [99], Moroccan coast [100] or South American coast [72].

The original data on antiviral activities of algal constituents go back more than 50 years to the observation that seaweed extracts protected chicken embryos against influenza B and mumps [101]. During 1960s and 1970s, several studies were carried out which demonstrated antiviral effects associated to algal substances against other pathogenic agents [59, 102-104]. However, these observations did not generate much interest because the antiviral action of those compounds was considered to be largely nonspecific [68]. A growing expectation about these substances arose recently after the isolation from algae of compounds with antiviral activity against enveloped viruses such as human immunodeficiency virus [68, 93, 99, 105-117], herpes simplex virus type 1 and type 2 [59, 66-69, 71, 75, 78, 91, 100, 104, 107, 116, 118-142], influenza A virus [68, 107, 143], respiratory syncytial virus [68, 107, 143], simian immunodeficiency virus [143], pseudorabies virus [122] or human cytomegalovirus [66, 68, 107, 122, 143].

Red Macroalgae

The Rhodophyta are a large assemblage of between 2500 and 6000 species in about 670 largely marine genera [144] that predominate along the coastal and continental shelf areas of tropical, temperate and cold-water regions [145].

Red algae are an interesting source of biologically active compounds including antiviral ones. For this reason, extensive farming and natural harvest of red algae occurs in numerous areas of the world. Despite different substances can be isolated from these algae, such as terpenes [108, 118], glycolipids [110, 142], lectins [99, 112, 114, 115, 117, 146-149] or phenolic compounds [130], their ability to synthesize polysaccharides is the most interesting property of red seaweeds. Polysaccharides from red seaweeds include different sulfated galactans [68, 75, 78, 93, 100, 107, 109, 113, 122, 128, 131, 132, 141, 150], sulfated rhamnans or mannans [67, 111, 119-121, 139, 140, 143], agars [73, 151, 152] and carrageenans [66, 69, 123, 124, 129, 133-135, 150, 153, 154].

Sulfated galactans are the major extracellular polysaccharides produced by red seaweeds. They essentially consist of linear chains of alternating 3-linked β-D-galactopyranosyl (G units) and 4-linked α-galactopyranosyl residues, which are classified either as carrageenans if the 4-linked α-galactopyranosyl units are in the D-configuration (D unit) or agarans if the 4-linked α-galactopyranosyl units are in the L-configuration (L unit). In these galactans, the D and L units may exist in the 3,6- anhydrogalactopyranosyl form (DA and LA, respectively) [155]. A third group of galactans, namely the DL-hybrids [156], contains G units linked to both, D and L units [156-160]. *Mannans* are polysaccharides with a backbone chain of β-1,4-linked mannose units. They comprise linear or branched polymers [161]. In some algae species, linear mannan seems to replace cellulose as the main cell wall glycan [162]. *Agars* are typically low in sulfate ester substitution, but those from numerous sources are rich in methyl ether or pyruvate acetal substitution. Conversely, *carrageenans* (name derived from the Irish coastal town of Carragheen) are comparatively rich in sulfate ester substitution but poor in methyl ether substitution, and rarely contain significant levels of pyruvate acetal substitution [163]. Three main forms of carrageenans have been identified: kappa, iota, and lambda. They differ from each other in sulfation degree, solubility and gelling properties [164, 165].

The clinical use of polysaccharides is limited by their high molecular weight [166], however they offer a number of important features as candidate antiviral agents: they are potent specific inhibitors of viral replication at micromolar concentrations, inhibit syncytium formation and cell-to-cell adhesions [167-169], are not cytotoxic, and selection for drug resistance *in vitro* is very low [113, 169, 170].

In general, the antiviral effect of algal compounds can be attributed to an inhibitory action on the initial attachment of the virus to the host cells, and is thought to be mediated by interactions of compounds with positively charged domains of the viral envelope glycoproteins involved in the attachment of the virus to the surface of the host cells [68, 127, 152, 171]. The antimicrobial activity of these compounds is determined by their chemical structure including the degree of sulfation, molecular weight, constituent sugars, conformation and dynamic stereochemistry [77, 152, 169]. Although there is not a total agreement [172], it is known that both the degree of sulfation and the distribution of sulfate groups are the most important factors on which the antiviral activity of these substances depends. Algal compounds with low degrees of sulfation are generally inactive [152], while more highly sulfated ones appear to inhibit virus adsorption [153, 173].

Compounds from Red Algae with Antiviral Activity

Table **1** includes the main extracts and/or substances isolated from red seaweeds which have shown to have antiviral activity against a wide spectrum of viruses including important human pathogenic agents such as human immunodeficiency virus [68, 93, 99, 105-117], herpes simplex virus [59, 66-69, 71, 75, 78, 91, 100, 104, 107, 116, 118-142], vesicular stomatitis virus [59, 66, 68, 104, 107, 118], cytomegalovirus [66, 68, 107, 122, 143], dengue virus [128, 132, 133, 150], vaccinia virus [59, 66, 68, 104, 107, 153], influenza virus [68, 107, 174], and others [66, 68, 69, 103, 107, 122-124, 129, 134, 135, 143, 146-148, 153, 154]. All species tested are red algae belonging to class Florideophyceae. A meticulous description about the compounds cited in Table **1** and their properties can be consulted in the next pages.

Florideophyceae. Bonnemaisoniales. Bonnemaisoniaceae

Asparagopsis Armata is the only species of family Bonnemaisoniaceae (order Bonnemaisoniales) which antiviral activity has been screened in.

Asparagopsis Armata

The ontogenesis of the Mediterranean invasive species Asparagopsis armata is an alternation of morphologically dissimilar gametic, carposporic, and tetrasporic reproductive phases which produce complex sulfated galactans composed of galactose:anhydrogalactose:sulfates in molar ratios of 1:0.01:1.23, 1: 0.04:0.47 and 1:0.01:1.13, respectively [176]. These peculiar polymers of 1,3- and 1,4-linked galactose units, containing uronic acids (3.5±15.9% dry wt.) and in which D-galactose content (77.6±92.6% of total galactose) exceeds L-galactose content, agree neither with ideal carageenan- nor agar-type polysaccharides.

Several extracts or components from this alga have been demonstrated to possess potent antiviral activity against herpes simplex virus and human immunodeficiency virus.

i. Herpes Simplex Virus

Different extracts from Asparagopsis Armata, of which the main effective components are polysaccharides, have important antiherpetic effect; however there are significant differences in relation to their potency. Water extract (EC_{50} = <2.5 µg mL^{-1}) from Asparagopsis Armata has a higher anti-HSV-1 effect than methanolic (EC_{50} = 7.7 µg mL^{-1}), dichloromethane (EC_{50} = 22.8 µg mL^{-1}) or chloroforme-methanol (EC_{50} = 40.9 µg mL^{-1}) extracts. Likewise, it is the less cytotoxic one: the percentages of Vero cell destruction are 18.4% for the aqueous extract (CC_{50} = >250 µg mL^{-1}), 67.6% for the methanolic extract (CC_{50} = 142.4 µg mL^{-1}), 56.8% for the chloroforme-methanol extract (CC_{50} = 157.1 µg mL^{-1}) and 62.3% for the dichloromethane extract (CC_{50} = 119.1 µg mL^{-1}) [100].

ii. Human Immunodeficiency Virus

Gametic and tetrasporic galactans extracted from Asparagopsis Armata inhibit human immunodeficiency virus type 1 replication at concentrations of 10 and 8 µg mL^{-1}, respectively. However, the carposporic polysaccharide is ineffective, even at concentrations of 100 µg mL^{-1} [93].

The mechanism of anti-human immunodeficiency virus action is generally attributed to the inhibition of virus attachment to the cell surface by ionic interactions between polysaccharides and cells. In general, preincubation of sulfated polysaccharides with cell rather than virus is necessary to get an effective inhibition of the attachment [177], however this is not the case for galactans from Asparagopsis Armata, since an inhibition is observed when the polysaccharide is added after or during infection but not before infection [93]. This time of action suggests an inhibition of an early step of human immunodeficiency virus infection, probably on the reverse transcription step [93].

Florideophyceae. Ceramiales. Ceramiaceae

Species of family Ceramiaceae (order Ceramiales) which antiviral activity has been screened in include: Ceramium Rubrum, Georgiella Confluens, and Griffthsia sp.

Ceramium Rubrum

Ceramium rubrum has antiviral properties against influenza virus and herpes simplex virus strains [100, 174].

i. Influenza Virus

The water extract from the red marine alga Ceramium rubrum considerably inhibits the reproduction of a range of influenza viruses (type A and B) *in vitro* and *in ovo*. The virus-inhibitory effect is selective, dose-related and strain-specific, with selectivity indices (SI) ranged from 9.5 to 68.3. A/Rostock is the most susceptible strain tested to inhibition (SI = 54.7). The inhibition affects adsorption as well as the intracellular steps of viral replication [174].

ii. Herpes Simplex Virus

Extracts from the red marine alga Ceramium Rubrum inhibit also the reproduction of some representative herpes simplex virus strains (type 1 and type 2). Concretely, water, methanolic, chloroforme-methanol, and dichloromethane extracts exhibit anti-HSV-1 activity with EC_{50} ranging from < 2.5 (methanolic) to >250 µg mL-1 (chloroforme-methanol). The water extract is more effective (EC_{50} = 12.4 µg mL^{-1}) and non cytotoxic than the other extracts: the percentages of Vero cell destruction are 14.2% for the aqueous extract (CC_{50} = >250 µg mL^{-1}), 66.2% for the methanolic extract (CC_{50} = 134 µg mL^{-1}), 57.4% for the chloroforme-methanol extract (CC_{50} = 178.4 µg mL^{-1}) and 66.2% for the dichloromethane extract (CC_{50} = 61.8 µg mL^{-1}). It is thought that the main effective components in these extracts are polysaccharides [100].

The inhibitory effect associated to the aqueous extract is selective, however SI are low (4.9-10.8). Herpes simplex virus type 1, strain KOS is the most susceptible to inhibition (SI = 10.8). The extract exhibits a direct inactivating effect on extracellular herpes simplex virus type 1, strain KOS. The herpes simplex virus-inhibitory activity of Ceramium extract is due mainly to its virucidal effect since EC_{50} is not statistically distinguishable from MIC_{90} (0.8-1.2 mg mL^{-1} and 1.4 mg mL^{-1} respectively) [174].

Table 1. Extracts and Compounds Isolated from Red Algae in Which Antiviral Activity has been Studied. Viruses Sensitive to the Extracts/Compounds are Highlighted in Bold Black, whereas the Insensitive Ones Appear in Grey

Species	Compounds isolated	Activity	References
Asparagopsis Armata	Water, methanolic, dichloromethane and chloroforme-methanol extracts (polysaccharides)	**Herpes simplex virus type 1**	[100]
	Galactans	**Human immunodeficiency virus type 1**	[93]
Ceramium Rubrum	Water extracts	**Influenza virus type A** **Influenza virus type B**	[174]
	Water, methanolic, dichloromethane and chloroforme-methanol extracts (polysaccharides) (polysaccharides)	**Herpes simplex virus type 1** **Herpes simplex virus type 2**	[100] [174]
Georgiella Confluens	Agarans	Herpes simplex virus	[163]
Griffithsia sp.	Lectins (griffithsin)	**Human immunodeficiency virus type 1**	[99] [112] [114] [115] [117] [146] [178]
		SARS (severe acute respiratory syndrome)-related coronavirus	[146] [147]
		Hepatitis C virus	[148]
		Herpes simplex virus	[149]
	Methanol-toluene extracts	Herpes simplex virus type 1 Vesicular stomatitis virus	[91]
Cryptopleura Ramosa	Agarans	**Herpes simplex virus type 1** **Herpes simplex virus type 2**	[151]
Acanthophora Spicifera	Agarans	**Herpes simplex virus type 1** **Herpes simplex virus type 2**	[73] [152]
Alsidium Corallinum	Methanolic and chloroforme-methanol extracts	Herpes simplex virus type 1	[100]

(Table 1) contd.....

Species	Compounds isolated	Activity	References
Boergeseniella Thuyoides	Sulfated polysaccharides	**Human immunodeficiency virus type 1**	[116]
	Sulfated polysaccharides	**Herpes simplex virus type 1**	[116]
	Water, dichloromethane and chloroforme-methanol extracts	**Herpes simplex virus type 1**	[100]
Bostrychia Montagnei	Fractions obtained of the raw water extract	**Herpes simplex virus type 1** **Herpes simplex virus type 2**	[127]
Halopithys Incurvus	Water, methanolic, dichloromethane and chloroforme-methanol extracts (polysaccharides)	**Herpes simplex virus type 1**	[100]
Laurencia Microcladia	Methanol-toluene extracts	Herpes simplex virus type 1 Vesicular stomatitis virus	[91]
Laurencia Pelagosae	Methanol-toluene extracts	Herpes simplex virus type 1 Vesicular stomatitis virus	[91]
Laurencia Venusta	Terpene (venustatriol)	**Herpes simplex virus type 1** **Vesicular stomatitis virus**	[146]
Lophosiphonia Subadunca	Methanol-toluene extracts	Herpes simplex virus type 1 Vesicular stomatitis virus	[91]
Osmundaria Obtusiloba	Glycolipids	**Herpes simplex virus type 1**	[172]
Polysiphonia Denudata	Water extracts	**Herpes simplex virus type 1** **Herpes simplex virus type 2**	[126]
Polysiphonia Subulifera	Methanol-toluene extracts	Herpes simplex virus type 1 Vesicular stomatitis virus	[91]
Pterosiphonia Complanata	Water, methanolic, dichloromethane and chloroforme-methanol extracts (polysaccharides)	**Herpes simplex virus type 1**	[100]
Symphyocladia Latiuscula	Methanolic extracts Bromophenols	**Herpes simplex virus type 1**	[130]
Amphiroa Beauvoisii	Methanol-toluene extracts	Herpes simplex virus type 1 Vesicular stomatitis virus	[91]

(Table 1) contd…..

Species	Compounds isolated	Activity	References
Amphiroa Cryptarthrodia	Methanol-toluene extracts	Herpes simplex virus type 1 Vesicular stomatitis virus	[91]
Amphiroa Rigida	Methanol-toluene extracts	Herpes simplex virus type 1 Vesicular stomatitis virus	[91]
Corallina Elongate	Methanol-toluene extracts	**Herpes simplex virus type 1** **Vesicular stomatitis virus**	[91]
Corallina Granifera	Methanol-toluene extracts	Herpes simplex virus type 1 Vesicular stomatitis virus	[91]
Corallina Officinalis	Sulfated xylogalactans	Herpes simplex virus type 1	[175]
Jania Adhaerens	Methanol-toluene extracts	Herpes simplex virus type 1 Vesicular stomatitis virus	[91]
Jania Rubens	Methanol-toluene extracts	Herpes simplex virus type 1 Vesicular stomatitis virus	[91]
Lithophyllum Expansum	Methanol-toluene extracts	**Herpes simplex virus type 1** **Vesicular stomatitis virus**	[91]
Lithophyllum Corallioides	Methanol-toluene extracts	Herpes simplex virus type 1 Vesicular stomatitis virus	[91]
Lithothamnion Lichenoides	Methanol-toluene extracts	Herpes simplex virus type 1 Vesicular stomatitis virus	[91]
Lithothamnion Valens	Methanol-toluene extracts	Herpes simplex virus type 1 Vesicular stomatitis virus	[91]
Mesophyllum Lichenoides	Methanol-toluene extracts	Herpes simplex virus type 1 Vesicular stomatitis virus	[91]
Spongites Hauckii	Methanol-toluene extracts	Herpes simplex virus type 1 Vesicular stomatitis virus	[91]
Spongites Ramulosa	Methanol-toluene extracts	Herpes simplex virus type 1 Vesicular stomatitis virus	[91]
Gelidiella Ramellosa	Methanol-toluene extracts	Herpes simplex virus type 1 Vesicular stomatitis virus	[91]
Gelidium Attenatum	Methanolic and chloroforme-methanol extracts	Herpes simplex virus type 1	[100]
Gelidium Pulchellum	Water, methanolic, dichloromethane and chloroforme-methanol extracts (polysaccharides)	**Herpes simplex virus type 1**	[100]

(Table 1) contd…..

Species	Compounds isolated	Activity	References
Gelidium Pusillum	Water, methanolic, dichloromethane, chloroforme-methanol, methanol-toluene extracts	**Herpes simplex virus type 1**	[100]
		Vesicular stomatitis virus	[91]
Gelidium Sesquipedale	Water and dichloromethane extracts	Herpes simplex virus type 1	[100]
Gelidium Spinulosum	Water, methanolic and dichloromethane extracts (polysaccharides)	**Herpes simplex virus type 1**	[100]
Pterocladia Capillacea	Sulfated galactans	**Cytomegalovirus** **Herpes simplex virus type 1** **Herpes simplex virus type 2** **Pseudorabies virus**	[122]
Constantinea Simplex	Water extracts	**Coxsackie B5 virus** Murine cytomegalovirus Encephalomyocarditis virus **Herpes simplex virus type 2** **Herpes simplex virus type 1** Semliki Forest virus **Vaccinia virus** **Vesicular stomatitis virus**	[103, 104]
Farlowia Mollis	Water extracts (polysaccharides)	Adenovirus type 7 Coxsackie B5 virus Echo-6-virus Encephalomyocarditis virus **Herpes simplex virus type 1** **Herpes simplex virus type 2** Japanese B encephalitis virus Murine cytomegalovirus Poliovirus type 2 Rhinovirus type 2 Respiratory syncytial virus Semliki Forest virus Sindbis virus **Vaccinia virus** **Vesicular stomatitis virus** Western equine encephalitis virus	[59, 104]

(Table 1) contd…..

Species	Compounds isolated	Activity	References
Gigartina Aciculaire	Lambda-carrageenans	Adenovirus type 2 Coxsackie B4 virus **Cytomegalovirus** **Herpes simplex virus type 1** **Herpes simplex virus type 2** **Human immunodeficiency virus type 1** Parainfluenza virus type 3 Poliovirus type 1 Reovirus type 1 **Sindbis virus** **Vesicular stomatitis virus** **Vaccinia virus**	[66]
		Hepatitis A virus	[154]
Gigartina Atropurpurea	Polysaccharides (caraageenan)	**Herpes simplex virus type 1** **Herpes simplex virus type 2**	[141]
Gigartina Pistillata	Lambda-carrageenans	Adenovirus type 2	[66]
		Coxsackie B4 virus **Cytomegalovirus** **Herpes simplex virus type 1** **Herpes simplex virus type 2** **Human immunodeficiency virus type 1** Parainfluenza virus type 3 Poliovirus type 1 Reovirus type 1 **Sindbis virus** **Vaccinia virus** **Vesicular stomatitis virus**	[66]
		Hepatitis A virus	[154]
Gigartina Skottsbergii	Lambda-carrageenans Upsilon/nu-carrageenans Kappa/iota-carrageenans	**Herpes simplex virus type 1** **Herpes simplex virus type 2**	[69] [70] [123] [124] [129] [135]
		Human herpesvirus 6	[134]
Gigartina Tenella	Glycolipids	**Human immunodeficiency virus type 1**	[110] [211]

(Table 1) contd…..

Species	Compounds isolated	Activity	References
Hypnea Musciformis	Water, methanolic, dichloromethane and chloroforme-methanol extracts (polysaccharides)	**Herpes simplex virus type 1**	[100]
Callophyllis Variegata	Galactans	**Dengue virus type 2** **Herpes simplex virus type 1** **Herpes simplex virus type 2**	[132]
Kallymenia Requienii	Methanol-toluene extracts	**Herpes simplex virus type 1** **Vesicular stomatitis virus**	[91]
Peyssonnelia sp.	Terpenes	**Human immunodeficiency virus type 1** **Human immunodeficiency virus type 2**	[108]
Peyssonnelia Bornetii	Methanol-toluene extracts	Herpes simplex virus type 1 Vesicular stomatitis virus	[91]
Peyssonnelia Rosa-Marina	Methanol-toluene extracts	Herpes simplex virus type 1 Vesicular stomatitis virus	[91]
Peyssonnelia Rubra	Methanol-toluene extracts	Herpes simplex virus type 1 Vesicular stomatitis virus	[91]
Peyssonnelia Squamaria	Methanol-toluene extracts	Herpes simplex virus type 1 Vesicular stomatitis virus	[91]
Gymnogongrus Griffithsiae	Kappa/iota/nu carrageenans	Dengue virus type 1 **Dengue virus type 2** **Dengue virus type 3** **Dengue virus type 4**	[150]
	Sulfated galactans	**Herpes simplex virus type 1** **Herpes simplex virus type 2**	[75]
Gymnogongrus Torulosus	Galactans	**Dengue virus type 2** **Herpes simplex virus type 2**	[128]
Phyllophora Crispa	Methanol-toluene extracts	Herpes simplex virus type 1 Vesicular stomatitis virus	[91]
Stenogramme Interrupta	Kappa/iota carrageenans Lambda carrageenans	**Herpes simplex virus type 1** **Herpes simplex virus type 2**	[125]

(Table 1) contd…..

Species	Compounds isolated	Activity	References
Agardhiella Tenera	Sulfated galactans	Coxsackie B4 virus **Cytomegalovirus** **Herpes simplex virus type 1** **Herpes simplex virus type 2** **Human immunodeficiency virus type 1** **Human immunodeficiency virus type 2** **Influenza virus A** Influenza virus B Junin virus Poliovirus type 1 Reovirus type 1 **Respiratory syncytial virus** **Sindbis virus** Tacaribe virus **Vaccinia virus** **Vesicular stomatitis virus**	[68] [107]
Eucheuma Cottonii	Kappa-carrageenans	Adenovirus type 2 Coxsackie B4 virus **Cytomegalovirus** **Herpes simplex virus type 1** **Herpes simplex virus type 2** **Human immunodeficiency virus type 1** Parainfluenza virus type 3 Poliovirus type 1 Reovirus type 1 **Sindbis virus** **Vaccinia virus** **Vesicular stomatitis virus**	[66]
		Hepatitis A virus	[154]
Eucheuma Spinosa	Iota-carrageenans	Adenovirus **Encephalomyocarditis virus** **Herpes simplex virus type 1** **Herpes simplex virus type 2** Measles virus Poliovirus **Semliki Forest virus** **Swine fever virus** **Vaccinia virus** Vesicular stomatitis virus	[153]
		Hepatitis A virus	[154]

(Table 1) contd.....

Species	Compounds isolated	Activity	References
Meristiella Gelidium	Iota/kappa/nu carrageenans	**Dengue virus type 2** **Herpes simplex virus type 2**	[133]
Sphaerococcus Coronopifolius	Polysaccharides	**Human immunodeficiency virus type 1**	[116]
		Herpes simplex virus type 1	[100] [116]
	Methanol-toluene extracts	Herpes simplex virus type 1 Vesicular stomatitis virus	[91]
Gracilaria Corticata	Sulfated polysaccharides	**Herpes simplex virus type 1** **Herpes simplex virus type 2**	[71] [138]
Gracilaria Salicornia	Water extracts	**Herpes simplex virus type 2**	[137]
Cryptonemia Crenulata	Galactans	**Dengue virus type** 1 **Dengue virus type 2** **Dengue virus type 3** **Dengue virus type 4** **Herpes simplex virus type 1** **Herpes simplex virus type 2**	[150] [75]
Grateloupia Filicina	Sulfated galactans	**Human immunodeficiency virus type 1**	[113]
	Amylose	**Herpes simplex virus type 2**	[136]
Grateloupia Indica	Sulfated galactans	**Herpes simplex virus type 1** **Herpes simplex virus type 2**	[78]
Grateloupia Longifolia	Sulfated galactans	**Human immunodeficiency virus type 1**	[113]
Tricleocarpa Oblongata	Methanol-toluene extracts	Herpes simplex virus type 1 Vesicular stomatitis virus	[91]
Nothogenia Fastigiata	Xylomannans	**Cytomegalovirus** **Human immunodeficiency virus type 1** **Human immunodeficiency virus type 2** **Influenza virus A** **Influenza virus B** **Junin virus** **Respiratory syncytial virus** **Simian immunodeficiency virus** **Tacaribe virus**	[143]

(Table 1) contd.....

Species	Compounds isolated	Activity	References
		Herpes simplex virus type 1 **Herpes simplex virus type 2**	[67] [119] [120] [121]
Scinaia Hatei	Sulfated xylomannans	**Herpes simplex virus type 1** **Herpes simplex virus type 2**	[139]
Schizymenia Binderi	Sulfated galactans	**Herpes simplex virus type 1** **Herpes simplex virus type 2**	[131]
Schizymenia Dubyi	Glucuronogalactans	**Human immunodeficiency virus type 1**	[109]
Schizymenia Pacifica	Sulfated polysaccharides	**Human immunodeficiency virus type 1**	[105] [106]
Plocamium Cartilagineum	Water, methanolic and chloroforme-methanol extracts Sulfated galactans	**Herpes simplex virus type 1** **Herpes simplex virus type 2**	[100] [141]
Botryocladia Botryoides	Methanol-toluene extracts	Herpes simplex virus type 1 Vesicular stomatitis virus	[91]
Sebdenia Polydactyla	Sulfated xylomannans	**Herpes simplex virus type 1**	[140]

Georgiella Confluens

Polysaccharides isolated from Georgiella Confluens are highly methylated agarans and have low content of 3,6-anhydrogalactose. Furthermore, they bear xylose single stubs linked at position 4 of the β-D-galactose, and sulfated (12.6% of total sulfate) mainly (~8-9%) at position 3 of the α-L-galactose, with lesser amounts of sulfation at position 4 of the β-D-galactose (~3-4%). Their antiviral properties have been tested but there is no proof about it [163].

Griffthsia sp.

Griffithsin is a lectin with a relative molecular mass of 13 kDa, consisting of 121-amino-acid*. It was originally isolated from an aqueous extract of the red alga *Griffithsia* sp. found in the coastal waters off New Zealand [99]. It has been

*The identity of its residue 31 is still unknown. The only information available up to now concerning this residue is: i) it does not match any of the 20 standard amino acids [99]; ii) its molecular mass is 151.05 [99]; iii) its functional role is indistinct, because it is known that the substitution of the residue 31 by other amino-acid (*e.g.* alanine) does not diminish the antiviral activity nor binding ability (to high mannose glycan structures) of the lectin as compared to the properties of the native lectin [178, 179].

purified and produced recombinantly in *Escheria coli* [99, 112, 180] and Nicotiana plants [146]. Furthermore, recently smaller peptides have been obtained from the griffithsin (known as grifonins), which appear to have similar biological functions to the naturally occurring lectin [179]. Griffithsin shows limited homology (less than 30% identity) to proteins such as jacalin [181], heltuba [182] or artocarpin [183], all members of the β-prism-I family of lectins [184, 185]. Griffithsin exists exclusively as a dimer and has a domain-swapped structure in which two β-strands of one monomer combine with 10 β-strands of the other monomer to form a β prism of three four-stranded sheets [146, 178, 186]. Each monomer (or subunit) of griffithsin contains three binding sites, orientated as an equatorial triangle, that have high affinity for mannose residues [185, 186] which cover the surfaces of virus [99].

Both native and recombinant griffithsin display potent and broad antiviral activity against human immunodeficiency virus type 1 [114, 115]. It is >1000-fold higher than the activities reported for several monosaccharide-specific lectins, such as Myrianthus holstii lectin [187]. Recently, it has been reported to be also active against other viruses, including coronavirus that causes severe acute respiratory syndrome (SARS), termed the SARS-related coronavirus [146, 147] and hepatitis C virus [148]. Intriguingly, griffithsin has also been shown to have *in vitro* activity against herpes simplex virus [149], in spite of there are controversial evidence about it [91].

i. Human Immunodeficiency Virus

At present, griffithsin is possibly the most potent and broad-spectrum human immunodeficiency virus entry inhibitor found in natural sources [99, 112]. Several authors [99, 188] have shown that it exhibits antiviral activity at lower concentrations than that reported previously for most antiviral proteins from natural sources. Griffithsin neutralizes human immunodeficiency virus type 1 by binding to high-mannose glycans on the viral envelope glycoproteins [99, 114, 115, 146, 178], so inhibiting cell fusion and transmission of human immunodeficiency virus at low nanomolar concentrations without cytotoxicity [99, 112]. Concretely, it binds to viral coat glycoproteins (gp120, gp41, gp160) and blocks the binding of gp120 to CD4 [189] thereby interfering with the structural transitions involved in receptor and co-receptor (CCR5, CXCR4 or both for some strains) docking and virus entry into human cells [190-192]. The high antiviral potency of this lectin has been correlated to its capacity to bind multiple glycans simultaneously [146, 178].

Griffithsin potently inhibits different subtypes of human immunodeficiency virus type 1, such as A, B, C clades [114, 115], in spite of glycosylation patterns between different human immunodeficiency virus type 1 clades vary [193] which play an important role in the antiviral activity of carbohydrate-binding proteins such as griffithsin. In this way, it is known that N-glycosylations on position 234 (N234) [115], 295 (N295) [115, 117] and 448 (N448) [117] in human immunodeficiency virus type 1 clade C virus are crucial binding sites for griffithsin and their absence decreases its antiviral potency. Likewise, antiviral effect of griffithsin is influenced by the administration of other drugs. Ferir *et al.* [194] published that the combination of griffithsin with tenofovir, maraviroc or enfuvirtide increases the antiviral potency of the lectin.

Taken together these data suggest that griffithsin may be a potential candidate for prophylactic use as an anti-human immunodeficiency virus microbicide. In addition to its remarkably high potency: i) it has excellent physicochemical properties, it is stable over a satisfactory pH and temperature range, both necessary properties if it must remain active in the human body for hours or be stored without refrigeration [112]; ii) the onset of its antiviral activity is rapid; iii) in spite of griffithsin has not yet been tested in human clinical trials, it is thought that it is not cytotoxic to human cells even at relatively high concentrations [195], because of griffithsin targets high-mannose arrays that are present on all human immunodeficiency virus envelope glycoproteins, are uncommon in mammalian cells [196, 197]. O'Keefe *et al.* [114] have demonstrated that griffithsin produced in the tobacco-like plant Nicotiana benthamiana is not mitogenic, has a good safety profile in the rabbit vaginal irritation model (the Gold Standard preclinical safety test for vaginal products), and shows no induction of pro-inflammatory chemokines and cytokines in human cervical explants.

ii. SARS-Related Coronavirus

Griffithsin inhibits replication and cytopathy of the SARS-related coronavirus [146]. Griffithsin displays activity against this virus at nanomolar-range levels [147]. The molecular target through which griffithsin appears to mediate its anticoronavirus activity is the surface envelope glycoprotein spike (S). Griffithsin binds directly to S *via* interaction with oligosaccharide moieties [147]. The affinity between griffithsin and SARS-related coronavirus (stoichiometry of 3:1) is weaker than that between griffithsin and human immunodeficiency virus gp120 (stoichiometry of ~10:1). This difference in the affinity for griffithsin between the two envelope glycoproteins is likely responsible for the difference seen in the antiviral activity of griffithsin against human immunodeficiency virus (0.048 to 0.63 nM) [99] and SARS-related coronavirus (48 to 94 nM) [147].

iii. Hepatitis C Virus

Similar to that commented for human immunodeficiency virus, the antiviral activity of griffithsin against hepatitis C virus is mediated by its binding to glycans present on the virus. Griffithsin prevents hepatitis C virus infection of Huh-7 hepatoma cells at nanomolar-range levels and also interferes with direct cell-to-cell transmission of hepatitis C virus, because of it avoids the attachment of the virus to its receptor CD81 [148]. These results indicate that griffithsin may be a novel molecule for the prevention of graft reinfection in hepatitis C virus-infected liver transplant patients.

Florideophyceae. Ceramiales. Delesseriaceae

Cryptopleura Ramosa is the only species of family Delesseriaceae (order Ceramiales) which antiviral activity has been screened in.

Cryptopleura Ramosa

Cryptopleura Ramosa is an alga widely distributed in the North Atlantic and the Mediterranean. Carlucci *et al.* [151] have isolated a sulfated compound from extracts of this alga. It is a low-molecular-weight (2.8 kDa) agaran which has a sulfate content of 35.2% and shows a high antiviral activity (1.6-4.2 $\mu g\ mL^{-1}$). This sulfated agaran is a selective inhibitor of herpes simplex virus types 1 and 2 replication in kidney epithelial cells (Vero cells) and cells of neural origin (astrocytes). It is thought that its effects are mediated by an inhibitory action on virus adsorption.

Florideophyceae. Ceramiales. Rhodomelaceae

Species of family Rhodomelaceae (order Ceramiales) which antiviral activity has been screened in include: Acanthophora Spicifera, Alsidium Corallinum, Boergeseniella Thuyoides, Bostrychia Montagnei, Halopithys Incurvus, Laurencia Microcladia, Laurencia Pelagosae, Laurencia Venusta, Lophosiphonia Subadunca, Osmundaria Obtusiloba, Polysiphonia Denudate, Pterosiphonia Complanata, and Symphyocladia Latiuscula.

Acanthophora Spicifera

Agarans isolated from the red seaweed Acanthophora Spicifera show a very selective and potent antiviral activity against herpes simplex virus types 1 and 2 with EC_{50} ranging from 0.6 to >50 μg mL^{-1} [152]. In general, those compounds that elute in the range of 0.75-1.0 M of NaCl (C-3, H-2, H-3, and W-4) show higher antiviral activity and have percentages of sulfate in the range of 18.2-25.1% than those elute with smaller ionic strength (between 0.25 and 0.5 M) and which have low percentages of sulfate (6.9–19.2%) [73].

As in other sulfated polysaccharides the high molecular weights and degree of sulfation are determinants of activity. Nevertheless, when the percentage of sulfate is very high, the molecular weight (if above a limit) becomes less important [151]. In relation to agarans isolated from Acanthophora Spicifera, increased amounts of methoxylated galactoses and/or xylose as single stubs at random in the chain, seem be deleterious for the activity. The few data produced in the agaran sulfate field suggest that all the sulfate groups, in different positions of the agaran backbone, could contribute to the low inhibitory activity of these galactans [73].

The antiviral activity of these sulfated seaweed polysaccharides are based on the formation of formally similar complexes that block the interaction of the viruses with the cells [152]. The initial contact between an enveloped virus and the host cell occurs by the ionic interaction between positively charged regions of the viral external glycoproteins and the negatively charged substituents of the cell surface.

The initial step is the binding of viral glycoprotein C (gC), and in some cases glycoprotein B (gB), to cell-surface heparan sulfate [198-200].

Alsidium Corallinum

There is little evidence about antiviral properties of compounds from Alsidium Corallinum. The only study carried out up to now reveals that extracts from Alsidium Corallinum (methanolic and chloroforme-methanol extracts) have not antiherpetic effect *in vitro* [100].

Boergeseniella Thuyoides

Polysaccharides from Boergeseniella Thuyoides composed of galactose, 3,6-anhydrogalactose, uronics acids, sulfate in ratios of 25.4, 16.0, 3.2, 7.6% (w/w) inhibit *in vitro* replication of encapsulated virus [100, 116]. Extracts from Boergeseniella Thuyoides have antiviral properties against human immunodeficiency virus and herpes simplex virus.

i. Human Immunodeficiency Virus

Polysaccharides from Boergeseniella Thuyoides inhibit *in vitro* replication of the human immunodeficiency virus at concentrations of 12.5 μg mL^{-1}. The adsorption step of herpes simplex virus type 1 to the host cell seems to be the specific target for polysaccharide action. It is quite possible that polysaccharides could affect the virus-cell attachment by spreading a three-dimensional gel network over the whole of the cell surface. This structural modification would entail envelope alteration and concealing of virus-specific receptors sites [116]. Such a mechanism would prevent adsorption of the viruses to the cell surface and hence penetration and replication. Bouhlal *et al.* [116] suggest that they exert a direct inhibitory effect on human immunodeficiency virus type 1 replication by controlling the appearance of the new generations of virus and potential virucidal effect.

ii. Herpes Simplex Virus

Sulfated polysaccharides from Boergeseniella Thuyoides confer total protection (100%) against herpes simplex virus type 1 as determined in a virus plaque reduction assay in Vero cells (EC_{50} = 17.2 μg mL^{-1}), but with low selectivity (SI =

14.5) [116]. This antiherpetic effect is also seen when extracts from this alga are tested. Concretely, water extract (EC_{50} = 12.6 μg mL^{-1}) from Boergeseniella Thuyoides has a higher antiviral effect than dichloromethane (EC_{50} = 26.2 μg mL^{-1}) or chloroforme-methanol (EC_{50} = 35 μg mL^{-1}) extracts. Furthemore, it exhibits an insignificant cytotoxic effect as compared to the other 2 extracts: the percentages of Vero cell destruction are 15.1% for the aqueous extract (CC_{50}=>250 μg mL^{-1}), 46.8% for the chloroforme-methanol extract (CC_{50} = >250 μg mL^{-1}) and 62.2% for the dichloromethane extract (CC_{50} = 151 μg mL^{-1}) [100].

Bostrychia Montagnei

Fractions obtained by anion-exchange chromatography of the raw extract (B4-B6) have low activity against herpes simplex virus type 1 (13.1-25.7 μg mL^{-1}) and herpes simplex virus type 2 (12.4-46.2 μg mL^{-1}), while others (B1-B3) are not active. The inhibitory effect of these compounds takes place only when they are added during the adsorption period. The activity could be correlated with the sulfate content and the molecular weights (22.0-4.0% and 34-43.7 kDa) in the active fractions and (11.2-16.2% and 5.6-31.3 kDa) in the nonactive ones [127]. Concretely, in relation to the sulfate content it is known that the 3-linked β-D-galactopyranosyl units of agarans from Bostrychia Montagnei [201] carry partial sulfation on C-2 (2.1-7.7%), C-4 (11.6-18.4%), and C-6 (12.4–20.2%), whereas approximately 50-60% of the 4-linked units have complete sulfation on C-3, with minor amounts of 2- and 6-sulfation (0.8-2.2% and 2.8-5.2%, respectively).

Halopithys Incurvus

Extracts from Halopithys Incurvus have significant anti-HSV-1 activity. The main effective components in these extracts are polysaccharides. Bouhlal *et al.* [100] have observed that water extract from this alga has a higher antiviral effect and is less cytotoxic (EC_{50} = 75.9 μg mL^{-1}; percentage of Vero cell destruction is 28.7%; CC_{50} = >250 μg mL^{-1}) than methanolic (EC_{50} = 83.5 μg mL^{-1}; percentage of Vero cell destruction is 89.3%; CC_{50} = 26.7 μg mL^{-1}), dichloromethane (EC_{50} = 36 μg mL^{-1}; percentage of Vero cell destruction is 67.9%; CC_{50} = 99.8 μg mL^{-1}) or chloroforme-methanol (EC_{50} = 87.7 μg mL^{-1}; percentage of Vero cell destruction is 71.9%; CC_{50} = 98.8 μg mL^{-1}) extracts.

Laurencia Microcladia

Laurencia Microcladia shows no antiviral activity either against herpes simplex virus type 1 cultured in kidney cells of monkey or vesicular stomatitis virus in kidney cells of hamster [91].

Laurencia Pelagosae

The only research carried out to study antiviral activity of compounds from Laurencia Pelagosae has demonstrated that extracts of this alga have no antiviral activity either against herpes simplex virus type 1 cultured in kidney cells of monkey or vesicular stomatitis virus in kidney cells of hamster [91].

Laurencia Venusta

There is little evidence about antiviral properties of compounds from Laurencia Venusta. However Sakemi *et al.* [118] have demonstrated that venustatriol, a triterpene tetracyclic ether isolated from this alga, is effective against vesicular stomatitis virus and herpes simplex virus type 1.

Lophosiphonia Subadunca

Up to now, the only study carried out about antiviral activity associated with compounds from Lophosiphonia Subadunca demonstrates that extracts of this alga lack antimicrobial activity against herpes simplex virus type 1 cultured in kidney cells of monkey and vesicular stomatitis virus in kidney cells of hamster [91].

Osmundaria Obtusiloba

Glycolipids from macroalgae Osmundaria Obtusiloba exhibit potent antiviral activity against acyclovir-sensible and -resistent herpes simplex virus type 1 (Viral Inhibition Index (VII) values in the range 0.75- 2.35 and 2.5-4.5, respectively) [172].

Polysiphonia Denudata

The water extract from the red marine alga Polysiphonia Denudata selectively inhibits the reproduction of herpes virus types 1 and 2 in cell cultures (EC_{50} = 8.7

to 47.7 mg mL^{-1}). The virus-inhibitory effect is dose-related, strain-specific and depended on virus inoculum. The inhibition affects adsorption as well as the intracellular stages of viral replication. The presence of the extract throughout the whole replicative cycle is necessary for the full expression of the antiviral effect. In higher concentrations (MIC_{90} = 6.5 mg mL^{-1}) the extract exhibits strong extracellular virus inactivating activity [126].

Polysiphonia Subulifera

Extracts of Polysiphonia Subulifera have no antiviral activity either against herpes simplex virus type 1 cultured in kidney cells of monkey or vesicular stomatitis virus in kidney cells of hamster [91].

Pterosiphonia Complanata

Extracts from Pterosiphonia Complanata, of which the main effective components are polysaccharides, have important antiherpetic effect; however there are significant differences in relation to their potency among the distinct extracts. Water extract (EC_{50} = 10.4 μg mL^{-1}) from this red alga has a higher antiviral effect against herpes simplex virus type 1 that methanolic (EC_{50} = 18.1 μg mL^{-1}), dichloromethane (EC_{50} = 23.9 μg mL^{-1}) or chloroforme-methanol (EC_{50} = 53.8 μg mL^{-1}) extracts. These extracts are very cytotoxic (percentages of Vero cell destruction >61.3%) [100].

Symphyocladia Latiuscula

Bromophenols (such as 2,3-dibromo-4,5-dihydroxybenzylalcohol), known antioxidants [202] and antimicrobial [203] agents, are the major constituents of the red alga Symphyocladia Latiuscula. Extracts from this alga as well as their constituents (bromophenols) might provide a basis for developing new anti-herpes simplex virus type 1 agents [130]. The methanol extract of Symphyocladia Latiuscula and its fractions exhibit antiviral activities against herpes simplex type 1 *in vitro* without cytotoxicity. The major component, 2,3,6-tribromo-4,5-dihydroxybenzyl methyl ether (TDB) of a CH_2Cl_2-soluble fraction (that is the most potent (IC_{50} value of 7.73 mg mL^{-1})) is active against wild type herpes simplex virus type 1, as well as phosphonoacetic acid (PAA)-resistant herpes simplex virus type 1 and thymidine kinase deficient herpes simplex virus type 1 (IC_{50} values of 5.48, 4.81 and 23.3 mg mL^{-1}, respectively). These results support the notion that these compounds exert antiviral activities through a different mechanism from that of acyclovir. The therapeutic effectiveness of the methanol extract and TDB from Symphyocladia Latiuscula has been further examined in BALB/c mice that were cutaneously infected with herpes simplex virus type 1 strain 7401H. Three daily oral administrations of the MeOH extract (600 mg/kg/day) and TDB (20 mg/kg/day) significantly delays the appearance of score 2 skin lesions (local vesicles) and limits the development of further score 6 (mild zosteriform) lesions in infected mice without toxicity compared with controls. In addition, TDB suppresses virus yields in the brain and skin. Therefore TDB should be a promising anti-herpes simplex virus agent.

Florideophyceae. Corallinales. Corallinaceae.

Species of family Corallinaceae (order Corallinales), which antiviral activity has been screened in include: Amphiroa Beauvoisii, Amphiroa Cryptarthrodia, Amphiroa Rigida, Corallina elongate, Corallina granifera, Corallina officinalis, Jania Adhaerens, Jania Rubens, Lithophyllum expansum, Lithothamnion corallioides, Lithophyllum lichenoides, Lithothamnion valens, Mesophyllum Lichenoides, Spongites Hauckii, and Spongites Ramulosa.

Amphiroa Beauvoisii

The only research carried out to study antiviral activity of compounds from Amphiroa Beauvoisii has demonstrated that extracts of this alga have no antiviral activity either against herpes simplex virus type 1 cultured in kidney cells of monkey or vesicular stomatitis virus in kidney cells of hamster [91].

Amphiroa Cryptarthrodia

There is little evidence about antiviral properties of compounds from Amphiroa Cryptarthrodia. However Ballesteros *et al.* [91] have demonstrated that extracts of this red alga have no antiviral activity either against herpes simplex virus type 1 cultured in kidney cells of monkey or vesicular stomatitis virus in kidney cells of hamster.

Amphiroa Rigida

Extracts of the red alga Amphiroa Rigida show no antiviral activity either against herpes simplex virus type 1 cultured in kidney cells of monkey or vesicular stomatitis virus in kidney cells of hamster [91].

Corallina Elongate

There is little evidence about antiviral properties of compounds from Corallina Elongate. The only study carried out up to now reveals that extracts of this alga show antiviral activity against herpes simplex virus type 1 cultured in kidney cells of monkey and vesicular stomatitis virus in kidney cells of hamster [91].

Corallina Granifera

The main groups of constituent of the marine red seaweed Corallina Granifera are hydrocarbons, alcohols, carbonyl compounds, acids and their esters, terpenes [204]. Antiviral activity of extracts from this alga has been tested against herpes simplex virus and vesicular stomatitis virus, but positive results have not been demonstrated [91].

Corallina Officinalis

The structure of compounds extracted from the calcareous red seaweed Corallina Officinalis has been characterized by methylation, desulfation-methylation, and ethylation analysis [205]. Two sulfated xylogalactans from this alga [206], with low percentages of total sulfate (6.4% and 12.5%), and partial sulfation on C-6 of the A-units, and C-2 and C-3 of the B-units have been identified. Their antiviral activity has been studied but no positive effect against human virus has been observed [175].

Jania Adhaerens

Extracts of the alga Jania Adhaerens show no antiviral activity either against herpes simplex virus type 1 cultured in kidney cells of monkey or vesicular stomatitis virus in kidney cells of hamster [91].

Jania Rubens

Antiviral activity of extracts from the red alga Jania Rubens has been tested against herpes simplex virus type 1 cultured in kidney cells of monkey and vesicular stomatitis virus in kidney cells of hamster, but positive results have not been demonstrated [91].

Lithophyllum Expansum

There is little evidence about antiviral properties of compounds from Lithophyllum Expansum. The only study carried out up to now reveals that extracts of this alga shows antiviral activity against herpes simplex virus type 1 cultured in kidney cells of monkey and vesicular stomatitis virus in kidney cells of hamster [91].

Lithothamnion Corallioides

Lithothamnion Corallioides has no antiviral activity either against herpes simplex virus type 1 cultured in kidney cells of monkey or vesicular stomatitis virus in kidney cells of hamster [91].

Lithophyllum Lichenoides

Antiviral activity of extracts from the red alga Lithophyllum Lichenoides has been tested against herpes simplex virus type 1 cultured in kidney cells of monkey and vesicular stomatitis virus in kidney cells of hamster, but positive results have not been demonstrated [91].

Lithothamnion Valens

The only research carried out to study antiviral activity of compounds from Lithothamnion Valens has demonstrated that extracts of this alga have no antiviral activity either against herpes simplex virus type 1 cultured in kidney cells of monkey or vesicular stomatitis virus in kidney cells of hamster [91].

Mesophyllum Lichenoides

Extracts of the red alga Mesophyllum Lichenoides have no antiviral activity either against herpes simplex virus type 1 cultured in kidney cells of monkey or vesicular stomatitis virus in kidney cells of hamster [91].

Spongites Hauckii

The only research about the antiviral activity of compounds from Spongites Hauckii has been carried out by Ballesteros *et al.* [91]. They have observed that extracts of this alga have no antiviral activity either against herpes simplex virus type 1 cultured in kidney cells of monkey or vesicular stomatitis virus in kidney cells of hamster [91].

Spongites Ramulosa

Spongites Ramulosa shows no antiviral activity either against herpes simplex virus type 1 cultured in kidney cells of monkey or vesicular stomatitis virus in kidney cells of hamster [91].

Florideophyceae. Gelidiales. Gelidiaceae.

Species of family Gelidiaceae (order Gelidiales) which antiviral activity has been screened in include: Gelidiella Ramellosa, Gelidium Attenatum, Gelidium Pulchellum, Gelidium Pusillum, Gelidium Sesquipedale, Gelidium Spinulosum, and Pterocladia Capillacea.

Gelidiella Ramellosa

Antiviral activity of extracts from the red alga Gelidiella Ramellosa has been tested against herpes simplex virus type 1 cultured in kidney cells of monkey and vesicular stomatitis virus in kidney cells of hamster, but positive results have not been demonstrated [91].

Gelidium Attenatum

Antiviral properties of methanolic and chloroforme-methanol extracts from Gelidium Attenatum have been studied but no antiherpetic effect *in vitro* has been observed [100].

Gelidium Pulchellum

Bouhlal *et al.* [100] have demonstrated that extracts from Gelidium Pulchellum have significant antiviral properties, with polysaccharide as one of the main effective components. Water extract (EC_{50} = 31.7 µg mL^{-1}) from Gelidium Pulchellum has a higher anti-HSV-1 effect than methanolic (EC_{50} = 16.1 µg mL^{-1}), chloroforme-methanol (EC_{50} = >250 µg mL^{-1}) or dichloromethane (EC_{50} = 245.4 µg mL^{-1}) extracts. Furthermore, it is significantly less cytotoxic than the others: the percentages of Vero cell destruction are 47.3% for the aqueous extract (CC_{50} = >250 µg mL^{-1}), 91.5% for the methanolic extract (EC_{50} = 15.7 µg mL^{-1}), 81.5% for the chloroforme-methanol extract (EC_{50} = 65 µg mL^{-1}) and 78.6% for the dichloromethane extract (EC_{50} = 100.3 µg mL^{-1}).

Gelidium Pusillum

Antiviral activity of extracts from Gelidium Pusillum has been tested against herpes simplex virus and vesicular stomatitis virus. Whereas Bouhlal *et al.* [100] have observed that the dichloromethanolic extract from Gelidium Pusillum has a higher antiherpetic effect (EC_{50} = 60.6 µg mL^{-1}; percentage of Vero cell destruction = 33%; CC_{50} = >250 µg mL^{-1}) than the methanolic extract (EC_{50} = 36.4 µg mL^{-1}; percentage of Vero cell destruction = 90.5 %; CC_{50} = 35.8 µg mL^{-1}), no antiviral activity against herpes simplex virus type 1 and vesicular stomatis virus has been reported by Ballesteros *et al.* [91] testing a methanol-toluene extract from this alga.

Gelidium Sesquipedale

Bouhlal *et al.* [100] have tested antiviral activity of extracts from Gelidium Sesquipedale, and they have constated that dichloromethane and aqueous extracts from this alga have not antiherpetic effect *in vitro*.

Gelidium Spinulosum

Extracts from Gelidium Spinulosum have significant antiviral activity, with polysaccharide as one of the main effective components. It has been observed that water extract (EC_{50} = 37.6 μg mL^{-1}) from this alga has a higher anti-HSV-1 effect than methanolic (EC_{50} = 70.5 μg mL^{-1}) or dichloromethane (EC_{50} = 22.7 μg mL^{-1}) extracts. Furthermore, it is significantly less cytotoxic than the others: the percentages of Vero cell destruction are 25.2% for the aqueous extract (CC_{50} = >250 μg mL^{-1}), 83.1% for the methanolic extract (CC_{50} = 40.1 μg mL^{-1}) and 61% for the dichloromethane extract (CC_{50} = 197 μg mL^{-1}) [100].

Pterocladia Capillacea

Despite Bouhlal *et al.* [100] have observed that different extracts from Pterocladia Capillacea (water, methanolic, dichloromethane and chloroforme-methanol) have not antiherpetic virus effect *in vitro*, other authors have demonstrated the opposite effect [122].

The sulfated galactan S1 isolated from Pterocladia Capillacea is a sulfated compound (~27% sulfate) constituted by 4-linked α -L-galactose 3-sulfate (B-units) with lesser amounts of 3-linked β-D-galactose 6-sulfate (A-units) [207]. It is a selective antiviral compound against herpes simplex virus types 1 and 2, human cytomegalovirus and pseudorabies virus at concentrations ranging 3.2-12 μg mL^{-1} [122]. S1 is effective in inhibiting virus replication independent of the host cell origin. In fact, although there is a slightly increasing potency of S1 for the tested cell lines in the order: baby hamster kidney cells (BHK-21 cells) > African green monkey kidney cells (Vero cells) > human epidermoid cancer cells (HEp-2), in the three systems S1 acts as a potent inhibitor of herpes simplex virus type 1 production. Available data suggest that the mode of action of S1 could be attributable to an inhibition of initial virus attachment to the host cell, concretely blocking the interaction between the viral glycoprotein gC and the cellular heparan sulfate proteoglycans [198, 199, 208].

Florideophyceae. Gigartinales. Dumontiaceae

Species of family Dumontiaceae (order Gigartinales) which antiviral activity has been screened in include: Constantinea Simplex and Farlowia Mollis.

Constantinea Simplex

Extracts from the marine alga Constantinea Simplex, probably polysaccharides [103], possess antiviral properties [103].

i. Herpes Simplex Virus

Extracts inhibit the replication of herpes simplex virus, being the herpes simplex virus type 1 clearly less susceptible (six to sevenfold) to the action of these natural compounds than the herpes simplex virus type 2. Intriguingly, viral inhibition is greater with pretreatment than with post-treatment of cell cultures (mouse embryo fibroblasts). This effect has also been observed *in vivo*. When mice inoculated with herpes simplex virus type 2 begin the therapy after viral inoculation the mean time of death is not shortened, in contrast to the observed when the therapy is administered previously to the inoculation [104]. The prophylactic (but not therapeutic) antiviral activity of these compounds seriously limits their potential use in treatment of human herpes simplex virus infections.

ii. Other Viruses

Other viruses that are susceptible to extracts from this alga, although in minus degree, include the coxsackie B5 virus [103], the vaccinia virus and the vesicular stomatitis virus [104]. On the contrary encephalomyocarditis virus, Semliki Forest virus, and murine cytomegalovirus are not affected by them [104].

Farlowia Mollis

Extracts from the marine red alga Farlowia Mollis, which have been suggested to be polysaccharides [103], inhibit virus replication *in vitro*.

i. Herpes Simplex Virus

Deig *et al.* [59] and Richards *et al.* [104] have observed that extracts from Farlowia Mollis inhibit herpes simplex virus replication (herpes simplex virus type 2 five to tenfold more susceptible than the herpes simplex virus type 1) in cells such as human embryonic lung, Vero monkey kidney, hamster kidney and mouse embryo fibroblast cells, pretreated with them. It is thought that the extracts may conduct their action coating or blocking cell receptor sites required for herpesvirus infection [59].

ii. Other Viruses

Treatment with extracts from Farlowia Mollis is also effective against other viruses: vaccinia virus and vesicular stomatitis virus. However, they do not affect the activity of encephalomyocarditis virus, Semliki Forest virus, murine cytomegalovirus, coxsackie B5, echo-6, polio 2, rhino 2, respiratory syncytial, adeno 7, vaccinia, vesicular stomatitis, Japanese B encephalitis, Western equine encephalitis, and Sindbis viruses [59, 104].

Florideophyceae. Gigartinales. Gigartinaceae.

Species of family Gigartinaceae (order Gigartinales) which antiviral activity has been screened in include: Gigartina Aciculaire, Gigartina Atropurpurea, Gigartina Pistillata, Gigartina Skottsbergii, and Gigartina Tenella.

Gigartina Aciculaire

Lambda-carrageenans from Gigartina Aciculaire are potent inhibitors of herpesviruses including herpes simplex virus type 1 (MIC = 1.6-4.5 $\mu g\ mL^{-1}$), herpes simplex virus type 2 (MIC = 1.5 $\mu g\ mL^{-1}$) and cytomegalovirus (MIC = 0.3 $\mu g\ mL^{-1}$) [66]. Likewise, lambda-carrageenans are active against vesicular stomatitis virus (MIC = 0.2-4 $\mu g\ mL^{-1}$), sindbis virus (MIC = 2 $\mu g\ mL^{-1}$), human immunodeficiency virus type 1 (MIC = 1.9 $\mu g\ mL^{-1}$) [66] and hepatitis A virus (SI = >222) [154]. Furthermore, vaccinia virus is also inhibited but only at relatively high concentrations of the polysaccharides (MIC = 16 $\mu g\ mL^{-1}$). On the other hand, replication of adenovirus type 2, coxsackie B4 virus, poliovirus type

1, parainfluenza virus type 3 and reovirus type 1 is not affected by these carrageenans (MIC = >200 μg mL^{-1}, MIC = >400 μg mL^{-1}, MIC = >400 μg mL^{-1}, MIC = >4 μg mL^{-1}, and MIC = >4 μg mL^{-1}, respectively) [66].

It is noteworthy that these carrageenans hold great promise for the treatment of cytomegalovirus and human immunodeficiency virus type 1 infections, which is particularly advantageous for patients with acquired immunodeficiency syndrome who are prone to both infections and in whom the same compound may be used not only to suppress the causative agent (human immunodeficiency virus type 1) but also to prevent or suppress exacerbations of opportunistic infections caused by cytomegalovirus.

Gigartina Atropurpurea

The polysaccharides isolated from Gigartina Atropurpurea (kappa-2 type carrageenan and unusual lambda-type carrageenan) possess good antiviral activity against herpes simplex virus types 1 and 2, particularly the lambda-type carrageenan isolated from the tetrasporophyte form of Gigartina Atropurpurea. The kappa-2 type carrageenan isolated from the gametophyte form of Gigartina Atropurpurea has more modest activity. Both of them are more effective against herpes simplex virus type 2 than against herpes simplex virus type 1 (EC_{50} values ranging from 0.7 to 2.4 μg mL^{-1} for herpes simplex virus type 2 and from 1.5 to 5.4 μg mL^{-1} for herpes simplex virus type 1). Since these compounds have no antiviral activity *per se*, their action involves inhibition of virus adsorption. They form stable virus-sulfated compound complexes where binding is not reversible and hence the sites on the viral envelope required for virus attachment to host cells are occupied by the polysaccharides [141].

Gigartina Pistillata

Lambda-carrageenans from Gigartina Pistillata are potent inhibitors of herpes viruses including herpes simplex virus type 1 (MIC = 1.6-4.5 μg mL^{-1}), herpes simplex virus type 2 (MIC = 1.5 μg mL^{-1}) and cytomegalovirus (MIC = 0.3 μg mL^{-1}) [66]. Likewise, lambda-carrageenans are active against vesicular stomatitis virus (MIC = 0.2-4 μg mL^{-1}), sindbis virus (MIC = 2 μg mL^{-1}), human immunodeficiency virus type 1 (MIC = 1.9 μg mL^{-1}) [66] and hepatitis A virus (SI = >222) [154]. This activity points to their potential as drugs for the chemotherapy of virus infections. Furthermore, vaccinia virus is also inhibited but only at relatively high concentrations of the polysaccharides (MIC = 16 μg mL^{-1}).

On the other hand, replication of adenovirus type 2, coxsackie B4 virus, poliovirus type 1, parainfluenza virus type 3 and reovirus type 1 is not affected by these carrageenans (MIC= >200 μg mL^{-1}, MIC= >400 μg mL^{-1}, MIC= >400 μg mL^{-1}, MIC= >4 μg mL^{-1}, and MIC= >4 μg mL^{-1}, respectively) [66].

Gigartina Skottsbergii

Carrageenans isolated from the red seaweed Gigartina Skottsbergii have been identified as potent and selective inhibitors of herpes simplex virus types 1 and 2 *in vitro* [69, 123, 124, 129, 135] and *in vivo* [129, 135]. More recently, evidence has emerged to show that these polysaccharides also produce marked inhibition of human herpesvirus 6 replication [134], although their effects have been less studied and characterized.

Lambda-type (1T1), upsilon/nu-type (1C3) and kappa/iota-type (1C) carrageenans are effective inhibitors of herpes simplex virus types 1 and 2 replication, as determined by a virus yield inhibition assay, in astrocytes [70, 124] as well as in Vero cells [69, 70, 123, 124, 129] and foreskin fibroblasts [69, 70]. The IC_{50} is in the range of 0.4-4.1 μg mL^{-1} for the 3 types of cells and both serotypes [123, 124]. Furthermore, no cytotoxicity is detected at concentrations of up to 1,000 μg mL^{-1}, indicating high SI for these compounds [69, 124].

Different inhibitory activity among the 3 structural types of carrageenans has been observed. Lambda-type (1T1) and upsilon/nu-type (1C3) carrageenans are most potent inhibitors of herpes simplex virus types 1 and 2 than kappa/iota-type carrageenans (1C) [69, 123]. Carlucci *et al.* [123] have pointed to the carrageenan 1C3 as the compound that has the best relationship between antiviral efficacy and lacks of cytotoxicity. These discrepant results have led to several authors to wonder if 1T1 and 1C3 carrageenans should retain their antiviral activity in *in vivo* conditions [129, 135]. Carlucci *et al.* [129] evaluated the protective efficacy of 1T1 in a murine model of herpes simplex virus type 2 and they observed that a single topical administration of 1T1 shortly before infection of mice with herpes simplex virus type 2 protected 9 out of 10 mice from herpes simplex virus type 2-induced lesions and mortality, compared with only 10% survival in control mice. In addition, 1T1 produced a total blockade in virus shedding in the vaginal secretions. When 1T1 pre-treatment was reinforced with a second dose 2 h after infection, total protection was observed even when the prophylactic administration had taken place at 60 min before infection. It has been suggested that the irreversible virucidal action of 1T1 against herpes virus might be responsible of its protective effect against virus replication and mortality following vaginal herpes simplex virus type 2 infection. On the other hand, Pujol *et al.* [135] tested the protective effect of 1C3 in a murine model of intraperitoneal herpes simplex virus type 1 infection and they constated that 1C3 administered immediately after herpes simplex virus type 1 infection increased the survival rate and delayed the mean day of death.

Mode of action studies have shown that the main target of the antiviral action of the carrageenans isolated from this alga is the initial binding of herpes simplex virus to the host cell [69], by interference with the interaction of the virion glycoprotein gC and/or gB with heparan sulfate residues of proteoglycans, the primary virus receptor on the cell surface [209, 210]. However, the interaction of 1T1 seems to be somewhat different from that of 1C1 and 1C3, in that the lambda-carrageenan 1T1 is able to inactivate virion particles at concentrations near the virus yield-inhibitory IC_{50}, whereas for the other two carrageenans, virucidal activity is only observed at concentrations highly exceeding the antiviral concentrations. The divergence in chemical structure among the carrageenans can explain their different behavior. Concretely, three main dissimilarities in the primary structure of 1T1 as compared with 1C1 and 1C3 have been described [123]: the molar ratio of galactose to 3,6-anhydrogalactose is 1:0.03, 1:0.64 and 1:0.37 for 1T1, 1C1 and 1 C3, respectively; the position of the sulfate group in the β-D-galactose residues is on C-2 in 1T1 and on C-4 in 1C1 and 1C3; and the content of α-D-galactose 2,6-disulfate residues is higher in 1T1.

Gigartina Tenella

KM043, a glycolipid isolated from the marine red alga Gigartina Tenella, belongs to the 6-sulfo-α-D-quinovopyranosyl-(1→3′)-1′,2′-diacylglycerol class of compounds. It has been shown to have significant anti-human immunodeficiency virus effect. It strongly and selectively inhibits mammalian DNA polymerase α, DNA polymerase β, terminal deoxynucleotidyl transferase, and human immunodeficiency virus-reverse transcriptase type 1 with IC_{50} values of 0.25, 0.38, 3.6, and 11.2 μM, respectively [110, 211]. The sulfo group [212] and the eicosapentanoic acid [213, 214] in KM043 are important for inhibitory activity.

Florideophyceae. Gigartinales. Hypneaceae.

Hypnea Musciformis is the only species of family Hypneaceae (order Gigartinales) which antiviral activity has been screened in.

Hypnea Musciformis

Extracts from Hypnea Musciformis, principally polysaccharides, have significant antiviral effect. Bouhlal *et al.* [100] have constated that the anti-HSV-1 effect associated to the water extract (EC_{50} = 23.5 μg mL^{-1}) is more potent that the effects which have methanolic (EC_{50} = 6.5 μg mL^{-1}), dichloromethane (EC_{50} = >250 μg mL^{-1}) or chloroforme-methanol (EC_{50} = 51.4 μg mL^{-1}) extracts. Furthermore, it is significantly less cytotoxic than the others: the percentages of Vero cell destruction are 10.6 % for the aqueous extract (CC_{50} = >250 μg mL^{-1}), 61.4% for the methanolic extract (CC_{50} = 140.1 μg mL^{-1}), 57 % for the chloroforme-methanol extract (CC_{50} = 205.5 μg mL^{-1}) and 49.48 % for the dichloromethane extract (CC_{50} = >250 μg mL^{-1}).

Florideophyceae. Gigartinales. Kallymeniaceae.

Species of family Kallymeniaceae (order Gigartinales) which antiviral activity has been screened in include: Callophyllis Variegate and Kallymenia Requienii.

Callophyllis Variegata

The potent antiviral activity and the low cytotoxicity associated to compounds from Callophyllis Variegata indicate that they can be considered very promising antiviral agents. Several galactans extracted from this red seaweed show potent antiviral activity against herpes simplex types 1 and 2 and dengue type 2 viruses, with values of IC_{50} ranging from 0.10 to 2.19 μg mL^{-1}. Some of them are even effective against acyclovir-resistant variants of herpes simplex virus (0.35-0.47 μg mL^{-1}) [132]. In relation to herpes simplex virus type 1, the inhibitory effect of these sulfated polysaccharides appears to be based mainly on its ability to interfere with the replication cycle of virus, in particular with the initial attachment of the virus to the target cell. The structure of these compounds indicates potential to prevent virus infection, since they fulfill features such as adequate molecular weight and sulfate on the 2-position of the 3-linked unit and on the 2-position of the 4-linked unit in the diads G2S→DA2S and G2S,4S→DA2S [152]. In the diad G2S→D2S,3S,6S sulfation in the 2-position of the 3-linked unit and on the 6-position of the 4-linked unit is consistent with the sulfation of the minimal binding domain to the virus in kappa-carrageenan [152]; however, the influence of sulfation on the 3-position remains uncertain.

Kallymenia Requienii

Up to now, the only study carried out about antiviral activity associated with compounds from Kallymenia Requienii demonstrates that extracts of this alga have antiviral activity either against herpes simplex virus type 1 cultured in kidney cells of monkey and vesicular stomatitis virus in kidney cells of hamster [91].

Florideophyceae. Gigartinales. Peyssonneliaceae.

Species of family Peyssonneliaceae (order Gigartinales) which antiviral activity has been screened in include: Peyssonnelia Bornetii, Peyssonnelia Rosa-Marina, Peyssonnelia Rubra, and Peyssonnelia Squamaria.

Peyssonnelia sp.

Peyssonol A and B are two natural compounds of the sesquiterpene hydroquinone group with biogenesis based on the farnesyl and hydroquinone precursors [215]. These inhibitors are structurally related to other compounds such as avarol, avarone derivatives [216] and illimaquinone [217]. Peyssonol A and B are isolated from algae Peyssonnelia sp. and are potent inhibitors of the RNA-dependent DNA polymerase activity of both human immunodeficiency virus types 1 and 2 reverse transcriptases (RTs). Both compounds inhibit more than 80% of the RNA-dependent DNA polymerase activity of the enzyme at a final inhibitor concentration of 20 μM. Peyssonol A and B strongly inhibit the poly(rA)n.oligo(dT)12-18-directed DNA synthesis of human immunodeficiency virus type 1 RT (IC_{50} = 6.4 and 4.3 μM, respectively). The response of human immunodeficiency virus type 2 RT to the inhibitors is somewhat different. In general, human immunodeficiency virus type 2 RT is less sensitive to peyssonols A and B and the responses of the 2 DNA-polymerizing activities of this enzyme to both inhibitors is less pronounced relative to human immunodeficiency virus type 1 RT. Thus, 50% inhibition of the human immunodeficiency virus type 2 RT-associated RNA-directed DNA synthesis is achieved at about 21 μM peyssonol A and at about 15 μM peyssonol B [108].

The inhibition of the DNA polymerase activities is independent of the nature of the template primers used. Peyssonol A binds the enzyme at sites different from the binding sites of both substrates, dTTP and poly(rA)n.oligo(dT)12-18, since its mode of inhibition is noncompetitive with respect to dTTP and varies from a noncompetitive (at low concentrations of peyssonols A) to a linear-mixed (at higher concentrations) with respect to the template primer. This is partially true for peyssonol B, which is noncompetitive with respect to only dNTP, but is competitive with respect to the template primer. Since peyssonol B and the template primer bear no apparent structural resemblance, the competitive pattern of inhibition can be explained by an indirect steric hindrance or by the overlap of the inhibitor and the substrate distinct binding sites of the enzyme. In relation to peyssonol B, the pattern of the steady-state kinetics with respect to dTTP varies from noncompetitive at low concentrations of peyssonol B to linear-mixed at higher concentrations. As in the case of peyssonol A, peyssonol B and dTTP bind the enzyme independently at different sites. Peyssonol B binds RT with higher affinity than dTTP. Alternatively, the binding of the inhibitor to a distinct site induces conformational changes that distort the binding of the template primer. Furthermore, both peyssonol A and peyssonol B interfere with the direct binding of the RT to the template primer, offering an explanation for the mechanism of the enzymne inhibition [108].

Peyssonnelia Bornetii

Extracts of the alga Peyssonnelia Bornetii show no antiviral activity either against herpes simplex virus type 1 cultured in kidney cells of monkey or vesicular stomatitis virus in kidney cells of hamster [91].

Peyssonnelia Rosa-Marina

Antiviral properties of extracts from Peyssonnelia Rosa-marina have been studied but no anti-hespes simplex virus type 1 or anti-vesicular stomatitis virus effect *in vitro* has been observed [91].

Peyssonnelia Rubra

Antiviral activity of extracts from the red alga Peyssonnelia Rubra has been tested against herpes simplex virus type 1 cultured in kidney cells of monkey and vesicular stomatitis virus in kidney cells of hamster, but positive results have not been demonstrated [91].

Peyssonnelia Squamaria

Extracts of the alga Peyssonnelia Squamaria show no antiviral activity either against herpes simplex virus type 1 cultured in kidney cells of monkey or vesicular stomatitis virus in kidney cells of hamster [91].

Florideophyceae. Gigartinales. Phyllophoraceae.

Species of family Phyllophoraceae (order Gigartinales) which antiviral activity has been screened in include: Gymnogongrus Griffithsiae, Gymnogongrus Torulosus, Phyllophora Crispa, and Stenogramme Interrupta.

Gymnogongrus Griffithsiae

Several structural types of carrageenans from Gymnogongrus Griffithsiae have shown a potent antiviral activity against enveloped viruses.

i. Dengue Virus

Kappa/iota/nu carrageenan G3d, a natural sulfated polysaccharide isolated from the red seaweed Gymnogongrus Griffithsiae [75] has been assayed for its antiviral action against the four serotypes of dengue virus [150]. The antiviral activity of the sulfated polysaccharide is dependent on the viral serotype (order of susceptibility from higher to lower: dengue virus type 2 > dengue virus type 3 > dengue virus type 4 > dengue virus type 1). G3d is an effective and selective inhibitor of dengue virus type 2. It inhibits dengue virus type 2 multiplication in Vero cells (IC_{50} value 0.9 μg mL^{-1}), whereas the IC_{50} values for the reference polysaccharides heparin and dextran sulfate (DS8000) are 1.9 and 0.9 μg mL^{-1}, respectively. On the other hand, dengue virus type 3 and dengue virus type 4 are significantly less susceptible to the polysulfate (IC_{50} value for dengue virus type 3 = 14.2 μg mL^{-1}; IC_{50} value for dengue virus type 4 = 29.3 μg mL^{-1}) and dengue virus type 1 is not susceptible to the compound. Similar results are observed when different types of host cells are used (human hepatoma cells and foreskin fibroblasts, besides Vero cells). G3d is an effective inhibitor of dengue virus type 2 and dengue virus type 3 in the human hepatoma cells and foreskin fibroblasts cells although with higher antiviral effectiveness against the serotype dengue virus type 2.

G3d is active only when added together with the virus or early after infection (1 hour). It is thought that virus adsorption and internalization are the main targets of this compound. This is a surprising result about the mode of action of polysulfates, since most studies on enveloped viruses have established that these compounds act by preventing predominantly the first stage of virion binding to cell receptor [68, 152]. In fact, a study carried out by Talarico *et al.* [75] demonstrated that this compound inhibits the viral attachment but it lacks any subsequent effect.

ii. Herpes Simplex Virus

Sulfated galactans isolated from Gymnogongrus Griffithsiae have *in vitro* activity against herpes simplex virus (values of EC_{50} ranging from 0.5 to 5.6 μg mL^{-1}) as determined in a virus plaque reduction assay in Vero cells. They have levels of effectiveness similar to that achieved by the reference compounds of known antiherpetic activity (heparin and dextran sulfate) [66], showing a broad spectrum of antiviral activity against herpes simplex virus types 1 and 2 [75]. Antiviral activity of these polysulfates is correlated with the degree of sulfation [68, 218], the degree of polymerization and the position of sulfate groups on the polymer backbone [75]. The mode of action of these compounds could be mainly ascribed to an inhibitory effect on virus adsorption, the first step of the replicative cycle.

Gymnogongrus Torulosus

Pujol *et al.* [128] have identified DL-galactan hybrids isolated from the red seaweed Gymnogongrus Torulosus with *in vitro* antiviral properties against herpes simplex virus type 2 and dengue virus type 2. These compounds are very active against both viruses with IC_{50} values in the range 0.6-16 μg mL^{-1} for herpes simplex virus type 2 and 0.19-1.7 μg mL^{-1} for dengue virus type 2. These galactans achieve full inhibitory activity when they are present during virus adsorption period, suggesting that the mode of action of these compounds is an interference in the binding of the surface envelope glycoprotein with the cell receptor.

Phyllophora Crispa

There is little evidence about antiviral properties of compounds from Phyllophora Crispa. The only study carried out up to now reveals that extracts of this alga shows antiviral activity against herpes simplex virus type 1 cultured in kidney cells of monkey and vesicular stomatitis virus in kidney cells of hamster [91].

Stenogramme Interrupta

Polysaccharides from cystocarpic (polysaccharide C) and tetrasporic (polysaccharide T) Stenogramme Interrupta show antiviral effects against different strains of herpes simplex virus [125]. Polysaccharides from cystocarpic Stenogramme Interrupta are of the kappa-/iota-carrageenan type while the polysaccharides from tetrasporic Stenogramme Interrupta are of lambda-carrageenan type [219]. The polysaccharide T is the most active polysaccharide isolated from Stenogramme Interrupta against herpes simplex virus (IC_{50} values = 0.65-2.88 μg mL^{-1}), whereas the polysaccharide C is slightly less effective than polysaccharide T (IC_{50} values = 1.9-9.33 μg mL^{-1}). However, both polysaccharides show a wide spectrum of action against the two serotypes of herpes simplex virus, including acyclovir resistant variants. In general, the strains of herpes simplex virus type 2 are more sensitive to the antiviral effect of polysaccharides isolated from Stenogramme Interrupta than is herpes simplex virus type 1. The antiherpetic activity of these polysaccharides is similar to that reported for the lambda- and kappa-/iota-carrageenans obtained from Gigartina Skottsbergii [123].

Polysaccharide T and C do not exert a direct virucidal effect on herpes simplex virus but are true antiviral agents interfering the replication cycle of herpes simplex virus. Specifically, the main target for polysaccharides T and C action in the replicative cycle is the virus attachment to the host cell, interfering with the initial binding of the viral glycoprotein gC to the cellular heparan sulfate proteoglycans. Caceres *et al.* [125] showed that the IC_{50} values for polysaccharides T and C vary in relation to the time when they are added: *Polysaccharide T.* IC_{50} = 2.56 μg mL^{-1} when polysaccharide only at adsorption and 0.65 μg mL^{-1} when polysaccharide at adsorption and post-adsorption; *polysaccharide C.* IC_{50} = 6.81 μg mL^{-1} when polysaccharide only at adsorption and 1.90 μg mL^{-1} when polysaccharide at adsorption and post-adsorption. If the carrageenans are added only after adsorption, they are no longer effective even at a concentration of 50 μg mL^{-1}.

Florideophyceae. Gigartinales. Solieriaceae.

Species of family Solieriaceae (order Gigartinales) which antiviral activity has been screened in include: Agardhiella Tenera, Eucheuma Cottonii, Eucheuma Spinosa, and Meristiella Gelidium.

Agardhiella Tenera

Sulfated galactans from the red seaweed Aghardhiella Tenera are active against several viruses [68, 107].

i. Human Immunodeficiency Virus

They provide protection against human immunodeficiency virus type 1 and human immunodeficiency virus type 2 at a concentration 10-fold higher than the concentration at which dextran sulfate (reference compound) [66] protects the cells (IC_{50} = 0.5 and 0.05 mg mL^{-1} for human immunodeficiency virus types 1 and 2, respectively) [68, 107]. Galactans block the binding of human immunodeficiency virus type 1 to the host cells (IC_{50} approximately 40.0 µg mL^{-1}). The inhibition of virus binding by galactans can be ascribed to a direct interaction of the compound with the human immunodeficiency virus envelope glycoprotein gp120.

ii. Other Viruses

Sulfated galactans are also active against other enveloped viruses (herpesviruses, togaviruses, arenaviruses, myxoviruses and rhabdoviruses) [68, 107]. They are particularly potent against herpes simplex virus type 1, herpes simplex virus type 2, cytomegalovirus and vaccinia virus. Concretely, their inhibitory effect on the replication of herpes simplex virus type 1 (IC_{50} = 0.7 µg mL^{-1}) and vaccinia virus (IC_{50} = 7 µg mL^{-1}) is higher than that obtained by dextran sulfate (MW5000) (IC_{50} = 2 µg mL^{-1} and IC_{50} = 200 µg mL^{-1}, respectively), whereas herpes simplex virus type 2 (galactan sulfate. IC_{50}= 2.5 µg mL^{-1}; dextran sulfate. IC_{50} = 1.4 µg mL^{-1}) and cytomegalovirus (galactan sulfate. IC_{50} = 4 µg mL^{-1}; dextran sulfate. IC_{50} = 0.4 µg mL^{-1}) are less sensitive. Sulfated galactans have also an inhibitory effect against RNA viruses. They are very active against Sindbis virus (IC_{50} = 11 µg mL^{-1}), influenza virus A (IC_{50} = 4 µg mL^{-1}), respiratory syncytial virus (IC_{50} = 4 µg mL^{-1}) and vesicular stomatitis virus (IC_{50} = 14 µg mL^{-1}). They inhibit these viruses at a concentration that is equal to or lower than the concentration at which dextran sulfate inhibits these viruses (IC_{50} = 150 µg mL^{-1}; IC_{50} = 14 µg mL^{-1}; IC_{50} = 14 µg mL^{-1}; IC_{50} = 14 µg mL^{-1}, respectively). On the contrary, galactans are not active against influenza virus B (IC_{50} = >200 µg mL^{-1}), poliovirus type 1 (IC_{50} = >200 µg mL^{-1}), coxsackie B4 virus (IC_{50} = >200 μg mL^{-1}), reovirus type 1 (IC_{50} = >100 μg mL^{-1}), Junin virus (IC_{50} = >100 μg mL^{-1}) and Tacaribe virus (IC_{50} = >100 μg mL^{-1}) at concentrations that are significantly lower than the cytotoxicity threshold. The inhibitory effects of galactans on enveloped viruses other than human immunodeficiency virus, such as herpes simplex virus, respiratory syncytial virus, vesicular stomatitis virus and influenza A virus, can also be attributed to inhibition of virus binding to the host cells.

Eucheuma Cottonii

Kappa-carrageenans isolated from Eucheuma Cottonii have a broad-spectrum antiviral activity [66, 154]. They are potent inhibitors of herpesviruses including herpes simplex virus type 1 (MIC = 3.7-15 μg mL^{-1}), herpes simplex virus type 2 (MIC = 2 μg mL^{-1}) and cytomegalovirus (MIC = 2.8 μg mL^{-1}). Likewise, kappa-carrageenans are active against vesicular stomatitis virus (MIC = 0.3-7 μg mL^{-1}), sindbis virus (MIC = 7 μg mL^{-1}), human immunodeficiency virus type 1 (MIC = 12 μg mL^{-1}) and hepatitis A virus (SI = >10). Furthermore, vaccinia virus is also inhibited but only at relatively high concentrations of the polysaccharides (MIC = 36 μg mL^{-1}).

However, kappa-carrageenans are inactive against adenovirus type 2 (MIC = >200 μg mL^{-1}), coxsackie B4 virus (MIC = >400 μg mL^{-1}), poliovirus type 1 (MIC = >400 μg mL^{-1}), parainfluenza virus type 3 (MIC = >40 μg mL^{-1}) and reovirus type 1 (MIC = >40 μg mL^{-1}).

Eucheuma Spinosa

Iota-carrageenans isolated from Eucheuma Spinosa show potent inhibitory effect on the replication of herpes simplex virus type 1 (CPE_{50} = 2 μg mL^{-1}), herpes simplex virus type 2 (CPE_{50} = 10 μg mL^{-1}), hepatitis A virus (SI = >400), Semliki Forest virus (CPE_{50} = 10 μg mL^{-1}), vaccinia virus (CPE_{50} = 10 μg mL^{-1}), swine fever virus (CPE_{50} = 10μg mL^{-1}) and naked viruses like encephalomyocarditis virus (CPE_{50} = 10 μg mL^{-1}) [153, 154]. On the contrary, these carrageenans are devoid of any activity against vesicular stomatitis virus (CPE_{50} = >200μg mL^{-1}), measles virus (CPE_{50} = >200μg mL^{-1}), poliovirus (CPE_{50} = >200μg mL^{-1}) and adenovirus (CPE_{50} = >200μg mL^{-1}) [153].

It is thought that antiviral activity of these carrageenans is attributed to the inhibition of a step in virus replication subsequent to viral internalization but prior to the onset of late viral protein synthesis [153].

Meristiella Gelidium

Compounds from Meristiella gelidium are significant antiviral agents.

i. Herpes Simplex Virus

Carrageenans isolated from Meristiella Gelidium are among the most potent sulfated polysaccharides obtained from red seaweeds according to their inhibitory activity against herpesvirus [152]. de SF-Tischer *et al.* [133] showed that galactans from Meristiella Gelidium (M1, M3 and M3a), which are iota/kappa/nu-hybrid carrageenans with the former one in higher proportion, exhibit antiherpetic activity, with IC_{50} values in the range 0.04-0.06 μg mL^{-1}. The antiviral action and selectivity index of these compounds are higher than the reference substances heparin (IC_{50} = 0.6 μg mL^{-1}) and DS 8000 (IC_{50} = 0.6 μg mL^{-1}) and the polysaccharides from other red algae, such as Gymnogongrus Griffithsiae [75]. Bearing in mind that the selectivity index against herpes simplex virus type 2 for the most active fraction isolated (M3a) is 25,000, this carrageenan may be considered as a promising agent for the treatment of genital herpes simplex virus type 2 infections.

ii. Dengue Virus

Besides their antiherpetic activity, the carrageenans M1, M3 and M3a also have inhibitory action against dengue virus type 2. However, the inhibitory action against dengue virus type 2 is lower than that detected against herpes simplex virus type 2. The range of IC_{50} against dengue virus type 2 is 0.14-1.6 μg mL^{-1}. Again, the galactans derived from Meristiella Gelidium are more effective inhibitors of dengue virus type 2 if compared with reference polysaccharides (IC_{50} for heparin = 1.9 μg mL^{-1} and IC_{50} for DS8000 = 0.9 μg mL^{-1}) [133].

Florideophyceae. Gigartinales. Sphaerococcaceae.

Sphaerococcus Coronopifolius is the only species of family Sphaerococcaceae (order Gigartinales) which antiviral activity has been screened in.

Sphaerococcus Coronopifolius

Polysaccharides from Sphaerococcus Coronopifolius composed of galactose, 3,6-anhydrogalactose, uronics acids and sulfate in ratios of 33.1, 11.0, 7.7 and 24.0% (w/w) inhibit *in vitro* replication of encapsulated virus [116]. These compounds have antiviral properties against human immunodeficiency virus [116] and herpes simplex virus [100, 116], but not against vesicular stomatitis virus [91].

i. Human Immunodeficiency Virus

Polysaccharides from Sphaerococcus Coronopifolius inhibit *in vitro* replication of the human immunodeficiency virus at concentrations of 12.5 $\mu g\ mL^{-1}$. The adsorption step of virus to the host cell seems to be the specific target for polysaccharide action. It is quite possible that polysaccharides could affect the virus-cell attachment by spreading a three-dimensional gel network over the whole of the cell surface. This structural modification would entail envelope alteration and concealing of virus-specific receptors sites. Such a mechanism would prevent adsorption of the viruses to the cell surface and hence penetration and replication. Bouhlal *et al.* [116] suggest that these polysaccharides exert a direct inhibitory effect on human immunodeficiency virus type 1 replication by controlling the appearance of the new generations of virus and potential virucidal effect.

ii. Herpes Simplex Virus

Despite Ballesteros *et al.* [91] found no antiherpetic activity associated to extracts from Sphaerococcus Coronopifolius, other studies have demonstrated the opposite effect. Polysaccharides from this alga confer total protection against herpes simplex virus type 1 as determined in a virus plaque reduction assay in Vero cells (EC_{50} = 4.1 $\mu g\ mL^{-1}$), although with low selectivity index (SI = 61) [116]. Furthermore, Bouhlal *et al.* [100] found antiherpetic activity associated to extracts from this alga. They observed that the water extract from Sphaerococcus

Coronopifolius has a higher antiviral effect (EC_{50} = 4.4 μg mL^{-1}) than methanolic (EC_{50} = 21.4 μg mL^{-1}), dichloromethane (EC_{50} = >250 μg mL^{-1}) or chloroforme-methanol (EC_{50} = 25.4 μg mL^{-1}) extracts. Furthermore, it is significantly less cytotoxic than the others: the percentages of Vero cell destruction are 11.1 % for the aqueous extract (CC_{50} = >250 μg mL^{-1}), 92.7% for the methanolic extract (CC_{50} = 3.3 μg mL^{-1}), 85.3 % for the chloroforme-methanol extract (CC_{50} = 48.5 μg mL^{-1}) and 45 % for the dichloromethane extract (CC_{50} = >250 μg mL^{-1}).

Florideophyceae. Gracilariales. Gracilariaceae

Species of family Gracilariaceae (order Gracilariales) which antiviral activity has been screened in include: Gracilaria Corticata and Gracilaria Salicornia.

Gracilaria Corticata

Antiviral properties of extracts from Gracilaria Corticata have been studied [71, 138]. Mazunder *et al.* [71] analyzed the antiviral activity of three soluble polysaccharides from Gracilaria Corticata collected from the shorelines of India, WE2NGF, Au2 and AAu2. They observed that WE2NGF, a high molecular weight galactan having sulfate group at C-6 of L-galactose and C-4 of D-galactose units, possesses a marked antiherpetic activity with IC_{50} values of 0.19 and 0.24 mg mL^{-1} for herpes simplex virus types 1 and 2, respectively. The other 2 fractions, Au2 (floridean starch) and AAu2 (agar polymer), are less active for both serotypes of herpes virus, with IC_{50} ranging from 27.5 to 50.0 mg mL^{-1}, than WE2NGF. An explanation for these results may be the fact that WE2NGF has a higher amount of sulfate ester groups and a higher molecular weight than the two other fractions tested. As it was previously commented, antiviral activity of sulfated seaweed polysaccharides depends on the degree of sulfation and molecular weight of the polysaccharide [138, 152, 220]. The antiviral activity increases with the degree of sulfation and molecular weight. Likewise the distribution of sulfate groups along polymer chain and the conformational flexibility of this chain for adopting a definite shape that might be required during the formation of polysaccharide-virus complex is an important aspect [119].

The mechanism of action of the WE2NGF could be attributed to inhibition of virus adsorption, interfering with the interaction of viral glycoproteins with the negatively charged heparan sulfate receptors present in the cell membrane [71]. Since WE2NGF lacks cytotoxicity, it may be a potential anti-herpes simplex virus drug candidate.

On the other hand, Chattopadhyay *et al.* [138] analyzed 6 water-extracted polysaccharides of Gracilaria Corticata: WE (water extract), F3· (subfraction with galactose, 6-*O*-methyl galactose, 3,6-anhydrogalactose and xylose residues as neutral sugars, characteristic of agar type molecule), WES1, WES2, F3S1 and F3S2 (all of them hyper sulfated derivatives). They observed that the 6 compounds have anti-herpes simplex virus activity with IC_{50} from 1.1 to 27.4 μg mL^{-1}. The inhibition against herpes simplex virus type 2 (1.7-14.6 μg mL^{-1}) is slightly higher when compared with that obtained against herpes simplex virus type 1 (3.7-27.4 μg mL^{-1}). F3S1 and F3S2 (hypersulfated F3 derivatives) are very selective herpes simplex virus inhibitors with selectivity indices in the range 617.3-877.7. Sulfate group located at C-4 of (1→3)-linked galactopyranosyl residues of the native galactan, seems to be very important for the anti-herpetic activity of these compounds.

Gracilaria Salicornia

The antiviral effect of Gracilaria Salicornia has been tested for the first time in 2007 [137]. The water crude extract of Gracilaria Salicornia, which is heat stable, has antiviral activity against herpes simplex virus type 2. It prevents the initial stages of herpes simplex virus type 2 replication such as adsorption and attachment of the virus to the host cell (extract at concentration 140-170 μg mL^{-1}; IC_{50} = 82-99.3 μg mL^{-1}). Furthermore it also exhibits a reasonable effect on inhibition of virus replication after attachment of herpes simplex virus type 2 to the monkey kidney cells (extract at concentration 190 μg mL^{-1}; IC_{50} = 8114-128 μg mL^{-1}). So, water soluble extract of Gracilaria Salicornia could be a good choice for natural antiherpetic compound development.

Florideophyceae. Halymeniales. Halymeniaceae

Species of family Halymeniaceae (order Halymeniales) which antiviral activity has been screened in include: Cryptonemia Crenulata, Grateloupia Filicina, Grateloupia Indica, and Grateloupia Longifolia.

Cryptonemia Crenulata

Polysulfates isolated from Cryptonemia Crenulata deserve consideration as virus entry inhibitors. Antidengue and antiherpetic activities associated to these natural compounds have been described.

i. Dengue Virus

DL-galactan hybrid C2S-3, a natural sulfated polysaccharide isolated from the red seaweed Cryptonemia Crenulata [75], has been assayed for its antiviral action against the four serotypes of dengue virus [150]. The antiviral activity of the sulfated polysaccharide is dependent on the viral serotype (order of susceptibility from higher to lower: dengue virus type 2 > dengue virus type 3 > dengue virus type 4 > dengue virus type 1). C2S-3 is an effective and selective inhibitor of dengue virus type 2. It inhibits dengue virus type 2 multiplication in Vero cells (IC_{50} value 1 μg mL^{-1}), whereas the IC_{50} values for the reference polysaccharides heparin and dextran sulfate (DS8000) are 1.9 and 0.9 μg mL^{-1}, respectively. On the other hand, dengue virus type 3 and dengue virus type 4 are significantly less susceptible to the polysulfate (IC_{50} value for dengue virus type 3, 13.9 μg mL^{-1}; IC_{50} value for dengue virus type 4 could not be estimated) and dengue virus type 1 is not susceptible to the compound. Similar results are observed when different types of host cells are used (human hepatoma cells and foreskin fibroblasts, besides Vero cells). C2S-3 is an effective inhibitor of dengue virus type 2 and dengue virus type 3 in human hepatoma cells and foreskin fibroblasts cells although with higher antiviral effectiveness against the serotype dengue virus type 2.

C2S-3 is active only when added together with the virus or early after infection (1 hour). It is thought that virus adsorption and internalization are the main targets of this compound [150, 221]. As it was commented in relation to polysaccharides from Gymnogongrus Griffithsiae, this is a surprising result about the mode of action of polysulfates, since most studies on enveloped viruses have established that these compounds act by preventing predominantly the first stage of virion binding to cell receptor [68, 152]. In fact, a previous study on the anti-herpetic activity of C2S-3 demonstrated that this compound is inhibitor of viral attachment but it lacks any subsequent effect [75].

ii. Herpes Simplex Virus

Sulfated galactans isolated from Cryptonemia Crenulata have *in vitro* activity against herpes simplex virus, exhibiting a more effective antiviral action and higher selectivity indices than the reference compounds (heparin and dextran sulfate) [75]. Furthermore, they show also a significant protective effect *in vivo* against herpes simplex virus type 2 vaginal infection, suggesting the potential use of this low cost product and easy to obtain in large quantities, for prophylaxis of virus infection. Antiviral activity of these polysulfates is correlated with the degree of sulfation [68, 218], the degree of polymerization and the position of sulfate groups on the polymer backbone [75]. Herpes simplex virus adsorption is the main target for the antiviral effect of these compounds, which mainly interfere with the interaction virion glycoprotein-heparan sulfate residues of sulfated galactans.

Grateloupia Filicina

Compounds isolated from Grateloupia Filicina have shown to have antiviral activity [113, 136].

i. Human Immunodeficiency Virus

Sulfated galactans isolated from Grateloupia Filicina cause potent inhibition of human immunodeficiency virus type 1 at micromolar concentrations when added at the time of infection or 2 h post-infection (EC_{50} = 0.006-0.004 μM, EC_{90} = 0.60-0.33 μM) [113]. This antiviral activity is comparable with dextran sulfate (EC_{50} = 0.001 μM, EC_{90} = 0.19-0.21 μM). The potency of the antiviral activity of these compounds is related with the sulfate content. Wang *et al.* [113] observed that the galactans GFP and GLPE with sulfate contents of 25.7% and 18.5%, respectively are significantly more potent than the GLP with a very low sulfate content.

It is likely that post-infection activity involves inhibition of early post absorption steps such as virus internalization and inhibition of cell-to-cell transmission in successive cycles of replication [113]. These findings together with observed low cytotoxicity and high selectivity indices (SI = 550->1667) are of relevance to the potential use of these natural compounds as virucidal vaginal formulations.

ii. Herpes Simplex Virus

Amylose extracted from Grateloupia Filicina by water distilling and ethanol sedimentation has a prominenent role against herpes simplex virus type 2 (IC_{50} = 5.80 microg mL^{-1}). The antivirus activity happens in the stage of herpes simplex virus type 2 binding, adsorption and ingression with Vero cell [136].

Grateloupia Indica

Sulfated galactans (F3 and GiWE) of Grateloupia Indica are potent inhibitors of herpes simplex virus types 1 and 2, with values of IC_{50} ranging from 0.25 to 0.31 μg mL^{-1}. Their antiherpetic activity spectrum includes acyclovir-resistant variants (B2006 and Field; IC_{50} ranging from 0.12 to 0.89 μg mL^{-1}) and syncytial variants (1C3-syn 13-8 and 1C3-syn 14-1; IC_{50} ranging from 0.32 to 1.06 μg mL^{-1}) of herpes simplex virus type 1. The antiviral effect of these polysaccharides is linked to the anionic features of the molecules, given mainly by the high amount of sulfate groups [78].

Sulfated galactans from Grateloupia Indica represent very potent antiherpetic compounds (SI = 943-7083) among the diverse types of natural sulfated polysaccharides tested for antiviral activity [152]. They show a higher inhibitory effect when compared with reference sulfated polysaccharides such as dextran sulfate 8000 (>92 to >1754 μg mL^{-1}) and heparin (>110 to > 1887 μg mL^{-1}) [78].

The inhibitory effect of these sulfated polysaccharides is based mainly on their ability to interfere with the replication cycle of herpes simplex virus. Concretely, the mode of antiviral action of these compounds is attributed predominantly to inhibition of virus binding to the cells [78]. This mechanism is the most frequently used by polysaccharides with antiviral effects [69, 75, 131, 151].

Galactans from Grateloupia Indica lack of virucidal activity. This finding is in accordance with other studies that report most algal sulfated galactans are not able to produce significant virion inactivation [71, 75, 131]. Kappa-carrageenans from Gigartina Skottsbergii, which possess potent inactivating properties against herpes simplex virus type 1 [69] are, however, an exception.

Grateloupia Longifolia

Sulfated galactans obtained from Grateloupia Longifolia cause potent inhibition of human immunodeficiency virus type 1 at micromolar concentrations when added at the time of infection or 2 h post-infection (EC_{50} = 0.011-0.002 μM, EC_{90} = 0.89-0.36 μM) [113]. This antiviral activity is comparable with dextran sulfate (EC_{50} = 0.001 μM, EC_{90} = 0.19-0.21 μM). The potency of the antiviral activity of these compounds is related with the sulfate content. Wang *et al.* [113] observed that the galactans GFP and GLPE with sulfate contents of 25.7% and 18.5%, respectively are significantly more potent than the GLP with a very low sulfate content.

It is likely that post-infection activity involves inhibition of early post absorption steps such as virus internalization and inhibition of cell-to-cell transmission in successive cycles of replication [113]. These findings together with their observed low cytotoxicity and high selectivity indices (SI = 187->5000) are of relevance to the potential use of these natural compounds as virucidal vaginal substances.

Florideophyceae. Nemaliales. Galaxauraceae

Tricleocarpa Oblongata is the only species of family Galaxauraceae (order Nemaliales) which antiviral activity has been screened in.

Tricleocarpa Oblongata

Ballesteros *et al.* [91] have tested antiviral activity of extracts from Tricleocarpa Oblongata, and they have constated that these compounds have no antiviral activity either against herpes simplex virus type 1 cultured in kidney cells of monkey or vesicular stomatitis virus in kidney cells of hamster.

Florideophyceae. Nemaliales. Scinaiaceae

Species of family Scinaiaceae (order Nemaliales) which antiviral activity has been screened in include: Nothogenia Fastigiata and Scinaia Hatei.

Nothogenia Fastigiata

Sulfated polysaccharides (xylomannans) isolated from Nothogenia Fastigiata inhibit efficiently the replication of human cytomegalovirus, respiratoroy syncytial virus, influenza A and B viruses, Junin and Tacaribe viruses, simian immunodeficiency virus [143] and herpes simplex virus type 1 (F, KOS, B-2006 and Field) and type 2 (G) [67, 119-121] in different cell lines (hamster kidney cells, African green monkey kidney cells and human epidermoid cancer cells). The potent inhibitory effect of these polysaccharides against high doses of virus represents a significant advantage for them with respect to other compounds only active against low viral inocula [120].

On the other hand, sulfated xylomannans obtained from this red seaweed are only weakly active against human immunodeficiency virus type 1 and human immunodeficiency virus type 2 (IC_{50}= ~10 μg mL^{-1}) [143]. However, they have been noted to be among the most characteristic marine metabolites with significant anti-human immunodeficiency virus activity [111].

Xylomannans afford significant inhibition if they are added to the cell cultures simultaneously with virus inoculums, but have no effect when they are added after infection (1 hour). Analysis of the early events of the viral replicative cycle shows that the antiviral effect of these polysaccharides is due to a specific inhibition of virus attachment to the host cell whereas virus internalization is not impaired [121, 143].

This antiviral activity of the xylomannans from Nothogenia Fastigiata can be explained on the basis of a flexible backbone, molecular size, content and distribution of sulfate groups and of the single stubs of β-(1 → 2)-linked D-xylose

[67, 218]. In relation to this effect, it is known that the ability to block the virus receptors does not depend directly on the primary structure as the backbone acts as carrier of the sulfate groups [218, 222, 223]. The sulfated polymer-virus "complex" is stabilized when a cooperative mechanism [224] of interaction between the sulfate groups and the positive virus receptors is involved, explaining the variation of antiviral activity with the sulfate content [67, 119, 121] and the molecular weight [67, 119]. The most adequate distribution of the sulfate groups for the mannan antiviral activity is that of the cell surface heparan sulfate receptors. The N-sulfation and the 6-O-sulfation of the α-D-glucosamine residues of heparan sulfate play a key role for viral binding [225]. Thus, those polysaccharides with a sulfate distribution structurally resembling the negative charge distribution of the binding sites of heparan sulfate competitively inhibit viral binding. Likewise, it is known the differential activity of an antiviral sulfated polysaccharide against several viruses (*e.g.* herpes simplex virus *versus* human immunodeficiency virus) is related to the topographycal distribution of the receptors on these viruses [218].

Scinaia Hatei

Sulfated xylomannans present in the red seaweed Scinaia Hatei, which contain a backbone of α-(1→3)-linked D-mannopyranosyl residues substituted at 2, 4 and 6 positions with single stubs of β-D-xylopyranosyl residues, have potent antiviral activity against herpes simplex virus types 1 and 2, as determined in a virus plaque reduction assay in Vero cells (IC_{50} values in the range of 0.6-4.6 μg mL^{-1}). The inhibitory effect of this type of polysaccharides against herpesviruses is very specific (SI in the range of >2000 – >654) [139].

The inhibitory effect detected by the plaque reduction assay is linked to the anionic features of the macromolecules [68, 152, 226]. Sulfate groups located at C-4 of α-(1→3)-linked D-mannopyranosyl units are very important for the anti-herpetic activity of this polymer [139]. It is thought that antiviral activity of sulfated xylomannans is mainly due to interference with some step of the herpes simplex virus multiplication cycle, and probably it is related to the inhibition of virus binding to the cells [77-79].

Florideophyceae. Nemastomatales. Schizymeniaceae

Species of family Schizymeniaceae (order Nemastomatales) which antiviral activity has been screened in include: Schizymenia Binderi, Schizymenia Dubyi, and Schizymenia Pacifica.

Schizymenia Binderi

Water-soluble polysaccharides from Schizymenia Binderi, considered as agaran-carrageenan hybrids, with predominance of a carrageenan backbone, have a highly selective antiviral activity against diverse strains of human herpes viruses [131]. They inhibit strains of both serotypes (herpes simplex virus types 1 and 2) to approximately the same extent, and are highly effective against strains of herpes simplex virus type 1 resistant to acyclovir (EC_{50} = 0.18-0.76 μg mL^{-1}; SI = 1316-5556). They exhibit a more effective antiviral action and selectivity indices higher than dextran sulfate 8000 indicating that the content of the sulfate groups and sulfation at position O-6 in dextran sulfate are not determinant factors on antiviral activity. Furthermore, these sulfated galactans have an antiviral effectiveness slightly superior to other sulfated galactans of algal origin, such as those compounds derived from Schizymenia Dubyi [109], Pterocladia Capillacea [122], Cryptopleura Ramosa [151], Nothogenia Fastigiata [121] and Bostrychia Montagnei [127].

Polysaccharides from Schizymenia Binderi exert a true antiviral action against herpes simplex virus, interfering with its multiplication in infected cells. Concretely, herpes simplex virus adsorption is the main target for the antiviral effect of these polysaccharides. Bearing in mind that both serotypes of herpes simplex virus use the heparan sulfate residues of cellular proteoglycans as the primary receptor for virion binding and adsorption [227], thus sulfated galactans of Schizymenia Binderi would exert its inhibitory effect by interference with the interaction of herpes simplex virus-heparan sulfate [131].

Schizymenia Dubyi

Water-soluble sulfated glucuronogalactans from Schizymenia Dubyi cause potent inactivation of human immunodeficiency virus type 1 [109]. Evaluation of the anti-human immunodeficiency virus type 1 effect of these polysaccharides indicates that syncitia formation and human immunodeficiency virus-associated reverse transcriptase *in vitro* are completely suppressed with 5 μg mL^{-1} of galactan extracted from Schizymenia Dubyi collected from April to July. This high anti-human immunodeficiency virus type 1 activity corresponds with a decrease in L-galactose, viscosity and sulfate content of the polysaccharide.

Schizymenia Pacifica

Sulfated polysaccharides isolated from Schizymenia Pacifica, which consist of galactose (73%), 3,6-anhydrogalactose (0.65%), and sulfonate (20%) and have a molecular weight of approximately 2,000,000, have been demonstrated to have significant antiviral activity [105, 106]. These compounds similar to lambda-carrageenans and with activity comparable to that of iota- and kappa-carrageenans, selectively inhibit the reverse transcriptase activity of human immunodeficiency virus in a dose-dependent fashion [106]. It seems that sulfate residues might play a key role in the inhibition of reverse transcriptase, because this enzyme can be inhibited by virtue of competition between the sulfated side chains of the polysaccharides and the template primer for a site on the enzyme [228]. Furthermore, these polysaccharides suppress the human immunodeficiency virus replication in human immunodeficiency virus-infected MT-4 cells. Nakashima *et al.* [106] counted a total of 127 plaques per dish in the control dishes, and 100, 60, 11, and 1 plaques per dish in the dishes containing 0.5×10^4, 1×10^4, 2×10^4, and 4×10^4 IU of polysaccharides per ml, respectively.

Florideophyceae. Plocamiales. Plocamiaceae

Plocamium Cartilagineum is the only species of family Plocamiaceae (order Plocamiales) which antiviral activity has been screened in.

Plocamium Cartilagineum

Complex sulfated compounds isolated from Plocamium Cartilagineum show good antiviral activity against herpes simplex virus types 1 and 2 [100, 141]. However they are more effective against herpes simplex virus type 2 ($IC_{50} = 2.4 \pm 1.5$ μg mL^{-1}) than against herpes simplex virus type 1 (5.4 ± 1.3 μg mL^{-1}). Furthermore, the extraction method used to obtain compounds from this alga is a very important factor. In this way, Bouhlal *et al.* [100] found that the water extract from Plocamium Cartilagineum (EC_{50} = 6.4 μg mL^{-1}) has a higher antiviral effect than methanolic (EC_{50} = 23.2 μg mL^{-1}) or chloroforme-methanol (EC_{50} = 27.4 μg mL^{-1}) extracts. Furthemore, it exhibits an insignificant cytotoxic effect as compared to the other 2 extracts: the percentages of Vero cell destruction are 4.81% for the aqueous extract (CC_{50} = >250 μg mL^{-1}), 85.2% for the methanolic extract (CC_{50} = 28.7 μg mL^{-1}) and 88.1 % for the chloroforme-methanol extract (CC_{50} = 64.3 μg mL^{-1}).

Complex sulfated galactans isolated from Plocamium Cartilagineum have no antiviral activity *per se*, so their action involves inhibition of virus adsorption. They form stable virus-sulfated compound complexes where binding is not reversible and hence the sites on the viral envelope required for virus attachment to host cells are occupied by the sulfated compounds [141].

Florideophyceae. Rhodymeniales. Rhodymeniaceae

Botryocladia Botryoides is the only species of family Rhodymeniaceae (order Rhodymeniales) which antiviral activity has been screened in.

Botryocladia Botryoides

Antiviral activity of extracts from the red alga Botryocladia Botryoides has been tested against herpes simplex virus type 1 cultured in kidney cells of monkey and vesicular stomatitis virus in kidney cells of hamster, but positive results have not been demonstrated [91].

Florideophyceae. Sebdeniales. Sebdeniaceae

Sebdenia Polydactyla is the only species of family Sebdeniaceae (order Sebdeniales) which antiviral activity has been screened in.

Sebdenia Polydactyla

Sulfated xylomannans isolated from Sebdenia Polydactyla show strong activity against herpes simplex virus type 1 (IC_{50} values are in the range 0.35-2.8 μg mL^{-1})

and lack cytotoxicity at concentrations up to 1,000 μg mL^{-1}. The most potent polysaccharide isolated from this alga has 0.6 sulfate groups per monomer unit and contains a backbone of α -(1-->3)-linked D-mannopyranosyl residues substituted at position 6 with a single stub of β-D-xylopyranosyl residues [140]. The degree of sulfation largely influences the *in vitro* anti-herpes simplex virus type 1 activity associated to these polysaccharides.

CONCLUSIONS

Virus infection is one of the major threats for human health. In this way, smallpox has been recognized as one of the most lethal and devastating viral infections. The exposure to viruses can be minimized through strict adherence to sanitation and personal hygiene practices and the use of physical barriers. However, even with such care, virus infection does occur, requiring treatments by antiviral agents. The lack of effective vaccines and/or therapies for several viral infections, and the rapid emergence of viral mutans, which acquire resistance to drugs, have urged a growing need for developing new therapeutic agents to treat viral diseases.

Natural products are the most consistent and successful source of drugs. Approximately, 50% of the drugs introduced since 1994 are either natural products or derived from natural products. Likewise, many other drugs are derived from the use of natural products during the discovery process. It is also important to highlight the success of these natural products from the financial point of view. It has been estimated that the combined annual sales from 9 drugs developed as results of natural compounds are over US $16 billion. Despite this evidence, their potential use in drug discovery has been undervalued. In fact, less than 10% of the world's biodiversity has been tested for biological activity.

The medical uses of red algae date back thousands of years in China. However, modern medicine is "just now" discovering how they can be used to treat and prevent viral infections. In fact, red marine algae are one of many alternative medicine treatments that have experienced a rapid growth in popularity in recent years. The present review provides evidence of numerous red algae-derived compounds with antiviral properties which operate both outside and within our infected cells. They inhibit the initial attachment of DNA and RNA viruses to the host cells as well as different intracellular steps of viral replication. The main effective components in these extracts are polysaccharides (galactans, mannans, agars and carrageenans). The promising results for these compounds could be related to their action against virus specific targets and their selective interaction with them. Both aspects are important bearing in mind that polysaccharides lack acute and long-term toxicity against the host and they are effective at micromolar concentrations. In the light of these results, we reckon that the possibilities of discovering new drugs from natural products to reduce viral infection rates are encouraging.

Up to now, most of studies on marine-derived viral inhibitors have been carried out in *in vitro* conditions or in mouse model systems. Although evidence for clinical efficacy has also been discussed in numerous publications, successful randomized double blind placebo controlled trials are still rare. Recently promising results were published for carrageenan [229, 230]. Thus, conducting clinical trials are expected to contribute to the generation of new drugs from such natural products. In spite of the advantages of these products (greater chance of finding physiologically active compounds, fewer side effects in comparison to orthodox medical drugs, and high probability of positive synergistic effects), we must be conscious that drug development and the new technologies must go hand in hand. In this way, gene expression profile studies employing microarray technology have helped to identify molecular targets of the biological activity. Likewise, computer-aided drug design, biochip, transgenic and RNA interference technology have increased the knowledge of molecular signaling processes. Understanding the effectiveness of compounds with antiviral actions against the different types of disease-causing human viruses will be important to maximize the effectiveness of treating patients with these natural products.

ACKNOWLEDGEMENTS

There are no acknowledgments to be made to this manuscript.

CONFLICT OF INTEREST

The authors confirm that this chapter content has no conflict of interest.

REFERENCES

[1] Breitbart M, Rohwer F. Here a virus, there a virus, everywhere the same virus? Trends Microbiol 2005; 13(6): 278-84.

[2] Suttle CA. Viruses in the sea. Nature 2005; 437(7057): 356-61.

[3] Edwards RA, Rohwer F. Viral metagenomics. Nat Rev Microbiol 2005; 3(6): 504-10.

[4] Baltimore D. Expression of animal virus genomes. Bacteriol Rev 1971; 35(3): 235-41.

[5] Pringle CR. Virus taxonomy--1999. The universal system of virus taxonomy, updated to include the new proposals ratified by the International Committee on Taxonomy of Viruses during 1998. Arch Virol 1999; 144(2): 421-9.

[6] Lynch JP 3rd, Fishbein M, Echavarria M. Adenovirus. Semin Respir Crit Care Med 2011; 32(4): 494-511.

[7] Karasneh GA, Shukla D. Herpes simplex virus infects most cell types *in vitro*: clues to its success. Virol J 2011; 8: 481.

[8] Mosca F, Pugni L. Cytomegalovirus infection: the state of the art. J Chemother 2007; 19 Suppl 2: 46-8.

[9] Paran N, Sutter G. Smallpox vaccines: New formulations and revised strategies for vaccination. Hum Vaccin 2009; 5(12): 824-31.

[10] Corcoran A, Doyle S. Advances in the biology, diagnosis and host-pathogen interactions of parvovirus B19. J Med Microbiol 2004; 53(Pt 6): 459-75.

[11] Comins C, Heinemann L, Harrington K, Melcher A, De Bono J, Pandha H. Reovirus: viral therapy for cancer 'as nature intended'. Clin Oncol (R Coll Radiol) 2008; 20(7): 548-54.

[12] Patel M, Steele AD, Parashar UD. Influence of oral polio vaccines on performance of the monovalent and pentavalent rotavirus vaccines. Vaccine 2012; 30 Suppl 1: A30-5.

[13] Frieman M, Baric R. Mechanisms of severe acute respiratory syndrome pathogenesis and innate immunomodulation. Microbiol Mol Biol Rev 2008; 72(4): 672-85.

[14] Wasley A, Fiore A, Bell BP. Hepatitis A in the era of vaccination. Epidemiol Rev 2006; 28: 101-11.

[15] Salloum S, Tai AW. Treating hepatitis C infection by targeting the host. Transl Res 2012; 159(6): 421-9.

[16] Jose J, Snyder JE, Kuhn RJ. A structural and functional perspective of alphavirus replication and assembly. Future Microbiol 2009; 4(7): 837-56.

[17] Smit JM, Moesker B, Rodenhuis-Zybert I, Wilschut J. Flavivirus cell entry and membrane fusion. Viruses 2011; 3(2): 160-71.

[18] Kew OM, Sutter RW, de Gourville EM, Dowdle WR, Pallansch MA. Vaccine-derived polioviruses and the endgame strategy for global polio eradication. Annu Rev Microbiol 2005; 59: 587-635.

[19] Karavidas A, Lazaros G, Noutsias M, *et al.* Recurrent coxsackie B viral myocarditis leading to progressive impairment of left ventricular function over 8 years. Int J Cardiol 2011; 151(2): e65-7.

[20] Lichty BD, Power AT, Stojdl DF, Bell JC. Vesicular stomatitis virus: re-inventing the bullet. Trends Mol Med 2004; 10(5): 210-6.

[21] Du L, Zhou Y, Jiang S. Research and development of universal influenza vaccines. Microbes Infect 2010; 12(4): 280-6.

[22] McCarthy MK, Weinberg JB. Eicosanoids and respiratory viral infection: coordinators of inflammation and potential therapeutic targets. Mediators Inflamm 2012; 2012: 236345.

[23] Turner RB, Couch RB. Rhinoviruses: Parainfluenza Viruses: the viruses and their replication. In: Knipe DM, Howley PM, Eds. Fields Virology. Philadelphia: Lippincott, Williams & Wilkins 2007; pp. 1449-96.

[24] Gómez RM, Jaquenod de Giusti C, Sanchez Vallduvi MM, Frik J, Ferrer MF, Schattner M. Junín virus. A XXI century update. Microbes Infect 2011; 13(4): 303-11.

[25] Yanagi Y, Takeda M, Ohno S. Measles virus: cellular receptors, tropism and pathogenesis. J Gen Virol 2006; 87(Pt 10): 2767-79.

[26] Dumais N. HIV and AIDS - Updates on Biology, Immunology, Epidemiology and Treatment Strategies. Croatia: InTech; 2011.

[27] Kwon SY, Lee CH. Epidemiology and prevention of hepatitis B virus infection. Korean J Hepatol 2011; 17(2): 87-95.

[28] Seddon J, Bhagani S. Antimicrobial therapy for the treatment of opportunistic infections in HIV/AIDS patients: a critical appraisal. HIV AIDS (Auckl) 2011; 3: 19-33.

[29] Lease ED, Zaas DW. Update on infectious complications following lung transplantation. Curr Opin Pulm Med 2011; 17(3): 206-9.

[30] Bellini WJ, Rota PA. Biological feasibility of measles eradication. Virus Res 2011; 162(1-2): 72-9.

[31] Tomori O. From smallpox eradication to the future of global health: innovations, application and lessons for future eradication and control initiatives. Vaccine 2011; 29 Suppl 4: D145-8.

[32] Munro MHG, Luibrand RT, Blent JW. The search for antiviral and anticancer compounds from marine organisms. In: Scheur PJ, Ed. Bioorganic marine chemistry. Berlin: Springer Verliag 1987; pp. 93-176.

[33] Vlietinck AJ, De Bruyne T, Vanden Berghe DA. Plant substances as antiviral agents. Curr Org Chem 1997; 1: 307-44.

[34] Mayer AMS. Current marine pharmacology contributions to new drug development in the biopharmaceutical industry. Pharmaceutical News 2002; 9: 479-82.

[35] Sassi AB, Harzallah-Skhiri F, Bourgougnon N, Aouni M. Antiviral activity of some Tunisian medicinal plants against herpes simplex virus type 1. Nat Prod Res 2008; 22(1): 53-65.

[36] Mayer AM, Rodríguez AD, Berlinck RG, Hamann MT. Marine pharmacology in 2005-6: Marine compounds with anthelmintic, antibacterial, anticoagulant, antifungal, anti-inflammatory, antimalarial, antiprotozoal, antituberculosis, and antiviral activities; affecting the cardiovascular, immune and nervous systems, and other miscellaneous mechanisms of action. Biochim Biophys Acta 2009; 1790(5): 283-308.

[37] Kitazato K, Wang Y, Kobayashi N. Viral infectious disease and natural products with antiviral activity. Drug Discov Ther 2007; 1(1): 14-22.

[38] Fenical W, Paul VJ. Algae in medicine and pharmacology. Hydrobiol 1984; 116-117: 135-70.

[39] Faulkner DJ. Marine natural products. Nat Prod Rep 1986; 3(1): 1-33.

[40] Faulkner DJ. Marine natural products. Nat Prod Rep 1987; 4(5): 539-76.

[41] Faulkner DJ. Marine natural products. Nat Prod Rep 1988; 5(6): 613-63.

[42] Faulkner DJ. Marine natural products. Nat Prod Rep 1990; 7(4): 269-309.

[43] Faulkner DJ. Marine natural products. Nat Prod Rep 1991; 8(2): 97-147.

[44] Faulkner DJ. Marine natural products. Nat Prod Rep 1993; 10(5): 497-539.
[45] Faulkner DJ. Marine natural products. Nat Prod Rep 1994; 11(4): 355-94.
[46] Faulkner DJ. Marine natural products. Nat Prod Rep. 1996; 13(2): 75-125.
[47] Faulkner DJ. Marine natural products. Nat Prod Rep 1998; 15(2): 113-58.
[48] Faulkner DJ. Marine natural products. Nat Prod Rep 2000; 17(1): 7-55.
[49] Faulkner DJ. Marine natural products. Nat Prod Rep 2001; 18(1): 1-49.
[50] González del Val A, Platas G, Basilio A, *et al.* Screening of antimicrobial activities in red, green and brown macroalgae from Gran Canaria (Canary Islands, Spain). Int Microbiol 2001; 4(1): 35-40.
[51] Faulkner DJ. Marine natural products. Nat Prod Rep 2002; 19(1): 1-48.
[52] Selvin J, Lipton AP. Biopotentials of *Ulva fasciata* and *Hypnea musciformis* collected from the peninsular coast of India. J Mar Sci Tech 2004; 12(1): 1-6.
[53] Smit AJ. Medicinal and pharmaceutical uses of seaweed natural products: A review. J Appl Phycol 2004; 16: 245-62.
[54] Cardozo KH, Guaratini T, Barros MP, *et al.* Metabolites from algae with economical impact. Comp Biochem Physiol C Toxicol Pharmacol 2007; 146(1-2): 60-78.
[55] Karabay-Yavasoglu NU, Sukatar A, Ozdemir G, Horzum Z. Antimicrobial activity of volatile components and various extracts of the red alga Jania rubens. Phytother Res 2007; 21(2): 153-6.
[56] Salvador N, Garreta AG, Lavelli L, Ribera MA. Antimicrobial activity of Iberian macroalgae. Sci Mar 2007; 71(1): 101-13.
[57] Blunt JW, Copp BR, Munro MH, Northcote PT, Prinsep MR. Marine natural products. Nat Prod Rep 2010; 27(2): 165-237.
[58] O'Sullivan L, Murphy B, McLoughlin P, *et al.* Prebiotics from marine macroalgae for human and animal health applications. Mar Drugs 2010; 8(7): 2038-64.
[59] Deig EF, Ehresmann DW, Hatch MT, Riedlinger DJ. Inhibition of herpesvirus replication by marine algae extracts. Antimicrob Agents Chemother 1974; 6(4): 524-5.
[60] Lindequest U, Schweder T. Marine biotechnology. In: Rehm HJ, Reed G, Eds. Biotechnology. Weinheim: Wiley-VHC 2001, Vol. 10, pp. 441-84.
[61] Newman DJ, Cragg GM, Snader KM. Natural products as sources of new drugs over the period 1981-2002. J Nat Prod 2003; 66(7): 1022-37.
[62] Gul W, Hamann MT. Indole alkaloid marine natural products: an established source of cancer drug leads with considerable promise for the control of parasitic, neurological and other diseases. Life Sci 2005; 78(5): 442-53.
[63] Mayer AM, Hamann MT. Marine pharmacology in 2001--2002: marine compounds with anthelmintic, antibacterial, anticoagulant, antidiabetic, antifungal, anti-inflammatory, antimalarial, antiplatelet, antiprotozoal, antituberculosis, and antiviral activities; affecting the cardiovascular, immune and nervous systems and other miscellaneous mechanisms of action. Comp Biochem Physiol C Toxicol Pharmacol 2005; 140(3-4): 265-86.
[64] Yasuhara-Bell J, Lu Y. Marine compounds and their antiviral activities. Antiviral Res 2010; 86(3): 231-40.
[65] Gamal AAE. Biological importance of marine algae. Saudi Pharm J 2010; 18: 1-25.
[66] Baba M, Snoeck R, Pauwels R, de Clercq E. Sulfated polysaccharides are potent and selective inhibitors of various enveloped viruses, including herpes simplex virus, cytomegalovirus, vesicular stomatitis virus, and human immunodeficiency virus. Antimicrob Agents Chemother 1988; 32(11): 1742-5.

[67] Kolender AA, Pujol CA, Damonte EB, Matulewicz MC, Cerezo AS. The system of sulfated alpha-(1-->3)-linked D-mannans from the red seaweed Nothogenia fastigiata: structures, antiherpetic and anticoagulant properties. Carbohydr Res 1997; 304(1): 53-60.

[68] Witvrouw M, De Clercq E. Sulfated polysaccharides extracted from sea algae as potential antiviral drugs. Gen Pharmacol 1997; 29(4): 497-511.

[69] Carlucci MJ, Ciancia M, Matulewicz MC, Cerezo AS, Damonte EB. Antiherpetic activity and mode of action of natural carrageenans of diverse structural types. Antiviral Res 1999; 43(2): 93-102.

[70] Carlucci MJ, Scolaro LA, Damonte EB. Herpes simplex virus type 1 variants arising after selection with an antiviral carrageenan: lack of correlation between drug susceptibility and syn phenotype. J Med Virol 2002; 68(1): 92-8.

[71] Mazumder S, Ghosal PK, Pujol CA, Carlucci MJ, Damonte EB, Ray B. Isolation, chemical investigation and antiviral activity of polysaccharides from Gracilaria corticata (Gracilariaceae, Rhodophyta). Int J Biol Macromol 2002; 31(1-3): 87-95.

[72] Ponce NM, Pujol CA, Damonte EB, Flores ML, Stortz CA. Fucoidans from the brown seaweed adenocystis utricularis: extraction methods, antiviral activity and structural studies. Carbohydr Res 2003; 338(2): 153-65.

[73] Duarte ME, Cauduro JP, Noseda DG, *et al.* The structure of the agaran sulfate from Acanthophora spicifera (Rhodomelaceae, Ceramiales) and its antiviral activity. Relation between structure and antiviral activity in agarans. Carbohydr Res 2004; 339(2): 335-47.

[74] Ghosh P, Adhikari U, Ghosal PK, *et al. In vitro* anti-herpetic activity of sulfated polysaccharide fractions from Caulerpa racemosa. Phytochemistry 2004; 65(23): 3151-7.

[75] Talarico LB, Zibetti RG, Faria PC, *et al.* Anti-herpes simplex virus activity of sulfated galactans from the red seaweeds Gymnogongrus griffithsiae and Cryptonemia crenulata. Int J Biol Macromol 2004; 34(1-2): 63-71.

[76] Thompson KD, Dragar C. Antiviral activity of Undaria pinnatifida against herpes simplex virus. Phytother Res 2004; 18(7): 551-5.

[77] Adhikari U, Mateu CG, Chattopadhyay K, Pujol CA, Damonte EB, Ray B. Structure and antiviral activity of sulfated fucans from Stoechospermum marginatum. Phytochemistry 2006; 67(22): 2474-82.

[78] Chattopadhyay K, Mateu CG, Mandal P, Pujol CA, Damonte EB, Ray B. Galactan sulfate of Grateloupia indica: Isolation, structural features and antiviral activity. Phytochemistry 2007; 68(10): 1428-35.

[79] Mandal P, Mateu CG, Chattopadhyay K, Pujol CA, Damonte EB, Ray B. Structural features and antiviral activity of sulphated fucans from the brown seaweed Cystoseira indica. Antivir Chem Chemother 2007; 18(3): 153-62.

[80] d'Ayala GG, Malinconico M, Laurienzo P. Marine derived polysaccharides for biomedical applications: chemical modification approaches. Molecules 2008; 13(9): 2069-106.

[81] Hayashi K, Nakano T, Hashimoto M, Kanekiyo K, Hayashi T. Defensive effects of a fucoidan from brown alga Undaria pinnatifida against herpes simplex virus infection. Int Immunopharmacol 2008; 8(1): 109-16.

[82] Klisch M, Häder DP. Mycosporine-like amino acids and marine toxins--the common and the different. Mar Drugs 2008; 6(2): 147-63.

[83] de Souza ET, de Lira DP, de Queiroz AC, *et al.* The antinociceptive and anti-inflammatory activities of caulerpin, a bisindole alkaloid isolated from seaweeds of the genus Caulerpa. Mar Drugs 2009; 7(4): 689-704.

[84] Paniagua-Michel J, Capa-Robles W, Olmos-Soto J, Gutierrez-Millan LE. The carotenogenesis pathway *via* the isoprenoid-beta-carotene interference approach in a new strain of Dunaliella salina isolated from Baja California Mexico. Mar Drugs 2009; 7(1): 45-56.

[85] Cen-Pacheco F, Nordström L, Souto ML, Martín MN, Fernández JJ, Daranas AH. Studies on polyethers produced by red algae. Mar Drugs 2010; 8(4): 1178-88.

[86] Cabrita MT, Vale C, Rauter AP. Halogenated compounds from marine algae. Mar Drugs 2010; 8(8): 2301-17.

[87] Güven KC, Percot A, Sezik E. Alkaloids in marine algae. Mar Drugs 2010; 8(2): 269-84.

[88] Kellmann R, Stüken A, Orr RJ, Svendsen HM, Jakobsen KS. Biosynthesis and molecular genetics of polyketides in marine dinoflagellates. Mar Drugs 2010; 8(4): 1011-48.

[89] La Barre S, Potin P, Leblanc C, Delage L. The halogenated metabolism of brown algae (Phaeophyta), its biological importance and its environmental significance. Mar Drugs 2010; 8(4): 988-1010.

[90] Pallela R, Na-Young Y, Kim SK. Anti-photoaging and photoprotective compounds derived from marine organisms. Mar Drugs 2010; 8(4): 1189-202.

[91] Ballesteros E, Martin D, Uriz MJ. Biological activity of extracts from some mediterranean macrophytes. Bot Mar 1992; 35: 481-5.

[92] Bourgougnon N, Roussakis C, Kornprobst JM, Lahaye M. Effects *in vitro* of sulfated polysaccharide from Schizymenia dubyi (Rhodophyta, Gigartinales) on a non-small-cell bronchopulmonary carcinoma line (NSCLC-N6). Cancer Lett 1994; 85(1): 87-92.

[93] Haslin C, Lahaye M, Pellegrini M, Chermann JC. *In vitro* anti-HIV activity of sulfated cell-wall polysaccharides from gametic, carposporic and tetrasporic stages of the Mediterranean red alga Asparagopsis armata. Planta Med 2001; 67(4): 301-5.

[94] Blunden G, Barwell CJ, Fidgen KJ, Jewers K. A survey of some British marine algae for anti-influenza virus activity. Bot Mar 1981; 24(5): 267-72.

[95] Premnathan M, Chandra K, Bajpai SK, Kathiresan K. A survey of some Indian marine plants for antiviral activity. Bot Mar 1992; 35(4): 321-4.

[96] Hudson JB, Kim JH, Lee MK, DeWreede RE, Hong YK. Antiviral compounds in extracts of Korean seaweeds: evidence for multiple activities. J Appl Phycol 1999; 10(5): 427-34.

[97] Ahn MJ, Yoon KD, Kim CY, *et al.* Inhibition of HIV-1 reverse transcriptase and HIV-1 integrase and antiviral activity of Korean seaweed extracts. J Appl Phycol 2002; 14(5): 325-9.

[98] Hayashi K, Hayashi T, Ujita K, Takaishi Y. Characterization of antiviral activity of a sesquiterpene, triptofordin C-2. J Antimicrob Chemother 1996; 37(4): 759-68.

[99] Mori T, O'Keefe BR, Sowder RC 2nd, *et al.* Isolation and characterization of griffithsin, a novel HIV-inactivating protein, from the red alga Griffithsia sp. J Biol Chem 2005; 280(10): 9345-53.

[100] Bouhlal R, Riadi H, Bourgougnon N. Antiviral activity of the extracts of Rhodophyceae from Morocco. Afr J Biotechnol 2010; 9(46): 7968-75.

[101] Gerber P, Dutcher JD, Adams EV, Sherman JH. Protective effect of seaweed extracts for chicken embryos infected with influenza B or mumps virus. Proc Soc Exp Biol Med 1958; 99(3): 590-3.

[102] Burkholder PR, Sharma GM. Antimicrobial agents from the sea. Lloydia 1969; 32(4): 466-83.

[103] Ehresmann DW, Deig EF, Hatch MT, DiSalvo LH, Vedros NA. Antiviral substances from california marine algae. J Phycol 1977; 13(1): 37-40.

[104] Richards JT, Kern ER, Glasgow LA, Overall JC Jr, Deign EF, Hatch MT. Antiviral activity of extracts from marine algae. Antimicrob Agents Chemother 1978; 14(1): 24-30.

[105] Nakashima H, Kido Y, Kobayashi N, Motoki Y, Neushul M, Yamamoto N. Antiretroviral activity in a marine red alga: reverse transcriptase inhibition by an aqueous extract of Schizymenia pacifica. J Cancer Res Clin Oncol 1987; 113(5): 413-6.

[106] Nakashima H, Kido Y, Kobayashi N, Motoki Y, Neushul M, Yamamoto N. Purification and characterization of an avian myeloblastosis and human immunodeficiency virus reverse transcriptase inhibitor, sulfated polysaccharides extracted from sea algae. Antimicrob Agents Chemother 1987; 31(10): 1524-8.

[107] Witvrouw M, Este JA, Mateu MQ, *et al.* Activity of a sulfated polysaccharide extracted from the red seaweed Aghardhiella tenera against human immunodeficiency virus and other enveloped viruses. Antiviral Chem Chemotheraphy 1994; 5(5): 297-303.

[108] Loya S, Bakhanashvili M, Kashman Y, Hizi A. Peyssonols A and B, two novel inhibitors of the reverse transcriptases of human immunodeficiency virus types 1 and 2. Arch Biochem Biophys 1995; 316(2): 789-96.

[109] Bourgougnon N, Lahaye M, Quemener B, *et al.* Annual variation in composition and *in vitro* anti-HIV-1 activity of the sulfated glucuronogalactan from Schizymenia dubyi (Rhodophyta, Gigartinales). J Appl Phycol 1996; 8(2): 155-61.

[110] Ohta K, Mizushina Y, Hirata N, *et al.* Sulfoquinovosyldiacylglycerol, KM043, a new potent inhibitor of eukaryotic DNA polymerases and HIV-reverse transcriptase type 1 from a marine red alga, Gigartina tenella. Chem Pharm Bull (Tokyo) 1998; 46(4): 684-6.

[111] Tziveleka LA, Vagias C, Roussis V. Natural products with anti-HIV activity from marine organisms. Curr Top Med Chem 2003; 3(13): 1512-35.

[112] Emau P, Tian B, O'keefe BR, *et al.* Griffithsin, a potent HIV entry inhibitor, is an excellent candidate for anti-HIV microbicide. J Med Primatol 2007; 36(4-5): 244-53.

[113] Wang SC, Bligh SW, Shi SS, *et al.* Structural features and anti-HIV-1 activity of novel polysaccharides from red algae Grateloupia longifolia and Grateloupia filicina. Int J Biol Macromol 2007; 41(4): 369-75.

[114] O'Keefe BR, Vojdani F, Buffa V, *et al.* Scaleable manufacture of HIV-1 entry inhibitor griffithsin and validation of its safety and efficacy as a topical microbicide component. Proc Natl Acad Sci U S A 2009; 106(15): 6099-104.

[115] Alexandre KB, Gray ES, Lambson BE, *et al.* Mannose-rich glycosylation patterns on HIV-1 subtype C gp120 and sensitivity to the lectins, Griffithsin, Cyanovirin-N and Scytovirin. Virology 2010; 402(1): 187-96.

[116] Bouhlal R, Haslin C, Chermann JC, *et al.* Antiviral activities of sulfated polysaccharides isolated from Sphaerococcus coronopifolius (Rhodophytha, Gigartinales) and Boergeseniella thuyoides (Rhodophyta, Ceramiales). Mar Drugs 2011; 9(7): 1187-209.

[117] Huang X, Jin W, Griffin GE, Shattock RJ, Hu Q. Removal of two high-mannose N-linked glycans on gp120 renders human immunodeficiency virus 1 largely resistant to the carbohydrate-binding agent griffithsin. J Gen Virol 2011; 92(Pt 10): 2367-73.

[118] Sakemi S, Higa T. Venustatriol. A new, anti-viral, triterpene tetracyclic ether from Laurencia venusta. Tetrahedron Lett 1986; 27: 4287-90.

[119] Kolender AA, Matulewicz MC, Cerezo AS. Structural analysis of antiviral sulfated alpha-D-(1-->3)-linked mannans. Carbohydr Res 1995; 273(2): 179-85.

[120] Pujol CA, Coto CE, Damonte EB. [Determination of the antiviral activity of a naturally occurring sulfated xylomannan under various experimental conditions]. Rev Argent Microbiol 1995; 27(2): 91-8.
[121] Damonte EB, Matulewicz MC, Cerezo AS, Coto CE. Herpes simplex virus-inhibitory sulfated xylogalactans from the red seaweed Nothogenia fastigiata. Chemotherapy 1996; 42(1): 57-64.
[122] Pujolt CA, Errea MI, Matulewicz MC, Damontet EB. Antiherpetic activity of S1, an algal derived sulphated galactan. Phytother Res 1996; 10: 410-3.
[123] Carlucci MJ, Pujol CA, Ciancia M, *et al.* Antiherpetic and anticoagulant properties of carrageenans from the red seaweed Gigartina skottsbergii and their cyclized derivatives: correlation between structure and biological activity. Int J Biol Macromol 1997; 20(2): 97-105.
[124] Carlucci MJ, Scolaro LA, Damonte EB. Inhibitory action of natural carrageenans on herpes simplex virus infection of mouse astrocytes. Chemotherapy 1999; 45(6): 429-36.
[125] Cáceres PJ, Carlucci MJ, Damonte EB, Matsuhiro B, Zuñiga EA. Carrageenans from chilean samples of Stenogramme interrupta (Phyllophoraceae): structural analysis and biological activity. Phytochemistry 2000; 53(1): 81-6.
[126] Serkedjieva J. Antiherpes virus effect of the red marine alga Polysiphonia denudata. Z Naturforsch C 2000; 55(9-10): 830-5.
[127] Duarte ME, Noseda DG, Noseda MD, Tulio S, Pujol CA, Damonte EB. Inhibitory effect of sulfated galactans from the marine alga Bostrychia montagnei on herpes simplex virus replication *in vitro*. Phytomedicine 2001; 8(1): 53-8.
[128] Pujol CA, Estevez JM, Carlucci MJ, Ciancia M, Cerezo AS, Damonte EB. Novel DL-galactan hybrids from the red seaweed Gymnogongrus torulosus are potent inhibitors of herpes simplex virus and dengue virus. Antivir Chem Chemother 2002; 13(2): 83-9.
[129] Carlucci MJ, Scolaro LA, Noseda MD, Cerezo AS, Damonte EB. Protective effect of a natural carrageenan on genital herpes simplex virus infection in mice. Antiviral Res 2004; 64(2): 137-41.
[130] Park HJ, Kurokawa M, Shiraki K, Nakamura N, Choi JS, Hattori M. Antiviral activity of the marine alga symphyocladia latiuscula against herpes simplex virus (HSV-1) *in vitro* and its therapeutic efficacy against HSV-1 infection in mice. Biol Pharm Bull 2005; 28(12): 2258-62.
[131] Matsuhiro B, Conte AF, Damonte EB, *et al.* Structural analysis and antiviral activity of a sulfated galactan from the red seaweed Schizymenia binderi (Gigartinales, Rhodophyta). Carbohydr Res 2005; 340(15): 2392-402.
[132] Rodríguez MC, Merino ER, Pujol CA, Damonte EB, Cerezo AS, Matulewicz MC. Galactans from cystocarpic plants of the red seaweed Callophyllis variegata (Kallymeniaceae, Gigartinales). Carbohydr Res 2005; 340(18): 2742-51.
[133] de SF-Tischer PC, Talarico, LB, Noseda MD, *et al.* Chemical structure and antiviral activity of carrageenans from Meristiella gelidium against herpes simplex and dengue virus. Carbohydr Polym 2006; 63(4): 459-65.
[134] Naesens L, Bonnafous P, Agut H, De Clercq E. Antiviral activity of diverse classes of broad-acting agents and natural compounds in HHV-6-infected lymphoblasts. J Clin Virol 2006; 37 Suppl 1: S69-75.

[135] Pujol CA, Scolaro LA, Ciancia M, Matulewicz MC, Cerezo AS, Damonte EB. Antiviral activity of a carrageenan from Gigartina skottsbergii against intraperitoneal murine herpes simplex virus infection. Planta Med 2006; 72(2): 121-5.

[136] Zhu YM, Wang YF, Zhang MY, *et al.* [The study on the extraction and the antivirus activity of amylose extracted from Grateloupia filicina]. Zhong Yao Cai 2006; 29(3): 256-9.

[137] Zandi K, Salimi M, Sartavi K. *In vitro* antiviral activity of the red marine alga from Persian Gulf, Gracilaria salicornia, against herpes simplex virus type 2. J Biol Sci 2007; 7(7): 1274-7.

[138] Chattopadhyay K, Ghosh T, Pujol CA, Carlucci MJ, Damonte EB, Ray B. Polysaccharides from Gracilaria corticata: sulfation, chemical characterization and anti-HSV activities. Int J Biol Macromol 2008; 43(4): 346-51.

[139] Mandal P, Pujol CA, Carlucci MJ, Chattopadhyay K, Damonte EB, Ray B. Anti-herpetic activity of a sulfated xylomannan from Scinaia hatei. Phytochemistry 2008; 69(11): 2193-9.

[140] Ghosh T, Pujol CA, Damonte EB, Sinha S, Ray B. Sulfated xylomannans from the red seaweed Sebdenia polydactyla: structural features, chemical modification and antiviral activity. Antivir Chem Chemother 2009; 19(6): 235-42.

[141] Harden EA, Falshaw R, Carnachan SM, Kern ER, Prichard MN. Virucidal activity of polysaccharide extracts from four algal species against herpes simplex virus. Antiviral Res 2009; 83(3): 282-9.

[142] Mattos BB, Romanos MTV, de Souza LM, Sassaki G, Barreto-Bergter E. Glycolipids from macroalgae: potential biomolecules for marine biotechnology? Rev Bras Farmacogn Braz J Pharmacogn 2011; 21(2): 244-7.

[143] Damonte E, Neyts J, Pujol CA, *et al.* Antiviral activity of a sulphated polysaccharide from the red seaweed Nothogenia fastigiata. Biochem Pharmacol 1994; 47(12): 2187-92.

[144] Woelkerling WJ. An introduction. In: Cole KM, Sheath RG, Eds. Biology of the red algae. Cambridge: Cambridge University Press 1990; pp. 1-6.

[145] Lüning K, Ed. Seaweeds: Their environment, biogeography, and ecophysiology. New York: Wiley 1990.

[146] Ziółkowska NE, O'Keefe BR, Mori T, *et al.* Domain-swapped structure of the potent antiviral protein griffithsin and its mode of carbohydrate binding. Structure 2006; 14(7): 1127-35.

[147] O'Keefe BR, Giomarelli B, Barnard DL, *et al.* Broad-spectrum *in vitro* activity and *in vivo* efficacy of the antiviral protein griffithsin against emerging viruses of the family Coronaviridae. J Virol 2010; 84(5): 2511-21.

[148] Meuleman P, Albecka A, Belouzard S, *et al.* Griffithsin has antiviral activity against hepatitis C virus. Antimicrob Agents Chemother 2011; 55(11): 5159-67.

[149] Zeitlin L, Pauly M, Whaley KJ. Second-generation HIV microbicides: continued development of griffithsin. Proc Natl Acad Sci U S A 2009; 106(15): 6029-30.

[150] Talarico LB, Pujol CA, Zibetti RG, *et al.* The antiviral activity of sulfated polysaccharides against dengue virus is dependent on virus serotype and host cell. Antiviral Res 2005; 66(2-3): 103-10.

[151] Carlucci MJ, Scolaro LA, Errea MI, Matulewicz MC, Damonte EB. Antiviral activity of natural sulphated galactans on herpes virus multiplication in cell culture. Planta Med 1997; 63(5): 429-32.

[152] Damonte EB, Matulewicz MC, Cerezo AS. Sulfated seaweed polysaccharides as antiviral agents. Curr Med Chem 2004; 11(18): 2399-41.

[153] González ME, Alarcón B, Carrasco L. Polysaccharides as antiviral agents: antiviral activity of carrageenan. Antimicrob Agents Chemother 1987; 31(9): 1388-93.

[154] Girond S, Crance JM, Van Cuyck-Gandre H, Renaudet J, Deloince R. Antiviral activity of carrageenan on hepatitis A virus replication in cell culture. Res Virol 1991; 142(4): 261-70.

[155] Usov AI. Structural analysis of red seaweed galactans of agar and carrageenan groups. Food Hydrocoll 1998; 12(3): 301-8.

[156] Estevez JM, Ciancia M, Cerezo AS. DL-Galactan hybrids and agarans from gametophytes of the red seaweed gymnogongrus torulosus. Carbohydr Res 2001; 331(1): 27-41.

[157] Stortz CA, Cases MR, Cerezo AS. The system of agaroids and carrageenans from the soluble fraction of the tetrasporic stage of the red seaweed Iridaea undulosa. Carbohydr Polymers 1997; 34(1): 61-5.

[158] Chopin T, Kerin BF, Mazerolle R. Phycocolloid chemistry as taxonomic indicator of phylogeny in the Gigartinales, Rhodophyceae: A review and current developments using Fourier transform infrared diffuse reflectance spectroscopy. Phycological Research 1999; 47(3): 167-88.

[159] Takano R, Shiomoto K, Kamei K, Hara S, Hirase S. Occurrence of carrageenan structure in an agar from the red seaweed Digenea simplex (Wulfen) C. Agardh (Rhodomelaceae, Ceramiales) with a short review of carrageenan-agarocolloid hybrid in the Florideophycidae. Bot Mar 2003; 46(2): 142-50.

[160] Zibetti RG, Noseda MD, Cerezo AS, Duarte ME. The system of galactans from Cryptonemia crenulata (Halymeniaceae, Halymeniales) and the structure of two major fractions. Kinetic studies on the alkaline cyclization of the unusual diad G2S-->D(L)6S. Carbohydr Res 2005; 340(4): 711-22.

[161] Moreira LR, Filho EX. An overview of mannan structure and mannan-degrading enzyme systems. Appl Microbiol Biotechnol 2008; 79(2): 165-78.

[162] Painter TJ. Structural evolution of glycans in algae. Pure & Appl Chem 1983; 55(4): 677-94.

[163] Kolender AA, Matulewicz MC. Sulfated polysaccharides from the red seaweed Georgiella confluens. Carbohydr Res 2002; 337(1): 57-68.

[164] Morris ER, Rees DA, Thom D, Welsh EJ. Conformation and intermolecular interactions of carbohydrate chains. J Supramol Struct 1977; 6(2): 259-74.

[165] Michel G, Nyval-Collen P, Barbeyron T, Czjzek M, Helbert W. Bioconversion of red seaweed galactans: a focus on bacterial agarases and carrageenases. Appl Microbiol Biotechnol 2006; 71(1): 23-33.

[166] Boisson-Vidal C, Haroun F, Ellouali M, *et al.* Biological activities of polysaccharide from marine algae. Drugs Fut 1995; 20(12): 1237-49.

[167] Baba M, Pauwels R, Balzarini J, Arnout J, Desmyter J, De Clercq E. Mechanism of inhibitory effect of dextran sulfate and heparin on replication of human immunodeficiency virus *in vitro*. Proc Natl Acad Sci U S A 1988; 85(16): 6132-6.

[168] Pearce-Pratt R, Phillips DM. Sulfated polysaccharides inhibit lymphocyte-to-epithelial transmission of human immunodeficiency virus-1. Biol Reprod 1996; 54(1): 173-82.

[169] Lüscher-Mattli M. Polyanions--a lost chance in the fight against HIV and other virus diseases? Antivir Chem Chemother 2000; 11(4): 249-59.

[170] Cushman M, Golebiewski WM, Pommier Y, *et al.* Cosalane analogues with enhanced potencies as inhibitors of HIV-1 protease and integrase. J Med Chem 1995; 38(3): 443-52.
[171] Neyts J, Snoeck R, Schols D, *et al.* Sulfated polymers inhibit the interaction of human cytomegalovirus with cell surface heparan sulfate. Virology 1992; 189(1): 48-58.
[172] Marchetti M, Pisani S, Pietropaolo V, Seganti L, Nicoletti R, Orsi N. Inhibition of herpes simplex virus infection by negatively charged and neutral carbohydrate polymers. J Chemother 1995; 7(2): 90-6.
[173] Witvrouw M, Fikkert V, Pluymers W, *et al.* Polyanionic (*i.e.,* polysulfonate) dendrimers can inhibit the replication of human immunodeficiency virus by interfering with both virus adsorption and later steps (reverse transcriptase/integrase) in the virus replicative cycle. Mol Pharmacol 2000; 58(5): 1100-8.
[174] Serkedjieva J. Antiviral activity of the red marine alga Ceramium rubrum. Phytother Res 2004; 18(6): 480-3.
[175] Cases M. Estudio del sistema de polisacáridos del alga roja calcárea Corallina officinalis. Ph.D. thesis. Buenos Aires, Argentina: University of Buenos Aires 1995.
[176] Haslin C, Lahaye M, Pellegrini M. Chemical composition and structure of sulphated water-soluble cell-wall polysaccharides from the gametic, carposporic and tetrasporic stages of Asparagopsis armata Harvey (Rhodophyta, Bonnemaisoniaceae). Bot Mar 2000; 43(5): 475-82.
[177] McClure MO, Moore JP, Blanc DF, *et al.* Investigations into the mechanism by which sulfated polysaccharides inhibit HIV infection *in vitro.* AIDS Res Hum Retroviruses 1992; 8(1): 19-26.
[178] Giomarelli B, Schumacher KM, Taylor TE, *et al.* Recombinant production of anti-HIV protein, griffithsin, by auto-induction in a fermentor culture. Protein Expr Purif 2006; 47(1): 194-202.
[179] Ziółkowska NE, Wlodawer A. Structural studies of algal lectins with anti-HIV activity. Acta Biochim Pol 2006; 53(4): 617-26.
[180] Micewicz ED, Cole AL, Jung CL, *et al.* Grifonin-1: a small HIV-1 entry inhibitor derived from the algal lectin, Griffithsin. PLoS One 2010; 5(12): e14360.
[181] Aucouturier P, Mihaesco E, Mihaesco C, Preud'homme JL. Characterization of jacalin, the human IgA and IgD binding lectin from jackfruit. Mol Immunol 1987; 24(5): 503-11.
[182] Bourne Y, Zamboni V, Barre A, Peumans WJ, Van Damme EJ, Rougé P. Helianthus tuberosus lectin reveals a widespread scaffold for mannose-binding lectins. Structure 1999; 7(12): 1473-82.
[183] Jeyaprakash AA, Srivastav A, Surolia A, Vijayan M. Structural basis for the carbohydrate specificities of artocarpin: variation in the length of a loop as a strategy for generating ligand specificity. J Mol Biol 2004; 338(4): 757-70.
[184] Raval S, Gowda SB, Singh DD, Chandra NR. A database analysis of jacalin-like lectins: sequence-structure-function relationships. Glycobiology 2004; 14(12): 1247-63.
[185] Chandra N. Common scaffolds, diverse recognition profiles. Structure 2006; 14(7): 1093-4.
[186] Moulaei T, Shenoy SR, Giomarelli B, *et al.* Monomerization of viral entry inhibitor griffithsin elucidates the relationship between multivalent binding to carbohydrates and anti-HIV activity. Structure 2010; 18(9): 1104-15.
[187] Charan RD, Munro MH, O'Keefe BR, *et al.* Isolation and characterization of Myrianthus holstii lectin, a potent HIV-1 inhibitory protein from the plant Myrianthus holstii(1). J Nat Prod 2000; 63(8): 1170-4.

[188] O'Keefe BR. Biologically active proteins from natural product extracts. J Nat Prod 2001; 64(10): 1373-81.
[189] Alexandre KB, Gray ES, Mufhandu H, *et al.* The lectins griffithsin, cyanovirin-N and scytovirin inhibit HIV-1 binding to the DC-SIGN receptor and transfer to CD4(+) cells. Virology 2012; 423(2): 175-86.
[190] Berger EA, Murphy PM, Farber JM. Chemokine receptors as HIV-1 coreceptors: roles in viral entry, tropism, and disease. Annu Rev Immunol 1999; 17: 657-700.
[191] Kagiampakis I, Gharibi A, Mankowski MK, *et al.* Potent strategy to inhibit HIV-1 by binding both gp120 and gp41. Antimicrob Agents Chemother 2011; 55(1): 264-75.
[192] Alexandre KB, Gray ES, Pantophlet R, *et al.* Binding of the mannose-specific lectin, griffithsin, to HIV-1 gp120 exposes the CD4-binding site. J Virol 2011; 85(17): 9039-50.
[193] Zhang M, Gaschen B, Blay W, *et al.* Tracking global patterns of N-linked glycosylation site variation in highly variable viral glycoproteins: HIV, SIV, and HCV envelopes and influenza hemagglutinin. Glycobiology 2004; 14(12): 1229-46.
[194] Ferir G, Palmer KE, Schols D. Synergistic activity profile of griffithsin in combination with tenofovir, maraviroc and enfuvirtide against HIV-1 clade C. Virology 2011; 417(2): 253-8.
[195] Kouokam JC, Huskens D, Schols D, *et al.* Investigation of Griffithsin's Interactions with Human Cells Confirms Its Outstanding Safety and Efficacy Profile as a Microbicide Candidate. PLoS ONE 2011; 6(8): e22635.
[196] Balzarini J.Targeting the glycans of gp120: a novel approach aimed at the Achilles heel of HIV. Lancet Infect Dis 2005; 5(11): 726-31.
[197] Balzarini J, Van Damme L. Microbicide drug candidates to prevent HIV infection. Lancet 2007; 369(9563): 787-97.
[198] WuDunn D, Spear PG. Initial interaction of herpes simplex virus with cells is binding to heparan sulfate. J Virol 1989; 63(1): 52-8.
[199] Lycke E, Johansson M, Svennerholm B, Lindahl U. Binding of herpes simplex virus to cellular heparan sulphate, an initial step in the adsorption process. J Gen Virol 1991; 72(Pt 5): 1131-7.
[200] Shieh MT, WuDunn D, Montgomery RI, Esko JD, Spear PG. Cell surface receptors for herpes simplex virus are heparan sulfate proteoglycans. J Cell Biol 1992; 116(5): 1273-81.
[201] Duarte ME, Noseda MD, Cardoso MA, Tulio S, Cerezo AS. The structure of a galactan sulfate from the red seaweed Bostrychia montagnei. Carbohydr Res 2002; 337(12): 1137-44.
[202] Fujisawa S, Atsumi T, Kadoma Y, Sakagami H. Antioxidant and prooxidant action of eugenol-related compounds and their cytotoxicity. Toxicology 2002; 177(1): 39-54.
[203] Gungor E, Celen S, Azaz D, Kara H. Two tridentate Schiff base ligands and their mononuclear cobalt (III) complexes: Synthesis, characterization, antibacterial and antifungal activities. Spectrochim Acta A Mol Biomol Spectrosc 2012; 94: 216-21.
[204] De Rosa S, Kamenarska Z, Stefanov K, *et al.* Chemical composition of Corallina mediterranea Areschoug and Corallina granifera Ell. et Soland. Z Naturforsch C 2003; 58(5-6): 325-32.
[205] Cases MR, Stortz CA, Cerezo AS. Structure of the 'corallinans'--sulfated xylogalactans from Corallina officinalis. Int J Biol Macromol 1994; 16(2): 93-7.
[206] Cases MR, Stortz CA, Cerezo AS. Methylated, sulphated xylogalactans from the red seaweed Corallinaofficinalis. Phytochemistry 1992; 31: 3897-900.

[207] Errea MI, Matulewicz MC. Cold water-soluble polysaccharides from tetrasporic Pterocladia capillacea. Phytochemistry 1994; 37(4): 1075-8.
[208] Herold BC, WuDunn D, Soltys N, Spear PG. Glycoprotein C of herpes simplex virus type 1 plays a principal role in the adsorption of virus to cells and in infectivity. J Virol 1991; 65(3): 1090-8.
[209] Herold BC, Visalli RJ, Susmarski N, Brandt CR, Spear PG. Glycoprotein C-independent binding of herpes simplex virus to cells requires cell surface heparan sulphate and glycoprotein B. J Gen Virol 1994; 75(Pt 6): 1211-22.
[210] Tal-Singer R, Peng C, Ponce De Leon M, *et al.* Interaction of herpes simplex virus glycoprotein gC with mammalian cell surface molecules. J Virol 1995; 69(7): 4471-83.
[211] Ohta K, Mizushina Y, Hirata N, *et al.* Action of a new mammalian DNA polymerase inhibitor, sulfoquinovosyldiacylglycerol. Biol Pharm Bull 1999; 22(2): 111-6.
[212] Simbulan CM, Taki T, Tamiya-Koizumi K, *et al.* Sulfate- and sialic acid-containing glycolipids inhibit DNA polymerase alpha activity. Biochim Biophys Acta 1994; 1205(1): 68-74.
[213] Mizushina Y, Watanabe I, Ohta K, *et al.* Studies on inhibitors of mammalian DNA polymerase alpha and beta: sulfolipids from a pteridophyte, Athyrium niponicum. Biochem Pharmacol 1998; 55(4): 537-41.
[214] Mizushina Y, Tanaka N, Yagi H, *et al.* Fatty acids selectively inhibit eukaryotic DNA polymerase activities *in vitro*. Biochim Biophys Acta 1996; 1308(3): 256-62.
[215] Talpir R, Rudi A, Kashman Y, Loya Y, Hizi A. Three new sesquiterpene hydroquinones from marine origin. Tetrahedron 1994; 50(14): 4179-84.
[216] Loya S, Hizi A. The inhibition of human immunodeficiency virus type 1 reverse transcriptase by avarol and avarone derivatives. FEBS Lett 1990; 269(1): 131-4.
[217] Loya S, Tal R, Kashman Y, Hizi A. Illimaquinone, a selective inhibitor of the RNase H activity of human immunodeficiency virus type 1 reverse transcriptase. Antimicrob Agents Chemother 1990; 34(10): 2009-12.
[218] Witvrouw M, Desmyter J, De Clercq E. Antiviral portrait series: 4. Polysulfates as inhibitors of HIV and other enveloped viruses. Antiviral Chem Chemother 1994; 5(6): 345-59.
[219] Cáceres PJ, Faúndez CA, Matsuhiro B, Vasquez JA. Carrageenophyte identification by second-derivative Fourier transform infrared spectroscopy. J Appl Phycol 1997; 8(6): 523-7.
[220] Vlietinck AJ, De Bruyne T, Apers S, Pieters LA. Plant-derived leading compounds for chemotherapy of human immunodeficiency virus (HIV) infection. Planta Med 1998; 64(2): 97-109.
[221] Talarico LB, Duarte ME, Zibetti RG, Noseda MD, Damonte EB. An algal-derived DL-galactan hybrid is an efficient preventing agent for *in vitro* dengue virus infection. Planta Med 2007; 73(14): 1464-8.
[222] Sosa MA, Fazely F, Koch JA, Vercellotti SV, Ruprecht RM. N-carboxymethylchitosan-N,O-sulfate as an anti-HIV-1 agent. Biochem Biophys Res Commun 1991; 174(2): 489-96.
[223] Koizumi N, Sakagami H, Utsumi A, *et al.* Anti-HIV (human immunodeficiency virus) activity of sulfated paramylon. Antiviral Res 1993; 21(1): 1-14.
[224] Rees DA, Morris ER, Thorn D, Madden JK. Shapes and interactions of carbohydrate chains. In: Aspinall GO, Ed. The Polysaccharides. London: Academic Press 1982, Vol. 1, pp. 195-290.

[225] Herold BC, Gerber SI, Polonsky T, Belval BJ, Shaklee PN, Holme K. Identification of structural features of heparin required for inhibition of herpes simplex virus type 1 binding. Virology 1995; 206(2): 1108-16.

[226] McReynolds KD, Gervay-Hague J. Chemotherapeutic interventions targeting HIV interactions with host-associated carbohydrates. Chem Rev 2007; 107(5): 1533-52.

[227] Spear PG. Entry of alphaherpesviruses into cells. Semin Virol 1993; 4: 167-80.

[228] Hallinan FM, Lee SH, Rozee KR. Inhibition of reverse transcriptase by polyvinyl sulfate (PVS). Cancer Biochem Biophys 1981; 5(2): 97-101.

[229] Fazekas T, Eickhoff P, Pruckner N, *et al.* Lessons learned from a double-blind randomised placebo-controlled study with a iota-carrageenan nasal spray as medical device in children with acute symptoms of common cold. BMC Complement Altern Med 2012; 12(1): 147.

[230] Eccles R, Meier C, Jawad M, Weinmüllner R, Grassauer A, Prieschl-Grassauer E. Efficacy and safety of an antiviral Iota-Carrageenan nasal spray: a randomized, double-blind, placebo-controlled exploratory study in volunteers with early symptoms of the common cold. Respir Res 2010; 11: 108.

 Frontiers in Anti-Infective Drug Discovery, *Vol. 2*, **2014, 86-158**

CHAPTER 2

Development of Synthetic Antimicrobial Peptides as Therapeutic Agents to Treat Drug Resistant Bacterial and Fungal Infections

Rickey P. Hicks* and Tiffany D. Clark

Department of Chemistry, East Carolina University, Greenville, NC 27858, USA

Abstract: The continued evolution of multiple drug resistant organisms associated with common bacterial and fungal infections have become a critical and life threatening challenge facing modern medicine. To overcome this challenge new therapeutic agents that kill these organisms *via* novel mechanisms of action must be developed. Antimicrobial peptides offer several advantages as potential therapeutic agents against multiple drug resistant organisms. Their greatest advantage is their unique mechanism of action which involves first the disruption of the target's cell membrane followed by lysis of the cell thus causing cell death. However, natural antimicrobial peptides also have several inherent disadvantages these included low metabolic stability, lack of bacterial strain selectivity and toxicity toward human cells. In this chapter the development of synthetic antimicrobial peptides containing both natural and unnatural amino acids as well as peptidomimetics designed to address these disadvantages will be discussed. An overview of the physicochemical properties required for antimicrobial activity will be presented with emphasis on the logic of the process of designing new antimicrobial peptides. Specific examples of synthetic antimicrobial peptides will be presented to highlight the application of various approaches to address the issues of metabolic stability, increasing the selectivity for prokaryotic verses eukaryotic cells, as well as increasing bacterial strain selectivity and potency. In addition the chemical analysis methods of Circular Dichroism spectroscopy (CD), isothermal calorimetry (ITC) and fluorescence spectroscopy to monitor calcein induced leakage from liposomes will be discussed. These techniques provide physicochemical information concerning peptide-lipid interactions which provide critical insight for the design of therapeutically useful antimicrobial peptides.

Keywords: Antimicrobial peptides, unnatural amino acids, peptide-lipid interactions, peptidomimetics, β-peptides, organism selectivity, circular dichroism spectroscopy, isothermal calorimetry, mechanism of antibacterial activity.

***Address correspondence to Rickey P. Hicks:** Department of Chemistry, East Carolina University, Science and Technology Building, Greenville, NC, United States; Tel: 252 328-9702; Fax: 252 328-6210; E-mail: hicksr@ecu.edu

Atta-ur-Rahman / M. Iqbal Choudhary (Eds.)

INTRODUCTION

Globally over the past two decades there has been a dramatic increase in the emergence and spread of *multiple drug resistant pathogenic microorganisms* (MDROs) [1-4]. Many nosocomial clinical isolates such as *Acinetobacter*, *Staphylococcus* and *Pseudomonas* have developed resistance to the older generations of antibiotics many also exhibit reduced sensitivity to some of the newer classes of antibiotics [5-7]. One organism of major concern is the Gram positive bacteria *Staphylococcus aureus* which is the causative agent in a wide range of illnesses from skin infections to serious invasive infections including septicemia and endocarditis as well as metastatic infections [8-10]. Methicillin-resistant *Staphylococcus aureus* (MRSA) is a particular concern since it can resulted in the development of serve, life-threatening infections even in people without other serious medical conditions [8, 11-13]. Another organism of major concern is the Gram negative bacteria *Pseudomonas aeruginosa,* which is the leading cause of serve infections in cystic fibrosis patients [14]. It is also the third leading cause of serve hospital-acquired infections [15, 16]. Over 200,000 cases of hospital-acquired *P. aeruginosa* infections are reported each year in the United States alone [17, 18]. *P. aeruginosa* infections associated with chronic wounds and medical implants are also a critical concern [19-21]. The evolution of drug resistant strains of *P. aeruginosa* has been reported [16, 22-24] which has intensified the medical crisis associated with *P. aeruginosa* infections. The dramatic and continued evolution of drug resistant strains of bacteria has resulted in an international health care crisis [25-27], which has stimulated an intensive worldwide research effort to develop new classes of antibiotics which exhibit novel mechanisms of antibacterial activity [26, 28-33].

POTENTIAL SOLUTION TO THE PROBLEM: ANTIMICROBIAL PEPTIDES

The antibiotics which are currently approved by the U.S. Food and Drug Administration generally exhibit their activity by targeting an enzymatic or structural target specific to bacteria [34-37]. As a class, natural and synthetic antimicrobial peptides exhibit great potential as new therapeutic agents because of their novel mechanism of antibiotic activity, coupled with the difficulty bacteria have in developing resistance to them [4, 29, 38-44]. Antimicrobial peptides (AMP) have evolved in almost every class of living organisms as a host defense mechanism against invading micro-organisms including bacteria, fungi, protozoa and parasites [45-47]. AMPs have been isolated and characterized from almost all known classes of organisms including humans [48], amphibians [49], insects, mammals, birds, fish and plants [46]. These peptides are also considered to be key players in the host's innate immunity [43, 50-52]. AMP's are generally small (5-50 amino acid residues) highly positively charged (+3 to +9) [53] amphipathic peptides with well-defined regions of hydrophobicity and hydrophilicity [40, 54, 55]. There are four general structural classes of AMPs 1) β-sheet peptides with disulfide backbone linkages, 2) α-helical, 3) extended and 4) loop-structured [43, 56]. As of January 2009, more than 1330 [57] natural and synthetic antimicrobial peptides exhibiting a wide range of biological activity have been reported [58]. The most promising applications of AMPs thus far are focused on their clinical development as topical antibiotics [55].

MECHANISM OF ACTION

AMPs are broadly divided into two mechanistic classes, membrane-disruptors and non-membrane-disruptors [52, 59]. The absence of a specific target or receptor for membrane-disruptor AMP's is supported by the observation that analogs containing D-amino acid replacements don't exhibit reduced anti-bacteria activity [60]. Membrane-disruptors are divided into two sub-classifications based on biological activity: 1) cell selective and 2) non-selective [50]. Cell selective AMPs exhibit potent cytotoxic activity against bacterial cells while at the same time exhibiting low toxicity against mammalian cells. Non-selective AMPs exhibit cytotoxic activity against bacteria as well as mammalian cells. A large number of investigations have focused on the development of cell selective AMPs [50, 61, 63] with varying degrees of success. In general, hemolytic activity (the ability to kill or lysis red blood cells, which is a measure of human cell toxicity) has, in many cases been correlated with an AMP which exhibit structural features including hydrophobicity, amphipathicity and helicial properties [40, 64]. It has been shown that selective incorporation of D-amino acids, proline, peptoids and amino acids with differing hydrophobicity can reduce the resulting hemolytic activity by imparting changes in the secondary structure that will affect the amphipathicity and α-helicity of the peptide [50, 63, 65].

There are many excellent reviews discussing the structure-activity relationships and biological mechanisms of actions of naturally occurring AMPs, including the defensins, cathelicidins, cecropins, magainins and many others [40, 41, 47-49, 52, 66-71]. These AMPs will not be discussed in this chapter.

When an un-structured peptide binds to the surface of a membrane it induces a stable secondary structure onto the backbone of the peptide [72]. As a result of peptide binding a process of membrane thinning will begin and finally results in the disruption of the bacterial membrane by one of three general mechanisms. 1) Barrel stave mechanism:

In this mechanism the peptide is inserted into the membrane parallel to the normal plane of the membrane. 2) Toroidal pore mechanism: The peptide induces, upon binding to the lipid bilayer, pores causing a rearrangement of the lipid molecules so the polar head groups of the lipid line the surface of the pore. 3) Micellization mechanism: This mechanism forms lipid encapsulated peptides resulting in loss of membrane integrity [52, 64-66, 72-75]. The binding of AMPs to membranes of various chemical compositons is a complex equlibria involving the three separate phases; 1) solution, 2) interface-associated, and 3) oligomerization of the peptide during membrane insertion [41, 76, 77]. A cartoon representation of the three phases of binding are shown in Fig. **1**.

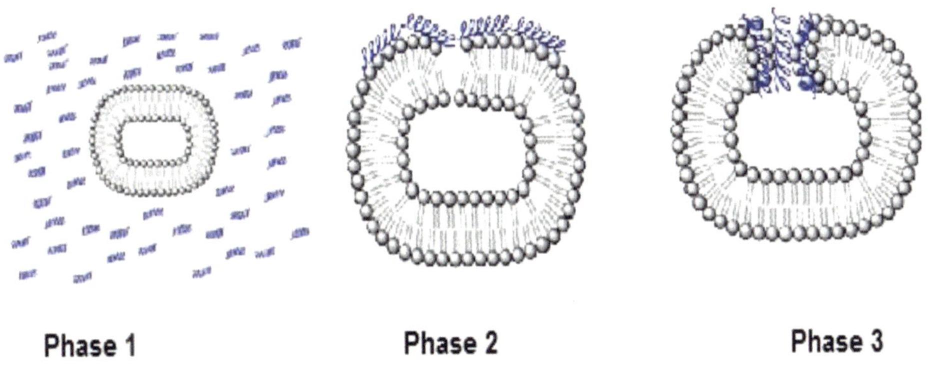

Figure 1: Cartoon representation of the three phases of AMP membrane binding.

The cartoon representation of the process through which binding of an AMP to a liposome occurs does not accurately describe the process. To better illustrate this process we conducted several molecular dynamics simulations in our laboratory. The binding of a single magainin 2 peptide (PDBID:2MAG) to the surface of a 4:1 1-Palmitoyl-2-Oleoyl-*sn*-Glycero-3-Phosphocholine (POPC) /1-Palmitoyl-2-Oleoyl-*sn*-Glycero-3-[Phospho-*rac*-(1-glycerol)] (POPG) lipid bilayer is shown in Fig. **2**. The electrostatic surface potential of the lipid is shown attracting magainin 2 to the surface of the lipid bilayer. This represents phase 2 of the binding process. In Fig. **3** three molecules of compound **23**, one of the peptides synthesized in our laboratory, are shown undergoing oligomerization in the early stages of membrane insertion. This represents early phase 3 of the bindng process.

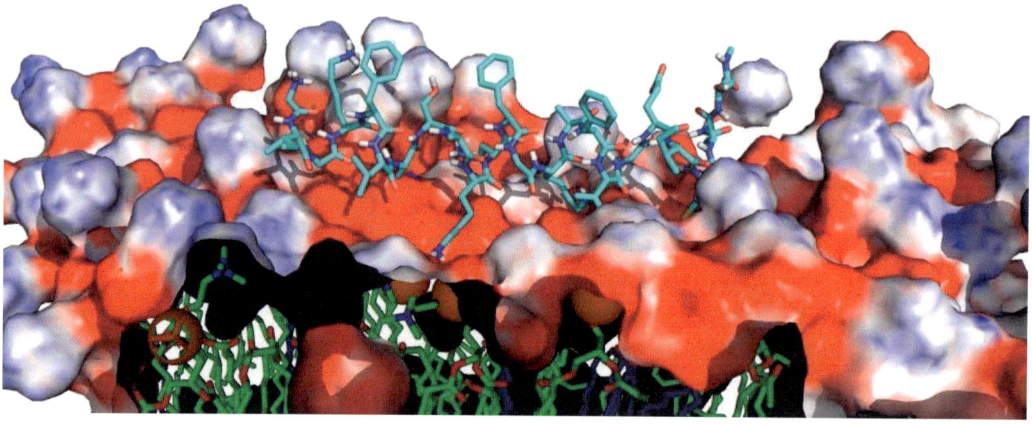

Figure 2: Molecular simulation of the binding of a single magainin 2 peptide (PDBID:2MAG) to the surface of a 4:1 POPC/POPG lipid bilayer. The electrostatic surface of the lipid is shown. Red indicates negative electrostatic potential. Blue indicates positive electrostatic potential. White indicates neutral electrostatic potential.

The selectivity of AMP's for prokaryotic *vs* eukaryotic cells is believed to be derived from the differences in the chemical compositions of their respective membranes [46, 78]. Bacterial cells contain a high percentage of negatively charged phospholipids while mammalian cells contain a much higher concentration of zwitterionic phospholipids in addition to cholesterol [30-33, 47, 79-81]. The electrostatic interactions that occur between the AMP(s) and the surface of the cell membrane are believed to be determinant for cell selectivity [4, 41, 82]. Hancock and co-workers [59] have extended this hypothesis to propose

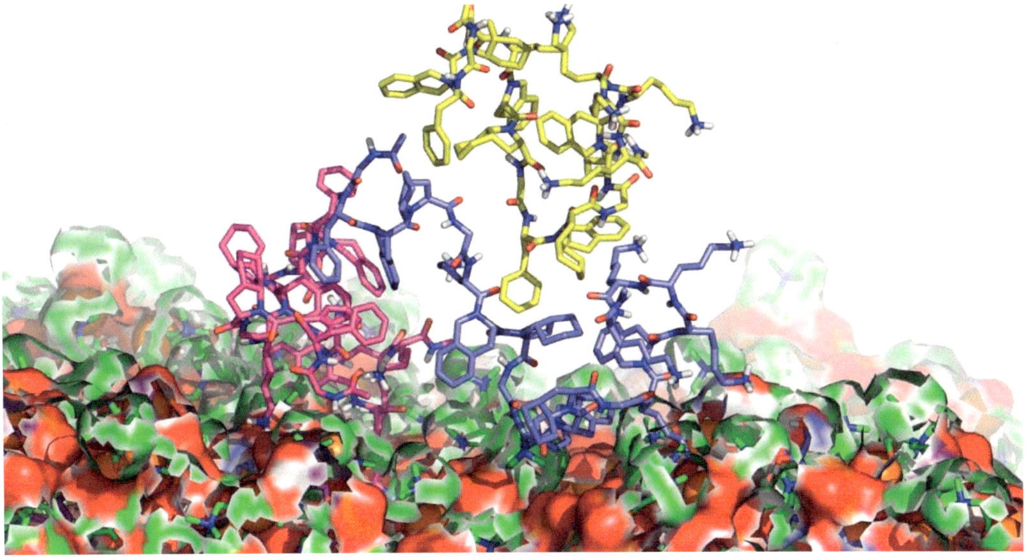

Figure 3: The molecular simulation of three molecules of compound **23** undergoing oligomerization and the early stages of membrane insertion with a 4:1 POPC/POPG lipid bilayer with part of the surface of the bilayer depicted.

the differences in membrane composition between different strains of bacteria are responsible for the diversity in the potency and selectivity exhibited by a particular AMP against different strains of bacteria. For example the following Gram positive strains contain different percentages of anionic lipids. For *Staphylococcus aureus,* 57% of the lipid composition of its' membrane is the anionic lipid 1-Palmitoyl-2-Oleoyl-*sn*-Glycero-3-[Phospho-*rac*-(1-glycerol)] (POPG), while for *Staphylococcus epidermidis,* has 90% of the lipid of its membrane is composed of POPG, and for *Bacillus subtilus* the percentage of POPG is reduced to 29% [83]. While the membranes of the Gram negative strains *Salmonella typimurium*, *Pesudomonas cepacia* and *Escherichia coli* contain only 33, 18 and 6 percent POPG respectively [83]. The membranes of *Klebsiella pneumoniae* and *Pseudomonas aeruginosa* contain 5 and 21 percent POPG respectively [42]. The membranes of many Gram-negative bacterial contain high concentrations of the zwitterionic lipid 1-Palmitoyl-2-Oleoyl-*sn*-Glycero-3-Phosphoethanolamine (POPE) instead of POPC. *Escherichia coli*, *Klebsiella pneumonia* and *Pseudomonas aeruginosa* contain 80, 82 and 60 percent of POPE respectively [42]. Other differences in the membrane composition between bacteria strains also exist including the presence of sterols, lipopolysaccharide, and peptidoglycan *etc.* [47]. Difference in structure, transmembrane potential and polarizability are also observed [46, 84]. The lipid bilayer of Gram positive bacteria is covered by a porous layer of peptidoglycan, while the structure of Gram negative bacteria is more complex with two lipid membranes containing, in addition to the normal lipids, lipopolysaccharides and porins (Fig. **4**) [46, 84]. The outer membrane of mycobacteria is the most complex of the three types consisting of a very thick mycolate-rich outer coat [85] which is very difficult to penetrate. There is a developing preponderance of evidence in the literature, supporting the concept that the selectivity and potency of a specific AMP is determined in a large measure by the chemical composition of the target membrane [59, 86]. Cartoon representations of Prokaryotic cell [87-90] membranes are shown in Fig. **4** and representations of Eukaryotic cell [92-96] membranes are shown in Fig. **5**.

POTENTIAL SHORTCOMING OF ANTIMICROBIAL PEPTIDES

As of June 2012, no AMP has been approved by the Food and Drug Administration for human use. The reason for this is a combination of factors including; low bioavailability, high cost of synthesis, moderate activity and relatively higher toxicity compared to conventional antibiotics and low metabolic stability [15, 97]. However, the potential advantages offered by antimicrobial peptides over conventional antibiotics has resulted in continued interest in the development of AMPs as therapeutic agents [70, 97]. The continued research into the development of AMPs into potentially therapeutically useful agents is fully justified, particularly in light of the lack of research by the pharmaceutical industry into expanding the collection of conventional antibiotics [97, 98]. For example investigations with model α-helical peptides have demonstrated that decreasing hydrophobicity, helicity and amphipathicity decreases hemolytic activity and thus reduces toxicity, while increasing the net positive charge increases antimicrobial activity [99]. It is the intent of this chapter to present an overview of some of the recent approaches used to design synthetic AMPs that address some of the inherent problems associated with naturally occurring AMPs, and therefore allow for the development of clinically useful AMPs.

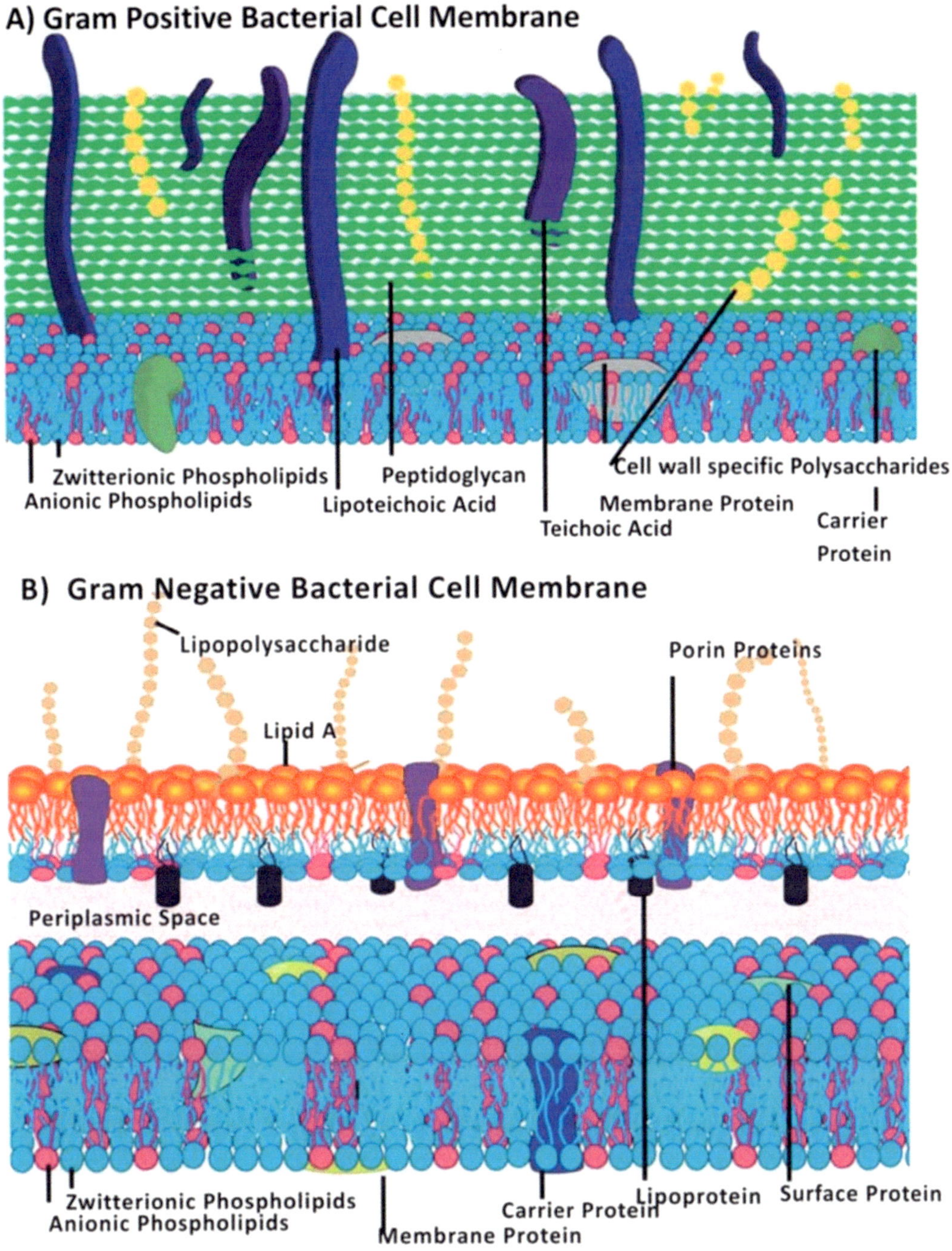

Figure 4: Our cartoon representations of Prokaryotic cell [87-91] membranes (Top) Gram Positive bacteria, (Bottom) Gram Negative bacterial.

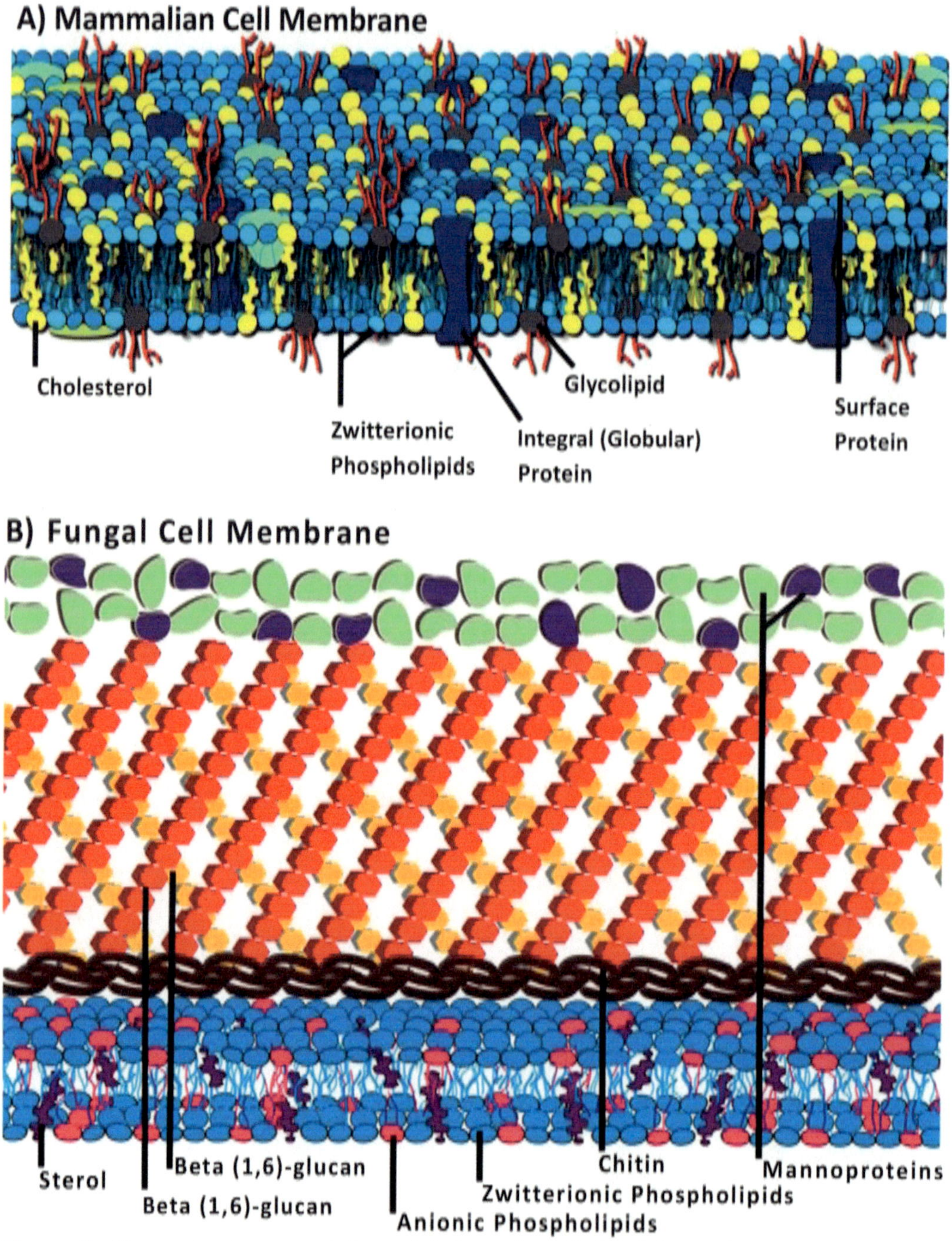

Figure 5: Our cartoon representation of Eukaryotic cell [92-96] membranes (Top) human, (Bottom) fungal.

DESIGN OF NOVEL SYNTHETIC ANTIMICROBIAL PEPTIDES

New Way to Look at Structure

Hicks and co-workers developed a series on AMPs based on the incorporation of unnatural amino acids into the primary sequence of a naturally occurring peptide [25]. These AMPs exhibited very different *in vitro* activity against *Staphylococcus aureus* and *Mycobacterium ranae* bacteria [25]. The results of a 3D-QSARs (Quantitative Structure Activity Relationship), study conducted by Bhonsle and co-workers indicated the physicochemical properties required for activity against *S. aureus* and *M. ranae* bacteria are different [100]. Bhonsle determined that there are five major physicochemical descriptors necessary to define the activity of these AMPs in the *S. aureus* QSAR model. These five physicochemical descriptors are: Jurs-Fractional-Positive-Surface-Area-3 (Jurs-FPSA-3), Jurs-Relative-Positive-Charge-Surface-area (Jurs-RPCS), Jurs-Differential-Positively-charged-Surface-Area-3 (Jurs-DPSA-3), Jurs-total-Solvent-Accessible-Surface-Area (Jurs-SASA) and Jurs-TotAl-hydrophobic-Surface-Area (Jurs-TASA) [100]. Five different physicochemical descriptors were necessary to define the activity of these AMPs in the *M. ranae* QSAR model. These descriptors are: sum-of-all-atomic-polarizabilities (Apol), Conformer Energy, Jurs-Partial-Positively-charged-Surface-Area-2 (Jurs-PPSA-2), Jurs-Relative-Negative-CharGe (Jurs-RNCG), and Jurs-Total-Polar-Surface-Area (Jurs-TPSA) [100]. These results support the hypothesis that for any particular AMP, organism selectivity and potency are controlled by the physicochemical interactions that occur between the AMP and the target cell membrane [100]. A method to visualize the role played by physicochemical properties is to compare the electrostatic surface potential maps of active and inactive analogues. In Fig. **6** the electrostatic potential surface maps of one active and one inactive analogue synthesized by Hicks and co-workers are shown [25]. The electrostatic surface potential map of the active analog, on the right, clearly shows that the electrostatic positive potential is located on predominately one face of the molecule while the other face is electrostatically neutral. The molecule is clearly amphipathic. The electrostatic surface potential map for the inactive analog, on the left, shows an even distribution of charge over the entire surface of the molecule, the molecule is therefore not amphipathic. Viewing these two analogues in this fashion helps to explain the differences in antibacterial activity. The reader may find this approach helpful in the design of new analogues.

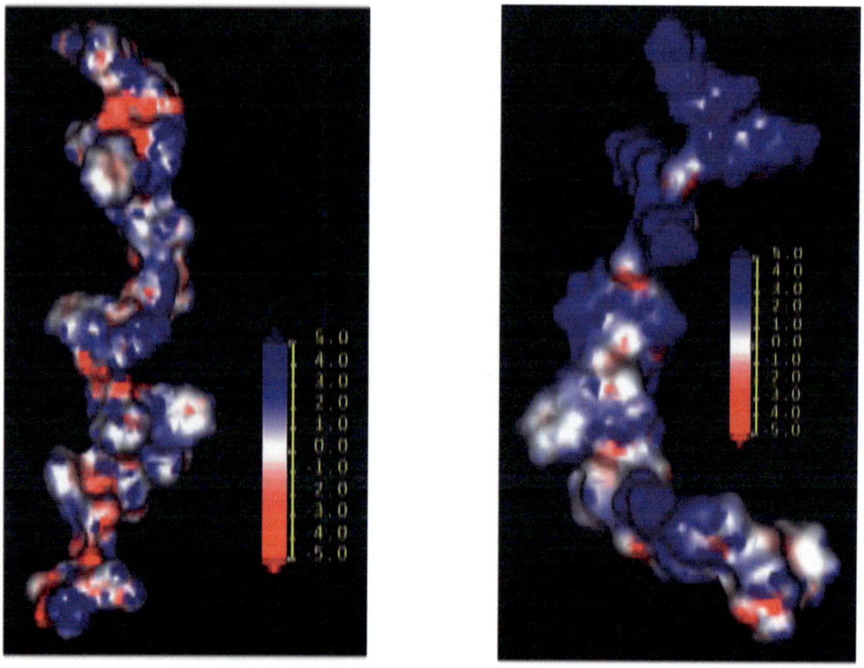

Figure 6: The electrostatic potential surface maps of one active and one inactive analogue synthesized by Hicks and co-workers are shown [25]. The electrostatic surface potential map of the active analog, on the right, clearly shows that the positive electrostatic potential is located on predominately one face of the molecule while the other face is electrostatically neutral. The molecule is clearly amphipathic. The electrostatic surface potential map for the inactive analog, on the left, show an even distribution of charge over the entire surface of the molecule, the molecule is therefore not amphipathic. Blue color indicates a positive electrostatic potential, Red indicates a negative electrostatic potential and White indicates a neutral electrostatic potential.

Reversed Sequence Synthetic Peptides

Gopal and co-workers have reported the synthesis and biological evaluation of a series of reversed sequence AMP with improved antibiotic activity [101]. The analogs developed by Gopal and co-workers are based upon the incorporation of the two amino acids Lys and Trp which are known to play important roles defining the interactions that occur between AMPs and bacterial membranes. Lys is the most commonly encountered basic amino acid in naturally occurring AMPs [101, 102]. Synthetic peptides containing Lys as the only basic residue placed on the polar face of an amphipathic structure have exhibited interesting antimicrobial activity as well as strong interactions with the anionic polar head groups found in the lipids of bacteria leading to organism selectivity [103-106]. For example the research group of Fernandez and co-workers [34] designed a synthetic AMP with the sequence $KWKKLLKKPLLKKLLKKLNH_2$ which exhibited very good *in vitro* activity against several strains of bacteria. Representative activity is listed in Table **1**. This peptide didn't exhibit hemolytic activity below 100 µM, thus it is considered a potential candidate for further therapeutic development [34].

The bulky indole side chain of Trp residues strongly interacts with the phospholipids found in bacteria cells and is therefore believed to be partially responsible for prokaryotic cell selectivity and toxicity [101, 107].

The approach used by Gopal and co-workers was to synthesize the analog WKWKWK $(WK)_3$ and the reversed sequence KWKWKW $(KW)_3$ and then to

Table 1: **Minimum Inhibitory Concentration (MIC) of the Peptide Developed by Fernandez and Co-Workers [34] Against Representative Strains of Bacteria and Fungi**

Organism	MIC (µM)
S. aureus	1.56
B. subtillis	0.78
P. aeruginosa	1.56
S. typhimurium	0.09
C. albicans	6.25
T. beigelii	3.25

compare the observed *in vitro* activity against selected strains of bacteria [101]. Reversed analogs are considered to exhibit similar structural and physiochemical properties to the original analog, however the amide bonds are inverted [101]. Fig. **7** shows a comparison of the sequence WKWK and the reversed sequence KWKW. When the two peptides are arranged so that the amino acid side chains line up the amide bonds are inverted. This results in changes in the hydrogen bonding pattern and the helical dipole moment of the peptide which can effect lipid binding [101]. This approach has been used to reduce the hemolytic activity associated with several antibiotic peptides [69, 108]. A representative sample of the antimicrobial activity of these two analogs is given in Table **2**. As seen in Table **2**, the reverse sequence generally resulted in an increase in antibacterial activity [101].

Table 2: Minimum Inhibitory Concentration (MIC) Values for the Peptide Developed by Gopal and Co-Workers [101]

Organism	MIC (µM) (WK)3	(KW)3
E. coli	256	64
S. typhimurium	16	16
P. aeruginosa	64	32
S. aureus	256	128
B. subtilis	128	64
C. albicans	32	16
T. beigelli	16	8

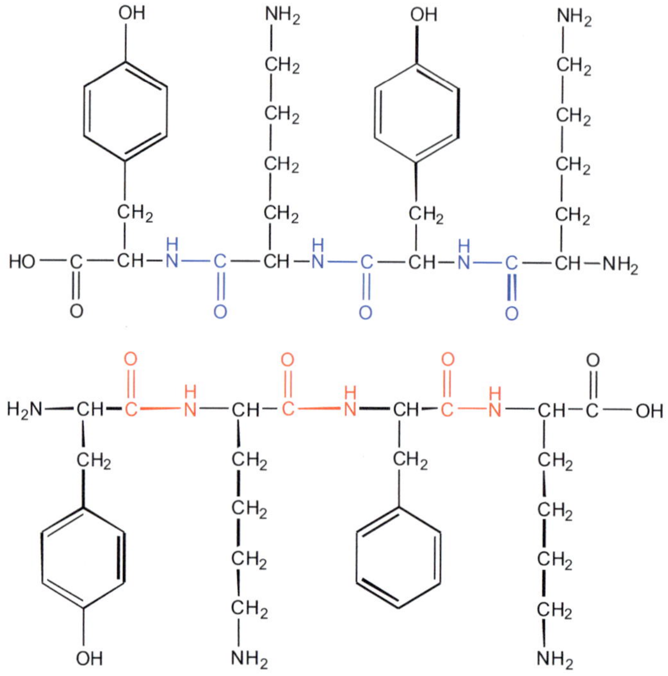

Figure 7: A comparison of the sequence WKWK and the reversed sequence KWKW. When the two peptides are arranged so that the amino acid side chains line up the amide bonds are inverted as indicated by the red and blue amide bonds.

β-Peptides and Peptoids

Changes in the conformational flexibility of the peptide backbone will affect the helicity and amphipathicity of the resulting AMP and thus affect lipid binding. Thus several modifications of the structural and resulting conformational properties of the traditional α-amino acid have been made. Included in these modifications are the β-peptides and peptoids. The insertion of an additional methylene unit between the C^{α} carbon and the nitrogen atom of an α-amino acid results in what is called a β-peptide [109]. A peptoid is obtained by relocating the side chain from the C^{α} carbon atom to the nitrogen atom [109].

A β-peptoid is obtained by the combined insertion of an additional methylene unit and the relocation of the side chain to the nitrogen atom [109]. Examples of these structures are given in Fig. **8**. The incorporation of peptoids into the peptidomimetic skeleton allows the compound to adopt conformations which would be highly unfavorable for peptides consisting of only α-or β-amino acids [109]. This is because the amide bonds of α and β amino acids are planar and adopt the *trans* configuration [109]. The incorporation of peptoids and β-peptoids greatly increases the available three-dimensional conformational space allowing these analogs to adopt new and novel conformations which may increase either organism selectivity, potency or both [109]. Seebach and co-workers [110] have discussed in detail the conformations adopted by linear and cyclic β-peptides this information is very useful in the design of novel β-peptides.

Examples of antimicrobial β-peptides include the following sequence alterations. DeGrado and co-workers reported the synthesis of a β-peptide (Fig. **9A**) based on the incorporation of multiple β-Lys and β-Leu residues exhibited a MIC value of 2.1 μM against *E. coli* [111]. Seebach and co-workers synthesized another β-peptide (Fig. **9B**) based on the incorporation of multiple β-Lys and β-Leu residues that exhibited a MIC value of 9.3 μM against *E. coli* [112]. Gellman and co-workers synthesized a β-peptide (Fig. **9C**) based on the incorporation of novel cyclic β-peptides that exhibited a MIC value of 6.3 μM against *E. coli* [113]. Gellman and co-workers have reported three cyclic β-peptides based on (*R,R*)-*trans*-2-aminocyclopentanecarboxylic acid that are useful in forming 12-helix structures that exhibit potent antibacterial activity [114]. β-peptides containing many of these building blocks have also exhibited antiviral activity [115].

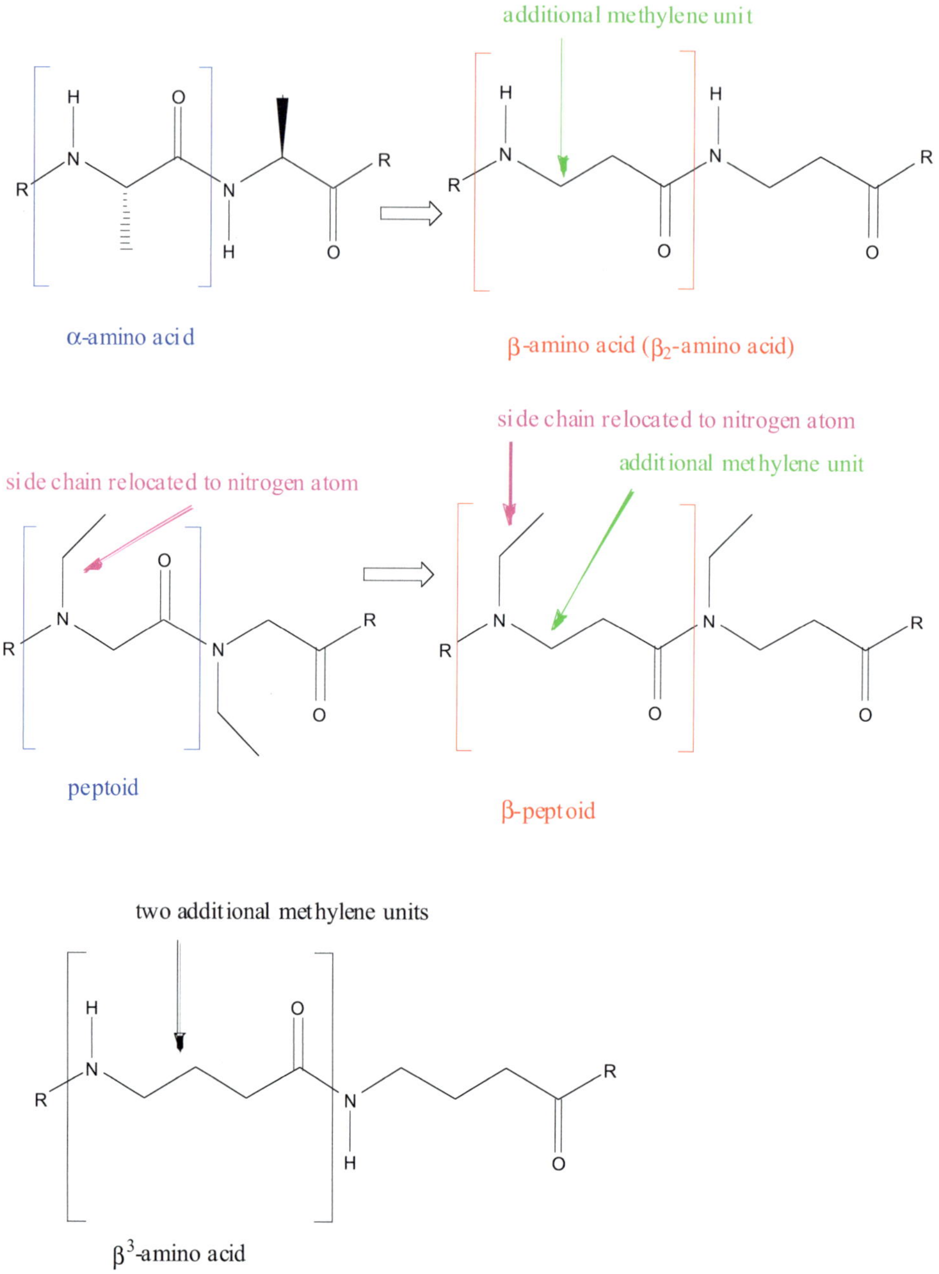

Figure 8: Example structures of α-peptides, β-peptides, peptoids and β-peptoids [109].

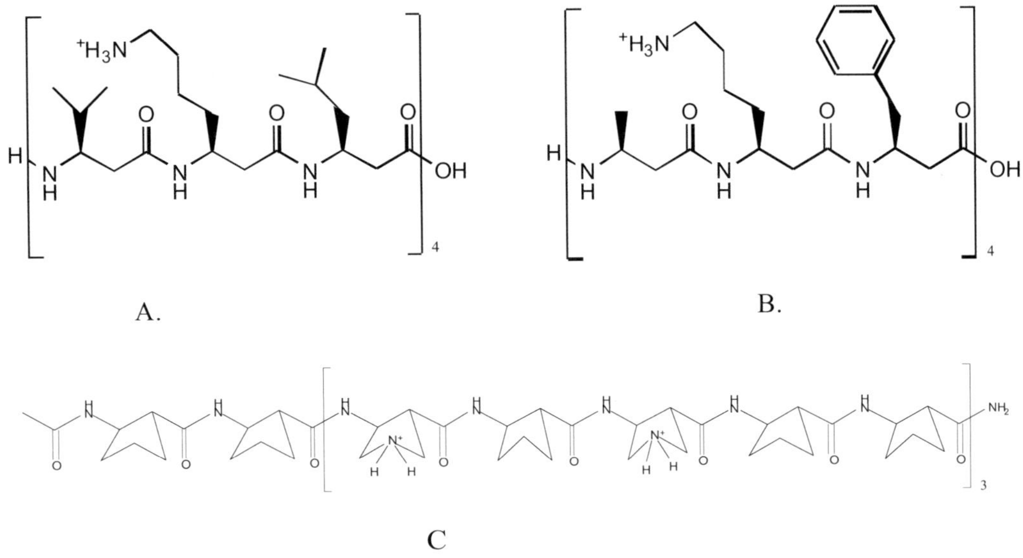

Figure 9: (**A**) DeGrado and co-workers reported the synthesis of a β-peptide based on the incorporation of multiple β-Lys and β-Leu residues [111]. (**B**) Seebach and co-workers synthesized another β-peptide based on the incorporation of multiple β-Lys and β-Leu residues [112]. (**C**) Gellman and co-workers synthesized a β-peptide based on the incorporation of novel cyclic β-peptides [113].

β-peptides disubstituted at the C^{α} carbon (referred to as $\beta^{2,2}$ amino acids) have been reported by Torfoss and co-workers and are given in Fig. **10** [116], these amino acids may also prove useful in the syntheses of antimicrobial agents.

Examples of antimicrobial β-peptoids include the following: Shuey and co-workers reported the synthesis of a β-peptoid (Fig. **11A**) that exhibited a MIC value of 53 μM against *E. coli* [117]. While Olsen and co-workers synthesized another β-peptoid (Fig. **11B**) that exhibited a MIC value of 2.8 μM against *E. coli* [118]. Haug and co-workers reported the synthesis and biological evaluation of a series of peptidomimetics which include the incorporation of β-(2,5,7-tri-*tert*-butylindol-3-yl)alanine [119]. These analogs exhibited very good *in vitro* MIC values against *E. coli, P. aeruginosa, S. aureus,* methicillin resistant *S. aureus* (MRSA), methicillin resistant *S. epidermidis* and glycopeptide resistant *S. aureus* [119]. One of these analogs LTX 109 (Fig. **12**) is currently in phase II clinical trials as a topical treatment for multiple drug resistant organism related infections [119, 120].

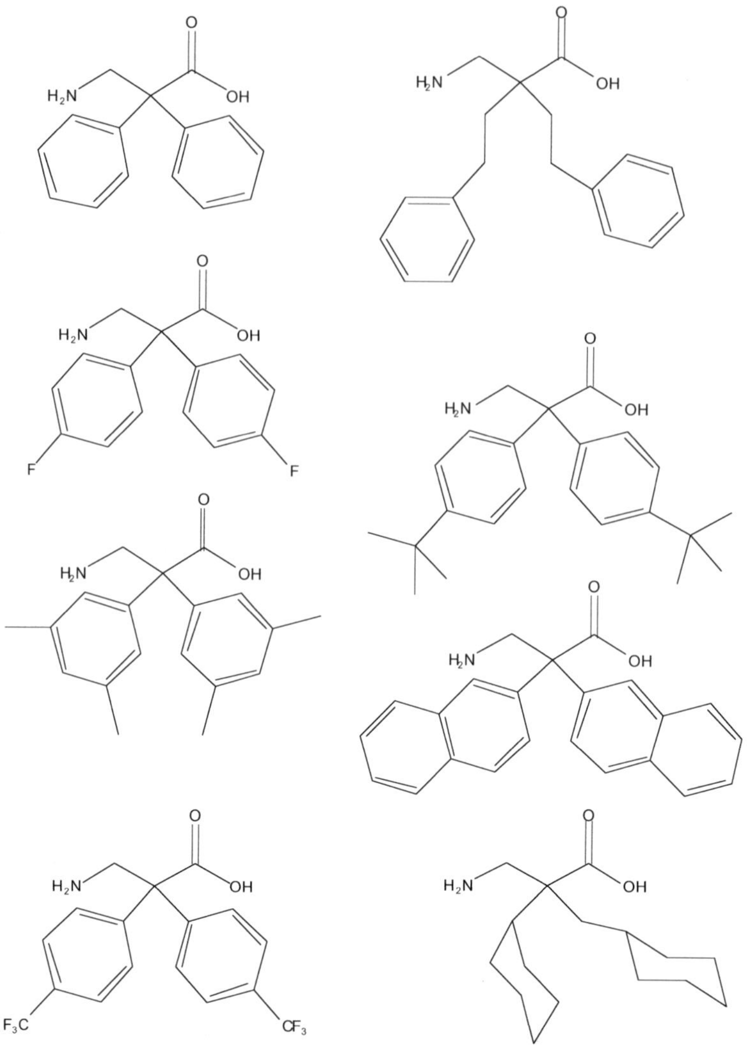

Figure 10: Torfoss and co-workers [116], reported these β-peptides disubstituted at the C^{α} carbon (referred to as $\beta^{2,2}$ amino acids).

Godballe and co-workers have published an excellent review on the incorporation of α-peptides, β^2-peptide, β^3-peptides and peptoids to control the physicochemical and structural properties of antimicrobial peptidomimetics [31]. Incorporation of the bulky peptiod residues shown in Fig. **10** will help to stabilize an α-helical structure in the resulting peptidomimetic [31]. The types of helical conformations possible from incorporation of these residues are given Table **3**, and the hydrogen bonding scheme stabilizing these helical structures are given in Fig. **13** [31, 112, 121-125].

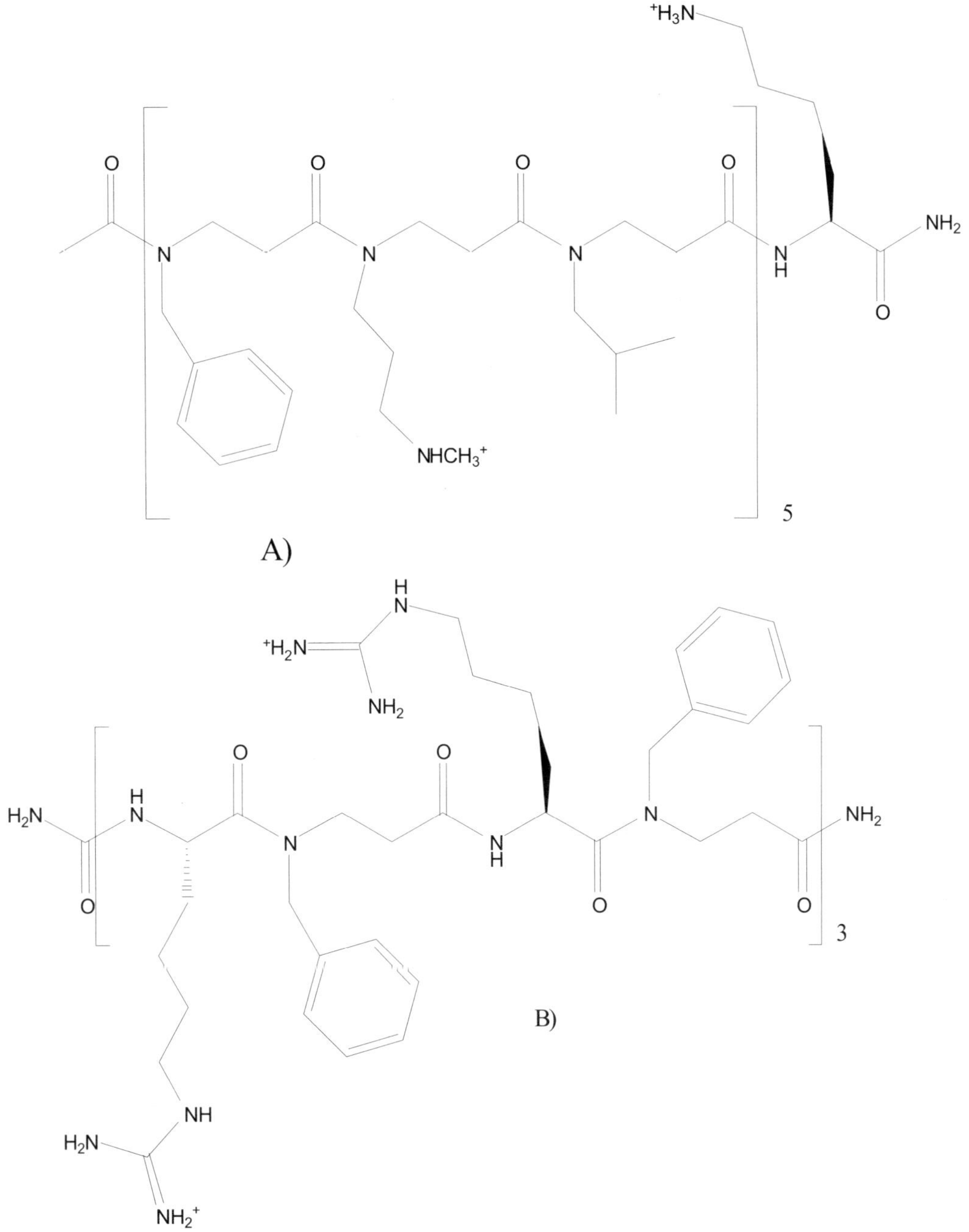

Figure 11: Examples of antimicrobial β-peptoids. (**A**) Shuey and co-workers reported the synthesis of this β-peptoid [117]. (**B**) Olsen and co-workers synthesized this β-peptoid [118].

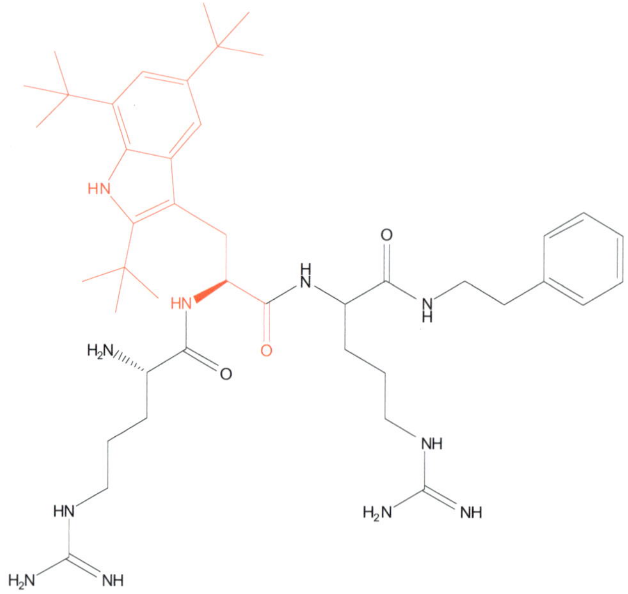

Figure 12: Haug and co-workers reported the synthesis and biological evaluation of a series of peptidomimetics which include the incorporation of β-(2,5,7-tri-*tert*-butylindol-3-yl)alanine highlighted in red [119].

Table 3: Types of Possible Helical Conformers Available to Peptidomimetics [31, 112, 121-125]

Amino Acid Type	Number of Atoms Per H-Bond Ring	Residues Per Turn
α	13-helix	3.6
α–β	11-helix	3
α–β	14/15-helix	4.5
β	6-ribbon	1.7
β	8-ribbon	2.2
β	10-helix	2.6
β	12-helix	2.7
β	14-helix	3,1
β	10/12-helix	2.7

Hybrid Peptides

In an effort to improve the therapeutic usefulness of naturally occurring antimicrobial peptides an approach was developed to take the amino acid sequences believed to be responsible for antimicrobial activity from two or more peptides and combined them together yielding what are referred to as hybrid peptides [43]. Fox and co-workers used sub-sequences from three naturally occurring AMPs, cecropin A, LL-37 and magainin 2 to design four new hybrid peptides [43]. All four analogs exhibited greater activity against *B. anthracis* (spores), *B. anthracis* (vegetative) and *B. cepacia* than the original natural AMPs [43].

Shin and co-workers reported the design, synthesis and biological evaluations of hybrid peptides obtained by combining regions of cecropin A with magainin 2 or from combining regions of cecropin A with melittin [126]. The cecropin A-magainin 2 analog combined residues 1-8 of the C-terminus of cecropin with residues 1-12 of the C-terminus of magainin 2 with a Leu replacement at position 16. This analog referred to as L-CA-MA (KWKLFKKIGIGKFLHLAKKF-NH_2) exhibited potent antibacterial and antitumor activity with reduced hemolytic activity [126]. The insertion of Gly-Ile or Gly-Pro dipeptides or a single Pro residue into the hinge region (GIGG shown in red) of L-CA-MA resulted in a dramatic loss of hemolytic activity without a concurrent reduction in the antibacterial and antitumor activity [126]. However for the following analogs CA(1-8)-MA(1-12), CA(1-8)-ME(1-12), Ca(1-13)-MA(1-13) and CA(1-13)-ME(1-13) the replacement of the tripeptide sequence Gly-Ile-Gly with the tripeptide sequence Gly-Pro-Gly resulted in a dramatic reduction in antibacterial, antitumor and hemolytic activity [126]. Replacement of the Leu at position 16 with the more hydrophobic residues of Phe or Trp increased the hemolytic activity of the new L-CA-MA analogs [126]. The conclusion reached by this study was the hydrophobicity at position 16 and the flexibility of the hinged region of the CA-MA and CA-ME hybrids are determinate in defining activity [126].

Structural Modification of Naturally Occurring AMPs

Structural activity relationship (SAR) studies have been conducted on many naturally occurring AMPs in an effort to increase the antimicrobial activity while concurrently reducing the toxicity. Findlay and co-workers have written an excellent review outlining the process of generating new AMPs based on naturally occurring scaffolding [33]. Huang and co-workers have also reviewed the relationships between structure and function of α-helical AMPs, this review is also an excellent source for guidance on the modification of existing AMP scaffolding [30].

The cathelicidins are a large family of naturally occurring peptides ranging in size from 12 to 80 amino acid residues [127]. Cathelicidin LL-37 is a human AMP derived from the 37 C-terminal residues of the human protein CAP-18 which exhibits broad spectrum antibacterial activity [128, 129]. Cathelicidin LL-37 has been shown to adopt an α-helical structure in the presence of lipids and micelles [127]. Dean and co-workers reported the design, synthesis and the biological activity of five analogs of cathelicidin LL-37 determining the importance of the ATRA motif for antimicrobial activity [127]. The amino acid sequence of these analogs and their activity against *S. aureus* are given in Table **4**. Also the peptide NA-CATH:ATRA1-ATRA1 inhibited the production of biofilms produced by *S. aureus* in the presence of salt [127].

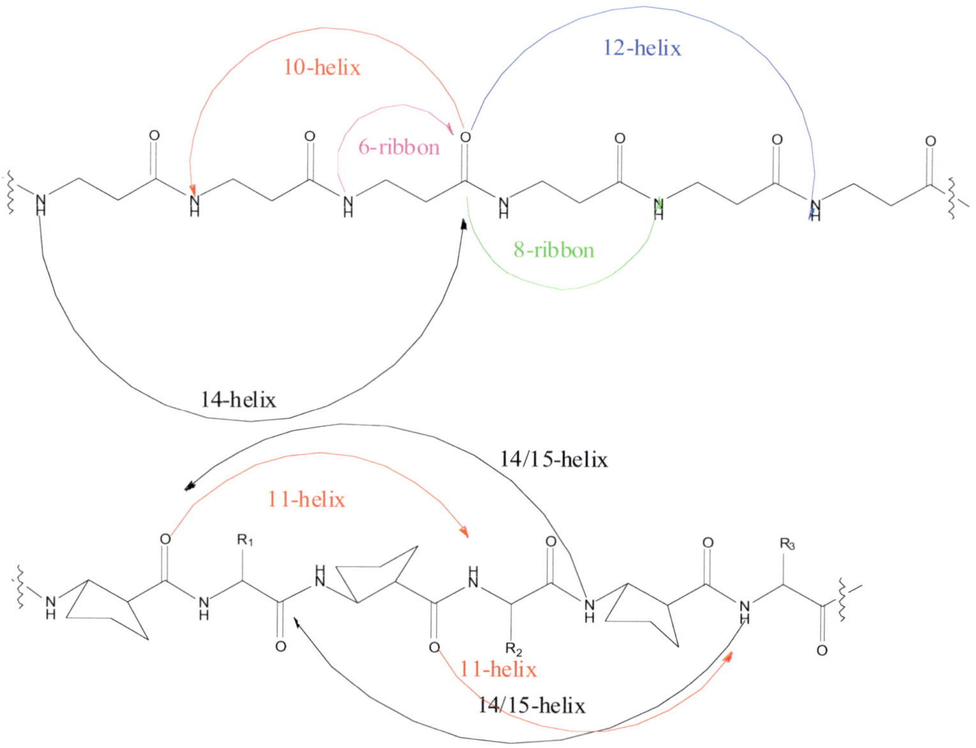

Figure 13: The hydrogen bonding scheme stabilizing the helical structures defined in Table **3** [31, 112, 121-125].

Sharma and co-workers designed and synthesized a 24 amino acid residue linear peptide and the corresponding di-Cys bridged cyclic peptide based on the putative lipopolysaccharide binding domain of the Indian mud crab, *Scylla serrata* [130]. The amino acid sequence of both peptides is TCHIRRKPKFRKFLYHE GKFWCP, the only difference between the two is one is linear while the other is cyclized *via* a disulfide bond between the Cys residues (shown in red) positioned at residues 2 and 23 [130]. Both peptides exhibited *in vitro* activity against *E. coli* and *P. aeruginosa* at concentrations below 64.64 μM [130].

Table 4: The Amino Acid Sequence of the Cathelicidin LL-37 Analogs Developed by Dean and Co-Workers [127] and their Activity Against *S. aureus*

Peptide	Amino Acid Sequence	*S. aureus* (EC_{50} μg/mL)
NA-CATH	KRFKKFFKKLKNSVKKRAKKFFKKPKVIGVTFPF	2.85
NA-CATH-ATRA1-ATRA1	KRFKKFFKKLKNSVKKRFKKFFKKLKVIGVTFPF	0.51
ATRA-1	KRFKKFFKKLK-NH_2	0.52
ATRA-1A	KRAKKFFKKLK-NH_2	0
ATRA-2	KRAKKFFKKPK-NH_2	18.0
LL-37	LLGDFFRKSKEKIGKEFKRIVQRIKDFLRNLVPRTES	1.27

Polymyxin B (PMB) is a mixture of cyclic decapeptides isolated from *Bacillus polymyxia* [131] which contains six L-2,4-diaminobutyic acid (Dab) residues. The 4-amino side chain of Dab [4] is acylated to the carbonyl of the C-terminal Thr^{10} residue [132]. Sato and co-workers reported the synthesis and biological evaluation of Polymyxin B analogs with fatty acyl modifications of the α-nitrogen of the Dab^{1} residue, these analogs exhibited potent and specific antibacterial activity against *P. aeruginosa* [132]. The amino acid sequences of these analogs and their antibacterial activity are given in Table **5**.

Peptides Obtained by Acid-Amide Substitutions

Ueno and co-workers developed a method for obtaining AMPs containing only natural amino acids using the method of acid-amide substitution, for example substituting a Gln residue for a Glu residue or an Asn residue for an Asp residue [133]. The rationale for this method is that substituting an acidic side chain such as Glu with its amide counterpart Gln will neutralize the negative charge and thus increases the overall positive charge of the AMP, thus increasing the antibacterial activity of the peptide [133]. In this investigation pro-regions of four different nematode cecropins (P1-P4) were selected for further study. There amino acids sequences and the corresponding substitutions are shown in Table **6**.

Table 5: Polymyxin B and the Analogs Developed by Sato and Co-Workers and their Minimum Inhibitory Concentration (nmol/mL) Against Gram Negative Bacteria [132]

Amino Acid Sequence	*E. coli*	*S. typhimurium*	*P. aeruginosa*
(PMB) Fa-Dab-Thr-Dab-Dab*-Dab-D-Phe-Leu-Dab-Dab-Thr*-	1	0.5	1
Thr-Dab-Dab*-Dab-D-Phe-Leu-Dab-Dab-Thr*-	>256	>256	128
Dab-Thr-Dab-Dab*-Dab-D-Phe-Leu-Dab-Dab-Thr*-	16	32	2
Ser--Dab-Dab*-Dab-D-Phe-Leu-Dab-Dab-Thr*-	64	64	1
Dab-Dab*-Dab-D-Phe-Leu-Dab-Dab-Thr*-	256	256	4
Ser-Dab*-Dab-D-Phe-Leu-Dab-Dab-Thr*-	>256	>256	2
Guanyl-Dab-Thr-Dab-Dab*-Dab-D-Phe-Leu-Dab-Dab-Thr*-	4	2	1
Guanyl-Thr-Dab-Dab*-Dab-D-Phe-Leu-Dab-Dab-Thr*-	2	2	1
Guanyl-Dab -Dab-Dab*-Dab-D-Phe-Leu-Dab-Dab-Thr*-	8	8	2
Guanyl-Dab-Dab*-Dab-D-Phe-Leu-Dab-Dab-Thr*-	16	16	2
Guanyl-Dab*-Dab-D-Phe-Leu-Dab-Dab-Thr*-	>256	>256	4
Guanyl-Dab-Guanyl-Dab*-Dab-D-Phe-Leu-Dab-Dab-Thr*-	16	32	0.5

*Indicates position of acylation cyclization.

Table 6: Acid Amide Substitution Peptides Developed by Ueno and Co-Workers [133]. The Basic Residues are Shown in Red. The Acid-Amide Substitutions are Highlighted in Yellow

Peptide	Sequence
NP1P	RRRFVAQQNAIHSRVSRQVPTLSNSV
P1P	RRRFVAEQDAIHSRVSREVPTLSDSV
NP2P	RRRFVVQQNTISPRLQVNQRFLPNSVQQI
P2P	RRRFVVQQDTISPRLEVDERFLPNSVQEQI
NP3P	RRRSVGQQNAIPSHIQVNKFFLRKPAKQHI
P3P	RRRSVGEEDAIPSHIEVNKFFLRKPAKEHI
NP4P	HRRSVAHQQQASLHVKTNQLPSPNTVRQQL
P4P	HRRSVAHQEEASLHVKTDELPSPNTVREQL

Peptides NP1P, NP2P and NP3P all exhibited significantly greater activity against a series of Gram positive and Gram negative bacteria than the starting pro-regions of the corresponding nematode cecropins [133]. Compound NP4P didn't exhibit any improvement in activity compared to compound P4 [133].

De Novo Design of Cationic AMPs

Based on the available knowledge of the structural and physicochemical requirements for antibacterial activity obtained from naturally occurring AMPs [41, 46, 52, 60, 62, 63, 65, 71, 80, 99, 134-136] many research groups have designed novel synthetic AMPs. Recent examples of this approach include the research of Thennarasu and co-workers who designed the synthetic peptide MSI-367 with the amino acid sequence of $(KFAKKFA)_3\text{-}NH_2$ [137]. This peptide contains only three amino acids, Lys, Ala and Phe. The minimum inhibitory concentrations for peptide MSI-367 against selected microbes are given in Table **7**. At concentrations comparable to the MIC values no hemolytic activity was observed [137]. However at higher concentration of approximately 40 μM 20% hemolysis of red blood cells was observed [137].

Table 7: Minimum Inhibitory Concentration (MIC) Values for the Peptide MSI-367 Developed by Thennarasu and Co-Workers [137]

Organism	MIC (μM)
E. coli	1.6
P. aeruginosa	2.8
S. aureus	1.6
C. albicans	25.8

Wiradharma and co-workers designed, synthesized and evaluated a series of short α-helical peptides with the following sequences, $(XXYY)_n$ where X= a hydrophobic residue, Y = a cationic residue and n = the number of repeating units [138]. Three analogs $(FFRR)_3$, $(LLRR)_3$ and $(LLKK)_3$ all containing three repeat units exhibited greater selectivity against bacterial cells than red blood cells compared to analogs containing two or four repeat units [138]. CD studies indicated that these analogs adopted a disordered conformation in aqueous solution, however they adopt an α-helical conformations in the presences of membrane model systems [138]. The propensity to adopt an α-helical structure increases with increasing the number of repeat units [138]. The minimum inhibitory concentrations against *B. subtitlis* and *C. albicans* as well as the 50% hemolytic concentrations (50% HC) of the analogs prepared by Wiradharma and co-workers are given in Table **8** [138].

Table 8: The Minimum Inhibitory Concentrations (MIC) As Well As the 50% Hemolytic Concentrations (HC_{50}) of the Analogs Prepared by Wiradharma and Co-Workers [138]

	MIC (mg/L)	(mg/L)	HC_{50}
Peptide	*B. subtilis*	*C. albicans*	
$(FFRR)_2$	125	>500	>500
$(LLRR)_2$	62.5	125	>500
$(LLKK)_2$	500	250	>500
$(FFRR)_3$	31.3	125	>500
$(AARR)_3$	>500	>500	>500
$(LLRR)_3$	15.6	500	>500
$(LLKK)_3$	31.3	125	>500
$(FFRR)_4$	20	>50	26
$(LLRR)_4$	10	>50	12
$(LLKK)_4$	10	>50	24

This data indicates to us that hydrophobicity, charge density (the hard positive charge of the Lys side chain verse the delocalized charge of the Arg side chain) and the number of repeating units determines the resulting activity against Gram positive bacteria, yeast as well as red blood cells for this series of peptides.

Glukhov and co-workers have designed, synthesized and evaluated a series of AMPs with the sequence KKKKKKAAXAAXAAXAA-NH_2 where X is either a Phe residue, or a Trp residue [139]. These AMPs exhibited very good antibacterial activity against *P. aerginosa* with very little hemolytic activity [139].

Juretic and co-workers have published an excellent review on the several computational methods that may be employed to design novel antimicrobial peptides [97].

Peptides Containing C^{α}-Tetra-Substituted α-Amino Acids

Of the available C^{α}-tetra-substituted α-amino acids, α–aminoisobutyric acid (Aib) is the most commonly employed and studied residue and it's allowed conformations are limited to constrained right and left-handed helical structures [140]. Grauer and Konig [141] have reported the synthesis of a series of novel C^{α}-tetra-substituted α-amino acids to reduce the conformational flexibility of a peptide, several of which are given in Fig. **14**. Incorporation of specific substituted C$^{\alpha}$-tetra-substituted α-amino acid derivatives into a peptide sequence can induce stable β-turns [142] or 3_{10} or α-helices [140, 141, 143]. Other commercially available C$^{\alpha}$ tetra-substituted α-amino acids are shown in Fig. **15**. Toniolo and co-workers have published an excellent review on the conformational preferences for C$^{\alpha}$ -tetra-substituted α-amino acids which are very helpful in the design of novel analogs [143].

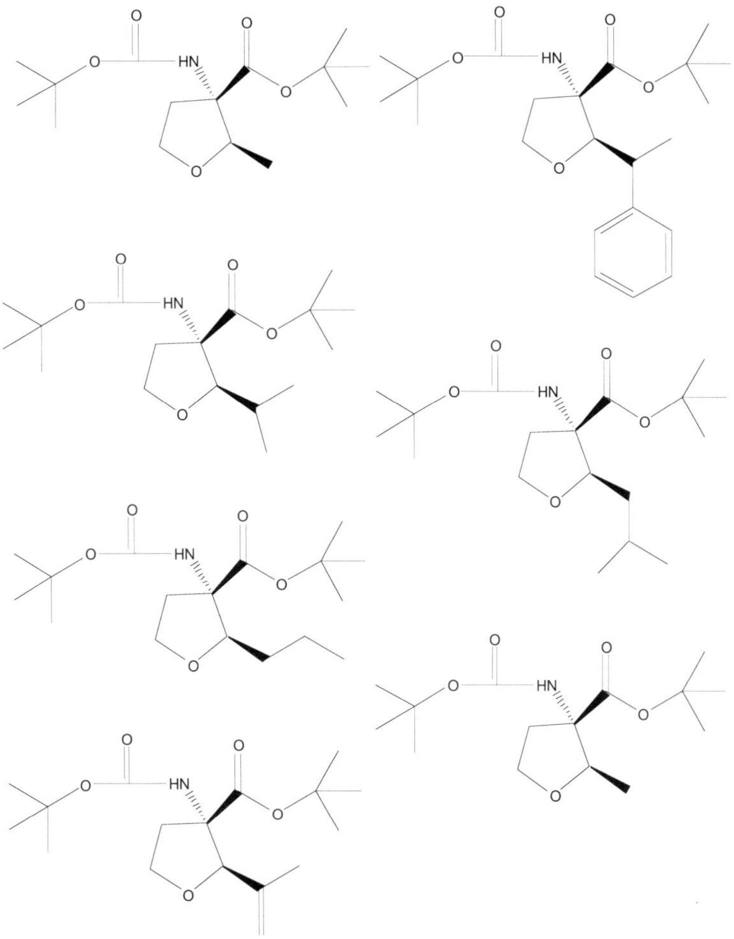

Figure 14: The series of novel C$^{\alpha}$ tetra-substituted α-amino acids reported by Grauer and Konig [141]. to reduce the conformational flexibility of the peptide backbone.

Taira and co-workers reported the synthesis and biological evaluation of three analogs based on multiple repeating units of the amino acid sequence Ac-(Aib-

Lys-Aib-Ala)$_n$-NH_2, where n= 3, 5 and 7 [144]. The CD spectra of peptide BRBA20 Ac-(Aib-Lys-Aib-Ala)$_5$-NH_2) exhibited characteristics associated with helical structures in the presence of both zwiterionic and anionic membrane model systems [144]. The Aib residue is an C^{α}-tetra-substituted α-amino acid (containing two methyl groups on the C^{α} carbon) and appears to be a strong inducer of helical structures [145]. The analogs where n=5 and 7 exhibit antibacterial activity against *E. coli* and *S. aureus*, the analog where n=3 was inactive against bacteria [144].

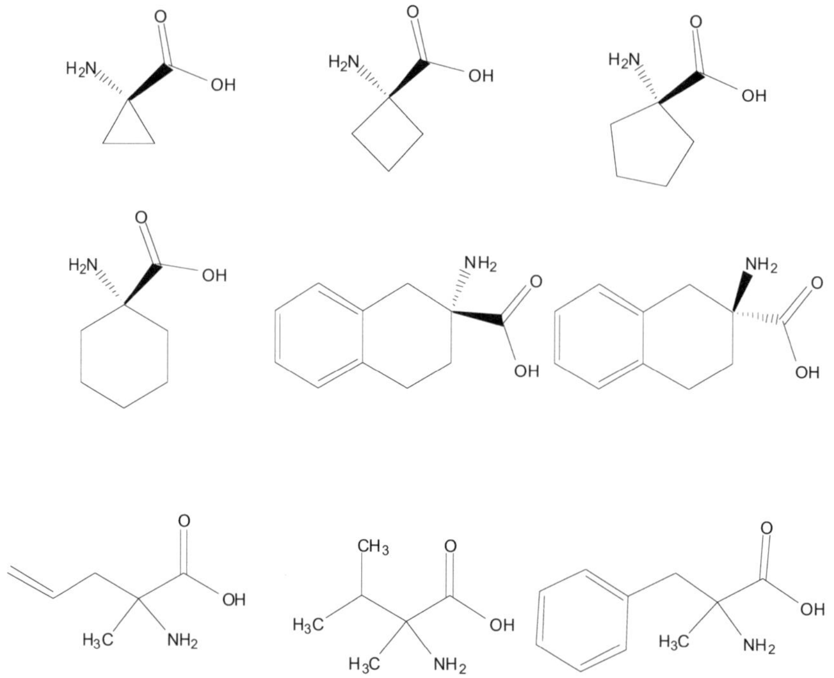

Figure 15: Commercially available C^{α} tetra-substituted α-amino acids.

Sambeth and Sussmuth reported the novel α,α- di-substituted amino acid shown in Fig. **16**. This amino acid was design to aid in the development of novel analogs of labyrinthopeptin A2 [146]. This compound has shown promise as a treatment for neuropathic pain [146]. However, this novel α,α- di-substituted amino acid due to its functionality may also be of interest to chemist designing novel antimicrobial agents.

Application of Unnatural Amino Acids

Incorporation of unnatural amino acids into a peptides primary sequence provides the peptide chemist with a "toolbox" of physicochemical properties that are not available in peptides containing only the 20 naturally occurring RNA encoded amino acids [140, 147-150]. This "toolbox" can be used to facilitate the development of novel peptides with specific physicochemical properties that have the ability to interact with the membranes of bacteria cells in novel ways [151]. Thus providing a methodology for the design of bacteria strain specific AMPs [152]. The application of unnatural amino acids for the development of peptide based drugs is growing in popularity because of the inherent increased metabolic stability [40, 81, 99, 149, 150] of unnatural amino acids as compared to the 20 naturally occurring RNA encoded amino acids. Unnatural amino acids include β-peptides, peptoids, tetra-substituted C^{α} α-amino acids, and backbone extended amino acids such as Gaba, 9-aminooctanoic acid, 10-aminodecanoic acid, 12-aminododecanoic acid and 16-aminopalmitic acid. The research conducted by Vasudev and co-workers [140] on the conformational analysis of backbone expanded amino acids, indicate that they can adopt various stable helical structures as well as stable β-sheets or other turn structures that are not obtainable with the 20 naturally occurring RNA encoded amino acids. Another class of unnatural amino acids is obtained by varying the number of $-CH_2-$ groups in side chains of the basic amino acids from 4 to 1. This modification will reduce the distance (the calculated distance is given in Table **9**) between the positive charge and the peptide backbone resulting in; a) less side chain flexibility during binding, and b) the positive charge density will reside closer to the peptide backbone. The effect of reducing the number of carbon atoms in the side chain on the distribution of the positive charge is shown in Fig. **17** comparing the electrostatic surface potential maps for the tripeptides Ala-X-Ala, where X= the charged residue [153-155]. Changing the number of carbon atoms in the side chain of the basic amino acid residue, also changes the overall hydrophobicity of the residue. The Combined Consensus Scale (CCS) (hydrophobicity) developed by Tossi and co-workers [156] for each residue is given in Table **9**. The natural basic amino acid Lys residue contains a four carbon side chain. The less common Orn residue contains a three carbon side chain while the unnatural basic amino acids Dab and Dpr contain a two carbon and one carbon side chain respectively.

Table 9: Basic Amino Acid Residues

Basic Amino Acid Residue	Number of Carbon Atoms	Distance [a]	CCS [b]
Drp	1	2.56	-9.3
Dab	2	2,98	-9.5
Orn	3	3.55	-9.0
Lys	4	4.76	-9.9

[a]Average distance in angstroms from peptide backbone to the positively charged nitrogen atom as calculated using ChemDraw 3D.
[b]Combined consensus scale hydrophobicity for each charge residue.

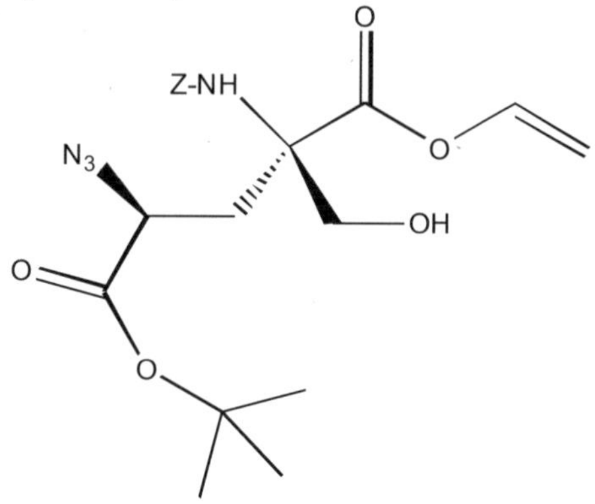

Figure 16: The novel α,α- di-substituted amino acid reported by Sambeth and Sussmuth. This residue has been reported to aid in the development of novel analogs of labyrinthopeptin A2 [146].

Other examples of commercially available unnatural amino acids are given in Fig. **18**.

ANTIMICROBIAL PEPTIDE-BIOFILM INTERACTIONS

Antimicrobial peptides have shown the potential to treat chronic and medical implant biofilm associated infections [157]. Dashper and co-worker reported that kappacin, an anionic AMP, isolated from bovine milk, inhibited the growth of several strains of oral cariogenic bacterial biofilms [158]. The work of Tao and co-workers showed that the AMP pleurocidin also exhibited the ability to inhibit the growth of several strains of oral cariogenic bacterial biofilms [159]. Leung and co-workers reported the highly cationic decapeptide with the amino acid sequence KKVVFKVKFK-NH_2 exhibited significant effects on the viability of mature oral biofilms [160]. Madhuri and co-workers reported that the AMP

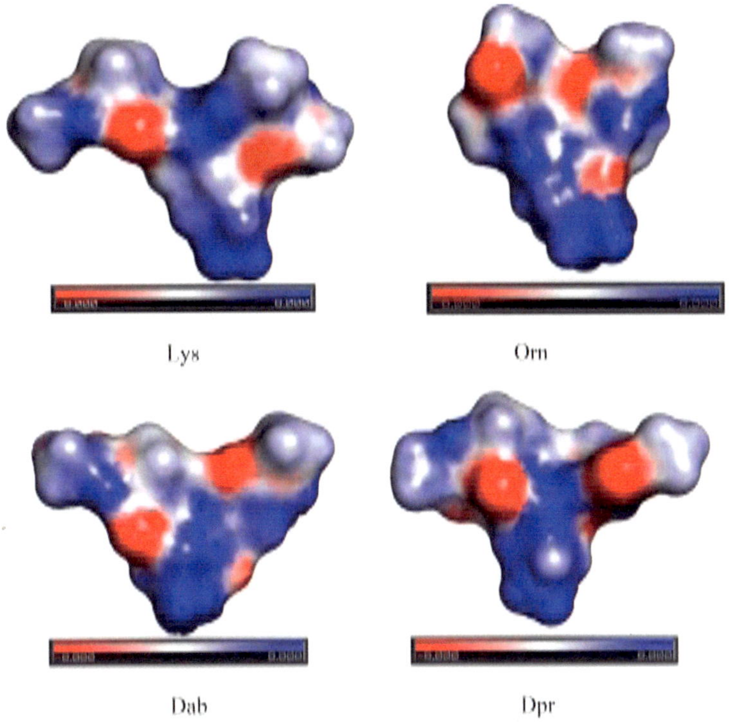

Figure 17: The electrostatic surface potential maps for the tripeptides, Ala-X-Ala, where X = Lys, Orn, Dab and Dpr. Negative electrostatic potential is indicated by a red color, positive electrostatic potential by a blue color. White indicates a neutral electrostatic potential. As the length of the side chains decreases the positive electrostatic potential merges into the peptide backbone indicated by the blue getting closer to the red color of the negative electrostatic potential of the amide bond oxygen [153-155].

α-melanocyte stimulating hormone exhibited antibacterial activity against *Staphylococcus aureus* biofilms [161]. Pompilio and co-workers reported several analogs of cathelicidin derived peptides exhibited activity against either *Pseudomonas aeruginosa* or *Staphylococcus aureus* biofilms, one peptide BMAP-28 exhibited activity against both [162]. Overhage and co-workers reported the human host defense peptide LL-37 inhibited the formation of *Pseudomonas aeruginosa* biofilms [19]. Kapoor and co-workers reported that a series of peptoids, (peptides containing unnatural amino acids and other organic structural subunits) exhibited activity against *Pseudomonas aeruginosa* biofilms [18]. The work of Mai *et al.* has shown that AMPs designed to target specific bacteria such as *Streptococcus mutans* are effective inhibitors of biofilm growth [163].

Flemming and co-workers reported a series synthetic antimicrobial peptidomimetics that exhibited superior antimicrobial activity against *Staphylococcal* biofilms compared to conventional antibiotics [164]. Their results confirm the hypothesis that synthetic antimicrobial peptidomimetics exhibit excellent potential as therapeutic agents for the treatment of biofilm associated bacterial infections [164]. Biofilms have extracellular polymeric substances including proteins and polysaccharides which increase the difficulty of membrane penetration by any antimicrobial agent including AMPs [20, 23, 165-167].

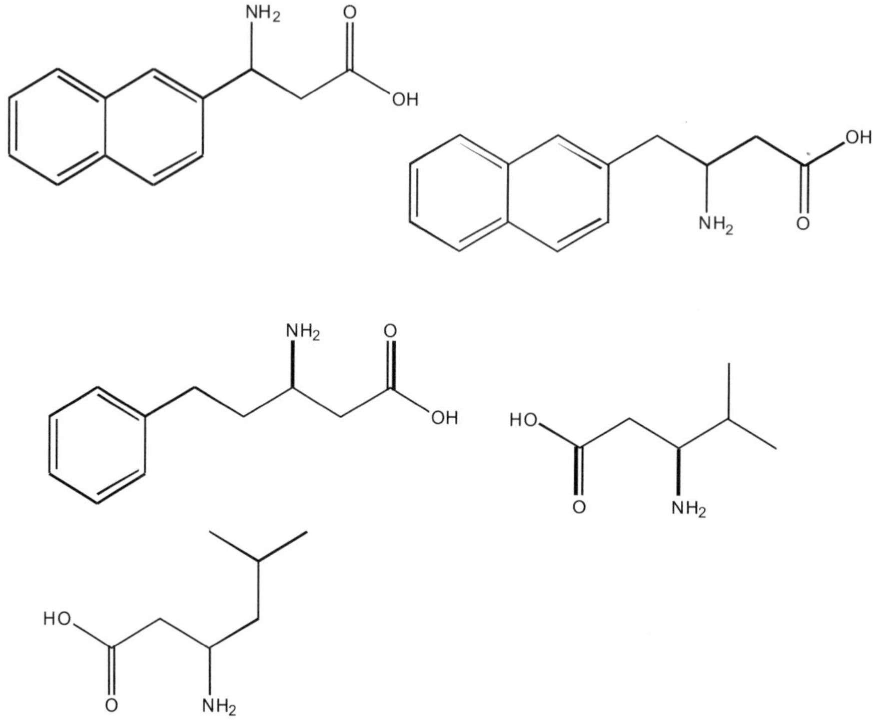

Figure 18: Examples of commercially available unnatural amino acids.

CASE STUDY: DESIGN OF AMPs CONTAINING UNNATURAL AMINO ACIDS

Selection of Model Natural Antimicrobial Peptide

Some AMP may exhibit broad spectrum antibacterial activity while others exhibit a very limited range of activity [43]. The potency and selectivity of an AMP are known to be associated with the physicochemical properties of conformation, net positive charge, and degree of amphipathicity [43, 152]. These factors must therefore be taken into consideration in the design of novel AMPs [152]. The first step in the *de novo* design of selective antimicrobial peptides incorporating unnatural amino acids involves selecting a naturally occurring antimicrobial peptide as a model. In this approach the primary amino acid sequence is not a major focus. However, knowledge of the secondary structure adopted by the peptide upon interacting with a zwitterionic and an anionic micelle or liposome and the resulting physiochemical surface properties is very critical for a successful outcome. It is a difficult process to sit down with a blank sheet of paper and design a series of potent selective antimicrobial peptides without an appropriate three-dimensional physicochemical model as a guide. Thus the starting point for such a design process is either to determine the structure using 2D-NMR and molecular modeling methods to determine the conformations of the SDS and DPC micelle bound antimicrobial peptide in your own laboratory [25] or use similar structural data reported in the literature. From these structures the electrostatic surface potential maps may be developed which provides visualization of the physicochemical properties of the molecule to be modeled [168].

In order to obtain the desired potency and for selectivity prokaryotic over eukaryotic cells it is critical that the peptide interact with zwitterionic and anionic membrane model systems *via* different mechanisms, *i.e.,* they must adopt different conformations upon binding to zwitterionic and anionic membrane models [99, 114, 169, 170]. The physicochemical properties that lead to different mechanisms of binding are not clearly understood [114]. However, factors such as hydrophobicity, structure, electronic charge, hydrophobic moment *etc.* appear to play major roles in defining selectivity [84, 100, 114, 170]. Therefore in this design methodology it is more important to focus on the overall shape of the molecule and the spatial distribution of physicochemical properties, such as charge density and hydrophobicity, than the amino acid composition of the primary amino acid sequence [25, 100].

Due to the molecular complexity and structural diversity of naturally occurring AMPs it is inherently difficult to design analogs with improved therapeutic efficacy [144]. Therefore, *de novo* design has become an established protocol for the systematic development of structure activity relationships to provide insight into physicochemical requirements for antibacterial activity [25, 100, 144, 171, 172].

Hicks and co-workers selected an analog of magainin-2 amide with three Ala replacements, ($Ala^{8,13,18}$) magainin-2 amide, as a model due to its activity against Gram positive and Gram negative bacteria, fungi and protozoa while concurrently exhibiting little mammalian cell toxicity [54]. The magainin family has been extensively investigated and has been characterized as α-helical amphipathic cell-selective membrane-disruptors [71, 82, 173]. For this investigation of ($Ala^{8,13,18}$) magainin-2 amide, DPC micelles [174] were selected as a simple model for zwitterionic lipids and SDS micelles [175] were selected as a simple model for anionic lipids. Two-dimensional NMR and molecular modeling [168] investigations indicated that ($Ala^{8,13,18}$)magainin-2 amide bound to DPC micelles adopts an α-helical structure involving residues 2 to 16 with the four C-terminal residues converging to a loose β-turn like structure, while ($Ala^{8,13,18}$) magainin-2 amide bound to SDS micelles adopts an α-helical structure involving residues 7 to 18 with the C- and N-terminal residues exhibiting a great deal of conformational flexibility. The most plausible explanation for ($Ala^{8,13,18}$) magainin-2 amide adopting different conformations on binding with SDS and DPC micelles is that different non-covalent (electrostatic and hydrophobic) interactions which are occurring between the surface of the peptide and the two micelle surfaces [168]. The observation of different binding conformations upon interaction with anionic and zwitterionic micelles and or liposomes is critical for the development of a cell-selective AMP [168, 169]. Using the NMR determined SDS and DPC micelle bound conformations of ($Ala^{8,13,18}$) magainin-2 amide, the electrostatic surface potential maps for these conformers were calculated indicating that the surface electron density of these peptides are very different and conformationally dependent [168].

The AMPs developed in this study incorporate three dipeptide units consisting of the conformationally restrained amino acids Tic (Tetrahydroisoquinoline-carboxylic acid) and Oic (Octahydroindolecarboxylic acid) into the peptides primary sequence. These dipeptide units induce regions of reduced flexibility into the peptide backbone and thus reducing the total conformational flexibility of the peptide during lipid binding. The basic skeleton of the Tic-Oic dipeptide based

AMP developed in our laboratory is given in Fig. **19**. Spacer #1, defines the distance between two Tic-Oic dipeptides units with either a hydrophobic residue or a charged residue (also called Spacer #2). Spacer #1 also plays a major role in characterizing the flexibility of any induced turn or helical structure by defining the intramolecule hydrogen bonding schemes available to the peptide backbone.

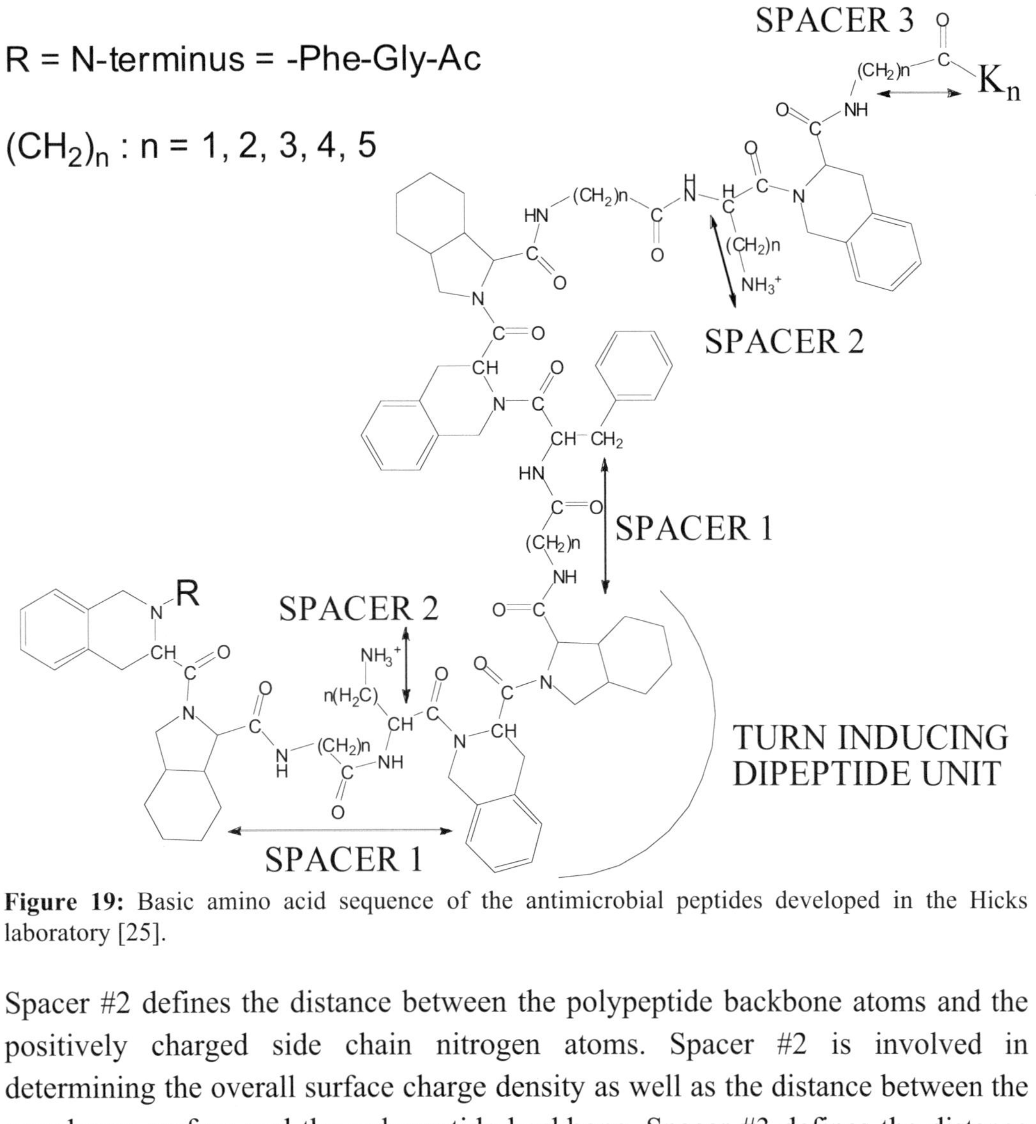

Figure 19: Basic amino acid sequence of the antimicrobial peptides developed in the Hicks laboratory [25].

Spacer #2 defines the distance between the polypeptide backbone atoms and the positively charged side chain nitrogen atoms. Spacer #2 is involved in determining the overall surface charge density as well as the distance between the membrane surface and the polypeptide backbone. Spacer #3 defines the distance between the last Tic residue and the cluster of Lys residues located at the C-terminus of the peptide. Spacer #3 is involved in providing additional conformational flexibility on surface binding. Over 80 analogs were synthesized and evaluated for biological activity against a variety of bacterial strains including; *Bacillus anthracis* AMES, *Francisella tularensis*, *Yersinia pestis*, *Brucella melitensis, Brucella abortus*, *Brucella suis*, *Acinetobacter baumanii, Staphylococcus aureus -(MRSA) Salmonella, typhimurium, Staphylococcus aureus* - Methicillin / Gentamicin / Tetracycline Resistant, *Bacillus subtillis,* and *Mycobacterium ranae,* at least one analog exhibited *in vitro* activity against each of these bacteria strain at a concentration of < 20 μM [25, 151, 176]. Many of these AMPs also exhibited very low *in vitro* hemolytic activity as well as a relatively high maximum tolerated dose in mice of 125 mg/kg [25]. These AMPs also exhibited excellent metabolic stability in pooled human liver microsomes for up to 60 minutes (unpublished results).

Studies have shown that the length of Spacer #1 defines how these AMPs interact with specific membrane models and thus defines organism selectivity and potency [169, 177]. The length of Spacer #2 plays a major role in defining how these compounds interact with membranes and thus their resulting biological activity. These peptides interact with anionic and zwitterionic membrane models *via* different mechanisms. From a therapeutic perspective, it is a critical observation that indicates it may be possible to obtain selectivity for bacterial cells *versus* mammalian cells. The properties of Spacer #2, (flexibility, charge density, hydrophobicity) seem to define organism selectivity and potency [178]. The effect of reducing the number of carbon atoms in the side chain of Spacer #2 on the electrostatic surface potential is shown in Fig. **17**. The effect of the changes in the electrostatic surface potential on antibacterial activity is highlighted with the activity against *B. anthracis* AMES, *S. aureus* (MRSA) and *Y. pestis.* The hydrophobicity of the Spacer #2, seems to play a major role in defining antibacterial activity against selected strains of Gram negative bacteria [178]. It has been demonstrated that the total number of positively charged residues located at the C-terminus of these AMPs has an effect on the observed organism selectivity and potency [179]. Also relocating the positive charge cluster from the C-terminus to the N-terminus plays a role in defining organism selectivity and potency [179]. Spacer #3 has been demonstrated to have little effect on the antibacterial activity, however it has a dramatic effect on metabolic stability in pooled liver microsomes [151]. A representative sample of the peptides synthesized by Hicks and co-workers is shown in Table **10** with their corresponding *in vitro* minimum inhibitory concentrations against select bacterial strains are given in Table **11** [151].

Table 10: Representative Amino Acid Sequences for the AMP Developed by HICKS and Co-Workers [15]

Comp #	Amino Acid Sequence
23	Ac-GF-Tic-Oic-GK-Tic-Oic-GF-Tic-Oic-GK-Tic-KKKK-CONH$_2$
29	Ac-Gaba-F-Tic-Oic-Gaba-K-Tic-Oic-Gaba-F-Tic-Oic-Gaba-K-Tic-KKKK-CONH$_2$
35	Ac-GF-F-Oic-GK-F-Oic-GF-F-Oic-GK-F-KKKK-CONH$_2$
36	Ac-βAla-F-Tic-Oic-βAla-K-Tic-Oic-βAla-F-Tic-Oic-βAla-K-Tic-KKKK-CONH$_2$
37	Ac-Ahx-F-Tic-Oic-Ahx-K-Tic-Oic-Ahx-F-Tic-Oic-Ahx-K-Tic-KKKK-CONH$_2$
38	Ac-F-Tic-Oic-K-Tic-Oic-F-Tic-Oic-K-Tic-KKKKKK-CONH$_2$
40	Ac-Gaba-F-Tic-Oic-Gaba-K-Tic-Oic-Gaba-F-Tic-Oic-Gaba-K-Tic-KKKKK-CONH$_2$
41	Ac-GF-Tic-Oic-GK-Tic-Oic-GF-Tic-Oic-GK-Tic-Orn-Orn-Orn-Orn-CONH$_2$
42	Ac-G-Fpa-Tic-Oic-GK-Tic-Oic-G-Fpa-Tic-Oic-GK-Tic-KKKK-CONH$_2$
43	Ac-GF-Tic-Oic-G-Orn-Tic-Oic-GF-Tic-Oic-G-Orn-Tic-Orn-Orn-Orn-Orn-CONH$_2$
45	Ac-GF-Tic-Oic-G-Dpr-Tic-Oic-GF-Tic-Oic-G-Dpr-Tic-Dpr-DprDpr-Dpr-CONH$_2$
46	Ac-βAla-Fpa-Tic-Oic-βAla-Dpr-Tic-Oic-βAla-Fpa-Tic-Oic–βAla-Dpr-Tic-Dpr-Dpr-Dpr-Dpr-CONH$_2$
50	Ac-GF-Tic-Oic-GK-Tic-Oic-GF-Tic-Oic-GK-Tic-βA-KKKK-CONH$_2$
52	Ac-GF-Tic-Oic-GK-Tic-Oic-GF-Tic-Oic-GK-Tic-Ahx-KKKK-CONH$_2$
53	Ac-GF-Tic-Oic-G-Dab-Tic-Oic-GF-Tic-Oic-G-Dab-Tic-Dab-Dab-Dab-Dab-CONH$_2$
56	Ac-GF-Tic-Oic-GR-Tic-Oic-GF-Tic-Oic-GR-Tic-RRRR-CONH$_2$
61	Ac-KKKK-GF-Tic-Oic-GK-Tic-Oic-GF-Tic-Oic-GK-Tic-CONH$_2$
62	Ac-GF-Oic-Oic-GK-Oic-Oic-GF-Oic-Oic-GK-Tic-KKKK-CONH$_2$
64	Ac-GF-Tic-Oic-GK-Tic-Oic-GF-Tic-Oic-GK-Tic-KKK-CONH$_2$

Small structural changes in an amino acid residue can lead to major differences in the observed biological activity of the resulting AMP. The difference between a Tic residue and a Phe residue is only one methylene group as shown in Fig. **20**. However it can result in a dramatic difference in biological activity as seen by the comparison of compounds **23** containing the Tic-Oic dipeptide and compound **35** which contains the Phe-Oic dipeptide. Compound **35** is several orders of magnitude more active (compared to compound **23**) against *Y. pesti, Brucella* *abortus, Brucella suis, B. anthracis,* and *Francisella tularensis* while being equally potent against *A. baumanii, S. aureus (MRSA), Burkholderia mallei,* and *Burkholderia pseudomallei.* A closer examination of the two amino acids reveals several major differences. First the additional methylene group of the Tic residue forms a bicyclic ring which is conformationally restrained and has greater steric bulk this is shown in Fig. **21**. The electrostatic surface potentials of both the Phe residue and the Tic residue incorporated into the tripeptides Ala-X-Ala are shown

Table 11: ***In Vitro*** **Activity MIC Activity (μM) Against Specific Bacterial Strains for the Compounds Synthesized by Hicks and Co-Workers [151]**

Comp #	*A. baumanii* ATCC 19606	*S. aureus* ATCC 33591 (MRSA)	*Y. pestis* CO92	*Brucella abortus* 2308	*Brucella suis* ATCC 23445	*B. anthracis* AMES	*Francisella tularensis* SCHU-S4	*Burkholderia mallei* ATCC 23444	*Burkholderia pseudomallei* BURK003 (1026b)
23	3.2	205	205	205	205	12.8	100	205	205
29	3.1	196	196	196	196	12.5	196	196	196
35	3.2	208	3.2	26.00	26.00	0.2	0.01	208	208
36	1.5	200	200	200	200	25	100	200	200
37	5.90	187	23.40	12	47	1.50	23.4	187	187
38	6.30	25.30	101	101	13.00	0.75	202	202	202
40	5.80	46.60	46.60	>186	93	0.71	186	186	186
41	6.50	52.40	26.20	209	13.00	0.81	104.80	209	209
42	3.10	101	202	202	202	12.60	202	202	202
43	6.60	53.00	26.50	106	106	0.82	106	212	212
45	3.60	114	228	228	228	14.80	228	228	228
46	3.40	109	219	219	219	6.80	219	219	219
50	6.20	199	199	199	199	12.40	199	199	199
52	3.00	196	48.90	196	196	48.90	196	196	196
53	3.40	220	220	220	220	6.80	220	220	220
56	5.98	96	192	192	192	5.98	192	192	192
61	12.80	102	13.10	51	25.60	0.40	51	204	204
62	3.20	207	207	207	207	26.00	104	207	207
64	6.70	54	27.00	27.00	>216	27.00	0.02	0.02	0.02

in Fig. **21** [153-155]. Clearly the conformational rigidity of the Tic residue isolates the negative electrostatic potential of the aromatic ring of the phenyl group more than that observed with the Phe residue and makes it more accessible to interact with the surface of the cell membrane.

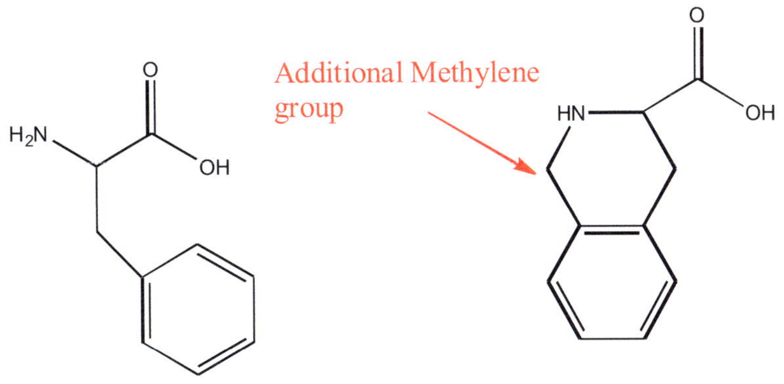

Phe Tic

Figure 20: Chemical structures for the amino acid residues Phe and Tic.

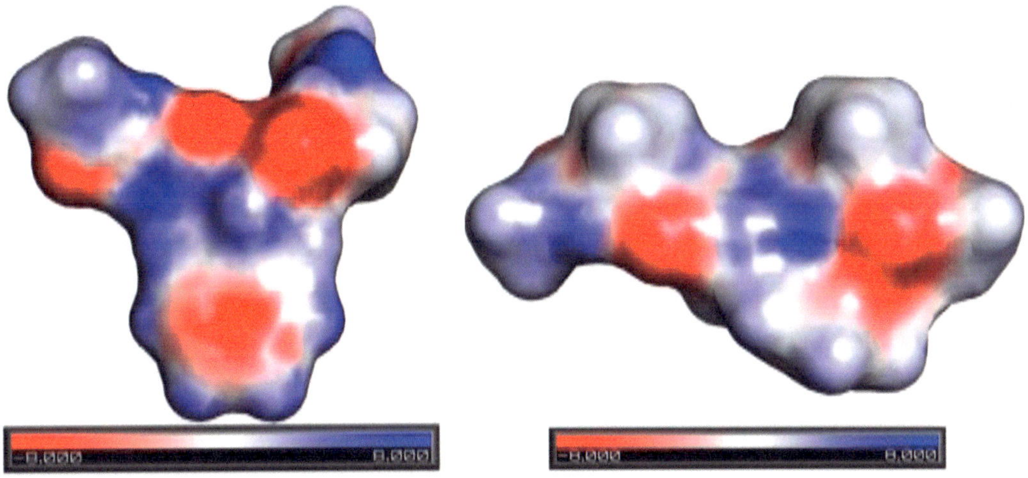

Tic Phe

Figure 21: The electrostatic surface potential maps for the tripeptides, Ala-Tic-Ala and Ala-Phe-Ala. Negative electrostatic potential is indicated by a red color, positive electrostatic potential by a blue color. White indicates a neutral electrostatic potential. The negative electrostatic potential of the aromatic ring of the Tic residue is more isolated than in the aromatic ring of the Phe residue [153-155].

The secondary amino acid residue Pro is known to play an important role in defining peptide secondary structure. The amino acid residue Oic is a bicyclic derivative of Pro obtained by the addition of four methylene units to form a second six membered ring. As seen in Fig. **22** which shows the electrostatic surface potentials for the tripeptides Ala-Pro-Ala and Ala-Oic-Ala the second ring adds steric bulk to the system and increases the hydrophobicity as well. As can be seen from Fig. **22** [153-155], the Oic residue presents a different surface to the membrane than does the Pro residue.

ANTIFUNGAL PEPTIDES

The need for new antifungal compounds has expanded with the number of immune-compromised patients such as those infected with AIDS, undergoing cancer treatment, and organ transplant recipients. These patients are at particularly high risk for fungal infections. Clinically relevant fungal species include but are not limited to: *Candida albicans* [180-186], *Fusarium solani*, *Saccharomyces cerevisiae* [183, 187], *Trichosporon beigelii* [182, 185], *Aspergillus fumigantus* [180, 183, 185, 186, 188], *Aspergillus nidulans* [183, 186], *Aspergillus flavus* [183, 186], *Cryptococcus neoformans* [180, 183-185, 189], *Fusarium solanij* [181, 183], *Scedosporium prolificans* [188], and *Pneumocystis carinii* [183]. Developing new antifungal therapies against these and other fungi is critical to improving the clinical outcomes for at risk patients. Given the need of new selective antimicrobial compounds that exhibit activity against multiple drug resistant organisms, antimicrobial peptides, specifically antifungal peptides (AFP), have the potential to be developed into therapeutically useful agents. Many of the naturally occurring peptides that have been identified as having antibacterial properties also have demonstrated *in vitro* antifungal activity. Antifungal peptides have been isolated from mammals, insects, amphibians, bacteria, and other fungi [180].

The limited collection of antifungal compounds presently available is wrought with dose limiting side effects associated with poor selectivity for fungal over mammalian cells. It is hypothesized that AFPs through their membrane disrupting properties improve cell permeability through the formation of pores or the inactivation of drug-efflux pumps [190].

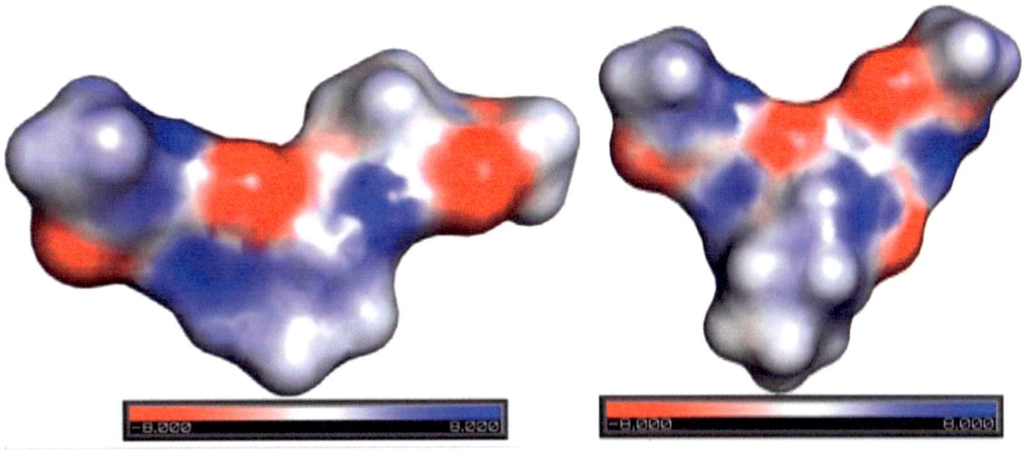

Pro Oic

Figure 22: The electrostatic surface potential maps for the tripeptides, Ala-Pro-Ala and Ala-Oic-Ala. Negative electrostatic potential is indicated by a red color, positive electrostatic potential by a blue color. White indicates a neutral electrostatic potential [153-155].

The majority of current antimycotics available for therapeutic use can be divided into four classes: azoles, polyenes (including those attached to lipids), echinocandins and peptidomimetics/AFPs [191]. Azoles function through the inhibition of an enzyme involved in ergosterol synthesis, a membrane component of fungal cell walls, which results in growth inhibition [192] (see Fig. **5B**). Polyenes interact with ergosterol specifically which results in membrane disruption leading to lysis and cell death [192]. Enchinocandins inhibit the synthesis of the glucan subunits by inhibiting the synthase enzyme [192]. Glucan is one of the essential subunits of the fungal cell wall (see Fig. **5B**) [193]. Despite the small molecule compounds available the development of resistance, toxicity, and the limited activity continue to restrict the utility of these molecules [191]. While most of the available antifungal compounds target the ergosterol of the fungal membrane there are a few drugs which use other mechanisms of action, primarily targeting intracellular organelles inhibiting the replication of the fungi [192].

While the latest generations of these small molecule drugs have improved activity many are fungistatic and not fungicidal against infectious fungi [183]. Additionally, the ease with which infectious fungi develop resistance and the toxic side effects limits the utility of the drugs available. Naturally occurring AFPs are able to provide a strong template for the development of novel antimycotics with a wide spectrum of antimicrobial activity with acceptable toxicity to the host organism [183]. The next few pages will discuss some of the design factors which have improved activity and selectivity, limited toxicity, and increased the overall therapeutic potential of AFPs.

FEATURES ASSOCIATED WITH ACTIVITY

Evidence suggests that the antifungal activity exhibited by AFPs is multifactorial without a single structural feature directly linked to antimycotic activity [183]. Here we will mention many of the factors which have demonstrated effect upon the activity of any given AFP. The diversity of fungi makes generalizations regarding activity difficult to compare and contrast. This is thus a limited perspective of structural features.

SEQUENCE

The amino acids contained in the AFP's primary sequence plays an important role in defining the activity of the peptide. Some of the standard amino acids associated with AFP activity include histidine, tryptophan, lysine, cysteine, arganine, serine, and proline amongst standard amino acids [181, 182, 186, 190, 194-196]. Attempts at developing peptidomimetics modeled from naturally occurring AFPs have primarily focused on manipulation of the peptide through the enrichment of the amino acid sequence with one or two selected residues such as histidine or lysine (see above mentioned residues which have been the target of such mutations) [194, 196]. Most AFPs presently known can be characterized based upon their amino acid composition. Typically they are composed of between 8 and 100 amino acids with weights between 5 and 4244 kDa [195]. Many of the naturally occurring AFPs are rather long in length resulting in limited commercial viability is limited by synthetic costs. Thus, the design of new AFPs should focus on peptides composed of 20 or fewer amino acids. Toward that end, investigations to identify smaller subunits of naturally occurring peptides responsible for antifungal activity are ongoing, followed by studies to improve activity [181, 189].

The lack of selectivity associated with D- and L-amino acids present in AMPs toward both human and other microbial organisms, suggests the stereospecificity of the AMPs does not play a role in their activity suggesting a lack of microbial receptors included in the mechanism of activity [47]. Given the diversity of structure AFPs and the lack of a specific receptor target, these peptides are amenable to incorporating nonstandard and unnatural amino acids to improve activity, protect from enzymatic breakdown, limit allergic potential, and improve their therapeutic potential.

AMPHIPATHICITY

Researchers have noted that those AMPs with predominantly antifungal activity tend to have amino acid sequences rich in polar neutral amino acids such as asparagine, cysteine, serine, and glutamine [47]. Scientists, having noted the structural properties associated with AFP activity have altered structural sequences in an effort to improve activity and selectivity with great success as evidenced by *in vitro* activity [181, 189, 196].

Much like the structural features associated with antibacterial activity, antifungal activity has been observed to benefit from the amphipathic nature of peptides by improving membrane peptide interaction. An increase in antimicrobial activity has been produced through greater hydrophobicity in the peptide sequence which has been accomplished through the substitution with hydrophobic amino acids leucine (L) and isoleucine (I) in some instances [181]. Incorporating nonstandard amino acids may provide an entirely new collection of AFPs to be developed into clinically useful drugs.

The charge associated with antifungal peptides has also been shown to affect the activity of the peptides. The net positive charge of the peptides enables binding to the negatively charged membranes of fungi mediated through electrostatic effects [181]. While much of the research has focused upon the cationic regions of an AFP, recent studies have demonstrated that the anionic charge also plays a critical role in antimycotic activity [187, 197]. Investigation into the functional role of charged residues within the naturally occurring AFP drosomycin has been undertaken. Drosomycin was originally isolated from *Drosophila melanogaster* and has the following peptide sequence: **D**CLSG**RYK**GPCAVWDNETC**RR** VCK**E**EGRSSGHCSPSL**K**CWCEGC.

Those residues identified to play a critical role in AFP activity have been noted with bold typeface, cationic residues are colored green while anionic residues are noted in cyan [187]. Looking at the electrostatic surface potential map (generated inn our laboratory) the amphipathic nature of the peptide is apparent (Fig. **23**). The electronegative residues are colored red while the electropositive residues are noted in blue, neutral regions are white. It is evident that one end of the peptide (the northern side relative to the paper) displays predominantly electronegative residues while the electropositive residues are more distributed in clusters throughout the remainder of the peptide.

Looking at the residues found to be requisite for *in vitro* activity (Fig. **23B**) [153-155] with the drosomycin peptide the cationic residues noted in green are well distributed across the peptide without having a large single concentration of charge aggregated together within the sequence. Additionally, the anionic residues noted in cyan (Fig. **23B**) are required for AFP activity demonstrating it isn't just the cationic charge necessary for activity; the amphiphatic nature of the peptide is the initial driving force between the peptide and the electrostatic surface of the membrane surface.

DEGREE OF STRUCTURE FORMATION

Much like the secondary structure associated with antibacterial activity, anti-fungal activity is also closely correlated with peptide conformation and the secondary structure adopted by the peptide plays a critical role in the interaction with the target membrane [86, 181, 184, 189]. While many peptides lack a well-defined structure in solution the electrostatic effect of polar molecules (either polar solvent in *in vitro* experiments, a model membrane, or cell membranes) can precipitate more formal secondary structure development.

Common structures associated with AFP activity include α - helix, β -turn and random coils (Fig. **24**) [86, 181, 182, 184, 189]. Analysis of the structures found

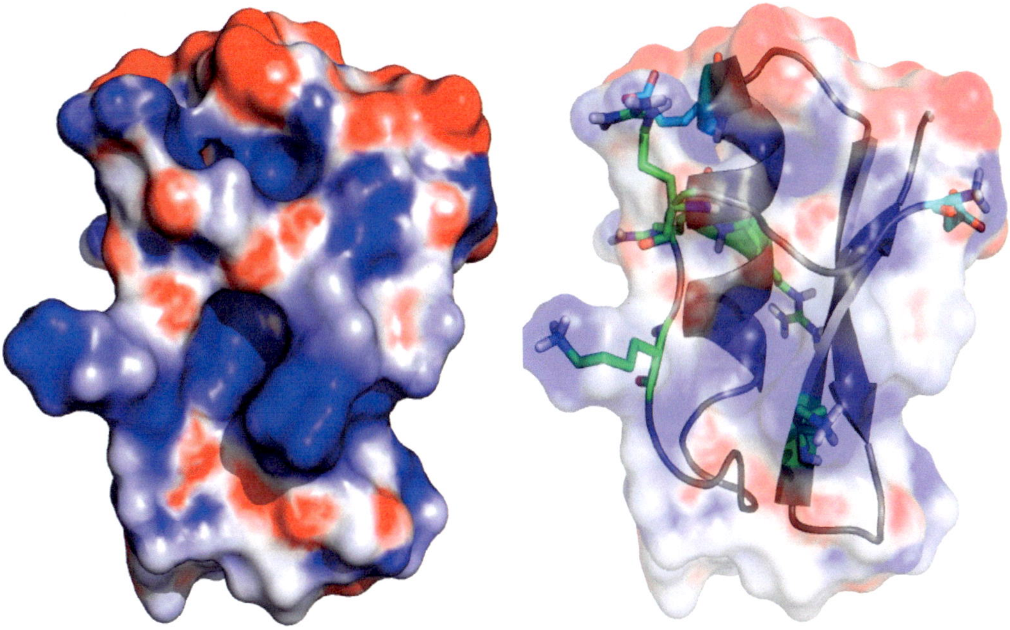

Figure 23: Drosomycin (PDB: 1MYN) with the electrostatic surface potential. Cationic residues are noted in green and anionic residues are noted in cyan (**A**) on Left shows the electrostatic surface only, (**B**) on Right shows the ribbon structure of the peptide under the electrostatic surface potential.

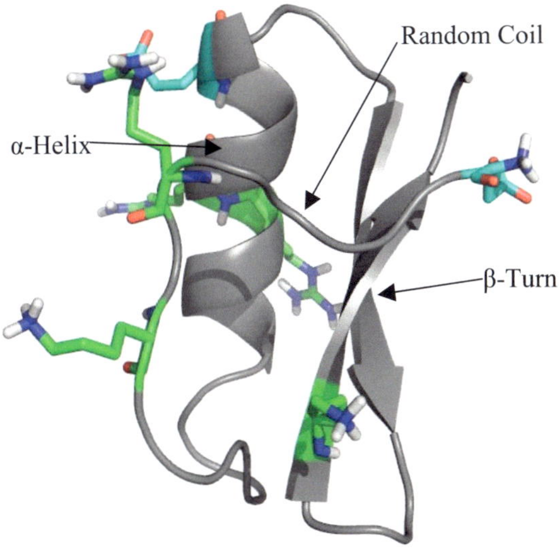

Figure 24: Drosomycin (PDB: 1MYN) cartoon highlighting the cationic (green) and anionic (cyan) residues. Drosomycin has a mixed secondary structure depicted as beta sheet, random coil or alpha helix.

in antifungal peptides present in the literature have concluded AFPs are predominantly random coils with α- helical shape being the second most common structure [47, 186]. The alpha helical structure is usually adopted by linear cationic AFPs when placed in a hydrophobic environment while the β -sheet typically results from the formation of disulfide bonds with cysteine residues [183]. The secondary structure adopted by AFPs extends beyond the traditional linear peptides to include circular modifications in an effort to avoid proteolysis [184, 189, 195, 196]. The specificity of the peptides to their cellular targets suggests the secondary structure of the peptide is a contributing factor attributed to AFP organism specificity at the cellular level. The amphipathic nature of the peptide having a polar hydrophilic portion of the folded peptide as well as a hydrophobic portion able to partition into the membrane improve activity profiles. The orientation of the peptide relative to the membrane is expected to be diverse; however, the electrostatic attraction between peptide and membrane encourage close proximity between the two. The polar face of the peptide is able to interact with the polar head groups of the membrane while the movement associated with the lipids interacting with the membrane may allow the incorporation of the hydrophobic face of the peptide into the hydrophobic region of the bilayer (Fig. **25**)

MECHANISM OF ACTION

The association between the AFP and the membrane surface is critical much like the association with bacterial membranes. Given the diversity of AFPs as one would expect there are several mechanisms through which they exert their antifungal activity. While the mechanism of action at the atomic level has been poorly defined beyond the three mechanisms: barrel & stave, torroidal pore, and carpet (Fig. **1**), customarily associated with AMP activity several groups have undertaken additional groupings based upon the method of membrane disruption.

AFPs which are selective must target the unique properties of the fungal membrane while avoiding the mammalian membrane to avoid toxicity. One aspect of the fungal membrane which distinguishes it from the mammalian membrane is the inclusion of chitin, a polysaccharide which is the structural component found in the cell walls of the fungi and other organisms (insects and arthropods). Several hundred repeating units of glucosamine and acetylglucosamine comprise this portion of the membrane (Fig. **26**) [198]. There are other aspects of the cell membranes which distinguish the fungal from the mammalian membrane such as the mannoproteins and the slight difference between cholesterol and the ergosterol of the fungi [185].

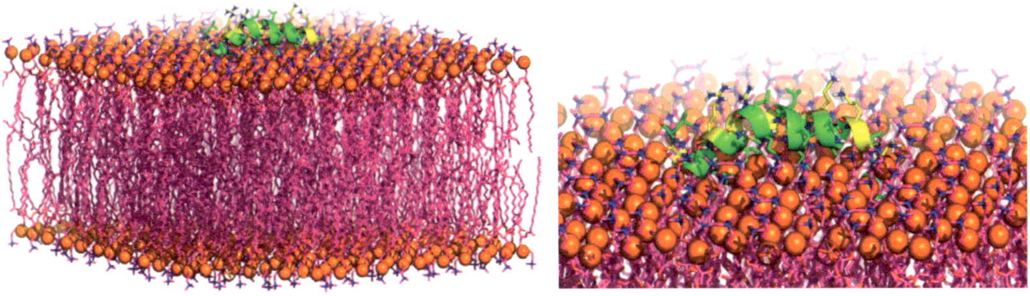

Figure 25: Zwitterionic membrane of POPC lipids with the antifungal peptide spinigerin (PDBID: 1ZRV) Polar residues are noted with yellow carbon atoms.

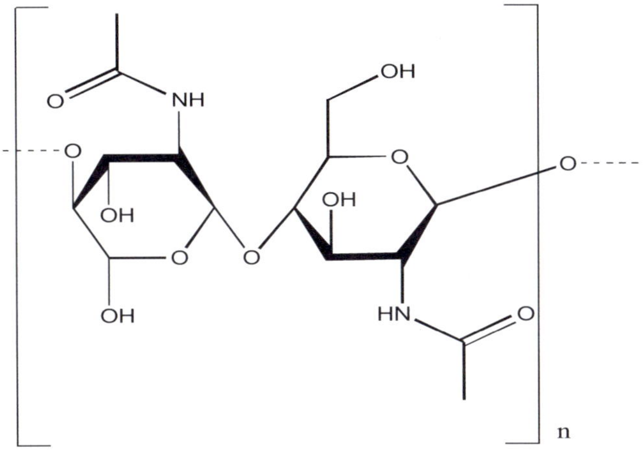

Figure 26: Glucosamine and acetylglucosamine repeat several hundred times to create the fungal cell wall structural component chitin [198].

A strong case can be made for the importance of electrostatic interactions occurring between an AFP and the membrane surface, peptides have been identified which do not appear to function through this mechanism [47]. Many AFPs have been identified as having cell lysis be the primary mode of action through which they exert their antimycotic activity. Additionally, using AFPs to destabilize the fungal membrane makes them great candidates to be an adjuvant to some of the already available antifungal small molecules [180, 183, 189]. The disruption of the membrane surface allows better permeability of drug to the small molecule intercellular target allowing for a lower, less toxic dose of drugs which may be prohibitively toxic at therapeutic doses when administered alone.

One of the new antimycotic compounds is sordarin (Fig. **27**) and its derivatives. Sordarin is unique because it is one of the only compounds which specifically target protein synthesis a challenging target due to the large overlap with mammalian synthase [185]. Blocking translation elongation factor 2 which is specific to fungi provides selective targeting of infectious cells over those of the host [185]. Presently derivatives of this compound are still in *in vitro* testing with high hopes of reaching the clinic in the future [199].

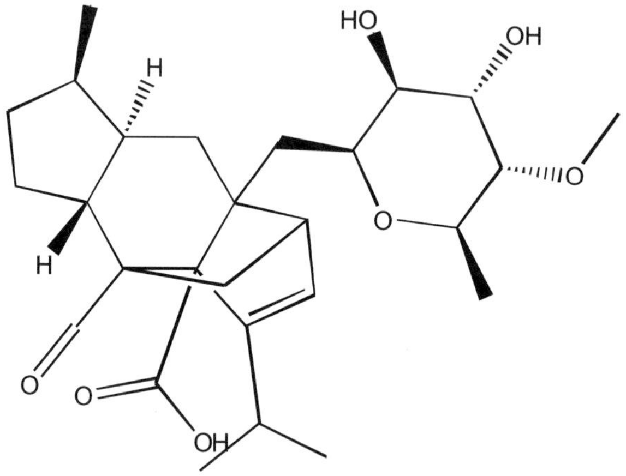

Figure 27: Sordarin a small antimycotic which acts by targeting fungal protein synthesis enzymes [185].

CLINICAL UTILITY OF AFPs

Despite the rather modest activity profiles of naturally occurring AFPs they may still have clinical utility. Numerous studies have demonstrated a synergistic effect upon systemic treatment with the AFPs in addition to some of the traditional small molecule antifungal agents [180, 183, 185]. AFPs are able to provide better toxicity profiles relative to the traditional small molecules used for the treatment of systemic fungal infections. The toxicity is often determined based upon an

AFP's ability to lyse human red blood cells (RBC) and inhibit the proliferation of human keratinocytes [181].

Despite the shrinking collection of antimycotic drugs, which retain their activity despite the constantly evolving fungi with multi-drug resistance, relatively modest effort has been expended toward further therapeutic development. The challenges of poor selectivity and the resulting toxicity continue to plague the small molecule efforts toward antifungal development paving the way for AFP commercialization. AFPs are not without their own limitations. Poor oral availability, potential for proteolytic cleavage along with the expense of synthesis and storage has limited the commercial viability of these biologic therapies. Incorporating nonstandard and unnatural amino acids into the peptide sequences could offer improved selectivity and help avoid the *in vivo* proteolysis improving bioavailability [184].

METHODS

Preliminary Evaluation

Once the peptide(s) have been synthesized and purified their potential as antimicrobial peptides must be evaluated. The *in vitro* screening against several strains of microbes is final validation of the antimicrobial activity of the new compounds. However, in most chemical research laboratories these assays are not readily available. Therefore samples must be submitted to commercial research organizations or collaborators for biological evaluation. This process can take 4-6 weeks to obtain results and depending on the number of peptides and assays to be tested, this can prove to be a relatively expensive and labor intensive operation. Therefore, the use of CD spectroscopy and calcein leakage studies as a first evaluation of new peptides should be considered. If the CD spectra of the peptides do not exhibit different conformations in membrane model systems than they do in buffer, it is most likely that they are not interacting with the membrane models, and therefore, it is unlikely they will interact with the membrane of a microbe. This indicates that the peptide is most likely biologically inactive [151, 152, 169, 177, 178]. The results from the calcein leakage assays are critical in determining if the peptide has the potential to disrupt a cell membrane and to induce cell lysis

[151, 177, 200]. Failure to induce calcein leakage, however, does not mean that the peptide will exhibit no antimicrobial activity, but rather that any observed *in vitro* activity is derived as a result of interacting with an intracellular target.

As pointed out by several researchers in order to develop AMPs as potential therapeutic agents it is critical to develop an understanding of the basis for the different interactions that occur between the AMP and zwitterionic and anionic lipids [40, 201, 202]. To accomplish this goal a combination of CD spectroscopy, Isothermal Titration Calorimetry (ITC) and induced calcein fluorescence leakage experiments maybe employed to investigate the binding interactions these new peptides experience with models of the membranes of mammalian and bacterial cells. Large unilamellar vesicles (LUVs) and Small unilamellar vesicles (SUVs) consisting of 1-Palmitoyl-2-Oleoyl-*sn*-Glycero-3-Phosphocholine (POPC) are often used as a simple model for the zwitterionic membranes of mammalian cells and membrane models consisting of (4:1 or 3:1) 1-Palmitoyl-2-Oleoyl-*sn*-Glycero-3-Phosphocholine (POPC) / **1**-Palmitoyl-2-Oleoyl-*sn*-Glycero-3-[Phospho-*rac*-(1-glycerol)] (Sodium Salt)) (POPG) are often used as a simple model for the anionic membranes of bacteria cells [203]. LUVs are selected instead of SUVs for calcein leakage and ITC studies because they are considered to be more closely related to biological membranes as they are not subject to the increased curvature stress associated with SUVs [204, 205], which as a result, decreases the stability of SUVs [205-207]. Understanding what physicochemical properties differentiate between binding with zwitterionic and anionic LUVs is critical in the development of these compounds as organism selective antibacterial drugs. In addition, often the interactions that occur between the peptide and anionic (SDS) and zwitterionic (DPC) micelles are investigated to isolate the surface binding interaction of these peptides from the aggregation and pore forming interactions that occur when binding to lipids. Also if NMR investigations are to be considered micelles are the model system of choice.

The first step of the binding process is the attraction of the positively charged AMP to the proximity of the surface of the negatively charged membrane by electrostatic interactions, therefore increasing the local concentration of the AMP near the surface of the membrane relative to the bulk solution [82, 204, 208]. The second major step in the process is thought to be actual binding of the AMP to the surface of the membrane [52, 209]. During the binding step the AMP will initially orient itself such that its long axis is parallel to the surface of the membrane. With the AMP localized near the polar head groups of the lipids, their hydrophobic side chains may insert into the hydrophobic core of the lipid bilayer. This state is commonly referred to as the S-state (surface bound state) [52, 209]. The work of Huang and co-workers has shown that the S-state binding leads to a thinning of the membrane and once a "critical peptide to lipid ratio" [210, 211] is reached membrane disruption and pore formation is initiated [210-212]. At this critical concentration the AMPs are believed to self assemble to form complexes of 4-6 AMPs [52, 209]. These oligomeric complexes [210] are thought to then insert into the hydrophobic core so that the long axis of the peptide is now oriented perpendicular to the membrane surface and the peptide is now in the I-state (inserted state) [52, 209]. This reorientation may be driven either entropically by the hydrophobic effect or enthalpically by Van-der-Waals Forces [213].

Preparation of POPC and POPC/POPG SUVs

LUVs or SUVs comprised of POPC were selected as a simple zwitterionic bilayer models whereas LUVs or SUVs consisting of 4:1 POPC/POPG were selected as a simple anionic bilayer models [203]. LUVs were selected instead of SUVs for calcein leakage and ITC studies because they are considered to be more closely related to biological membranes since LUVs are not subject to the increased curvature stress associated with SUVs [204, 205], which as a result decrease the stability of SUVs [205-207]. Understanding what physicochemical properties differentiate between binding with zwitterionic and anionic LUVs is critical in the development of these compounds as organism selective antibacterial drugs [40].

The appropriate amount of dry POPC or 4:1 POPC/POPG (mol to mol) was weight out to yield a final lipid concentration of 35 mM. The lipid was dissolved in chloroform and vortexed for 3 minutes. The sample was dried under nitrogen for four hours and under high vacuum overnight. The lipid was then hydrated with 2 mL of buffer (40 mM sodium phosphate, pH = 6.8) and vortexed extensively. SUVs were prepared by sonication of the milky lipid suspension using a titanium tip ultra-sonicator (Qsonica Sonicators model Q55) for approximately 40 minutes in an ice bath until the solution became transparent. The titanium debris was removed by centrifugation at 14,000 rev./min for 10 minutes using an Eppendorf table top centrifuge [204]. Final lipid concentration used for CD studies was 1.75 mM.

A defined amount of dried POPC or 4:1 POPC/POPG (mol to mol) was weight out and suspended in buffer (40 mM sodium phosphate, pH = 6.8) and spun for 30 minutes resulting in a total lipid concentration of 1.75 mM for CD studies and 35 mM for ITC studies. Large unilamellar vesicles (LUVs) were prepared by extrusion using a Mini-Extruder (Avanti Polar Lipid Inc) [214, 215]. The solution was extruded through a 100 nm pore size polycarbonate membrane 21 times. After extrusion the LUVs were allowed to "rest" for at least two hours before use to allow equilibration to occur. The final lipid concentration was calculated based on the weight of the dried lipid [169, 204, 208, 216-218]. Previously Kennedy and co-workers reported the preparation of LUVs using this procedure resulted in a homogeneous population of LUVs with >95% of the particles falling into the particle size range of 70-100 nm [219]. Kennedy and co-workers have also previously shown by ^{31}P NMR that these LUVs are unilamellar [219].

LUVs for Dye Release Experiments

A defined amount of dried POPC or 4:1 POPC/POPG LUVs (mol to mol) was weighed and suspended in a calcein-containing buffer (70mM calcein, 10mM Bis-Tris, 150mM NaCl, 1mM EDTA, pH=7.1, the pH was corrected using 3mM NaOH and the final lipid concentration was calculated based on dilution). The resulting solution was vortexed for one minute (5 times). The calcein-encapsulated LUVs were extruded using the same technique as above. Following extrusion the unencapsulated calcein was removed by gel filtration on a Sephadex G50 column (eluent: buffer containing 10 mM Bis-Tris, 150 mM NaCl, 1 mM EDTA, pH =7.1) The fraction containing calcein-encapsulated liposomes was collected and retained for fluorescence studies [135, 169, 204, 208, 216-218, 220, 221]. Prior to use each batch of calcein encapsulated LUVs were subjected to a self-quenching efficiency test. The self-quenching efficiency (Q) for each lipid suspension was set at a minimum value of 80% before it could be used in these investigations. The Q value was calculated using the following equation: $Q = (1 - (F_0/F_T)) \times 100\%$ where F_0 and F_T are the background fluorescence of the lipid suspension and the total fluorescence after the addition of a solution of 10% Triton X, respectively [174, 202, 222, 223]. Fig. **28** illustrates the appearance of the gel filtration on a Sephadex G50 column used to remove the unencapsulated calcein, Fig. **29** illustrates visually the results of the self-quenching efficiency (Q) test.

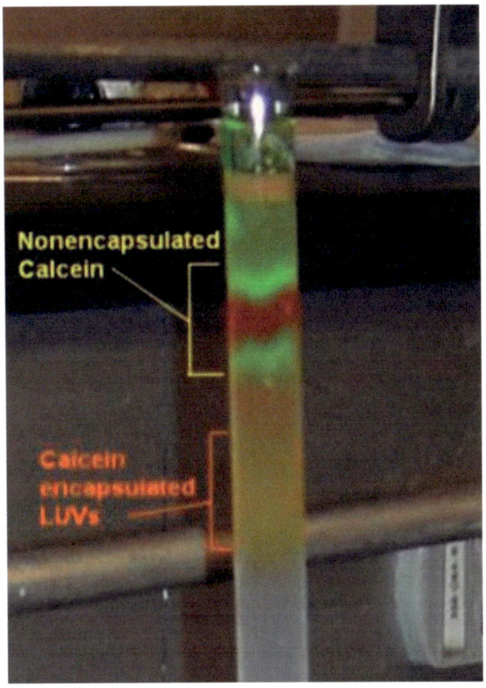

Figure 28: Close-up and labeled picture of the Sephadex G50 column used to remove the unencapsulated calcein.

Circular Dichroism

CD spectroscopy is very sensitive and its use to monitor conformational changes in peptides and proteins which has been well documented [205, 224, 225]. Traditionally SUVs have been employed almost exclusively to investigate the binding of peptides and proteins with lipids in CD studies in order to minimize the contribution of light scattering on the spectra [205, 226]. As pointed out by the independent work of Schmidt and co-workers [227] and Wong and co-workers [228], SUVs due to high vesicle curvature are metastable and produce "anomalous peptide partitioning [205-207]". However, the work of Ladokhin and co-workers have shown that undistorted CD studies can be obtained in the presence of up to 3 mM LUVs above 200 nm and in the presence of 7 mM LUVs above 215 nm [205]. In this study we are employing both SUV's and LUV's to investigate the binding interactions that occur between these AMPs and a zwitterionic and an anionic liposome. In addition, in this investigation we used anionic (SDS) and zwitterionic (DPC) micelles to isolate and investigate the surface binding interaction of these peptides from the aggregation and pore forming interactions that occur upon binding to lipids.

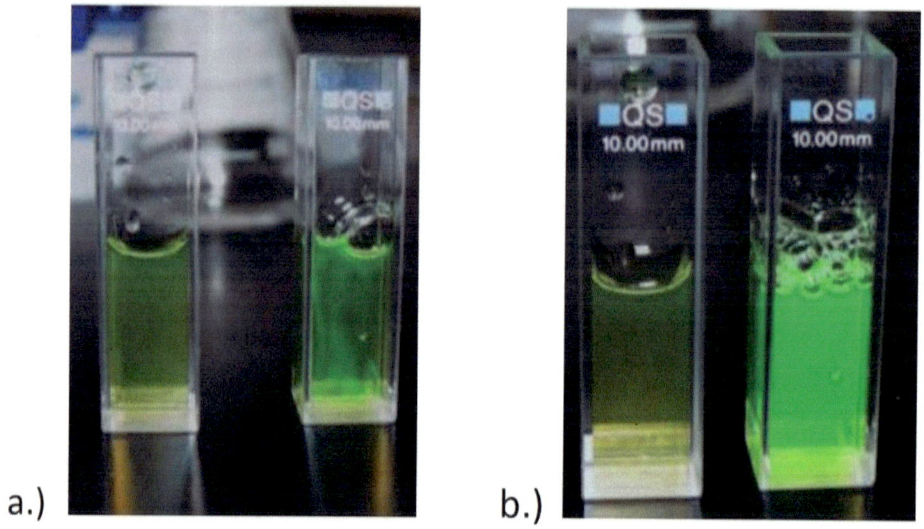

Figure 29: Comparison of concentrated calcein encapsulated LUVs (left in each picture) and concentrated calcein encapsulated LUVs after the addition of 10% (v/v) TritonX-100. **a**) Addition of 10% TritonX-100 with little mixing. **b**) Addition of 10% TritonX-100 after mixing.

In the analysis of CD data it must be noted that the spectrum of a peptide represents the linear combination of a number of different conformers [224, 229]. This is particularly true when liposomes are used as there are several different peptide-liposome interactions possible depending on the peptide to lipid ratio. Changes in the intensity or shape of the CD spectrum of a peptide in the presence of a liposome indicate that the peptide is adopting different conformations upon interacting with that particular liposome as compared to another environment such as a buffer [224, 229]. Due to the high percentage of unnatural amino acids incorporated into the peptides under investigation here, no quantitative estimation of secondary structural features are possible.

Peptide solutions of 75 μM dissolved in 40mM phosphate buffer (pH=6.8) were used in these investigations. Binding studies were conducted using SUV and LUV preparations consisting of 1.75 mM POPC or 4:1 POPC/POPG in 40 mM phosphate buffer (pH = 6.8) with peptide concentrations of 100 μM. For the binding studies in the presence of micelles, 100 μM peptide was used with either 80 mM DPC or SDS in 40 mM phosphate buffer (pH = 6.8). All CD spectra were obtained by acquiring 8 scans on a JASCO J-815 CD Spectrometer using a 0.1 mm cylindrical quartz cell (Starna Cells, Atascadero, CA) from 260 to 195 nm at 20 nm/min, 1 nm bandwidth, data pitch 0.2 nm, response time 2.0 sec and 5 mdeg sensitivity at room temperature (~25°C). Contributions due to micelles and LUVs and SUVs were eliminated by subtracting the lipid spectra of the corresponding peptide-free solutions. All analysis of CD spectra was conducted after smoothing (with a means-movement function) and conversion to molar ellipticity using the JASCO Spectra Analysis program [169, 203, 214]. CD spectra that exhibited HT values of greater than 400 were not used due to excessive light scattering and / or absorption. Titration studies were conducted using concentrations of POPC or 4:1 POPC/POPG LUVs varying from 0.8 to 12 mM.

The CD spectra of compound **23** in the presence of both anionic and zwitterionic SUV and LUVs are shown in Fig. **30**. The spectra in the presence of anionic LUVs and SUV are different from the CD spectra in the presence of zwitterionic LUVs and SUVs this suggest that compound 23 is adopting different conformations on binding to the two different liposomes which suggest the possibility of organism selectivity [178].

Isothermal Titration Calorimetry

The application of ITC to the study of peptide membrane interactions is well documented in the literature [174, 215, 216]. In an ideal case, this technique allows for the complete analysis of the thermodynamic parameters (free energy, enthalpy, entropy, binding constants and heat capacity changes) associated with the binding

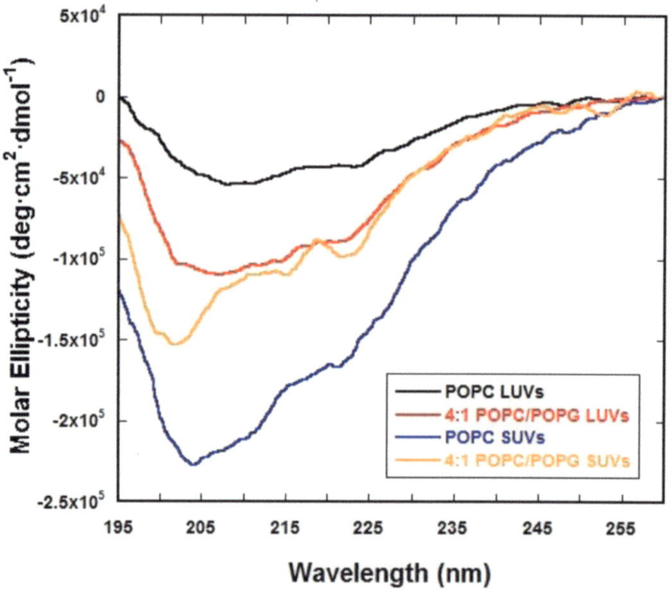

Figure 30: A Comparison of the CD spectra of compound 23 in the presence of 1.75 mM POPC LUVs, 1.75 mM POPC/POPG LUVs, 1.75 mM POPC SUVs, and 1.75 mM 4:1 POPC/POPG SUVs.

interactions of peptides to LUVs [216, 230]. The interaction of peptides with lipid vesicles are driven by three forces: the hydrophobic effect, the coil-helix transition and non-classical hydrophobic effect [201, 208]. Further, Wieprecht and co-workers [208] proposed that the binding of a peptide to a LUV is dependent on the global structural physicochemical properties including overall charge, hydrophobicity, and amphipathicity of the AMP. In the analysis of any peptide liposome binding data it must be remembered that of a large number of different conformational states are possible for each peptide and are in equilibrium with each other [213]. These states vary from bulk solution, to surface bound, various aggregations states and pore formation as well as the reverse processes [213]. The starting point for ITC experiments is to titrate minimal lipid into excess peptide. At the very beginning of the titration the equilibrium concentration of the peptide on the surface of the liposome is saturated and therefore favors pore formation (if these peptides do in fact form pores). The vast majority of the peptides under these circumstances would remain in solution. As the concentration of the lipid increases all possible states of the peptide-lipid binding process will exists. These include all liposome bound states, included monomeric, small to large clusters and peptides involved in pore formation.

A cartoon representation of this hypothesis is given in Fig. **31**. In our laboratory all data was acquired using a Microcal VP-ITC calorimeter (Microcal, Northampton, MA). All experiments were run in 40 mM sodium phosphate buffer, pH 6.8, at 25ºC. All solutions were degassed for approximately 10 minutes under vacuum before loading the reaction cell and syringe. For full titration experiments, 15 µL aliquots of 35 mM lipid solutions in buffer were titrated into 1.4 µL of peptide (100 - 200 µM). For binding single injection experiments, 15 µL of dilute samples of peptide (100-200 µM) were titrated into excess lipid (15-20 mM). A stirring speed of 220 rpm and injection duration of 30 sec were chosen to ensure sufficient mixing while keeping the baseline noise to a minimum. To ensure complete equilibration between injections, a delay of 700 sec between injections was used. The background heat of dilution was obtained by titrating LUVs into the reaction cell containing only buffer and was subtracted prior to analysis. Data was analyzed with Origin® software (version 7.0). ITC data collection was obtained in duplicate in an effort to ensure reproducibility [169, 204, 208, 214, 216-218].

There are two different models to consider when extracting thermodynamic data from ITC thermograms. The first and much simpler model, does not take into account the electrostatic interactions between the peptide and the membrane surface while the second considers these interactions [217]. The former model, and simplest of the two, involves the partitioning of the peptide between the aqueous phase and the lipid membrane, assuming equation 1 as determined by Wieprecht and Seelig [217] is a linear relationship:

$$X_b = K_p c_f \qquad \textbf{(1)}$$

where X_b is the molar ratio of membrane-bound peptide per lipid, c_f is the concentration of free peptide in solution and K_p is the partition coefficient. The second model takes into consideration electrostatic interactions. Given that the peptides under investigation are highly positively charged and the LUVs surface contains regions of positive and negative charge although the net charge of the POPC LUVs is neutral, the second model is the more relevant for our analysis. The membrane surface contains localized regions of negative charge therefore attracting the positively charged residues of the peptide. This results in an increase

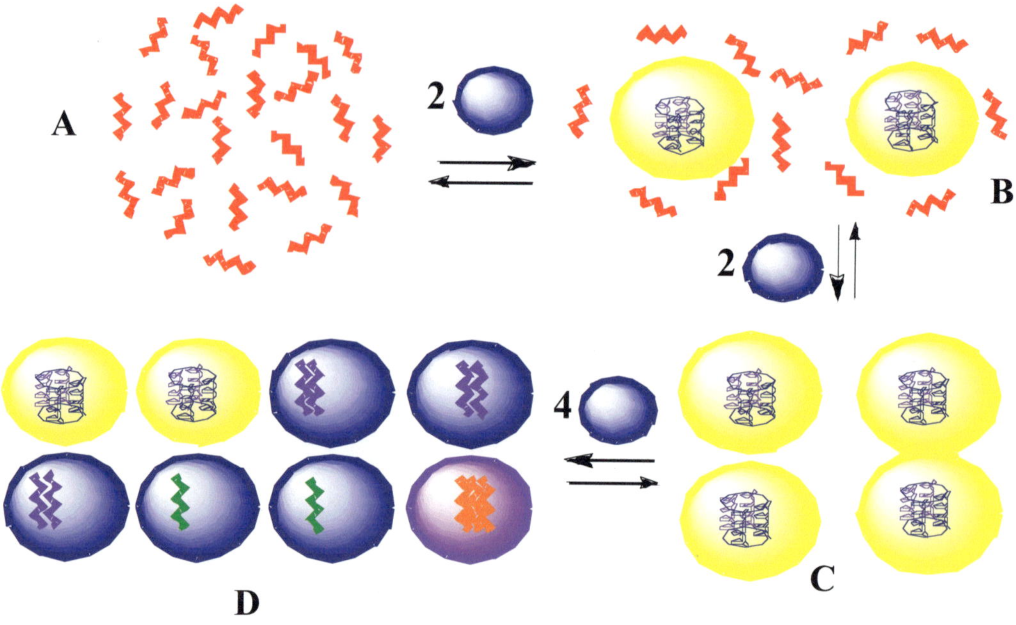

Figure 31: Cartoon representation of the effect of increasing liposome concentration on the possible liposome bound states of a AMP. Individual red helices represent peptide in buffer. Hexameric clusters of blue helices represent peptides involved in pore formation. Green helices represent monomeric surface bound peptide. Purple and orange clusters represent various sized aggregates of peptide bound to the surface of the liposome. All of the liposome bound peptides (both S-state and I-state) are in equilibrium with free peptide. Blue circles represent the liposome. **REGION A:** This region of the cartoon represents the peptide in buffer. **REGION B:** This region represents the effect of the addition of a small concentration of liposomes. The concentration of the peptide in buffer is higher than the concentration required to saturate the surface of the liposome. Thus pore formation will occur (if the peptide forms pores). **REGION C:** Represents the point when the concentration of the peptide exactly matches that required to completely saturates all the liposomes present. **REGION D:** In region D the concentration of the liposomes is higher than the concentration of the peptide required to saturate the liposomes so all possible states of the peptide are present in a complex equilibrium.

of peptide concentration at the surface of the membrane, c_m in comparison to the bulk solution, *c*f [213]. Therefore, equation 2 [134, 217, 231, 232], is more appropriate for the analysis of our data.

$$X_b = Kc_m \tag{2}$$

By plotting X_b *versus* c_m, K can finally be obtained as it is the slope of the line. Knowing K allows for the calculation of other thermodynamic data, including free energy (ΔG) and entropy (ΔS) from the following equations 3 and 4 [134, 217, 231, 232].

$$\Delta G^0 = -RT \ln 55.5K \quad \textbf{(3)}$$

$$\Delta G^0 = H - \Delta TS \quad \textbf{(4)}$$

Two example ITC thermograms are show in Fig. **32** for the titration of lipid into compound **23**. In the case of POPC liposomes titrated into compound **23** (Fig. **32A**) the thermogram is relatively simple showing an isotherm that displays a single endothermic phase. The slow linear change in the slope of the isotherm of the binding to zwitterionic POPC has been attributed by Andrushchenko and co-workers to the fact that electrostatic interactions do not play a critical function in the binding of the AMP to the liposome [233]. Previous ITC studies [234] have noted that an endothermic phase can be attributed to a combination of several events. These may include electrostatic interactions between the peptide and the membrane surface, disruption of polar head groups accompanied by reorganization of lipids on the surface of the membrane, disruption of the solvation spheres on both the peptide and the membrane surface and other less understood phenomena [234].

In contrast, the titration of **23** with mixed liposomes (Fig. **32B**) displays a more complex isotherm with two distinct phases. An endothermic phase is observed at low lipid to peptide ratios followed by an exothermic phase as the liposome concentration increases. Although this behavior is not very common it has been observed in other systems [235]. Andrushchenko and co-workers reported similar thermograms for mixed liposomes with tryptophan-rich cathelicidin antimicrobial peptides; tritrpo4 and tritrpo6 [233]. At low lipid to peptide ratios, this behavior has been attributed to processes such as pore formation [208], peptide aggregation [233], and changes in the phase properties of the lipids [236]. Binding of the peptide to the liposome surface is thought to occur at high lipid to peptide ratios [213]. The observed thermograms are very different indicating that compound 23 interacts with POPC (zwitterionic lipid) and 4:1 POPC/POPG (anionic lipid) through different mechanisms [169]. This data strongly suggest that the potential for organism electivity exist.

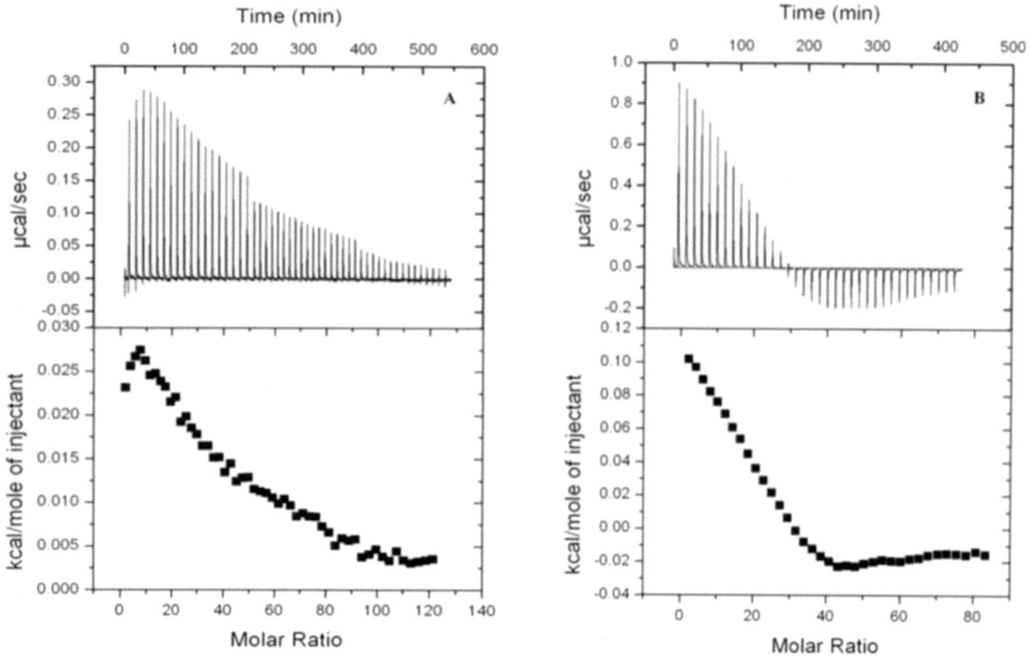

Figure 32: ITC data for the titration of 35 mM lipid into 0.2 mM compound **23**. Data was acquired using a Microcal VP-ITC calorimeter (Microcal, Northampton, MA). All experiments were run in 40 mM sodium phosphate buffer, pH 6.8, at a temperature of 25°C and a stirring speed of 220 rpm. Liposome was delivered in 15 μL injections at 700s intervals. (**A**) Titration of POPC into compound **23**. (**B**) Titration of mixed liposomes into compound **23**.

Calcein Leakage Assays

In our laboratory peptide induced calcein leakage was investigated using an ISS PC1 photon counting spectrofluorometer (ILC Technology) at an excitation wavelength of 494 nm and an emission wavelength of 518 nm. An aliquot of peptide (10-50 μL) in buffer (10 mM Bis-Tris, 150 mM NaCl, 1 mM EDTA, pH 7.2) was added to the cell containing LUVs (36.6 μM lipid concentration) to give an overall peptide concentration of 4-20 μM. The fluorescence intensity was measured every minute for the first 20 minutes of the experiment and then every 10 minutes until the emission intensity showed no further significant increase (approximately 90 minutes). One hundred percent leakage was determined with the addition of 50 μL of 10% (v/v) Triton X in distilled water. The apparent percent leakage was calculated using the following equation: % leakage = $[(F-F_0)/(F_T-F_0))]$ x 100%, where F_0 and F_T are the initial fluorescence before introduction of peptide and after the addition of Triton X, respectively [135, 169, 208, 214, 220, 221].

ACKNOWLEDGEMENTS

None declared.

CONFLICT OF INTEREST

The authors confirm that this chapter content has no conflict of interest.

REFERENCES

[1] Cookson, B.: Clinical significance of emergence of bacterial antimicrobial resistance in the hospital environment. *J. Appl. Microbiol.* **2005**, *99*, 989-96.

[2] Davies, J.: Inactivation of antibiotics and the dissemination of resistance genes. *Science* **1994**, *264*, 375-382.

[3] Schutze, G. E.; Kaplan, S. L.; Jacobs, R. F.: Resistant *pneumococcus*: a world-wide problem. *Infection* **1994**, *22*, 233-237.

[4] Lohner, K.: New strategies for novel antibiotics: peptides targeting bacterial cell membranes. *Gen. Physiol. Biophys.* **2009**, *28*, 105-116.

[5] Bonapace, C. R.; White, R. L.; Friedrich, L. V.; Bosso, J. A.: Evaluation of antibiotic synergy against *Acinetobacter baumannii*: a comparison with Etest, time-kill, and checkerboard methods. *Diagn. Microbiol. Infect. Dis.* **2000**, *38*, 43-50.

[6] Chait, R.; Craney, A.; Kishony, R.: Antibiotic interactions that select against resistance. *Nature* **2007**, *446*, 668-71.

[7] Drago, L.; De Vecchi, E.; Nicola, L.; Colombo, A.; Guerra, A.; Gismondo, M. R.: Activity of levofloxacin and ciprofloxacin in combination with cefepime, ceftazidime, imipenem, piperacillin-tazobactam and amikacin against different *Pseudomonas aeruginosa* phenotypes and *Acinetobacter*. *Chemotherapy* **2004**, *50*, 202-210.

[8] Kraus, D.; Peschel, A.: *Staphylococcus aureus* evasion of innate antimicrobial defense. *Future Microbiol.* **2008**, *3*, 437-451.

[9] Foster, T. J.: The *Staphylococcus aureus* superbug. *J. Clin. Invest.* **2004**, *114*, 1693-1696.

[10] Lowy, F. D.: *Staphylococcus aureus* infections. *N. Engl. J. Med.* **1998**, *339*, 520-532.

[11] Gross, M.; Cramton, S. E.; Gotz, F.; Peschel, A.: Key role of teichoic acid net charge in *Staphylococcus aureus* colonization of artifical surfaces. *Infection and Immunity* **2001**, *69*, 3423-3426.

[12] Thurlow, L. R.; Hanke, M. L.; Frotz, T.; Angle, A.; Aldrich, A.; Williams, S. H.; Engebretsen, I. L.; Bayles, K. W.; Horswill, A. R.; Kielian, T.: *Staphyococcus aureus* biofilms prevent macrophage phagocytosis and attenuate inflammation *in vivo*. *J. Immunology* **2011**, *www.jimmunol.org/cgi/doi/10.4049/jimmunol.1002794*.

[13] Chambers, H. F.; Delco, F. R.: Waves of resistance: *Staphylococcus aureus* in the antibiotic era. *Nat. Rev. Microbiol.* **2009**, *7*, 629-641.

[14] Rowe, S. M.; Miller, S.; Sorscher, E. J.: Cystic fibrosis. *N. Engl. J. Med.* **2005**, *352*, 1992-2001.

[15] Marr, A. K.; Gooderham, W. J.; Hancock, R. E. W.: Antibacterial peptides for therapeutic use: obstacles and realistic outlook. *Curr. Opin. Pharmacol.* **2006**, *6*, 468-472.

[16] Gooderham, W. J.; Bains, M.; McPhee, J. B.; Wiegand, I.; Hancock, R. E. W.: Induction by cationic antimicrobial peptides and involvement in intinsic polymyxin and antimicrobial peptide resistance, biofilm formation, and swarming motility of PsrA in *Pseudomonas aeruginosa*. *J. Bacteriol.* **2008**, *190*, 5624-5634.

[17] Lyczak, J. H.; Cannon, C. L.; Pier, G. B.: Establishment of *Pseudomonas aeurginosa* infection: lessions from a versatile opportunist. *Microbes Infect.* **2000**, *2*, 1051-1060.

[18] Kapoor, R.; Wadman, M. W.; Dohm, M. T.; Cryzewski, A. M.; Spormann, A. M.; DBarron, A. E.: Antimicrobial peptoids are effective against *Pseudomonas aeruginosa* biofilms. *Antimicrob. Agents Chemother.* **2011**, *55*, 3054-3057.

[19] Overhage, J.; Campisano, A.; Bains, M.; Torfs, E. C. W.; Rehm, B. H. A.; Hancock, R. E. W.: Human host defense peptide LL-37 prevents bacterial biofilm formation. *Infection and Immunity* **2008**, *76*, 4176-4182.

[20] Costerton, J. W.; Stewart, P. S.; Greenberg, E. P.: Bacterial biofilms a common cause of persistent infections. *Science* **1999**, *284*, 1318-1322.

[21] Dieter, R. S.: Coronary artery stent infection. *Catheter Cardiovasc. Interv.* **2004**, *62*, 281.

[22] Hancock, R. E. W.; Speert, D. P.: Antibiotic resistance in *Pseudomonas aeruginosa*: mechanisms and impact on treatment. *Drug Resist, Updat.* **2000**, *3*, 247-255.

[23] Chan, C.; L., B.; Deber, C.: Helix induction in antimicrobial peptides by alginate in biofilms. *J. Biological Chemistry* **2004**, *279*, 38749-38754.

[24] Chopra, L. E. A.: Treatment of health-care associated infections caused by Gram-negative bacteria: a consensus statement. *Lancet Infect. Dis.* **2008**, *8*, 133-139.

[25] Hicks, R. P.; Bhonsle, J. B.; Venugopal, D.; Koser, B. W.; Magill, A. J.: *De Novo* Design of Selective Antibiotic Peptides by Incorporation of Un-natural Amino Acids. *J. Med. Chem.* **2007**, *50*, 3026-3036.

[26] Bush, K.: Why it is important to continue antibacterial drug discovery. *ASM News* **2004**, *70*, 282-287.

[27] Klevens, R. M.; Edwards, J. R.; Richards, C. L.; Horan, T. C.; Gaynes, R. P.; Pollack, D. A.; Cardo, D. M.: Estimating Health Care-Associated Infections and Deaths in U.S. Hospitals, 2002. *Public Health Reports* **2007**, *122*, 160-166.

[28] Hart, G. "Drug resistance threatens to reverse medical progress.," World Health Organization, 2000.

[29] Shlaes, D. M.; Projan, S. J.; Edwards, J. E.: Antibiotic discovery: state of the state. *ASM News* **2004**, *70*, 275-281.

[30] Huang, Y.; Huang, J.; Chen, Y.: Alpha-helical cationic antimicrobial peptides:relationships of structure and function. *Protein Cell* **2010**, *1*, 143-152.

[31] Godballe, T.; Nilsson, L. L.; Petersen, P. D.; Jenssen, H.: Antimicrobial β-peptides and α-peptoids. *Chem. Biol. Drug Des.* **2011**, *77*, 107-116.

[32] Song, J.: What's new on the antimicrobial horizon? *Int. J. Antimicrob. Agents* **2008**, *32*, S207-S213.

[33] Findlay, B.; Zhanel, G. G.; Schweizer, F.: Cationic amphipiles, a new generation of antimicrobials inspired by natural antimicrobial peptide scaffold. *Antimicrobial Agents and Chemotherapy* **2010**, *54*, 4049-4058.

[34] Fernandez, D. I.; Sani, M.-A.; Gehman, J. D.; Hahm, K.-S.; Separovic, F.: Interactions of a synthetic Leu-Lys rich antimicrobial peptde with phospholipid bilayers. *Eur. Biophys. J.* **2011**, *40*, 471-480.

[35] Shakil, S.; Kham, R.; Khan, A. U.: Aminoglycosides *versus* bacteria: a description of the action resistance mechanism, and nosocomial battlegrouond. *J. Biomed. Sci.* **2008**, *15*, 5-14.

[36] Oliphant, C. M.; Green, G. M.: Quinolones: a comprehensive review. *Am. Fam. Physician* **2002**, *65*, 455-464.

[37] Hooper, D. C.: Nechanism of action of antimicrobials:focus on fluroquinolones. *Clin. Infect. Dis.* **2001**, *32*, S9-S15.

[38] Kamysz, W.: Are antimicrobial peptides an alternative for conventional antibiotics. *Nuclear Med. Reviews* **2005**, *8*, 78-86.

[39] Zhang, L.; Harris, S. C.; Falla, T. J.: *Therapeutic application of innate immunity peptides*; Horizon Bioscience: San Diego, 2005.

[40] Toke, O.: Antimicrobial peptides;new candidates in the fight against bacterial infections. *Biopolymers* **2005**, *80*, 717-735.

[41] Bechinger, B.: Insights into the mechanism of action of host defense peptides from biophysical and structural investigations. *J. Pept, Sci..* **2011**, *17*, 306-314.

[42] Epand, R. M.; Epand, R. F.: Bacterial membrane lipids in the action of antimicrobial agents. *J. Pept. Sci.* **2011**, *17*, 298-305.

[43] Fox, M. A.; Thwaite, J. E.; Ulaeto, D. O.; Atkins, T. P.; Atkins, H. S.: Design and characterization of novel hydrid antimicrobial peptides based on cecropin A, LL-37 and magainin II. *Peptides* **2012**, *33*, 197-205.

[44] Jang, S. A.; Kim, H.; Lee, J. Y.; Shin, J. R.; Kim, D. J.; Cho, J. H.; Kim, S. C.: Mechanism of action and specifity of antimicrobial peptides designed based on buforin IIb. *Peptides* **2012**, *34*, 283-289.

[45] Phoenix, D. A.; Harris, F.; Dennison, S.; Chatfield, L.; Sayed, Z.; Hussain, S.: *J. E. C. Qua L.* **2003**, *1*, 44-61.

[46] Dennison, S. R.; Wallace, J.; Harris, F.; Phoenix, D. A.: Amphiphilic α-helical antimicrobial peptides and their structure/function relationships. *Protein and peptide Letters.* **2005**, *12*, 31-39.

[47] Yeaman, M. R.; Yount, N. Y.: Mechanisms of antimicrobial pepitde action and resistance. *Pharmacological Reviews* **2003**, *55*, 27-55.

[48] Ganz, T.: Defensins: antimicrobial peptides of innate immunity. *Nature reviews, Immunology* **2003**, *3*, 710-720.

[49] Simmaco, M.; Mignogna, G.; Barra, D.: Antimicrobial peptides from amphibian skin: what do they tell us? *Biopolymers* **1999**, *47*, 435-450.

[50] Song, Y. M.; Park, Y.; Lim, S. S.; Yang, S.-T.; Woo, E.-R.; Park, S.; Lee, J. S.; Kim, J. I.; Hahm, K.-S.; Kim, Y.; Shin, S. Y.: Cell selectivity and mechanism of action of antimicrobial model peptides containing peptoid residues. *Biochemistry* **2005**, *44*, 12094-12106.

[51] Devine, D. A.; Hancock, R. E. W.: Cationic peptides: distribution and mechanisms of resistance. *Curr. Pharmaceutical Design* **2002**, *8*, 703-714.

[52] Brogden, K. A.: Antimicrobial peptides: pore formers or metabolic inhibitors in bacteria? *Nature Rev. Microbiol.* **2005**, *3*, 238-250.

[53] Hancock, R. E. W.: The therapeutic potential of cationic peptides. *Exp. Opin. Invest. Drugs* **1998**, *7*, 167-174.

[54] Zasloff, M.: Antimicrobial peptides of multicellular organisms. *Nature* **2002**, *415*, 389-395.

[55] Zhang, L.; Falla, T. J.: Host defense peptides for use as potential therapeutics. *Curr. Opin. Investig. Drugs* **2009**, *10*, 164-71.

[56] Oyston, P. C. F.; Fox, M. A.; Richards, S. J.; Clark, G. C.: Novel peptide therapeutics for treatment of infections. *J. Med. Microbio.* **2009**, *58*, 977-987.

[57] Wang, G.; Li, X.; Wang, Z.: APD2: the updated antimicrobial peptide database and its application in peptide design. *Nucleic Acids Res.* **2009**, *37*, D933-937.

[58] Khandelia, H. I., J. H.; Mouritsen, O. G. : The impact of peptides on lipid membranes. *Biochim. Biophys. Acta* **2008**, *1778*, 1528-1536.

[59] Powers, J.-P. S.; Hancock, R. E. W.: The relationship between peptide structure and antibacterial activity. *Peptides* **2003**, *24*, 1681-1691.

[60] Matsuzaki, K.: Why and how are peptide-lipid interactions utilized for self-defense. *Biochemica et Biophysica Acta* **1999**, *1462*, 1-10.

[61] Papo, N.; Shai, Y.: Effects of drastic sequence alteration and D-amino acid incorporation on the membrane binding behavior of lytic peptides. *Biochemistry* **2004**, *43*, 6393-6403.

[62] Dathe, M.; Meyer, J.; Beyerman, M.; Maul, B.; Hoischen, C.; Bienert, M.: General aspects of peptide selectivity towards lipid bilayers and cell membrane studied by variation of structural parameters of amphipathic α-helical model peptides. *Biochim, Biophys. Acta* **2002**, *1558*, 171-186.

[63) Chen, Y.; Mant, C. T.; Farmer, S. W.; Hancock, R. E.; Vasil, M. L.; Hodges, R. S.: Rational design of α-helical antimicrobial peptides with enhanced activities and specificity/therapeutic index. *J. Biol. Chem.* **2005**, *280*, 12316-12329.

[64] Oren, Z.; Hong, J.; Shai, Y.: *J. Biol. Chem.* **1997**, *272*, 14643-14649.

[65] Dathe, M.; Wiencek, J. M.: Structural features of helical antimicrobial peptides: their potential to modulate activity on model membranes and biological cells. *Biochimica et Biophysica Acta* **1999**, *1462*, 71-87

[66] Epand, R. M.; Vogel, H. J.: Diversity of antimicrobial pepitdes and their mechanisms of action. *Biochimica et Biophysica Acta* **1999**, *1462*, 11-28.

[67] Zucca, M.; Scutera, S.; Saba, V.: Antimicrobial peptides: New frontiers in the therapy of infections. In *Drug Development-A case study based insight into modern strategies*; Rundfeldt, C., Ed.; INTECH, 2011.

[68] Yang, D.; Chertov, O.; Oppenheim, J. J.: Participatiion of mammalian defensins and cathelicidins in antimicrobial immunity: receptors and activity of human defensins and cathelicidin (LL-37). *J. Leukocyte Biology* **2001**, *69*, 691-697.

[69] Ando, S.; Mitsuyasu, K.; Soeda, Y.; Hidaka, M.; Ito, Y.; Matsubara, K.; Shindo, M.; Uchida, Y.; Aoyagi, H.: Structure-activity relationship pf indolicidin, a Trp-rich antibacterial peptide. *J. Pept, Sci..* **2010**, *16*, 171-177.

[70] Bommarius, B.; Kalman, D.: Antimicrobial and host defense peptides for therapeutic use against multidrug-resistant pathogens: new hope on the horizon. *Drugs* **2009**, *12*, 376-380.

[71] Matsuzaki, K.: Magainins as paradigm for the mode of action of pore forming polypeptides. *Biochimica et Biophysica Acta* **1998**, *1376*, 391-400.

[72] Gottler, L. M.; Ramamoorthy, A.: Structure, membrane orientation, mechanism, and function of pexiganan-a highly potent antimicrobial peptide designed from magainin. *Biochimica et Biophysica Acta* **2009**, *1788*, 1680-1686.

[73] Wu, M.; Maier, E.; Benz, R.; Hancock, R. E. W.: Mechanism of interaction of different classes of cationic antimicrobial peptides with planar bilayers and with cyctoplasmic membrane of *Escherichia coli*. *Biochemistry* **1999**, *38*, 7235-7242.

[74] Epand, R. M.; Epand, R. F.: Modulation of membrane curvature by peptides. *Biopolymers* **2001**, *55*, 358-363.

[75] Henzler-Wildman, K. A.; Lee, D.-K.; Ramamoorthy, A.: Mechanism of lipid bilayer disruption by the human antimicrobial peptide LL-37. *Biochemistry* **2003**, *42*, 6545-6558.

[76] White, S. H.; Wimley, W. C.: Membrane protein folding and stability: physical principles. *Annu. Rev. Biophys. Biomol. Struct.* **1999**, *28*, 319-365.

[77] Bechinger, B.: Membrane association and pore formation by alpha-helical peptides. *Adv. Exp. Med. Biol.* **2010**, *677*, 24-30.

[78] Fernandez, D. I.; Gehman, J. D.; Separovic, F.: Membrane interactions of antimicrobial peptides from Australian frogs. *Biochemica et Biophysica Acta* **2009**, *1788*, 1630-1638.

[79] Papo, N.; Shai, Y.: New lytic peptides based on the D,L amphipathic helix motif preferentially kill tumor cells compared to normal cells. *Biochemistry* **2003**, *42*, 9346-9354.

[80] Leontiadou, H.; Mark, A. E.; Marrink, S. J.: Antimicrobial Peptides in Action. *J. Am. Chem. Soc.* **2006**, *128*, 12156-12161.

[81] Hancock, R. E. W.; Lehrer, R.: Cationic peptides: a new source of antibiotics. *Trends Biotechnol* **1998**, *16*, 82-88.

[82] Wenk, M. R.; Seelig, J.: Magainin 2 amide interaction with lipid membranes: calorimetric detection of peptide binding and pore formation. *Biochemistry* **1998**, *37*, 3909-3916.

[83] Lohner, K.; Prenner, E. J.: Differential scanning calorimetry and X-ray diffraction studie of the specificity of the interaction of antimicrobial peptides with membrane-mimetic systems. *Biochimica et Biophysica Acta* **1999**, *1462*, 141-156.

[84] Giangaspero, A.; Sandri, L.; Tossi, A.: Amphipathic α-helical antimicrobial peptides. *Eur. J. Biochem.* **2001**, *268*, 5589-5600.

[85] Azuma, I.; Yamamura, Y.; Tanaka, Y.; Kohsaka, K.; Mori, T.; Itoh, T.: Cell wall of Mycobacterium lepraemurium Strain Hawaii. *J. Bacteriology* **1973**, *113*, 515-518.

[86] Yeaman, N. R.; Yount, N., Y,: Mechanisms of antimicrobial peptide action and resistance. *Pharmacol. Rev.* **2003**, *55*, 27-55.

[87] http://www.google.com/imgres?hl=en&biw=1523&bih=586&tbm=isch&tbnid=58OF1BIs qdzY5M:&imgrefurl=http://xnet.rrc.mb.ca/davidb/complex.htm&docid=YQdO-am25QpiQ M&imgurl=http://faculty.ccbcmd.edu/courses/bio141/lecguide/unit1/prostruct/images/u1fig 10b.jpg&w=361&h=289&ei=MInkT7HEGIT69QSlqtz2CQ&zoom=1&iact=rc&dur=3&sig =109727374085822156413&page=1&tbnh=119&tbnw=149&start=0&ndsp=25&ved=1t:4 29,r:14,s:0,i:116&tx=61&ty=47.

[88] http://micro.digitalproteus.com/morphology2.php.

[89] http://www.sigmaaldrich.com/life-science/metabolomics/enzyme-explorer/learning-center/l ysing-enzymes.html.

[90] Dai, T.; Huang, Y.-Y.; Hamblin, M. R.: Photodynamic therapy for localized infections-State of the art. *Photodiagnosis and Photodynamic Therapy* **2009**, *6*, 170-188.

[91] http://en.wikibooks.org/wiki/Medical_Physiology/Cellular_Physiology/Cell_structure_and _Function.

[92] http://php.med.unsw.edu.au/cellbiology/index.php?title=Cell_Membranes_and_Compartments.
[93] http://people.csail.mit.edu/seneff/statins_muscle_damage_heart_failure.html.
[94] http://www.doctorfungus.org/thedrugs/antif_pharm.php.
[95] Katzung BG; Masters SB; AJ:, T.: *Basic and Clinical Pharmacology, 11th Edition.*
[96] Kartsonis, N. A.; Nielsen, J.; Douglas, C. M.: Caspofungin: the first in a new class of antifungal agents. *Drug Resistance Updates* **2003**, *6*, 197-218.
[97] Juretic, D.; Vukicevic, D.; Petrov, D.; Novkovic, M.; Bojovic, V.; Lucic, B.; Tossi, A.: Knowledge-based computational methods for identifying or design novel, non-homologous antimicrobial peptides. *Eur. Biophys. J.* **2011**, *40*, 371-385.
[98] Norrby, S. R.; Nord, C. E.; Finch, R.: Lack of development of new antimicrobial drugs: a potential serious threat to public health. *Lancelet Infect. Dis.* **2005**, *5*, 115-119.
[99] Conlon, J. M.; Al-Ghaferi, N.; Abraham, B.; Leprince, J.: Strategies for transformation of naturally-occurring amphibian antimicrobial peptides into therapeutically valuable anti-infective agents. *Methods* **2007**, *42*, 349-357.
[100] Bhonsle, J. B.; Venugopal, D.; Huddler, D. P.; Magill, A. J.; Hicks, R. P.: Application of 3D-QSAR for identification of descriptors defining bioactivity of antimicrobial peptides. *J. Med. Chem.* **2007**, *50*, 6545-6553.
[101] Gopal, R.; Kim, Y. J.; Seo, C. H.; Hahm, K.-S.; Park, Y.: Reversed sequence enhances antimicrobial activity of a synthetic peptide. *J. Pept, Sci..* **2011**, *17*, 329-334.
[102] Wang, Z.; Wang, G.: APD:the antimicrobial peptide database. *Nucl. Acid. Res.* **2004**, *32*, D590-D592.
[103] Papo, N.; Oren, Z.; Pag, U.; Sahl, S. G.; Shai, Y.: The consequence of sequence alterntion of an amphipathic alpha-helical antimicrobial peptide and its diastereomers. *J. Biol. Chem.* **2002**, *277*, 33913-33921.
[104] Gopal, R.; Park, S. C.; Ha, K. J.; Cho, S. J.; Kim, S. W.; Song, P. I.; Nah, J. W.; Park, Y.; Hahm, K.-S.: Effect of leucine and lysine substitution on the antimicrobial activity and evaluation of the mechanism of the HPA3NT3 peptides. *J. Pept, Sci..* **2009**, *15*, 589-594.
[105] ParK, Y.; Lee, D. G.; Jang, S. A.; Woo, E.-R.; Jeong, H. G.; Choi, C. H.; Hahm, K.-S.: A Leu-Lys rich antimicrobial peptide:activity and mechanism. *Biochemica et Biophysica Acta* **2003**, *1645*, 172-182.
[106] Epand, R. F.; Lehrer, R. I.; Waring, A.; Wang, W.; Maget-Dana, R.; Lelievre, D.; Epand, R. M.: Direct comparison of membrane interactions of model peptides composed of only Leu and Lys residues. *Biopolymers* **2003**, *71*, 2-16.
[107] Schibli, D. J.; RF, E.; Vogel, H. J.; M., E. R.: Typtophan-rich antimicrobial peptides: comparative properties and membrane interactions. *Biochem. Cell Biol.* **2002**, *80*, 667-677.
[108] Juvvadi, P.; Vunnam, S.; Merrifield, R. B.: Synthetic melittin, its enantio, retro, and retroenantio isomers and selected chimeric analogs:thier antibacterial, hemolytic and lipid bilayer action. *J. Am. Chem. Soc.* **1996**, *118*, 8989-8997.
[109] Olsen, C. A.: Beta-peptoid "foldamers" -why the additional methylene unit? *Peptide Science* **2011**, *96*, 561-566.
[110] Seebach, D.; Matthews, J. L.: β-peptides: a surpise at every turn. *Chem. Commun.* **1997**, 2015-2022.
[111] Hamuro, Y.; Schneider, J. P.; DeGrado, W. F.: *J. Am. Chem. Soc.* **1999**, *121*, 12200-12201.

[112] Arvidsson, P. I.; Ryder, N. S.; Weiss, H. M.; Gross, G.; Kretz, O.; Woessner, R.; Seebach, D.: Antibiotic and hemolytic activity of a beta(2)/beta(3) peptide capable of folding into a 12/10-helical secondary structure. *CHEM Bio. Chem.* **2003**, *4*, 1345-1347.

[113] Porter, E. A.; Wang, X.; Lee, S. H.; Weisblum, B.; Gellman, S. H.: Antibiotics: Non-haemolytic [beta] amino acid oligomer. *Nature* **2000**, *404*, 565.

[114] Porter, E. A.; Weisblum, B.; Gellman, S. H.: Mimicry of host-defense peptides by unnatural oligomers: antimicrobial β-peptides. *J. Am. Chem. Soc.* **2002**, *124*, 7324-7330.

[115] English, E. P.; Chumanov, R. S.; Gellman, S. H.; Compton, T.: Rational development of beta-peptide inhibitors of human cytomegalovirus entry. *J. Biol. Chem.* **2006**, *281*, 2661-2667.

[116] Torfoss, V.; Ausbacher, D.; de A.Cavalcanti-Jacobsen, C.; Hansen, T.; Brandsdal, B. O.; Havelkova, M.; Strom, M. B.: Synthesis of anticancer heptapeptides containing a unique lipophilic $\beta^{2,2}$ amino acid building block. *J. Pept, Sci..* **2012**, *18*, 170-176.

[117] Shuey, S. W.; Delaney, W. J.; Shah, M. C.; Scialdone, M. A.: Antimicrobial beta-peptoids by a block synthesis approach. *Bioorg. Med. Chem. Lett.*, **2006**, *16*, 1245-1248.

[118] Olsen, C. A.; Bonke, G.; Vedel, L.; Andsersen, A.; Witt, M.; Franzyk, H.; Jaroszewski, J. W.: Alpha-peptide/beta-peptoid chimeras. *Org. Lett.* **2007**, *9*, 1549-1552.

[119] Haug, B. E.; Stensen, W.; Kalaaji, M.; Rekdal, O.; Svenden, J. S.: Synthetic antimicrobial peptiidomimetics with therapeutic potential. *J. Med. Chem.* **2008**, *51*, 4306-4314.

[120] Isaksson, J.; Brandsdal, B. O.; Engqvist, M.; Flaten, G. E.; Svenden, J. S. M.; Stensen, W.: A synthetic antimicrobial peptidomimetic (LTX 109): Stereochemical impact on membrane disruption. *J. Med. Chem.* **2011**, *54*, 5786-5795.

[121] Seebach, D.; Ciceri, P. E.; Overhand, M.; Jaun, B.; Rigo, D.; Oberer, L.; Hommel, U.; Amstutz, R.; Widner, H.: Probing the helical secondary structure of short chain beta-peptides. *Helv. Chem. Acta* **1996**, *79*, 2043-2066.

[122] Seebach, D.; Gademann, K.; Schreiber, J. V.; Matthews, J. L.; Hintermann, T.; Oberer, L.; Hommel, U.; Widner, H.: Mixed beta-peptides: a unigue helical secondary structure in solution. *Helv. Chem. Acta* **1997**, *80*, 2033-2038.

[123] Cheng, R. P.; Gellman, S. H.; DeGrado, W. F.: beta peptides from strucutre to function. *Chem. Rev.* **2001**, *101*, 3219-3232.

[124] Goodman, C. M.; Choi, S.; Shandler, S.; DeGrado, W. F.: Foldamers as versatile frameworks for the design and evolution of function. *Nat. Chem. Biol.* **2007**, *3*, 252-262.

[125] Wu, Y. D.; Han, W.; Wang, D. P.; Gao, Y.; Zhao, Y. L.: Theoretical analysis of secondary structures of beta-peptides. *Acc. Chem. Res.* **2008**, *41*, 1418-1427.

[126] Shin, S. Y.; Kang, J. H.; Hahm, K.-S.: Structure-antibacterial, antitumor and hemolytic activity relationships of cecropin A-magainin 2 and cecropin A-melittin hybrid peptides. *J. Pept. Res.* **1999**, *53*, 82-90.

[127 Dean, S. N.; Bishop, B. M.; van Hoek, M. L.: Natural and synthetic cathelicidin peptide with antimicrobial and anti-biofilm activity against *staphylococcus aureus. BMC Microbiology* **2011**, *11*, 114-126.

[128] Gennaro, R.; Scocchi, M.; Merluzz, L.; Zanetti, M.: Biological characterization of a novel mammalian antimicrobial peptide. *Biochim, Biophys. Acta* **1998**, *1425*, 361-368.

[129] Balaban, N.; Cirioni, O.; Giacometti, A.; Ghiselli, R.; Braunstein, J. B.; Silvestri, C.; Mocchegiani, F.; Saba, V.; Scalise, G.: Treatment of *Staphylococcus aureus* biofilm infection by the quorum-sensing inhibitor RIP. *Antimicrob Agents Chemother* **2007**, *51*, 2226-2229.

[130] Sharma, S.; Yedery, R. D.; Patgaonkar, M. S.; Selvaakumar, C.; Reddy, K. V.: Antibacterial activity of a synthetic peptide that mimics the LPS binding domain of India mud crab, Scylla serrata anti-lipopolysaccharide factor (SsALF) also involved in the modification of vaginal immue functions through NF-kB signaling. *Microbial Pathogenesis* **2011**, *50*, 179-191.

[131] Ainsworth, G. C.; Brown, A. M.; Brownlee, G.: *Nature* **1947**, *160*, 263-264

[132] Sato, Y.; Shindo, M.; Sakura, N.; Uchida, Y.; Kato, I.: Novel des-fatty acyl-polymyxin B derivatives with *Pseudomonas aeruginosa*-specific antimicrobial activity. *Chem. Pharm. Bull* **2011**, *59*, 597-602.

[133] Ueno, S.; Minaba, M.; Nishiuchi, Y.; Taichi, M.; Tamada, Y.; Yamazaki, T.; Kato, Y.: Generation of novel cationic antimicrobial peptides from natural non-antimicrobial sequence by acid-amide substitution. *Annals of Clinical Microbiology and Antimicrobials* **2011**, *10*, 11.

[134] Beschiaschvili, G.; Seelig, J.: Melittin binding to mixed phosphatidylglycerol/phosphatidyl-choline membranes. *Biochemistry* **1990**, *29*, 52-58.

[135] Dathe, M.: Peptide Helicity and Membrane Surface Charge Modulate the Balance of Electrostatic and Hydrophobic Interactions with Lipid Bilayers and Biological Membranes. *Biochemistry* **1996**, *35*, 12612-12622.

[136] Shai, Y.; Oren, Z.: From "carpet" mechanism to *de novo* designed diastereomeric cell-selective antimicrobial peptides. *Peptides* **2001**, *22*, 1629-1641.

[137] Thennarasu, S.; Huang, R.; Lee, D. K.; Yang, P.; Maloy, L.; Chen, Z.; Ramamoorthy, A.: Limiting an antimicrobial peptide to the lipid-water interface enhances its bacterial membrane selectivity: A case study of MSI-367. *Biochemistry* **2010**, *49*, 10595-10605.

[138] Wiradharma, N.; Khoe, U.; Hauser, C. A. E.; Seow, S. V.; Zhang, S.: Synthetic cationic amphiphilic α-helical peptides as antimicrobial agents. *Biomaterials* **2011**, *32*, 2204-2212.

[139] Glukhov, E.; Burrows, L. L.; Deber, C.: Membrane interactions of designed cationic antimicrobial peptides: the two thresholds. *Biopolymers* **2008**, *89*, 360-371.

[140] Vasudev, P. G.; Chatterjee, S.; Shamala, N.; Balaram, P.: Structural chemistry of peptides containing backbone expanded amino acid residues: Conformational features of β φ and hydrid peptides. *Chemical Reviews* **2010**, *10.1021/cr100100x published online*.

[141] Grauer, A. A.; Konig, B.: Synthesis of new C^{α} tetrasubstituted a-amino acids. *Beilstein Journal of Organic Chemistry* **2009**, *5*, doi:10.3762/bjoc.5.5.

[142] Crisma, M.; Moretto, A.; De Zotti, M.; Formaggio, F.; Kaptein, B.; Broxtermen, Q. B.; Toniolo, C.: Turn stabilization in short peptides by C^{α}-methylated α-amino acids. *Biopolymers* **2005**, *80*, 279-293.

[143] Toniolo, C.; Crisma, M.; Formaggio, F.; Peggion, C.: Control of peptide conformation by the Thorpe-Ingold effect (C^{α}-tetrasubstitution). *Peptide Science* **2002**, *60*, 396-419.

[144] Taira, J.; Kida, Y.; Yamaguchi, H.; Kuwano, K.; Higashimoto, Y.; Kodama, H.: Modifications on amphiphilicity and cationicity of unnatural amino acid containing peptides for the improvement of antimicrobial activity against pathogenic bacteria. *J. Pept, Sci.*. **2010**, *16*, 607-612.

[145] Burgess, A. W.; Leach, S. J.: An obligatory alpha-helical amino acid residue. *Biopolymers* **1973**, 2599-2605.

[146] Sambeth, G. M.; Sussmuth, R. D.: Synthetic studies toward labionin, a new a,a-disubstituted amino acid from type III lantibotic labyrinthopeptin A2. *J. Pept, Sci.*. **2011**, *17*, 581-584.

[147] Goodman, M.; Shao, H.: Peptidomimetic building blocks for drug discovery:An overview. *Pure and Appl. Chem.* **1996**, *66*, 1303-1308.

[148] Hendrickson, T. L.; de Crecy-Lagard, V.; Schimmel, P.: Incorporation of nonnatural amino acids into proteins. *Annu. Rev. Biochem.* **2004**, *73*, 147-176.

[149] Ma, J. S.: Unnatural amino acids in drug discovery. *CHIMICA OGGI Chemistry Today* **2003**, 65-68.

[150] Oh, J. E.; Lee, K. H.: Synthesis of novel unnatural amino acid as a building block and its incorporation into an antimicrobial peptide. *Bioorganic & Medicinal Chemistry* **1999**, *7*, 2985-2990.

[151] Venugopal, D.; klapper, D.; Srouji, A.; Bhonsle, J. B.; Borschel, R.; Mueller, A.; Russell, A. L.; Williams, B. C.; Hicks, R. P.: Novel antimicribial peptides that exhibit activity against select agents and other drug resistant bacteria. *Bioorganic & Medicinal Chemistry* **2010**, *18*, 5137-5147.

[152] Hicks, R. P.; Russell, A. L.: Application of Unnatural Amino Acids to the *De Novo* Design of Selective Antibiotic Peptides. In *Unnatural Amino Acids: Methods and Protocols, Methods in Molecular Biology*; Pollegioni, L., Servi, S., Eds.; Springer, Science 2012; Vol. 794; pp 135-167.

[153] Dolinsky, T. J.; Czodrowski, P.; Li, H.; Nielsen, J. E.; Jensen, J. H.; Klebe, G.; Baker, N. A.; : PDB2PQR: Expanding and upgrading automated preparation of biomolecular structures for molecular simulations. *Nucleic Acids Res,* **2007**, *35*, W522-525.

[154] Dolinsky, T. J.; Nielsen, J. E.; McCammon, J. A.; Baker, N. A.: PDB2PQR: an automated pipeline for the setup, execution, and analysis of Poisson-Boltzmann electrostatics calculations. *Nucleic Acids Res,* **2004**, *32*, W665-667.

[155] Baker, N. A.; Sept, D.; Joseph, S.; Holst, M. J.; McCammon, J. A.: Electrostatics of nanosystems: application to microtubules and the ribosome. *Proc. Natl. Acad. Sci. USA* **2001**, *98*, 10037-10041.

[156] Tossi, A.; Sandri, L.; Giangaspero, A.: New consensus hydrophobicity scale extended to non-proteinogenic amino acids. In *Proceeding of the 27th European Peptide Symposium Sorrento*; Benedetti, E., Pedone, C., Eds.; Edizioni Ziino: Napoli, Italy, 2002.

[157] Park, S.-C.; Park, Y.; Hahm, K.-S.: The role of antimicrobial peptides in preventing multidrug-resistant bacterial infections and biofilms. *Int. J. Mol. Sci.* **2011**, *12*, 5971-5992.

[158] Dashper, S. G.; Liu, S. W.; Reynolds, E. C.: Antimicrobial peptides and their potential as oral therapeutic agents. *Int. J. Pept. Res.Therapetics* **2007**, *13*, 505-516.

[159] Tao, R.; Tong, Z.; Lin, Y.; Xue, Y.; Wang, W.; Kuang, R.; Wang, P.; Tian, Y.; Ni, L.: Antimicrobial and antibiofilm activity of pleurocidin against cariogenic microorganisms. *Peptides* **2011**, *32*, 1748-1754.

[160] Leung, K. P.; Crowe, T. D.; Abercrombie, J. J.; Molina, C. M.; Bradshaw, C. J.; Jensen, C. L.; Luo, Q.; Thompson, G. A.: Control of oral biofilm formation by antimicrobial decapeptides. *J. Dent. Res,* **2005**, *84*, 1172-1177.

[161] Madhuri; Shireen, T.; Venugopal, S. K.; Ghosh, D.; Gadepalli, R.; Dhawan, B.; Mukhopadhyay, K.: *In vitro* antimicrobial activity of alpha-melanocyte stimulating hormone against major human pathogen *Staphylococcus aureus*. *Peptides* **2009**, *30*, 1627-1635.

[162] Pompilio, A.; Scocchi, M.; Pomponio, S.; Guida, F.; Di Primio, A.; Fiscarelli, E.; Gennaro, R.; Di Bonaventura, G.: Antibacterial and anti-biofilm effects of cathelicidin peptides agains pathogens isolated from cystic fibrosis patients. *Peptides* **2011**, *32*, 1807-1814.

[163] Mai, J.; Tian, X.-L.; Gallant, J. W.; Merkley, N.; Biswas, Z.; Syvitski, R.; Douglas, S. E.; Ling, J.; Li, Y.-H.: A novel target-speciific, salt-resistant antimicrobial peptide against the cariogenic pathogen *streptococcus* mutans. *Antimicrob. Agents Chemother.* **2011**, *55*, 5205-5213.

[164] Flemming, K.; Klingenberg, C.; Cavanagh, J. P.; Sletteng, M.; Stensen, W.; Svenden, J. S.; Flaegstad, T.: High *in vitro* antimicrobial activity of synthetic antimicrobial peptidomimetics against *staphylococcal* biofilms. *J. Antimicrob. Chemother.* **2009**, *63*, 136-145.

[165] Marsh, P. D.: Dental plaque: biological significance of a biofilm and community life-style. *J Clin Periodontol.* **2005**, *32 Suppl 6*, 7-15.

[166] Sutherland, I. W.: Biofilm exopolysaccharides:strong and sticky framework. *Microbiology* **2001**, *147*, 3-9.

[167] Sutherland, I. W.: The biofilm matrix-an immobilized but dynamic microbial environment. *Trends Microbiol.* **2001**, *9*, 222-227.

[168] Hicks, R. P.; Mones, E.; Kim, H.; Koser, B. W.; Nichols, D. A.; Bhattacharjee, A. K.: Comparison of the conformation and electrostatic surface properties of magainin peptides bound to SDS and DPC micelles: Insight into possible modes on antimicrobial activity. *Biopolymers* **2003**, *68*, 459-470.

[169] Russell, A. L.; Kennedy, A. M.; Spuches, A.; Venugopal, D.; Bhonsle, J. B.; Hicks, R. P.: Spectroscopic and thermodynamic evidence for antimicrobial peptide membrane selectivity. *Chem. Phys. Lipids* **2010**, *163*, 488-497.

[170] Tossi, A.; Sandri, L.; Giangaspero, A.: Amphipathic a-helical antimicrobial peptides. *Biopolymers* **2000**, *55*, 4-30.

[171] Taira, J.; Furukawa, S.; Hatakeyama, T.; Aoyagi, H.; Kodama, H.: Modification of hydrophobic value and hydrophobic moment value of cationic model peptides for conversion of peptide-membrane interactions. *Bull. Chemm. Soc. Jpn.* **2008**, *81*, 733-739.

[172] Fernandez-Lopez, S.; Kim, H. S.; Choi, E. C.; Delgado, M.; Granja, J. R.; Khasanov, A.; Kraehenbuehi, K.; Long, G.; Weinberger, D. A.; Wilcoxen, K. M.; Ghadiri, M. R.: Antibacterial agents based on the cyclic D,L -a-peptide architecture. *Nature* **2001**, *412*, 452-455.

[173] Yang, L.; Weiss, T. M.; Lehrer, R. I.; Huang, H. W.: Crystallization of antimicrobial pores in membranes: magainin and protegrin. *Biochemical J.* **2000**, *79*, 2002-2009.

[174] Jing, W.; Hunter, H. N.; Hagel, J.; Vogel, H. J.: The structure of the antimicrobial peptide Ac-RRWWRF-NH_2 bound to micelles and its interactions with phospholipid bilayers. *J. Pept. Res.* **2003**, *61*, 219-229.

[175] Watson, R. M.; Woody, R. W.; Lewis, R. V.; Bohle, D. S.; Andreotti, A. H.; Ray, B.; Miller, K. W.: Conformational changes in pediocin AcH upon vesicle binding and approximation of the membrane-bound structure in detergent micelles. *Biochemistry* **2001**, *40*, 14037-14046.

[176] Russell, A., L.; Klapper, D.; Srouji, A. H.; Bhonsle, J. B.; Borschel, R.; Mueller, A.; Hicks, R. P.: The design of bacteria strain selective antimicrobial peptides based on the incorporation of unnatural amino acids. In *Antibacterial Agents/ Book 2*; Bobbarala, V., Ed.; InTech Publishing, 2012; Vol. ISBN 979-953-307-747-4.

[177] Russell, A. L.; Kennedy, A. M.; Spuches, A. M.; Gibson, W. S.; Venugopal, D.; Klapper, D.; Srouji, A. H.; Bhonsle, J. B.; Hicks, R. P.: Determining the Effect of the Incorporation of Unnatural Amino Acids into Antimicrobial Peptides on the Interactions with

Zwitterionic and Anionic Membrane Model Systems. *Chemistry and Physics of Lipids* **2011**, *164*, 740-758.

[178] Russell, A. L.; Williams, B. C.; Spuches, A.; Klapper, D.; Srouji, A. H.; Hicks, R. P.: The role played by charge density and proximity to the peptide backbone on the binding interactions that occur between Antimicrobial Peptides containing unnatural amino acids and zwitterionic and anionic liposomes. *Bioorganic Medicinal Chemistry,* **2012**, *20*, 1723-1739.

[179] Russell, A., L.; Spuches, A. M.; Williams, B.; Venugopal, D.; Klapper, D.; Srouji, A. H.; Hicks, R. P.: The effect of the placement and total charge of the basic amino acid clusters on antibacterial organism selectivity and potency′ *Bioorg. Med. Chem.* **2011**, *19*, 7008-7022.

[180] De Lucca, A. J.; Walsh, T. J.: Antifungal Peptides: Novel Therapeutic Compounds against Emerging Pathogens, *Antimicrob.l Agents Chemother.* **1999**, *43*, 1-11.

[181] Qi, X.; Zhou, C.; Li, P.; Xu, W.; Cao, Y.; Ling, H.; Chen, W. N.; Li, C. M.; Xu, R.; Lamrani, M.; Mu, Y.; Leong, S. S. J.; Chang, M. W.; Chan-Park, M. B.: Novel short antibacterial and antifungal peptides with low cytotoxicity: Efficacy and action mechanisms. *Biochem. Biophys. Res. Commun.* **2010**, *398*, 594-600.

[182] Sung, W. S.; Lee, D. G.; Pleurocidin-derived antifungal peptides with selective membrane-disruption effect, *Biochem. Biophys.l Res. Commun.* **2008**, *369*, 858-861.

[183] Matejuk, A.; Leng, Q.; Begum, M. D.; Woodle, M. C.; Scaria, P.; Chou, S.-T.; Mixson, A. J.: Peptide-based antifungal therapies against emerging infections. *Drugs Fut.* **2010**, *35*, 197-217.

[184] Moradi, S.; Soltani, S.; Ansari, A. M.; Sardari., S.: Peptidomimetics and their applications in antifungal drug. *Anti-Infective Agents Med. Chem.* **2009**, *8*, 327-344.

[185] Arikan, S.; R. J. H. New agents for treatment of systemic fungal infections *Expert Opinion on Emerging Drugs* **2000**, *5*, 135-160.

[186] Soltani, S.; Keymanesh, K.; Sardari, S.: *In silico* analysis of antifungal peptides. *J Expert Opin. Drug Discov.* **2007**, *7*, 837-847.

[187] Zhang, Z. T.; Zhu, S.: Functional role of charged residues in drosomycin, a Drosophila antifungal peptide,. *Develop. Compar. Immunol.* **2010**, *34*, 953-958.

[188] Landon, C.; Florent Barbault, F.; Legrain, M.; Menin, L.; Guenneugues, M.; Schott, V.; Vovelle, F.; Dimarcq, J.-L.: Lead optimization of antifungal peptides with 3D NMR structures analysis *Protein Sci.* **2004**, *13*, 703-713.

[189] Di Marino, S.; Scrima, M.; Grimaldi, M.; D'Errico, G.; Vitiello, G.; Sanguinetti, M.; De Rosa, M.; Soriente, A.; E., N.; D'Ursi, A. M.: Antifungal peptides at membrane interaction. *Eur. J. Med. Chem.* **2012**, *51*, 154-162.

[190] Brouwer, C. P. J. M.; Rahman, M.; Welling, M. M.; : Discovery and development of a synthetic peptide derived from lactoferrin for clinical use. *Peptides* **2011**, *32*, 1953-1963.

[191] De Brucker, K.; Cammue, B. P. A.; Thevissen, K.: Apoptosis-inducing antifungal peptides and proteins. *Biochem. Soc. Trans.,* **2011**, *39*, 1527-1532.

[192] Williams, D. A.; Lemke, T. L.: *Foye's principles of medicinal chemistry, ch36. Antifungal Drugs, 891-903.*

[193] Mulder, M. P. C.; Kruinjtzer, J. A. W.; Breukink, E. J.; Kemmink, J.; Pieters, R. J.; Liskamp, R. M. J.: Synthesis and evaluation of novel macrocyclic antifungal peptides. *Bioorg. Med. Chem.* **2011**, *19*, 6505-6517.

[194] Olivella, M. S.; Rodríguez, A. M.; Zacchino, S. A.; Somlai, C.; Penke, B.; Farkas, V.; Perczel, A.; Enriz, R. D.: New antifungal peptides. Synthesis, bioassays and initial structure prediction by CD spectroscopy. *Bioorganic & Medicinal Chemistry Letters* **2010**, *20*, 4808-4811.

[195] Bun Ng, T.; Wong, J. H.: A review of antifungal and antiviral Proteins. *Novel Therapeutic Agents from Plants* **2009**, 208-238.

[196] Jiang, Z.; Jan Kullberg, B.; van der Lee, H.; Vasil, A. I.; Hale, J. D.; Mant, C. T.; Hancock, R. E. W.; Vasil, M. L.; Netea, M. G.; Hodges, R. S.: Effects of Hydrophobicity on the Antifungal Activity of α-Helical Antimicrobial Peptides. *Chem.Biol. Drug Des.* **2008**, *72*, 483-495.

[197] Zhang, Z. T.; Zhu, S., Y.: Drosomycin an essential component of antifungal defence in drosophila. *Insect. Mol. Biol.* **2009**, *18*, 549-556.

[198] Martínez, J. P.; Falomir, M. P.; Gozalbo, D.: *Chitin: A Structural Biopolysaccharide*John Wiley & Sons, Ltd, 2009, 2009.

[199] Lass-Flörl, C.: Update in Drug Development, Antifungal. In *22nd European Congress of Clinical Microbiology and Infectious diseases (ECCMID)*. 2012.

[200] Medina, M. L.; Chapman, B. S.; Bolender, J. P.; Plesniak, L. A.: Transient vesicle leakage initiated by synthetic apoptotic peptides derived from the death domain of neurotrophin receptor p75NTR. *J. Pept, Sci.* **2002**, *59*, 149-158.

[201] Wieprecht, T.; Beyermann, M.; Seelig, J.: Binding of Antibacterial Magainin Peptides to Electrically Neutral Membranes: Thermodynamics and Structure. *Biochemistry* **1999**, *38*, 10377-10387.

[202] Mason, A. J.; Marquette, A.; Bechinger, B.: Zwitterionic phospholipids and sterols modulate antimicrobial peptide-induced membrane destabilization. *Biophysical J.* **2007**, *93*, 4289-4299.

[203] Bringezu, F.; Wen, S.; Dante, S.; Hauss, T.; Majerowicz, M.; Waring, A.: The insertion of the antimicrobial peptide dicynthaurin monomer in model membranes: thermodynamic and structural characterization. *Biochemistry* **2007**, *46*, 5678-5686.

[204] Wieprecht, T.; Apostolov, O.; Seelig, J.: Binding of the antibacterial peptide magainin 2 amide to small and large unilamellar vesicles. *Biophysical Chem.* **2000**, *85*, 187-198.

[205] Ladokhin, A. S.; Vidal, M. F.; White, S. H.: CD spectroscopy of peptides and proteins bound to large unilamellar vesicles. *J. Membrane Biol.* **2010**, *236*, 247-253.

[206] Seelig, J.; Ganz, P.: Nonclassical hydrophobic effect in membrane binding equilibria. *Biochemistry* **1991**, *30*, 9354-9359.

[207] Ladokhin, A. S.; Jayasinghe, S.; White, S. H.: How to measure and analyze tryptophan fluorescence in membranes properly, and why bother? *Anal. Biochem.* **2000**, *285*, 235-245.

[208] Wieprecht, T.; Apostolov, O.; Beyermann, M.; Seelig, J.: Membrane binding and pore formation of the antibacterial paprtide PGLa: thermodynamic and mechanistic aspects. *Biochemistry* **2000**, 442-452.

[209] Lee, D. G.; Park, Y.; Jin, I.; Hahm, K.-S.; Lee, H.-H.; Moon, Y.-H.; Woo, E.-R.: Structure-antiviral activity relationships of cecropin A-magainin 2 hybrid peptide and its analogues. *J. Peptide Sci.* **2004**, *10*, 298-303.

[210] Chen, F.-Y.; Lee, M.-T.; Huang, H. W.: Evidence for membrane thinining effect as the mechanism for peptide-induced pore formation. *Biophys. J.* **2003**, *84*, 3751-3758.

[211] Lee, M.-T.; Hung, W.-C.; Chen, F.-Y.; Huang, H. W.: Mechanism and kinetics of pore formation in membrane by water-soluble amphipathic peptides. *PNAS* **2008**, *105*, 5087-5092.

[212] Almeida, P. F.; Pokorny, A.: Mechanisms of antimicrobial, cytolytic, and cell-penetrating peptides: from kinetics to thermodynamics. *Biochemistry* **2009**, *48*, 8083-8093.

[213] Seelig, J.: Titration calorimetry of lipid-peptide interactions. *Biochimica et Biophysica Acta* **1997**, *1331*, 103-116.

[214] Wei, S.-T.: Solution Structure of a Novel Tryptophan-Rich Peptide with Bidirectional Antimicrobial Activity. *J. Bacteriol.* **2006**, *188*, 328-334.

[215] Hunter, H. N.; Jing, W.; Schibli, D. J.; Trinh, T.; Park, I. Y.; Kim, S. C.; Vogel, H. J.: The interactions of antimicrobial peptides derived from lysozyme with model membrane systems. *Biochimica et Biophysica Acta,* **2005**, *1668*, 175-189.

[216] Wieprecht, T.; Beyermann, M.; Seelig, J.: Thermodynamics of the coil a-helix transition of amphipathic peptides in a membrane environment: role of vesicle curvature. *Biophysical Chem.* **2002**, *96*, 191-201.

[217] Wieprecht, T.; Seelig, J.: Isothermal titration calorimetry for studying interactions between peptides and lipid membranes. In *Peptide-Lipid Interactions*; Simon, S. A., McIntosh, T. J., Eds.; Academic Press: San Diego, 2002; Vol. Current Topics in Membranes, ; pp 32-58.

[218] Wen, S.: Dicynthaurin (ala) Monomer Interaction with Phospholipid Bilayers Studied by Fluorescence Leakages and Isothermal Titration Calorimetry. *J. Phys. Chem.* **2007**, *111*, 6280-6287.

[219] Kennedy, A.; Hmel, P. J.; Seelbaugh, J.; Quiles, J. Q.; Hicks, R. P.; Reid, T. J.: Characterization of the main phase transition in 1,2-dipalmitoylphosphateidylcholine LUV's by 1H NMR. *J. Liposome Res.* **2002**, *12*, 221-237.

[220] Wieprecht, T.; Dathe, M.; Schumann, M.; Krause, E.; Beyermann, M.; Bienert, M.: Conformation and functional study of magainin 2 in model membrane environment using the new approach of systematic double D-amino acid replacement. *Biochemistry* **1996**, 10844-10853.

[221] Tamba, Y.; Yamazaki, M.: Single Giant Unilamellar Vesicle Method Reveals Effect of Antimicrobial Peptide Magainin 2 on Membrane Permeability. *Biochemistry* **2005**, *44*, 15823-15833.

[222] Benachir, T.; Lafleur, M.: Study of vesicle leakage induced by melittin. *Biochimica et Biophysica Acta* **1995**, *1235*, 452-460.

[223] Tachi T; Epand RF; Epand RM; K., M.: Position-dependent hydrophobicity of the antimicrobial magainin peptide affects the mode of peptide lipid interactions and selective toxicity. *Biochemistry* **2002** *41*, 10723-10731.

[224] Glattli, A.; Daura, X.; Seebach, D.; van Gunsteren, W. F.: Can one derive the conformational preference of a β-peptide from its CD spectrum. *JACS* **2002**, *124*, 12972-12978.

[225] Ladokhin, A. S.; Selsted, M. E.; White, S. H.: CD spectra of indolicidin antimicrobial peptides suggest turns, not polyproline helix. *Biochemistry* **1999**, *38*, 12313-12319.

[226] Huang, C. H.: Studies on phosphatidylcholine vesicles. Formation and physical characteristics. *Biochemistry* **1969**, *8*, 344-352.

[227] Schmidt, C. F.; Lichtenberg, D.; Thompson, T. E.: Vesicle-vesicle interactions in sonicated dispersions of dipalmitoylphosphatidylcholine. *Biochemistry* **1981**, *20*, 4792-4797.

[228] Wong, M.; Anthony, F. H.; Tillack, T. W.; Thompson, T. E.: Fusion of dipalmintoylphosphatidylcholine vesicles at 4 C. *Biochemistry* **1982**, *21*, 4126-4132.
[229] Berova, N.; Nakanishi, K.; Woody, R. W.: *Circular Dichroism Principles and Applications*; Wiley-VCH: New York, 2000.
[230] Thomas, C. J.; Surolia, N.; Surolia, A.: Kinetic and thermodynamic analysis of the interactions of 23-residue peptides with endotoxin. *J. Biol. Chem.* **2001**, *276*, 35701-35706.
[231] Seelig, J.; Nebel, S.; Ganz, P.; Bruns, C.: Electrostatic and nonpolar peptide-membrane interactions. lipid binding and functional properties of somatostatin analogs of charge z = +1 to z = +3. *Biochemistry* **1993**, *32*, 9714-9721.
[232] Beschiaschvili, G.; Seelig, J.: Peptide binding to lipid bilayers. binding isotherms and .zeta.-potential of a cyclic somatostatin analog. *Biochemistry* **1990** *29*, 10995-11000.
[233] Andrushchenko, V. V.; Aarabi, M. H.; Nquyen, L. T.; Prenner, E. J.; Vogel, H. J.: Thermodynamics of the interaction of tryptophan-rich cathelicidin antimicrobial peptides with model and natural membranes. *Biochimica et Biophysica Acta* **2008**, *1778*, 1004-1014.
[234] Abraham, T.; Lewis, R. N. A. H.; Hodges, R. S.; McElhaney, R. N.: Isothermal titration calorimetry studies of the binding of the antimicrobial peptide gramicidin S to phospholipid bilayer membranes. *Biochemistry* **2005**, *44*, 11279-11285.
[235] Jelokhani-Niaraki, M.; Hodges, R. S.; Meissner, J. E.; Hassenstein, U. E.; Wheaton, L.: Interaction of gramicidin S and its aromatic amino acid analoques with phospholipid membranes. *Biophys. J.* **2008**, *95*, 3306-3321.
[236] Epand, R. M.; Segrest, J. P.; Anantharamaiah, G. M.: Thermodynamics of the binding of human apolipoprotein A-1 to dimyristoylphosphatidylglycerol. *J. Biol. Chem.* **1990**, *265*, 20829-20832.

Frontiers in Anti-Infective Drug Discovery, Vol. 2, 2014, 159-223

CHAPTER 3

Natural Products as Anti-Infective Agents

Sidharth Chopra[1,*], Ellen D. Beaulieu[2] and Jeremiah P. Malerich[2]

[1]Central Drug Research Institute, Lucknow, UP, India; [2]SRI International, Biosciences Division, Menlo Park, CA, USA

Abstract: Natural products have historically been a rich source of the active ingredients of drugs, especially as anti-infective agents. Natural products provide valuable scaffolds for lead optimization since they are potent, soluble, bioavailable, targeted therapies for many indications. In the wake of a de-emphasis of natural product research in the private sector, the current pipeline for anti-infectives is dwindling. New technologies in natural product isolation, synthesis, and screening in the post genomic era have provided valuable new leads for drug discovery. This chapter describes anti-bacterial, anti-viral, and anti-parasitic therapeutics approved by the FDA since 2005 as well as compounds in clinical development that are natural products or are bioinspired. The chapter also describes new technologies that can accelerate the future discovery of natural anti-infectives.

Keywords: Natural products, MRSA, ESKAPE pathogens, drug discovery, antibiotic, anti-viral, influenza, HIV, anti-fungal, anti-malarial, endoperoxide, synthetic biology.

INTRODUCTION

Natural products hold a critical position in the history of medicinal treatment of disease, particularly microbial infection. While the role of natural products in drug discovery has shifted over the last generation, natural products remain a rich source of new therapeutic compounds and inspiration for medicinal chemists. In general we consider natural products to be discrete and well-characterized secondary metabolites, *i.e.*, biosynthetic compounds outside of the fundamental lipid, protein, carbohydrate, and nucleic acid pathways. This statement should be considered a generality and not a rigid definition.

***Address correspondence to Sidharth Chopra:** Department of Microbiology, Central Drug Research Institute, Lucknow-226022, India; Tel: +91-979 22 11636; E-mail: skchopra007@gmail.com

Atta-ur-Rahman / M. Iqbal Choudhary (Eds.)

Despite the historical success of natural products, advances in science and technology have brought wholly synthetic compounds to the fore of drug discovery. The rise of HTS capabilities enables discovery efforts to evaluate thousands to millions of compounds. These quantities are orders of magnitude larger than the number of natural products and analogs that can be isolated or synthesized. These large non-natural compound libraries are generated by combinatorial chemistry, which enables the rapid synthesis of related analogs. The synthesis of natural products typically requires many operations and is rarely amenable to parallel synthesis techniques. Their isolation from natural sources or from fermentation can be challenging in reproducibility and the high fidelity necessary for APIs. As such, pharmaceutical investment in isolation of new bioactive natural products has dwindled [1]. However, while the investment in natural products isolation may provide an inferior quantity of compounds to screen, investment is rewarded in the quality of those compounds. Natural products offer a richness of structural diversity. Natural products cover a larger region of chemical space than totally synthetic compounds from combinatorial approaches [2]. Furthermore, since they evolved in a natural context, they are predisposed to have favorable drug-like properties such as solubility and bioavailability. In Lipinski's rules, natural products routinely break the guidelines recognized for synthetic compounds, such as molecular weight and lipophilicity, and instead occupy an entirely separate category. For anti-infective indications, natural products are even more suitable. Secondary metabolites are nature's weapons in the chemical warfare between organisms for survival. With these considerations in mind, it is no surprise that over the period 1981-2010, 65% of anti-infective drugs approved by the FDA are natural products or natural product inspired [3].

This chapter reviews anti-infective drugs that have entered the market or clinical trials in the period 2005-2012 that are secondary metabolite themselves, direct derivatives of natural products, and analogs inspired by natural products. Two special sections describe examples of enabling technologies in natural product research: (1) a new strategy for identification of antibiotic natural products and (2) the use of synthetic biology to produce the first-line antimalarial artemisinin.

ANTI-BACTERIAL COMPOUNDS

Introduction

The discovery and development of antibiotics (*e.g.*, sulfonamides and β-lactams) in the early 1930s revolutionized healthcare. For the first time, potentially fatal bacterial infections could be treated. As with the earliest antibiotics, the majority of antibiotics discovered have been natural products or their synthetic derivatives. This chapter details the discovery and developments of newer natural products or bioinspired anti-infectives approved by the FDA since 2005. The earlier period has been well documented [4]. These are listed below based on their mechanism of action or microbial target.

Peptidoglycan Biosynthesis and Cell Membrane Integrity Inhibitors

Peptidoglycan biosynthesis is a bacterial process distinct from mammalian hosts. Clinical agents used to inhibit this process include glycolipodepsipeptides (ramoplanin), carbapenems (biapenem, ertapenem, doripenem, and tebipenem) and cephalosporins (ceftobiprole, ceftaroline, and CXA-101).

Ramoplanin-A_2, developed by Nanotherapeutics, is a glycolipodepsipeptide produced by *Actinoplanes* sp. (Fig. **1**) first described in 1984 by Gruppo Lepetit [5-9]. Ramoplanin-A_2 blocks bacterial cell wall biosynthesis by inhibiting the *N*-acetylglucosaminyltransferase-catalysed conversion of lipid intermediate I to lipid intermediate II prior to transglycosylation and transpeptidation reactions [10]. However, its mechanism of action is distinct from that of glycopeptides as it does not complex with the D-Ala–D-Ala sequence of cell wall precursors [10]. This compound has been evaluated in Phase II trials for both treatment of enteric infection from vancomycin-resistant enterococci and CD associated diarrhea, due to its lack of systemic absorption through oral dosage [11].

Teicoplanin (Targocid), developed by Sanofi-Aventis, is a glycopeptide antibiotic extracted from *Actinoplanes teichomyceticus* with a similar spectrum of activity to vancomycin. It inhibits bacterial cell wall synthesis at an orthogonal site from that of β-lactams. Therefore, teicoplanin is effective against MRSA, β-lactam resistant

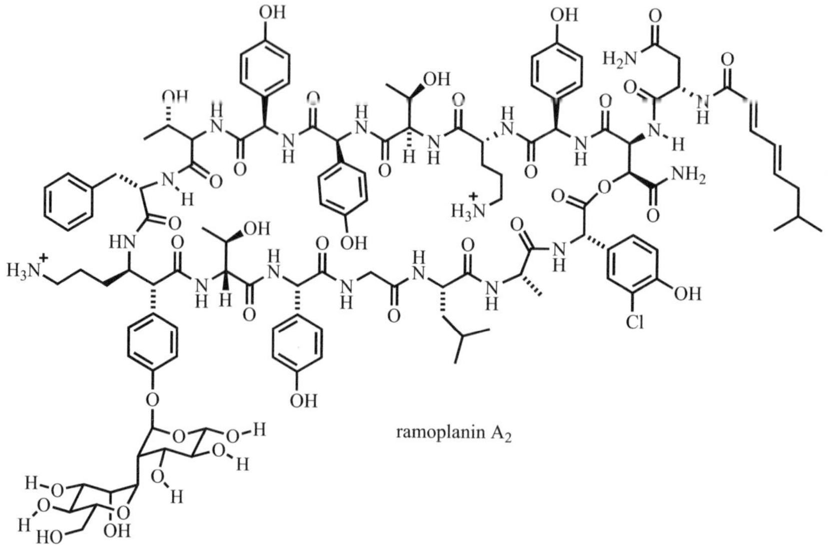

Fig. (1). Structure of ramoplanin A_2, a glycolipodepsiptide inhibitor of peptidoglycan biosynthesis.

streptococci, and *E. faecalis*, and it has comparable efficacy to vancomycin in curing pseudomembranous colitis caused by CD [12]. Teicoplanin does not show cross-resistance to β-lactam antibiotics, macrolides, aminoglycosides, tetracycline, rifampicin or chloramphenicol [13]. Chemically, teicoplanin consists of a mixture of several compounds, namely five major components (teicoplanins A_{2-1} to A_{2-5}, Fig. **2**) and 4 minor components (teicoplanins R_{S-1} to R_{S-5}) [14].

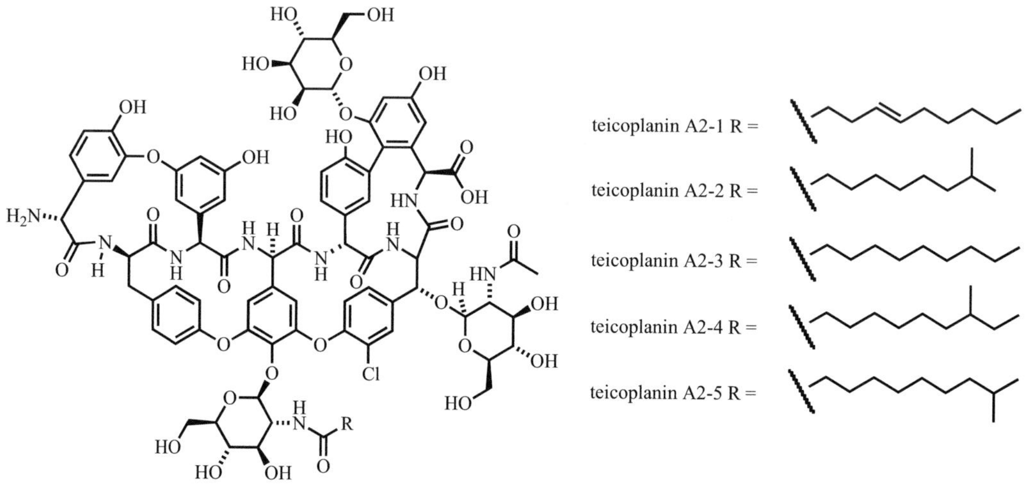

Fig. (2). Structures of the teicoplanins, a natural mixture of inhibitors of cell wall synthesis.

Biapenem, ertapenem, doripenem and tebipenem belong to the carbapenem class of antibiotics. These are synthetic derivatives of thienamycin, a secondary metabolite of *Streptomyces cattleya* (Fig. **3**) [15]. Biapenem (L-627) developed by Lederle is a parenteral carbapenem with potent activity against a wide panel of bacteria including anaerobes [16]. It is also stable to human renal dehydropeptidase I and therefore does not require the co-administration of a dehydropeptidase I enzyme inhibitor [17]. Ertapenem and doripenem are broad-spectrum carbapenems active against Gram-positive, Gram-negative, and anaerobic bacteria. Ertapenem was developed to improve carbapenem bioavailability. The compound has superior protein binding with concomitant increase in the half-life of the drug making it efficacious with once daily dosing [18]. Doripenem (S-4661) developed by Shinogi Company, Japan in collaboration with Johnson & Johnson is a potent agent against *P. aeruginosa* [19]. However, all the carbapenems are only available as parenteral formulations. To add to the diversity in the field, tebipenem pivoxil (L-084, ME1211), developed by Meiji Seika Kaisha (Japan), is a novel orally bioavailable carbapenem developed to treat drug-resistant *S. pneumonia* causing otolaryngologic and respiratory infections in pediatric patients [20]. Tebipenem pivoxil is a pro-drug of tebipenem to improve its intestinal absorption [21]. Tebipenem was approved for human use in Japan in 2009 but it yet to be approved in the US or Europe.

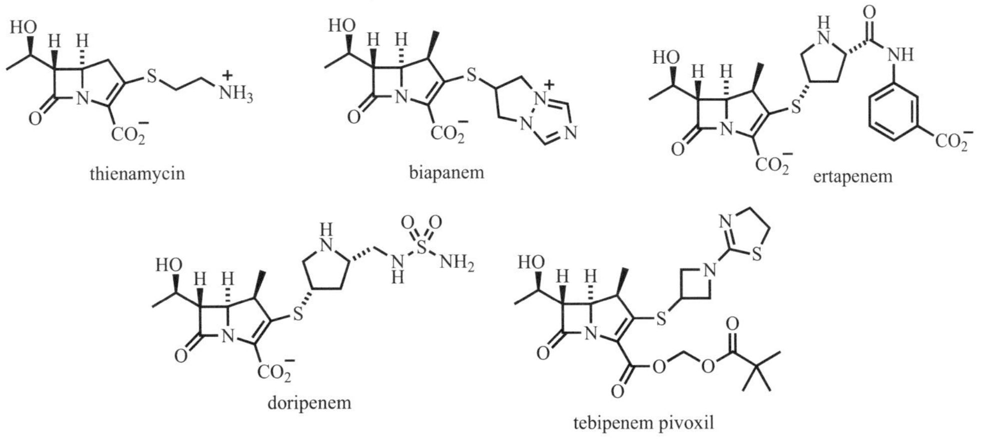

Fig. (3). Structures of carbapenem inhibitors of peptidoclycan synthesis.

Ceftobiprole, ceftaroline, and CXA-101 (Fig. **4**) are cephalosporins that were originally isolated from fungus *Acremonium* (previously known as

Cephalosporium). Ceftobiprole (Zeftera, RO0639141-000, BAL9141) discovered by Basiliea Pharmaceuticals and developed by Johnson & Johnson Pharmaceuticals, is a parenteral, extended spectrum cephalosporin currently in a Phase III clinical trial for treatment of CSSSI caused by Gram-positive and Gram-negative bacteria [22]. It was designed to be resistant to *S. aureus* β-lactamase and inhibits transpeptidation by penicillin binding proteins leading to cell death [23]. Ceftobiprole medocaril is a water-soluble prodrug developed to improve parenteral administration, which is then rapidly converted to ceftobiprole, diacetyl, and carbon dioxide [24].

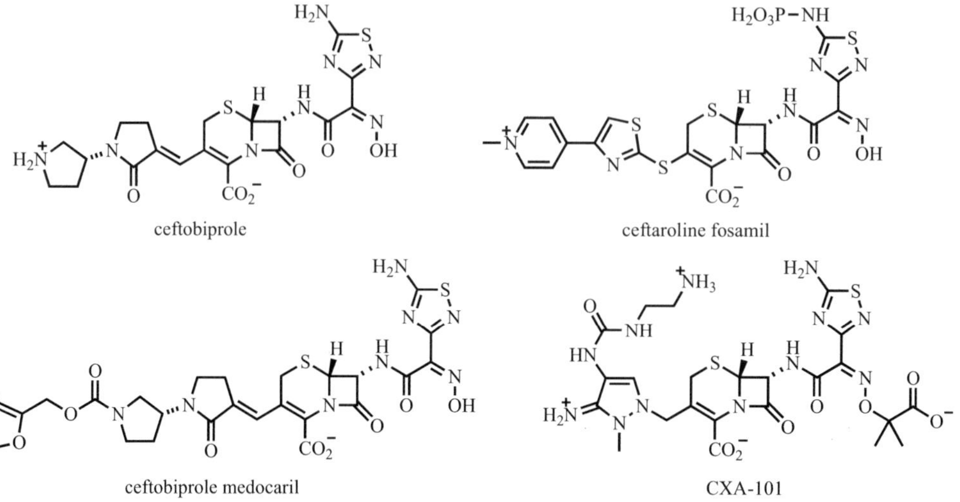

Fig. (4). Structures of cephalosporin inhibitors of cell wall biosynthesis.

Ceftaroline, (Teflaro, PPI-0903), developed by Forest Laboratories, is a novel, bactericidal, broad-spectrum oxyimino cephalosporin possessing a similar spectrum as ceftobiprole. It was evaluated in the clinic for treatment of ABSSI caused by susceptible Gram-positive and Gram-negative bacteria, including MRSA and for CABP caused by *Streptococcus pneumoniae*, MSSA, *Escherichia coli*, *Klebsiella pneumonia*, and *Klebsiella oxytoca* and was approved by the FDA in 2010 [25]. Ceftaroline binds to PBP2a (a MRSA specific PBP) for which most of the other β-lactams have low affinity [25]. The phosphate prodrug ceftaroline fosamil is rapidly converted to ceftaroline *in vivo* by plasma phosphatases. In a

Phase III clinical trial, it was noninferior to vancomycin and aztreonam in treating CSSSI [26].

Additionally, CXA-101, (FR264205, ceftolozane), developed by Cubist, is a novel cephalosporin for the treatment of complicated IAI caused by Gram-negative pathogens including MDR *Pseudomonas aeruginosa*, *E. coli*, and *Klebsiella pneumonia* [27]. CXA-101 possesses excellent anti-psuedomonal activity since it evades several resistance mechanisms employed by *P. aeruginosa* [28-30]. It has a similar spectrum of activity to other cephalosporins and is currently in a Phase III clinical trial for cUTI and cIAI as CXA-201, a combination of CXA-101 and tazobactam, a β-lactamase inhibitor [27].

Cell Membrane Inhibitors

After peptidoglycan biosynthesis, disruption of the cell membrane is one of the most common targets for antimicrobial drugs. A number of natural products target the cell membrane including PMX-30063, lotilibcin, XF-73, and PM181104 (Fig. **5**). One of the major advantages of membrane targeting drugs is their low propensity for resistance, which extends the therapeutic lifetime of the drug.

PMX-30063 (Brilacidin), jointly developed by University of Pennsylvania and PolyMedix, is a membrane active antimicrobial defensin-mimetic that is bactericidal against both Gram-positive and Gram-negative bacteria [31-34]. It is being investigated in an IV formulation for the treatment of MRSA [35, 36]. This compound was effective in Phase II clinical trials for the treatment of ABSSSI caused by *Staphylococcus aureus*, including MRSA [37]. It exhibited a very low propensity for resistance development [36].

Lotilibcin (WAP-8294A_2), developed by Rigen Pharmaceuticals, is a novel depsipeptide antibiotic and a major component of WAP-8294 antibacterial complex produced by Gram-negative bacteria *Lysobacter* sp. [38]. It has a narrow spectrum of activity but is a rapid bactericidal agent against MRSA infections, including SSSI, pneumonia, bacterial endocarditis, and ostemyelitis [39]. Lotilibcin damages the bacterial cell membrane putatively *via* interaction with phospholipids [40-42], and this novel mode of action and activity against resistant strains make it a valuable lead for clinical development. It is being developed in an IV formulation for a Phase I trial with Green Cross Corporation, Korea.

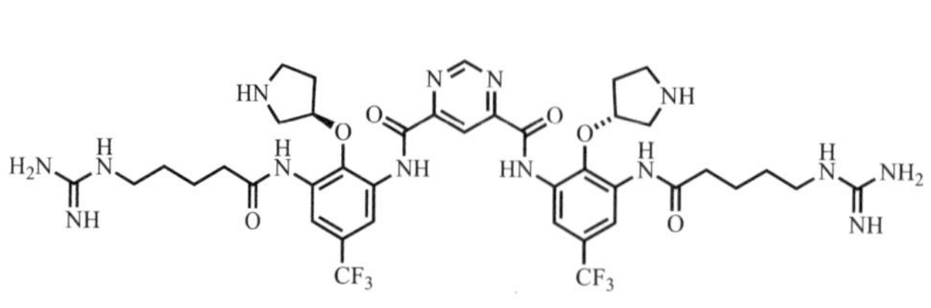

PMX 30063

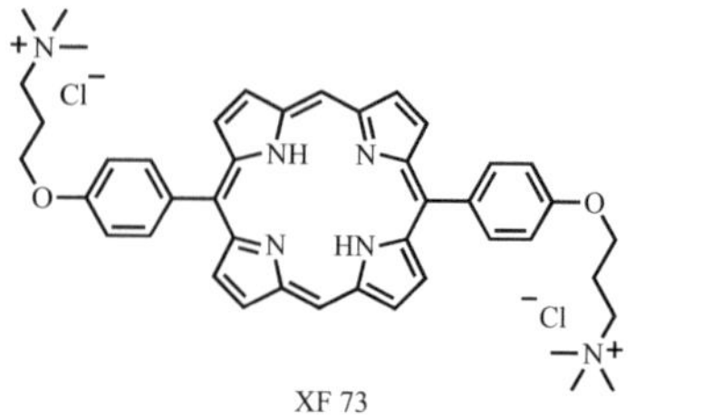

XF 73

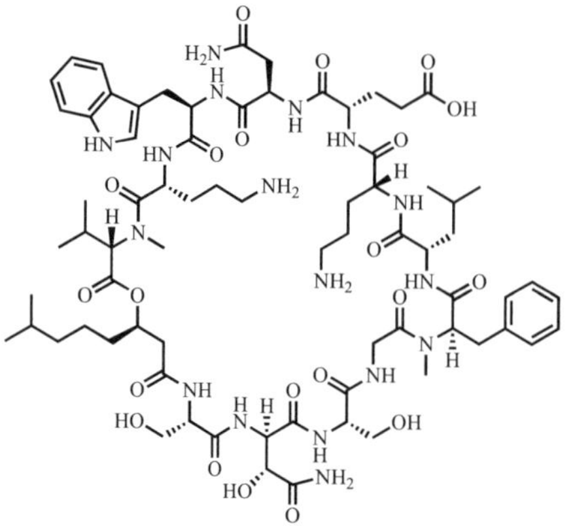

lotilibcin

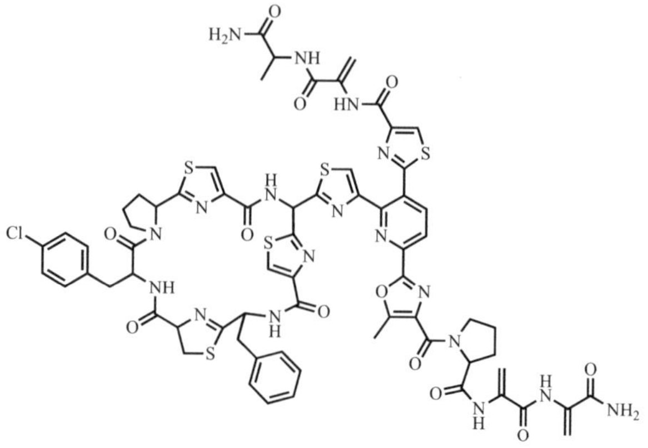

PM 181104
(stereochemistry not reported)

Fig. (5). Structures of cell membrane inhibitors.

XF-73, developed by Destiny Pharma, is a dicationic porphyrin derivative active against drug-resistant Gram-positive pathogens. XF-73 putatively perturbs the cytoplasmic membrane causing a rapid loss of potassium ions and ATP, disrupting the proper function of membrane-bound proteins [43-46]. This mechanism raises the barrier to resistance as viable resistant mutants are challenging to select even during prolonged laboratory subculture in the presence of compound [47]. The preclinical development program for XF-73 included evaluation as a treatment of ulcers, promotion of wound healing, and for CD infections [48, 49]. It was successfully evaluated in a Phase I trial for nasal decolonization of MRSA [50].

Interestingly, some of the antimicrobial natural products have dual modes of action targeting both the peptidoglycan biosynthesis and cell membrane integrity at the same time. These molecules include telavancin, dalbavancin and oritavancin, which are semisynthetic derivatives of vancomycin, a glycopeptide natural product, isolated from *Amycolatopsis orientalis* (Fig. **6**).

Telavancin (Vibativ), developed by Theravance, is a multivalent, semisynthetic derivative of vancomycin with a hydrophobic side chain attached to the vancosamine sugar. It both inhibits peptidoglycan biosynthesis and disrupts the cell membrane through depolarization [51]. Telavancin is rapidly bactericidal against clinically important bacteria including MRSA, VISA, and PRSP *in vitro* [52]. Unlike daptomycin, telavancin remains active *in vitro* in the presence of pulmonary surfactant [53]. The FDA approved telavancin for the treatment of CSSSI in 2009. Since it does not interact with other antibiotics or enzyme inhibitors, it can be used in combination therapy regimens [53]. Telavancin was granted limited approval by FDA in December 2012 for the treatment of CAP where no other alternatives are available.

Oritavancin, (LY333328), developed by Targanta Therapeutics, is a novel vancomycin derivative for treatment of serious Gram-positive infections. Oritavancin has a half-life of more than two weeks, making it efficacious in a single-dose regimen [54]. It is also is a potent inhibitor of stationary phase staphylococci. Like telavancin, oritavancin has no known drug-drug interactions with other antibiotics [54], and the two compounds share a similar mechanism of action [55]. Oritavancin is currently in Phase III development in a single dose regimen for the treatment of ABSSSIs, including those due to MRSA [56].

Dalbavancin, (BI397, Zeven), developed by Durata Therapeutics, is a vancomycin analog with an antimicrobial spectrum comparable to telavancin and oritavancin. Similar to oritavancin, it has a long half-life and can be effective in weekly dosing [57]. It also exhibits superior tissue penetration than other vancomycin derivatives. Although *in vitro* studies suggested that dalbavancin was effective against VRSA, the preponderance of *in vivo* evidence does not support this indication. Dalbavancin is currently in a Phase III trial for the treatment of ABSSSIs [58].

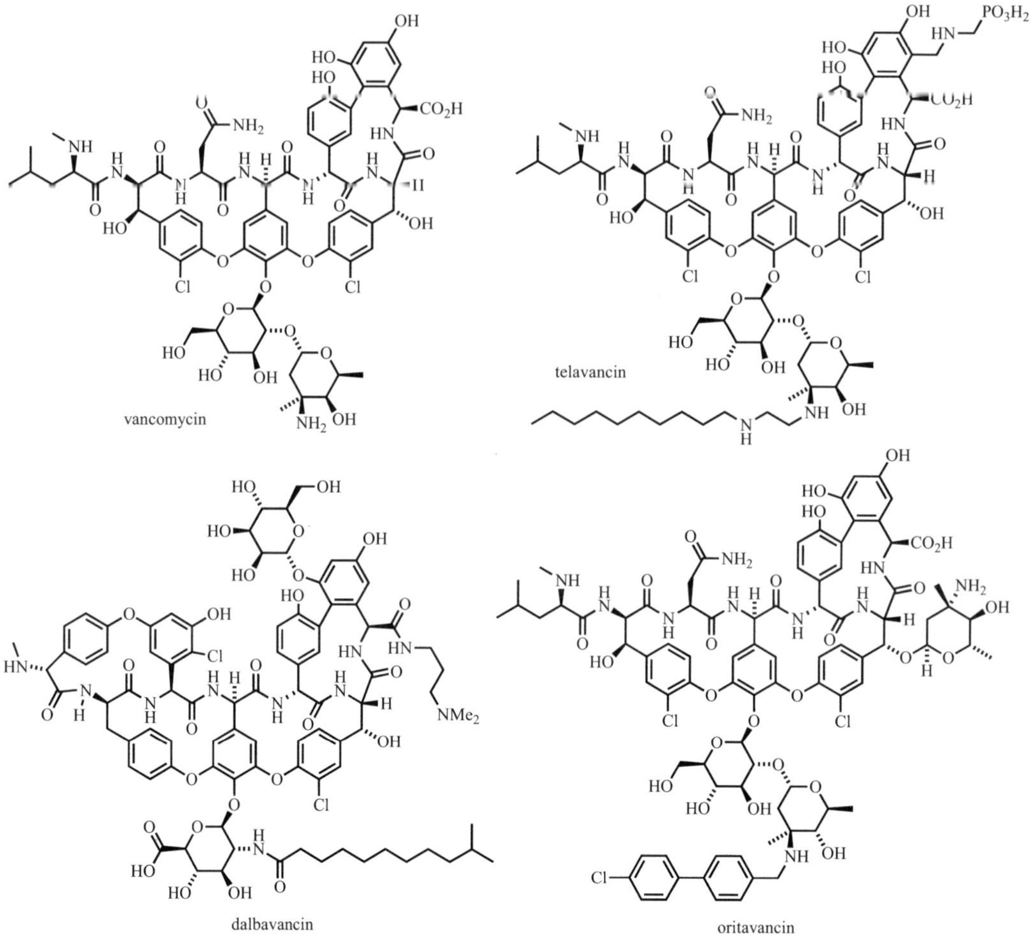

Fig. (6). Structures of glycopeptides with multiple modes of antibiotic activity.

DNA-Dependent RNA Polymerase Inhibitors

Bacterial DNA dependent RNA polymerase differs significantly from the mammalian counterpart, thus establishing it as an attractive novel target for identification of new antibiotics. This class includes fidaxomicin (Dificid, OPT-80 and PAR-101), developed by Optimer Pharmaceuticals. Fidaxomicin (Fig. 7) was the first in a new class of narrow spectrum macrocyclic drugs obtained from the actinomycete *Dactylosporangium aurantiacum* to be granted FDA approval in 2011 [59]. It was earlier reported as tiacumicin B, and a series of analogs were designed by Abbott Laboratories [60-62]. Fidaxomicin has an identical structure to the lipiarmycins and clostomicins, both of which belong to the macrolactone class [63-69]. These natural products were shown to inhibit the bacterial DNA-dependent RNA polymerase [69-72]. Recently, studies have shown that these macrolactones impede the *de novo* initiation of RNA synthesis through binding to the σ70-subunit region-3.2 and the RNA polymerase B-subunit switch-2 element, which controls the clamping of the promoter DNA in the RNA polymerase active-site cleft [73]. Fidaxomicin is non-systemic and bactericidal, and it has demonstrated selective eradication of CD with minimal disruption to the multiple species of bacteria that make up the normal, healthy intestinal flora [74, 75]. This is of particular importance because the maintenance of normal physiological conditions in the colon can reduce the probability of CD infection recurrence. Phase III trials with fidaxomicin showed that it was able to achieve a higher global cure rate than vancomycin with a lower recurrence rate, which was defined as no recurrence with 4 weeks [76, 77]. In addition to its activity against Gram-positive bacteria, fidaxomicin also showed good potency against drug resistant *Mycobacterium tuberculosis* [78].

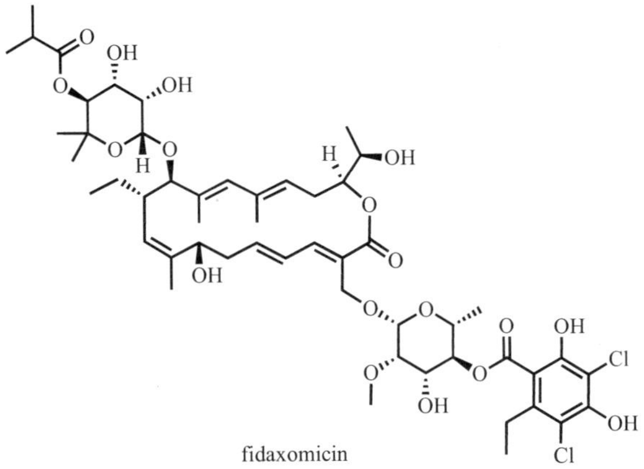

Fig. (7). Structure of fidaxomicin, a bacterial RNA-polymerase inhibitor.

Protein Synthesis Inhibitors

Since prokaryotic protein synthesis is distinct from that in eukaryotes, the bacterial synthetic machinery is a logical target for drug discovery. Inhibitors of protein synthesis include ribosomal inhibitors (tigecycline, TP-434, retapamulin,

BC-3781, ACHN-490, and ACT-179811) and peptide deformylase inhibitors (GSK1322322, actinonin, BB83698, and LBM-415).

Tigecycline (GAR936, Tygacil), developed by Wyeth Pharmaceuticals, is the first in the glycylcycline class to be approved for clinical use (Fig. 8) [79]. Tigecycline, a synthetic derivative of minocycline, was developed to specifically overcome bacterial mechanisms of tetracycline resistance. The compound evades efflux pumps such as Tet(A-E) (responsible for acquired resistance of Enterobacteriaceae and *Acinetobacter* spp to minocycline) and the Tet(K) pumps (confer resistance to tetracycline in staphylococci). Tigecycline also has a different binding orientation than other tetracyclines to bacterial ribosomes modified by the Tet(M) protein, a resistance mechanism common to Gram-positive cocci and *Neisseria* spp [80-82]. Tigecycline binds to the 30S ribosomal subunit with more potency than tetracycline and blocks entry of amino-acyl transfer RNA into the A site of the ribosome [82]. Tigecycline successfully completed Phase III trials for CSSSI where it was noninferior to an IV formulation of vancomycin/aztreonam [83]. A Phase III trial for complicated IAI also showed noninferiority to an IV formulation of imipenem/cilastatin [83-86]. Unlike orally available tetracyclines, tigecycline is administered parentally as a single dose. However, it still causes a similar side effect profile. Since it evades most classical mechanisms of tetracycline resistance, it has broad spectrum activity against multi-drug resistant strains of *Escherichia coli, Klebsiella, Enterobacter, Citrobacter spp., Acinetobacter spp., Bacteroides spp., Proteae, P. aeruginosa, Enterococci, Staphylococci* and *Streptococci* [87].

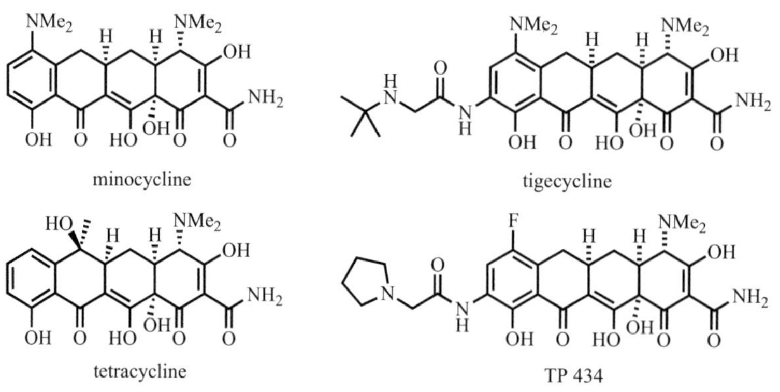

Fig. (8). Structures of tetracycline inhibitors of protein synthesis.

TP-434, developed by Tetraphase Pharmaceuticals, is a tetracycline derivative fluorinated at the C-9 position. This chemical modification confers protection against efflux and ribosomal resistance mechanisms, similar to the profile described for tigecycline [88]. It is a broad-spectrum agent against Gram-positives and Gram-negatives including some drug resistant pathogens. It is currently in Phase II trials to assess activity compared to ertapenem in Adult Community-Acquired Complicated IAI [89].

Retapamulin (SB-275833, Altabax, Altargo), developed by GlaxoSmithKline, is a member of the pleuromutilin family (Fig. **9**). It was originally isolated in the 1950's from *Clitopilus passeckerianus,* an edible mushroom [90]. Other members of this family including valnemulin and tiamulin have been approved for veterinary use, but retampulin is the first approved human therapeutic. It inhibits bacterial protein synthesis by binding to the 23S rRNA, blocking the peptidyl transferase component of the 50S subunit on the bacterial ribosome [91]. It also partially inhibits the binding of initiator tRNA substrate to the ribosomal P site. Retapamulin is a bacteriostatic drug that is active against resistant strains [92]. It is currently utilized as a topical formulation due to its low bioavailability. Retapamulin was approved in 2007 for treatment of impetigo due to MRSA or *S. pyogenes*.

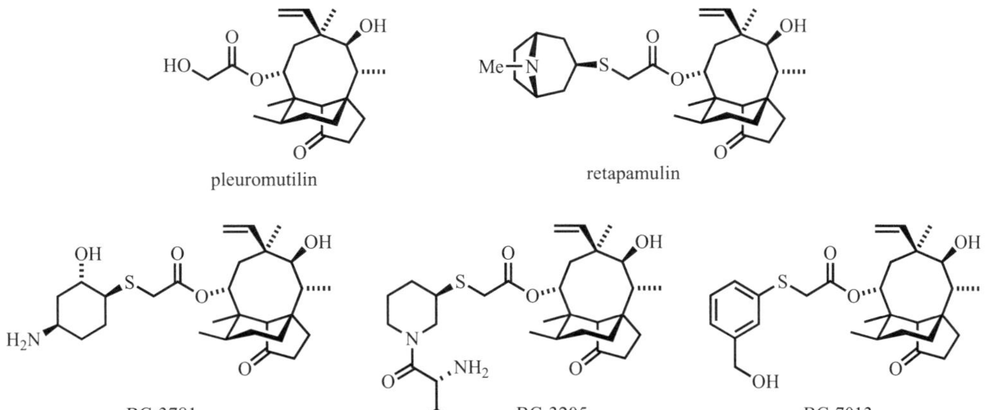

Fig. (9). Structures of pleuromutilin inhibitors of protein synthesis.

Recently there has been a major thrust, primarily by Nabriva Therapeutics, to discover bioavailable analogs of retapamulin for systemic application. BC-3781 is a promising systemic pleuromutilin with activity against MRSA, MDR *Streptococcus pneumonia*, and VRE. In recently completed Phase II trials for the treatment of serious MDR SSSI, it was noninferior to an IV formulation of vancomycin [93-95]. BC-7013 is in Phase I trial as a topical formulation for the treatment of uncomplicated SSSI [96]. BC-3205 is being developed as on orally available pleuromutilin [97, 98].

Pristinamycin is a naturally occurring mixture of two synergistic components produced by *Streptomyces pristinaespiralis* in a 30:70 ratio (Fig. **10**). Referred to as streptogramins, the two components of the pristinimycin mixture are pristinamycin I, a depsipeptide and pristinamycin II, a macrolide. These two inhibit protein synthesis by binding to the peptidyl transferase domain of the 50S

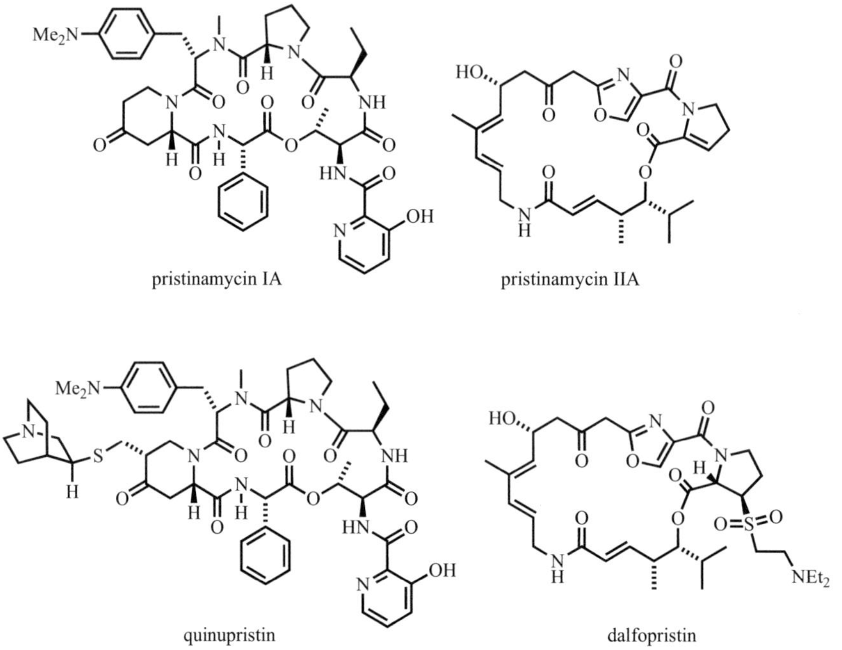

Fig. (10). Structures of the components of pristinamycin (pristinamycin IA and IIA) and synercid (quinupristin and dalfopristin).

subunit of the ribosome but have only modest activity when used as single agents [99]. They are only available as an oral formulation due to poor water solubility and are effective against MRSA and Streptococci. Even though the mixture contains a macrolide component, pristinamycin exhibits potent activity against erythromycin-resistant MRSA as pristinamycin I is still active [100].

Due to its poor solubility, pristinamycin's effectiveness in combating systemic infection is very limited. To improve bioavailability of the streptogramin combination, quinupristin and dalfopristin (Synercid) were developed by Rhone-Poulenc. Dalfopristin is a derivative of a group A streptogramin while quinupristin is a group B streptogramin. These two water-soluble streptogramins are administered in an injectable formulation at a 30:70 ratio [100]. Like pristinamycin I and II, they exhibit modest activity as single agents against MRSA but show synergistic bactericidal activity when used in this combination [101].

ACHN-490 (Plazomicin), developed by Achaogen, is an aminoglycoside antibiotic. It is a derivative of the aminoglycoside sisomicin, isolated from *Micromonospora* (Fig. **11**) [102]. Sisomicin is structurally related to gentamicin and is only active against Gram-positive bacteria. As extensive resistance to aminoglycosides has been well documented, Achaogen designed sisomicin derivatives that exhibited potent activity against aminoglycoside-resistant strains. Medicinal chemistry optimization identified ACHN-490 as a broad-spectrum agent active against MDR systemic Gram-negative bacteria including *E. coli* and MRSA [103, 104]. Recently, it was efficacious in Phase II clinical trial for treatment of urinary tract infections and pyelonephritis caused by MDR enterobacteriaece [103-105].

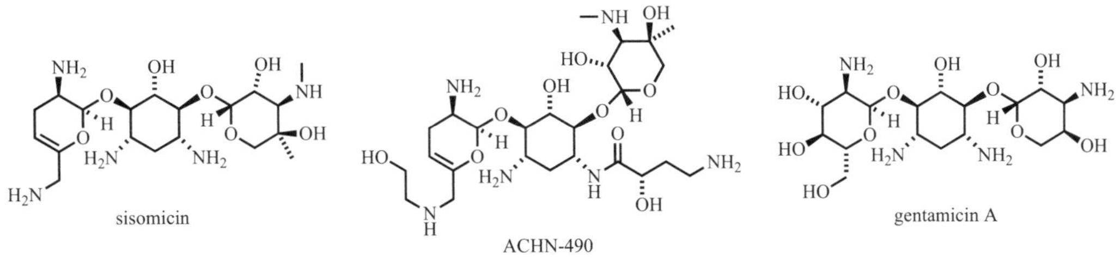

Fig. (11). Structures of aminoglycoside inhibitors of protein synthesis.

Telithromycin (HMR-3647, Ketek), developed by Sanofi-Aventis, is a macrolide antibiotic that was recently approved by the FDA [106]. It is a derivative of erythromycin, a macrolide originally isolated from *Saccharopolyspora erythraea* (Fig. **12**). Telithromycin strongly binds to 50S ribosomal subunit. It has potent activity against *Streptococcus pneumoniae, Haemophilus influenzae, Moraxella catarrhalis*, and *S. aureus,* including MDR isolates [107]. Telithromycin was approved by the FDA in 2004 for the treatment of respiratory infections.

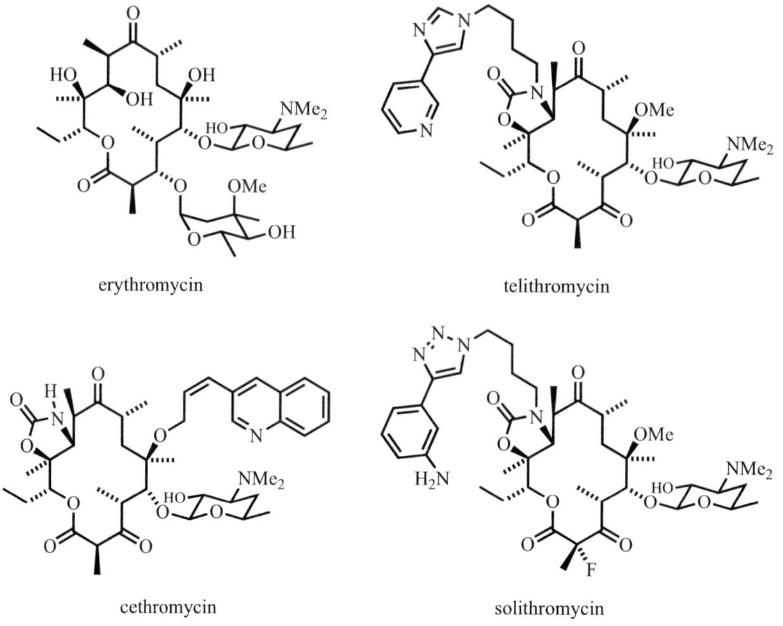

Fig. (12). Structures of macrolide inhibitors of protein synthesis.

Cethromycin (ABT-7730, Fig. **13**), developed by Abbott and Advanced Life Sciences, is an erythromycin analog developed for treatment of CAP caused by susceptible strains of *Streptococcus pneumoniae, Haemophilus influenzae, Staphylococcus aureus, Moraxella catarrhalis,* and *Legionella pneumophila.* It exhibits potent activity against *ermB* resistant strains of *Streptococcus pneumonia* [108].

Solithromycin (CEM-101, OP-1068), developed by Cempra, is also an erythromycin inspired macrolide (Fig. **13**) [109]. The drug inhibits drug-resistant Gram-positive and Gram-negative bacteria including macrolide resistant strains [110-113]. Unlike telithromycin, solithromycin is not associated with adverse side effects such as visual disturbances and exacerbations of myasthenia gravis [114,

115]. This difference is attributed to the absence of the pyridyl group present in telithromycin that may have off target binding to nicotinic acetylcholine receptors. Solithromycin was effective in a recently completed in a Phase II clinical trials for CABP [116]. It is utilized to treat community-acquired RTI and SSSI [117].

Peptide Deformylase Inhibitors

Peptide deformylase (PDF) is an essential gene in prokaryotes and absent in mammalian cells, thus making it an attractive antibacterial target. Since there is no approved drug that inhibits bacterial PDF, a first in class compound would be of significant clinical benefit and with investment potential for industry. The small peptide actinonin, isolated from *Streptomyces* sp NCIB 8845, was identified by Vicuron Pharmaceuticals [118-120]. The clinical development of actinonin was not pursued. Several derivatives of actinonin have been investigated in the clinic including GSK1322322, BB83698, and LBM-415 (Fig. **13**).

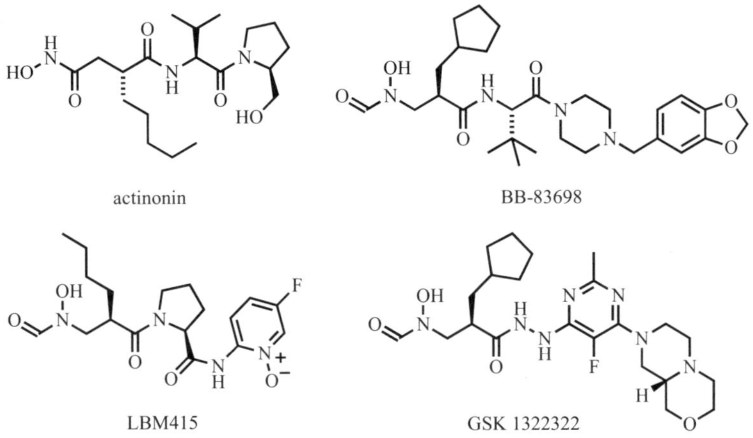

Fig. (13). Structures of hydroxamide peptidyl inhibitors of peptide deformylase.

BB-83698 developed by Oscient and LBM415 developed by Novartis were the first peptide deformylase inhibitors to reach Phase I trials, but further development was discontinued [121]. BB-83698, is a synthetic *N*-formyl hydroxylamine-based peptidomimetic that is a potent inhibitor (IC_{50} ~7 nM) of PDF [122]. The compound demonstrated oral, subcutaneous, and intravenous efficacy against *S. pneumoniae* and *S. aureus* in peritoneal, lung, and thigh infections [123, 124]. LBM415 was pursued in the clinic for the oral and parenteral treatment of RTI and SSSI caused by susceptible Gram-positive organisms. Its activity against Gram-negative organisms is much weaker [125]. Both of these agents exhibited bacteriostatic activity [126].

GSK1322322, developed by GlaxoSmithKline, is also a peptiodmimetic inhibitor of PDF. It is being pursued for the treatment of CBSSSI and hospitalized CAP caused due to MDR *Streptococcus pneumoniae* and MRSA [127, 128]. GSK1322322 was efficacious in a completed Phase II trial *versus* linezolid for the treatment of ABSSSIs [129].

Compounds with Complex or Unknown Mechanisms of Action

A number of natural products exhibit complex or undetermined modes of action. NVC-422 (Fig. **14**), developed by NovaBay Pharmaceuticals, is a more stable derivative of *N,N*-dichlorotaurine, a natural oxidant that plays an integral role in the immune system [130-133]. NVC-422 is a broad-spectrum agent for bacterial and viral pathogens including MDR *Staphylococcus aureus*, *Enterococcus faecium,* Gram-negative bacteria, *Candida albicans*, adenovirus, and herpes simplex virus. It is also effective against *S. aureus* in biofilms [134, 135]. NVC-422 was evaluated in a Phase II trial for prevention of urinary catheter blockade and encrustation [136]. It is also being tested for eye, ear, and sinus infections along with acne, impetigo, and other dermatological indications.

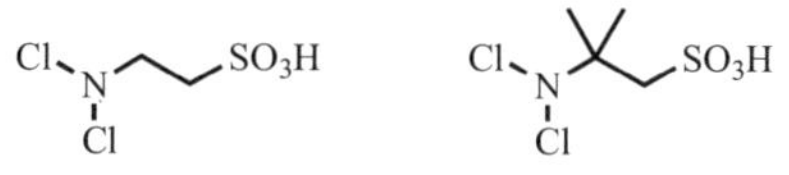

N,N-dichlorotaurine NVC-422

Fig. (14). Structures of chlorotaurines.

BAL30072, developed by Basiliea Pharmaceutica, is a novel monocyclic sulflactam derived from monobactam, which was isolated from *Chromobacterium violaceum* (Fig. **15**). BAL30072 exhibits potent antimicrobial activity against a broad range of Gram-negative bacteria, including MDR *P. aeruginosa*, *A. baumannii* and *K. pneumoniae*. It is stable against class B metallo-β-lactamases and an inhibitor of the class C β -lactamase [137]. BAL-30072 is currently undergoing a Phase I clinical trial to measure safety and tolerability after multiple IV infusions [138, 139].

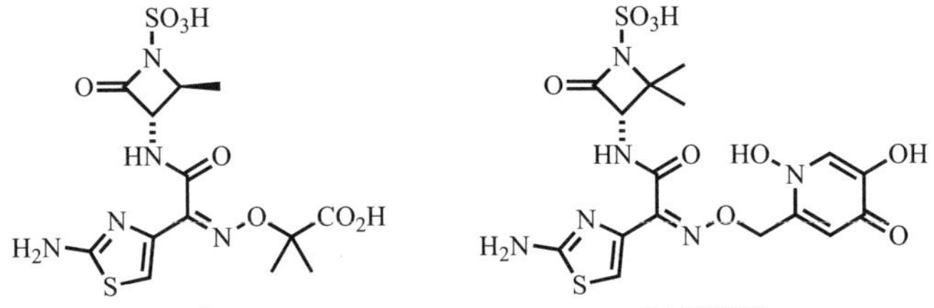

Fig. (15). Structures of sulflactam antibiotics.

Novel Screening Platforms for Natural Product Discovery

Researchers at Merck interested in developing new antibiotics with novel mechanisms of action developed new screening technologies for the identification of bioactive natural antibiotics. Recognizing that bacterial type II fatty acid biosynthesis (FASII) is both essential for bacterial survival and has significant difference in the structure and organization of enzymes from the humans [85, 140, 141], the discovery group developed screening assays to identify specific inhibitors of bacterial fatty acid synthesis [142, 143]. Their first report described a high throughput screening assay capable of measuring activity against multiple enzymes in the FASII pathway including FabD, FabF/B, FabG, FabA/Z, and FabI [143]. They have also developed a more selective cell-based assay to identify specific inhibitors of the condensing enzymes FabH/F [142]. This assay exploits the mechanism of antisense mRNA to FabH/F enzymes that reduces the *fabF/H* gene products thereby reducing the amount of FabF/H in the cell. This effect is known as RNA silencing. With less of the molecular target available, the cell is more sensitive to inhibitors of that molecular target. The Merck assay used this RNA silencing in bacterial strains expressing antisense mRNA of FabH/F enzymes to identify selective FabH/F inhibitors.

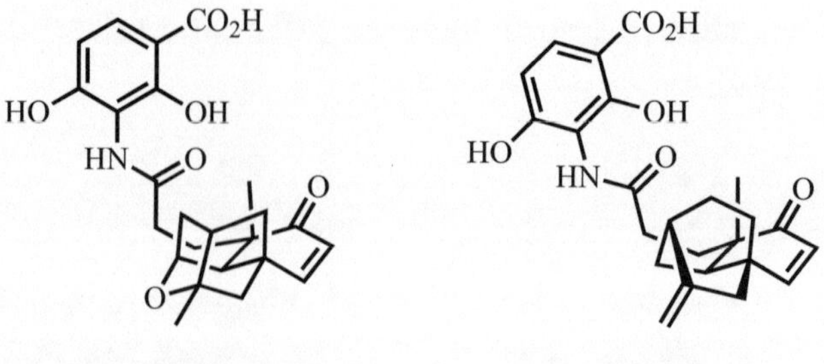

Fig. (16). Structures of bacterial FASII inhibitors.

Using their novel FASII HTS assays, investigators screened over 250,000 natural extracts from actinomycetes and fungi and identified the novel antibiotic platensimycin (Fig. **16**) [144, 145]. Platensimycin was isolated from a strain of the South African soil bacterium *Streptomyces platensis*. It exhibited broad-spectrum activity against Gram-positive bacteria by inhibiting the FabF/B condensing enzymes [145]. In fact, it is the only compound reported to interfere with the condensing enzymes that displayed broad-spectrum efficacy *in vivo* with no associated toxicity [145]. It also exhibited high activity against several antibiotic resistant strains resistant strains including MRSA, VISA, and VRE. A subsequent report described the isolation of platencin, a structurally related terpene isolated from *S. platensis* [146]. This natural product interferes with the FabH acyl carrier protein as well as the FabF condensing enzyme, the target of platensimycin.

Since their original publication, over 32 congeners of platensimycin and platencin have been described. Modifications to the terpenoid core are named as the A series [147-150] and modifications to the anilide portion are named as the B series [151, 152]. Compounds with complete elimination of the aromatic unit or a difference in length of the carbon chain have been named in a different way entirely [147, 148, 150, 153, 154]. Most of the analogs are likely oxidation products of cytochrome P450s following cyclization, and the addition of the polar hydroxyl group reduces the compounds' affinities for the hydrophobic pocket in FabF. Therefore, platensimycin and platencin remain the most potent members of the family. However, due to their high rate of clearance, they are only efficacious when dosed *via* continuous infusion, which is not viable as a dosing strategy for antibiotics [155]. The pharmacokintetic properties of this structural class must be improved if they are to be developed into a viable therapy.

ANTI-VIRAL COMPOUNDS

Compounds for Treatment of HIV/AIDS

The first protease inhibitor (PI) for the treatment of HIV was approved by the FDA in 1995 [156]. Since this introduction, many members in the PI class have been approved and used in conjunction with reverse transcriptase inhibitors to form the HAART approach used in AIDS chemotherapy. This regimen was a major advance in HIV/AIDS treatment and has radically decreased the incidence of AIDS-related deaths in industrialized nations [157]. PIs are expensive to synthesize and have toxicity associated with the high dosages required. The peptide-like structure of early PIs requires expensive syntheses and limits their bioavailability. These challenges contribute to the high cost of treatment. In addition, HAART regimens lack potency to combat multidrug-resistant strains thus leading to an increased rate of resistance to many approved therapies. The development of HAART treatment regimens for HIV infected individuals has had a dramatic improvement for the treatment options for HIV/AIDS. However, by coupling the requisite chronic treatment of infection and the large number of treatment-experienced patients, drug resistance is a major challenge [158, 159]. New anti-HIV therapeutics with novel mechanisms of action are needed to address the critical need.

Darunavir (UIC 94017, TMC 114), developed by Tibotec (Belgium), was designed to address the limitations among the approved PIs. Darunavir was designed to incorporate cyclic polyethers, a motif found in bioactive natural products such as the bis-THF motif seen in ginkolide B (Fig. **17**) [160]. This design element was to improve solubility of new PIs.

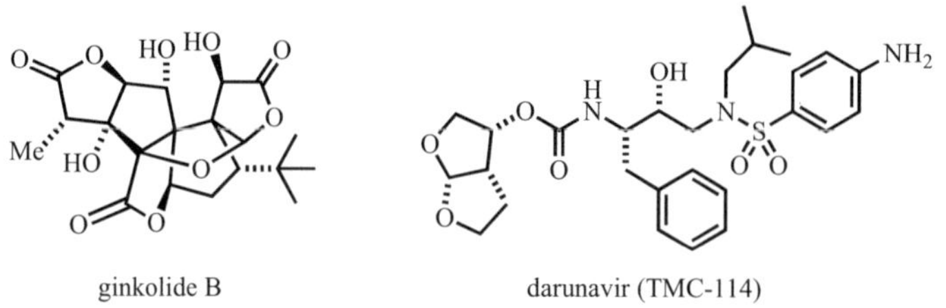

Fig. (17). Structures of ginkolide B and the compound it inspired, darunavir.

The main design goals were to produce potent non-peptidic protease inhibitors that mimic peptidic binding modes in the protease that also have increased bioavailability. The developers hypothesized that exploiting conformationally constricted heterocycles that mimic amino acid binding motifs of peptides would provide a more bioavailable compound. The cyclic ether motif was selected due to its prevalence in bioavailable bioactive natural products such as ginkolide B [160]. Co-crystal structures of 3(*S*)-THF urethane ligands showed their weak binding to the main chain Asp29 and Asp30, in the P_2 subsite of the protease [161]. The development of the bis-THF analogs improved potency by providing strong interaction with both Asp29 and Asp30 [162]. Through iterative rounds of optimization, the combination of the bis-THF as the P_2 binding motif with the *p*-aminosulfonamide as the $P_{2'}$ binding motif provided an exceptionally potent PI (K_i = 16 pM) anti-viral [163]. The dual binding motifs present in darunavir provide extensive hydrogen bonding in the enzyme active site backbone that improves its potency and its resistance profile. Darunavir showed a wide spectrum of activity against multi-PI resistant HIV-1 variants presumably because multiple mutations in the backbone would be required to completely disrupt its binding [164].

Darunavir was tested in combination with ritonavir and showed efficacy and good tolerability in treatment experienced patients in the Phase IIb POWER studies, achieving ≤ 50 copies HIV-1 RNA/ml of blood in 45-46% of patients [165]. The Phase III ARTEMIS efficacy study showed patients receiving darunavir/ritonavir in combination with nucleoside analogs tenofovir and emtricitabine showed higher rates of HIV-1 RNA suppression than the control arm with lopinavir/ritonavir at week 96 [166]. The MONET trial was designed to determine whether a darunavir/ritonavir could show noninferior efficacy to the triple arm darunavir/ritonavir with two nucleoside analogs in patients with less than 50 copies/mL of HIV-1 RNA [167]. The MONET was the first randomized trial of a ritonavir-boosted monotherapy approach that showed noninferior efficacy compared to the triple antiretroviral treatment arm. Darunavir was approved for use in combination with ritonavir by the FDA in 2006 [168].

Tipranavir (PNU-140690), developed by Pharmacia & Upjohn, is an analog of the natural product phenprocoumon. Screening of natural products and their derivatives at Upjohn revealed that phenprocoumon inhibited the HIV-1 protease. Phenprocoumon had a K_i = 1 μM against the protease (Fig. **18**) [169]. The related natural product warfarin was a known inhibitor of HIV replication [170]. Further studies indicated warfarin was a competitive inhibitor of the protease with a K_i = 3.3 μM [171]. Phenprocoumon and warfarin had each been used previously in humans and had high oral bioavailability with low clearance [172], making the 4-hydroxypyran-2-one scaffold a valuable lead for the development of a new non-peptidic PIs for HIV.

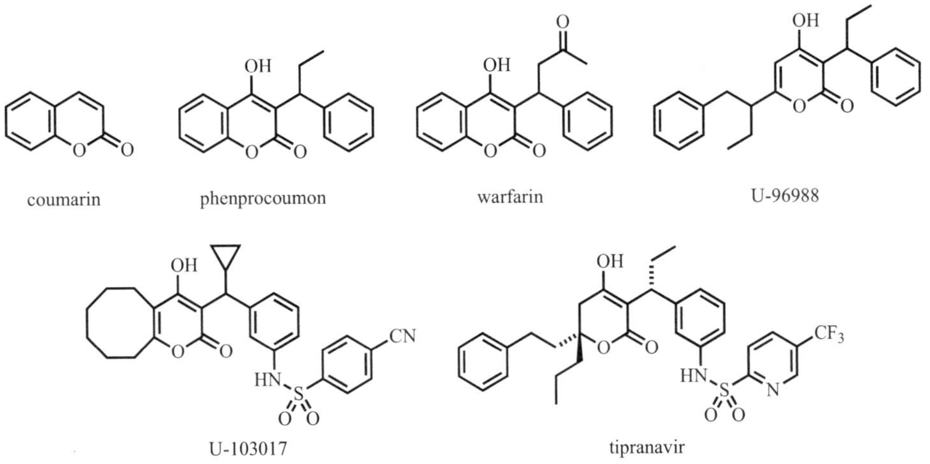

Fig. (18). Coumarin, the coumarin natural products phenprocoumon and warfarin, and synthetic pyrones inspired by them.

Iterative cycles of medicinal chemistry on phenprocoumon led to more potent compounds. The modification of the 4-hydroxycoumarin to 4-hydroxypyrone found in U-96988 led to enhanced binding (K_i = 38 nM) [169]. Adding a sulfonamide in the *meta* position (U-103017) significantly improved potency (K_i < 1 nM, IC_{50} = 1-2 μM) [173]. The fusion of the dihydropyrone with the sulfonamide substituent yielded the new analog tipranavir [174], a potent compound with excellent anti-viral activity (K_i = 8 pM, IC_{50} = 30 nM) [175].

These three lead compounds from Pharmacia & Upjohn that were advanced to clinical trials from their PI program. Tipranavir was evaluated in the RESIST trials 1 and 2 in combination with ritonavir (500 mg/200 mg, twice daily). In this study, a larger percentage of patients on the tipranavir/ritonavir regimen responded to treatment (33.6%) than a competitor protease with ritonavir regimen (15.3%). Patients on the tipranavir/ritonavir treatment also had greater increase in CD4 counts from baseline [176]. The superior immunological and virological response led the FDA to approve tipranavir in 2005 [177] and further approve its use for treatment-experienced pediatric patients in 2008 [178]. It is manufactured by Boehringer-Ingelheim. Due to its low drug-resistance profile, tipranavir in combination with ritonavir can be used as a salvage therapy in treatment experienced patients. However, due to its cytochrome P450 inhibitory properties, it can cause drug-drug interactions and has been associated with elevated cholesterol and triglyceride levels [179].

In 1994, the terpene betulinic acid (Fig. **19**) was isolated from the leaves of a rainforest plant and was shown to inhibit HIV replication (EC_{50} = 1.4 μM) [180]. Functionalization of betulinic acid identified bevirimat as a potent inhibitor of HIV viral replication in acutely infected H9 lymphocytes (EC_{50} < 0.34 nM) [181]. It was determined that the compound acts by interfering with Gag processing of the capsid precursor p25 to a mature capsid protein p24 resulting in the formation of non-infective virus particles [182]. Bevirimat was highly active against wild type clinical isolates (EC_{50} = 10.4 nM) with low toxicity (IC_{50} >25 μM) giving an excellent therapeutic index >2,500 [182]. Bevirimat was evaluated using the SCID-hu Thy/Liv mice infected both with wild type HIV-1 virus and an azidothymidine (AZT) resistant HIV-1 strain. The compound was orally bioavailable, reduced viral RNA load, and protected T cells from depletion [183]. Based on the promising *in vitro* and *in vivo* data, the FDA granted "Fast-Track" New Drug Development Status to bevirimat in December 2004.

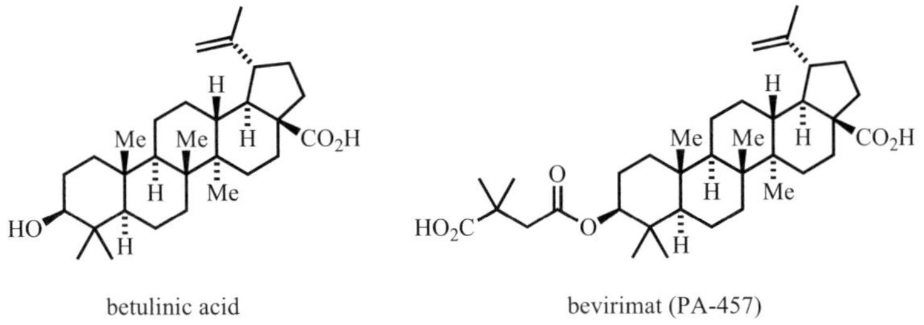

Fig. (19). Structure of betulinic acid and its semisynthetic derivative bevirimat, inhibitors of Gag processing in HIV.

In a Phase I study, bevirimat was safe in healthy volunteers in both single and escalating doses. It was well absorbed and had a long half-life of 60-80 h indicating it may be efficacious in a once daily dosing regimen [184]. A double blind Phase I and II study in HIV infected individuals who were treatment naïve using bevirimat as a monotherapy showed that bevirimat was effective and reduced viral load with once daily dosing [185]. A multicenter Phase II study showed that there were naturally occurring polymorphisms in codon position 369-371 in Gag that dictated a patient's response to bevirimat. Patients with the most commonly occurring amino acid residues glutamine-valine-threonine were likely to respond to bevirimat therapy, while patients with mutations at this position were less likely to respond [186, 187]. Later studies showed that a patient's response to bevirimat therapy can be predicted from genotype analysis of the p2 peptide which could be used to inform its future clinical administration [188]. In 2009, Myriad Genetics acquired the rights to the development of bevirimat but in 2010 announced discontinuation of further development in order to focus on their oncology portfolio [189].

Compounds for Treatment of Hepatitis B Virus

Entecavir (SQ-34676, BMS-200475), developed by Bristol-Myers Squibb, is a 2'-deoxyguanosine analog (Fig. **20**) identified as a potent inhibitor of HBV [190]. Guanine-based nucleosides inhibit transcription by binding the protein primer site in HBV [191]. Entecavir was 30-fold more active against HBV (EC_{50} = 3.75 nM) than the adenine analog (EC_{50} = 128 nM), and it was selective for activity against HBV when tested against a panel of DNA and RNA viruses [190]. Detailed mechanistic studies showed that entecavir inhibits all three steps in viral genome replication: priming, reverse transcription, and DNA-dependent DNA synthesis. Presumably, entecavir is converted to the triphosphate form (BMS-200475-TP) in the cell. Mechanistic studies showed that entecavir triphosphate strongly inhibits the polymerase (K_i = 3.2 nM). Its incorporation into the viral DNA led to chain termination after 2-3 additional nucleotides [192].

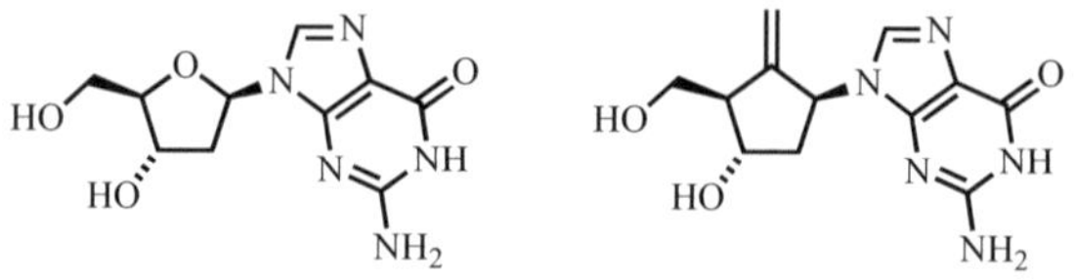

Fig. (20). 2'-Deoxyguanosine and its synthetic analog entecavir.

Entecavir was evaluated in a number of clinical studies. In these clinical studies, the HBeAg, a protein circulating in the bloodstream when the virus is actively replicating, can be used as an endpoint. A Phase II randomized study in patients both with and without HBeAg showed both 0.5 and 1.0 mg doses reduced the viral load in sera with no significant side effects [193]. A Phase II study was designed to determine the efficacy of entecavir in patients with resistance to lamivudine who are currently on lamivudine. After week 24 of this study, 79% of patients had undetectable HBV DNA by the branched DNA assay *versus* only 13% of patients who remained on lamivudine. 68% of patients on the entecavir regimen were able to normalize their ALT levels compared to only 6% in the lamivudine treatment group [194]. A two-year Phase III study of HBeAg positive patients with chronic hepatitis showed 81% of patients had a viral load below 300 copies per mL, undetectable levels, with entecavir *versus* only 39% with lamivudine [195, 196]. Entecavir was approved by the FDA in 2005 for the treatment of chronic HBV [197]. The treatment shows a low resistance rate and a high rate for virological suppression when compared to other current therapies [198]. It has also proven to be a safe long-term treatment for chronically ill patients [199, 200].

Telbivudine (β-L-thymidine, L-dT), developed by Idenix in partnership with Novartis, is a non-natural nucleoside anti-viral agent (Fig. **21**). Telbivudine was found to be a potent (EC_{50} = 0.19 μM) inhibitor of HBV replication. The nucleoside was inactive in screens against fifteen other DNA and RNA viruses, indicating it is a selective inhibitor of HBV [201]. Telbivudine also has an extremely safe toxicity profile. This compound was active in the woodchuck model for chronic HBV infection, inhibiting viral DNA replication throughout treatment [201]. Telbivudine targets the positive strand of HBV DNA, which may raise the barrier to resistance [202, 203].

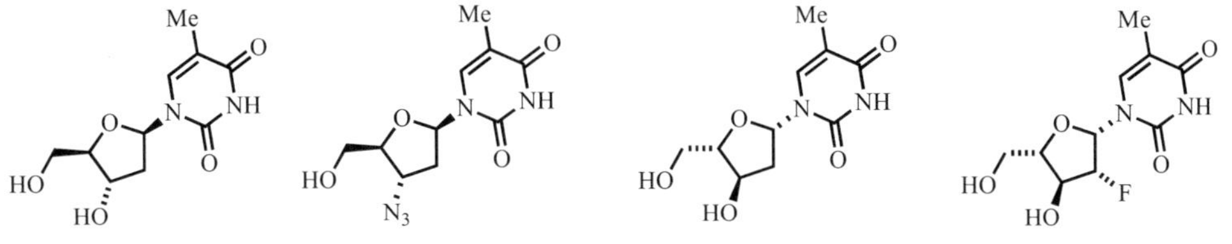

Fig. (21). Structure of thymidine and its synthetic analogs.

Telbivudine (Fig. **22**) was evaluated in the clinic by Idenix in partnership with Novartis under a development and commercialization agreement. The Phase IIb trial with telbivudine reduced HBV to undetectable levels below 200 particles per mL in 61% of patients *versus* only 32% who received lamivudine as the alternate treatment arm. Also, 86% of patients with the telbivudine treatment reduced their serum ALT levels, a marker for liver inflammation, to normal levels *versus* only 63% of patients in the lamivudine treatment arm [204]. The international Phase III GLOBE study enrolled 1370 patients at 135 centers worldwide. In this study, telbivudine was superior to lamivudine in reduction of HBV DNA levels and showed lower resistance. The overall response rate after one year of treatment was also greater for patients treated with telbivudine [205]. A further analysis of data from the GLOBE study revealed that non-detectable serum HBV levels after twenty four weeks of treatment with telbivudine was the strongest predictor of clinical outcome after two years of treatment [206]. Telbivudine was first approved for the treatment of HBV in 2006 [207].

Clevudine (L-FMAU, Fig. **22**), developed by a partnership between Bukwang Pharmaceuticals and Pharmasset, is a thymidine nucleoside analog under investigation for the treatment of chronic HBV [208]. The compound was found to be a potent inhibitor of HBV replication (EC_{50} in 2.2.15 cells = 0.10 μM) with a high anti-viral selectivity index (>2,000). Clevudine is a prodrug that is converted into its active triphosphate form by both cytosolic and mitochondrial kinases [209]. Mechanistic studies suggest that clevudine selectively inhibits the viral DNA polymerase, but the compound is not incorporated into cellular DNA [210].

The clinical development of clevudine was pursued by Bukwang Pharmaceuticals in South Korea. A double blind placebo controlled Phase III study in South Korea showed that clevudine decreased HBV infection in both HBeAg-positive and negative chronic HBV patients for the 24-week treatment period with no evidence for viral resistance [211, 212]. The drug was subsequently approved for use in Korea in 2006. A 48-week trial showed that clevudine was superior to lamivudine in suppressing viral replication without the emergence of resistance [213]. However, subsequent trial data at 48 weeks has shown a low rate of viral breakthrough [214-216]. Though no adverse events were reported in the clinical trials, there is now evidence that clevudine induces myopathy by the depletion of mitochondrial DNA in patients on long-term therapy [217-219]. The Korean Food and Drug Administration concluded that the myopathy associated with clevudine was not life threatening and is reversible, so they have approved continued use of clevudine [220]. Further study of long term compound administration in naive patients with chronic HBV has shown a rate of 6.9% for the adverse myopathy. Pharmasset elected to voluntarily halt their Phase III QUASH study in 2009 due to concerns over adverse events associated with the long term treatment of patients in Korea [221].

Compounds for Treatment of Influenza

Influenza is a viral respiratory illness that can cause hospitalization and death in susceptible populations. There are two treatment strategies for influenza including M2 ion channel inhibitors and NA inhibitors. M2 inhibitors like amantadine or rimantadine block this viral ion channel in an infected cell, preventing normal viral replication [222, 223]. However, M2 inhibitors are known to have a poor viral resistance profile causing them to be removed from first tier treatment strategy in the US until circulating flu strains regain susceptibility [224]. NA inhibitors bind the NA active site and prevent the release of viral progeny from the infected host cell, thereby preventing the spread of the virus. Without the action of NAs, the virus would be limited to a single cycle of replication. Therefore, NA inhibitors must be administered early to be effective [225].

The first two NA inhibitors to be licensed were zanamivir from Glaxo Wellcome and Biota (Relenza, FDA approval for treatment and prophylaxis, 1999) [225, 226] and oseltamavir from Hoffmann-LaRoche and Gilead Sciences (Tamiflu, FDA approval 1999) [227, 228]. Both compounds are analogs of the sialic acid derivative DANA (Fig. **23**). DANA is a known inhibitor of influenza NA (IC_{50} = 5-10 μM) [229]. A study of human isolates resistant to NA inhibitors suggests that viral susceptibility to NA inhibitors depends both on the NA structure but also on HA receptor-binding efficiency [230]. As of the 2007-2008, the CDC reported a marked increase in seasonal H1N1 isolates were resistant to oseltamivir, and by the 2008-2009 season, the number of oseltamivir-resistant influenza A (H1N1) isolates was almost 100% [231]. Zanamivir appears to have a higher barrier to resistance, but the nature of this property is unclear [232].

Laninamavir (R-125489, CS-8958), developed by Daiichi Sankyo, is a new NA inhibitor with activity against oseltamivir-resistant strains [233]. Esters of laninamivir including its octanoyl form (CS-8958) have a prolonged survival effect in the mouse model [234]. Laninamivir was potent against a panel of influenza strains including several pandemic H1N1 (IC_{50} = 0.41-1.55 nM), seasonal H1N1 (IC_{50} = 2.09 nM) [233], and H5N1 (IC_{50} = 0.32 - 2.1 nM) strains [235]. Laninamivir was less potent against H3N2 and influenza B than oseltamivir or zanamivir [233]. While laninamivir showed comparable *in vitro* efficacy to both zanamivir and oseltamivir, the prodrug laninamivir octanoate, CS-8958 showed superior *in vivo* efficacy with a single intranasal dose in several animal models for influenza [234-236]. The licensed drugs zanamivir (intranasal) and oseltamivir (oral) each require twice daily administration. Laninamivir octanoate, the prodrug, had a short half-life in lung tissue of 0.833 h, but the concentration of laninamivir in the lung spiked after intranasal administration and was retained in the lung for a much longer time ($t_{1/2}$ as long as 41.4 h) [234, 237]. Due to its superior exposure and high activity against susceptible and resistant strains of many NA subtypes, the prodrug laninamivir octanoate was advanced as a clinical candidate.

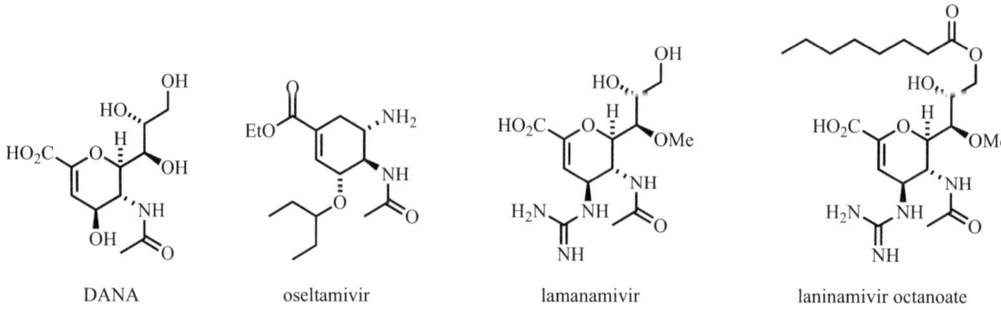

Fig. (22). DANA and its synthetic anti-influenza analogs.

Laninamivir octanoate was the first long acting neuraminidase inhibitor to be tested in the clinic. Phase I studies showed that a single dose of laninamivir octanoate provided sustained exposure to laninamivir with a $t_{1/2}$ in plasma of 3 days. There were no adverse events observed in any group [238]. A Phase II/III of pediatric patients was conducted as a double blind randomized trial with comparative treatment of oseltamivir during the 2008-2009 Japanese influenza season. During that season, nearly all circulating influenza strains were H1N1 with oseltamivir resistance (H274Y). The single intranasal dose of laninamivir octanoate showed significantly reduced time to alleviation of illness for oseltamivir resistant H1N1, but there was no significant difference in time to alleviation for H3N2 or influenza B infections [239]. The MARVEL study was a double-blinded active-controlled Phase III study in adults comparing a single intranasal dose with a twice daily oseltamivir regimen. The MARVEL study showed noninferior efficacy of laninamivir octanoate. Both the 20 and 40 mg/kg doses were well tolerated [240]. Japan approved the use of laninamivir octanoate (Inavir) in 2010 [241]. Daiichi Sankayo is teaming with Biota for clinical development in the US. Biota was awarded a $231 million dollar contract through the BARDA for the clinical development of laninamivir for the US market and support a new drug application [242].

Peramivir (RWJ-270201, BCX-1812), developed by BioCryst Pharmaceuticals, is a second DANA analog in development concurrently with laninamivir (Fig. **24**). Peramivir was designed using the co-crystal structures of both DANA and α/β-6-acetyl-amino-3,6-dideoxy-D-glycero-altro-2-nonulofuranosonic acid [243]. Peramivir was designed to occupy both of the hydrophobic pockets in the active site and act as a transition state mimic. The use of the cyclopentane scaffold dictates that the binding groups are positioned differently in the active site of the NA enzymes allowing the compound to retain activity against zanamivir-resistant strains with the E119G mutation (IC_{50} = 0.4-1.4 nM against 17 different influenza A strains) [243, 244]. Peramivir was evaluated against oseltamivir and ribavirin in one H1N1 and two H3N2 mouse models for infection and was inhibitory to all infections with a large therapeutic window [245].

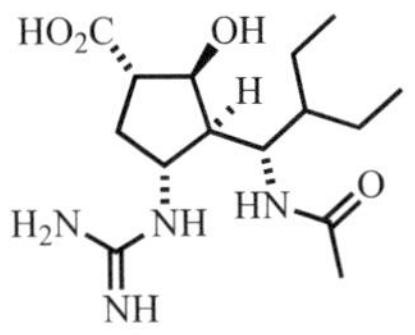

peramivir

Fig. (23). Structure of peramivir.

BioCryst Pharmaceuticals partnered with Shionogi & Co. for the development and commercialization of peramivir in Japan. Phase II studies showed that a single intravenous dose of peramivir at either 300 or 600 mg/kg significantly reduced time to alleviate symptoms when compared to placebo with comparable adverse event profile [246]. Both dose levels also were well tolerated in high-risk patients including those with chronic respiratory illness and those on immunosuppressives [247]. A Phase III randomized double-blind clinical trial comparing the use of a single intravenous dose of peramivir (300 or 600 mg) to twice daily oral dosing of oseltamivir (75 mg) was conducted in patients with seasonal influenza. This study showed that the single intravenous dose of peramivir was noninferior to the 5-day oseltamivir regimen, suggesting that this dosing regimen would be effective and could increase compliance [248]. Peramivir was approved in Japan for the treatment of influenza in adults and children older than 1 month of age and showed decreased time for fever reduction compared to zaninamivir and laninaimvir for some pediatric populations [249]. Peramivir is currently in development in the US under a $238.4 million dollar contract with BARDA. A Phase III study comparing the efficacy of peramivir to the standard of care in both adults and adolescents showed there was a statistically small difference between treatment with peramivir and the control group. As a result of this disappointing preliminary study analysis, Biocryst Pharmaceuticals elected to suspend the Phase III study in November 2012 [250].

Broad Spectrum Anti-Viral Agents

Ribavirin (Fig. **24**) is a purine nucleoside analog first synthesized in 1970 that can target both DNA and RNA viruses [251], the first broad-spectrum anti-viral agent approved for clinical practice. The compound can adopt many conformations in the active site of an enzyme and can target any enzyme that utilizes purine nucleosides or nucleoside phosphates as substrates or cofactors [252]. Ribavirin in combination with IFNα is currently the frontline treatment for HCV [253-256]. Despite its broad spectrum action, off target action has complicated its use in the clinic by causing several adverse side effects including dose-limiting hemolytic anemia and teratogenicity [257, 258].

Taribavirin (viramidine), developed by Valeant Pharmaceuticals International, is a ribavirin prodrug that has a different pharmacokinetic profile than the parent ribavirin. It was originally developed in 1973 to probe the hydrogen bonding characteristics of ribavirin by exchanging the carbonyl oxygen with a nitrogen in the pendant amide [259]. It has *in vitro* activity comparable with ribavirin, but *in vivo*, it acts as a prodrug and is converted into ribavirin by adenosine deaminase [260]. The enzyme-activated prodrug approach provides a good strategy to improve bioavailability and target specific tissue distribution. Adenosine deaminase has a wide distribution in human tissues and a high catalytic capacity. Studies with [^{14}C]taribavirin *versus* [^{14}C]ribavirin *via* oral dosing in rats and cynomolgus monkeys showed that taribavirin has a higher liver-targeting capacity making it a safer candidate for HCV therapy [261].

Valeant Pharmaceuticals International is leading the clinical development of taribavirin for HCV. Phase II studies comparing the safety and efficacy of taribavirin *versus* ribavirin in combination with pegylated IFN showed that taribavirin was as effective as ribavirin with lower incidence of anemia [262]. In a Phase III study comparing the efficacy of taribavirin (600 mg BID) *versus* ribavirin (1000 or 1200 mg/day) in combination with either pegylated IFNα-2a or 2b (180 μg), taribavirin met the primary safety endpoint, lowering anemia.

However, taribavirin failed to meet the primary efficacy endpoint of noninferiority to the standard of care with ribavirin [263, 264]. Post hoc analysis of the clinical data showed that higher exposure to taribavirin was critical to having sustained virological response suggesting that weight-based dosing would be critical to achieving efficacy endpoints. A Phase IIb study with weight-based dosing showed that 20-25 mg/kg reduced the rates of anemia while maintaining a good sustained virological response in treatment-naive patients with chronic HCV [265]. A new Phase III study with weight-based dosing will be required to show noninferiority of taribavirin to ribavirin in chronic HCV.

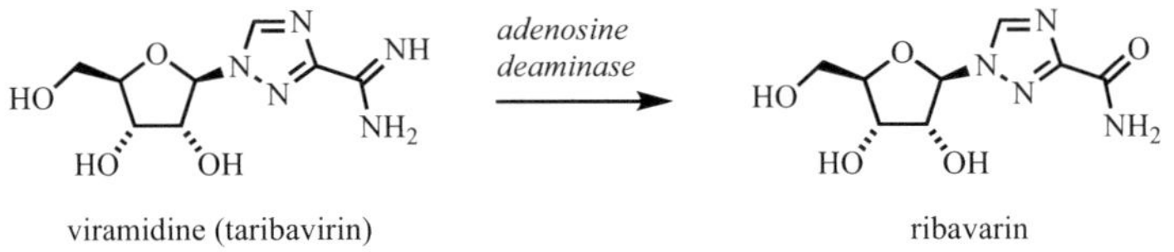

Fig. (24). Ribavirin and its prodrug taribavirin (viramidine).

ANTI-FUNGAL AGENTS

Anidulafungin (tradename Eraxis, previously LY303366) is a cyclic lipopeptide antifungal agent derived from the natural product echinocandin B (Fig. **25**). Echinocandin B was isolated from *Aspergillus nidulans* and identified as having antibiotic and antifungal properties [266] attributed to its ability to inhibit glucan synthesis, which is required for development of the fungal cell wall [267]. By targeting a pathway unique to the pathogen, lipopeptides are less toxic than other antifungal agents such as amphotericin B [268]. In their study of echinocandin B, researchers from Eli Lilly realized that the lipophilic side chain is necessary for activity, as the deacylated derivative was inactive [269]. Short lipophilic side chains were ineffective as well [270]. A 12-carbon lipophilic side chain regained moderate activity, and systematically extending the length of the side chain revealed 17-18 carbon chains to give the optimal activity. Incorporation of an aromatic ring in the lipophilic side chain reduced hemolytic toxicity associated with the parent echinocandin B. Further modification to cilofungin revealed that introducing a rigid, linear directionality to the side chain, either through incorporation of alkyne groups or a poly-phenyl series as seen in anidulafungin, improved antifungal activity. Anidulafungin was developed by Pfizer and gained

FDA approval in 2006. It is currently indicated for treatment of *Candida* infection. The compound also has activity against *Aspergillus* fungus [271] and in a 2007-2012 study was clinically evaluated as cotherapy with voriconazole [272].

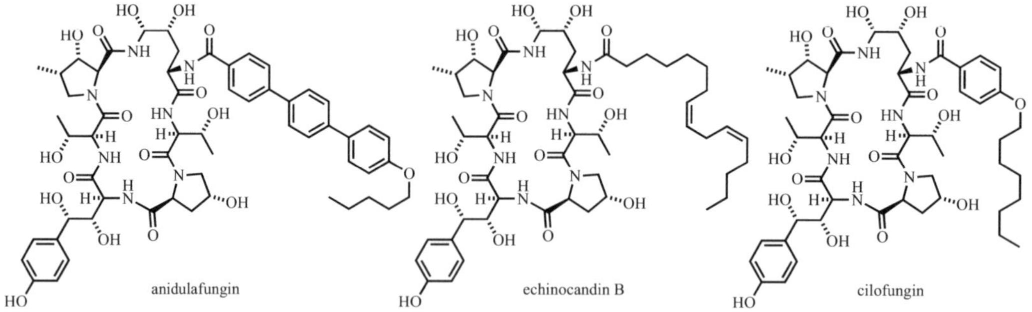

Fig. (25). Anidulafungin, its parent natural product echinocandin B, and congner cilofungin.

ANTI-MALARIAL AGENTS

Artemisinin (Fig. **26**) is the most potent antimalarial agent isolated from the Chinese medicinal herb *Artemisia annua* (sweet wormwood). Simple derivatives of artemisinin such as dihydroartemisinin, artemether, arteether, artesunate, and artelinic acid offer improved solubility, bioavailability, stability, and pharmacokinetic properties [273]. Artemisinin-based combination therapies are recommended by the World Health Organization as the first-line treatment for malaria [274, 275]. However, these semisynthetic therapeutics all suffer from the need to isolate artemisinin from its natural source. The low yield of extraction limits the compounds' utility for the large population at risk for malaria. Research in synthetic biology may enable the expanded use of artemisinin and its congeners (see below).

Inspired by the endoperoxide pharmacophore of artemisinin, medicinal chemists have expended significant effort designing simplified endoperoxides that are more synthetically tractable than the natural product [276]. Hoffmann-La Roche's endoperoxide arteflene entered Phase I and Phase II clinical trials, but its development was discontinued due to high recrudescence rates [277, 278]. In 2004, a multi-centered team from academia, non-governmental organizations, and the pharmaceutical industry identified the 1,2,4-trioxolanes (ozonides) surrounded by aliphatic ring systems as active antimalarial compounds [279]. Further optimization of physicochemical and biopharmaceutical properties afforded OZ277 as a clinical candidate. Following a Phase II clinical trial of a combination therapy of OZ277 and piperaquine [280], the Indian company Ranbaxy announced continued study of OZ277 in a Phase III clinical trial [281].

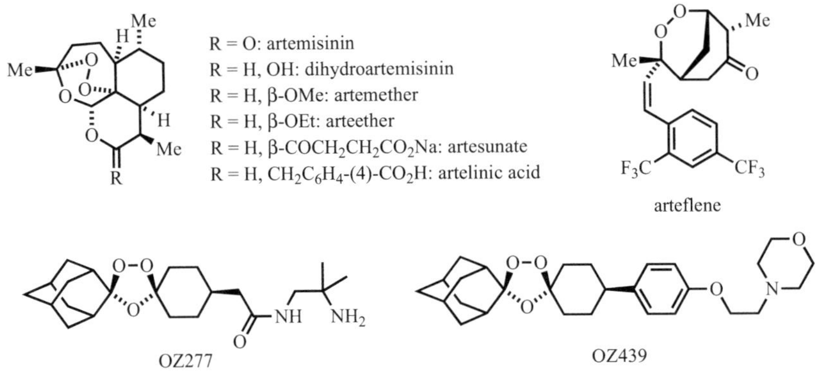

Fig. (26). Artemisinin, its semisynthetic derivatives, and drug candidates inspired by its pharmacophore.

The second-generation ozonide OZ439 was developed to improve the pharmacokinetic properties of OZ277 in hopes of reaching a single dose cure for uncomplicated malaria [282]. The nature of the 8′ substituent proved to be the key realization. Changing the 8′ group from an alkyl group, as in OZ277, to an aromatic ring, as in OZ439, resulted in a compound with 50-fold increase in stability to iron(II) mediated decomposition and 15-fold increased stability in whole blood. *In vivo* pharmacokinetic parameters including half-life and plasma concentration *vs* time increased substantially as well. A single 30 mg/kg dose of OZ439 cured >99% of mice in the *Plasmodium berghei* model, with no evidence of parasites 30 days after infection. The Phase I study concluded that OZ439 is safe and well tolerated in doses up to 1600 mg/kg in humans and should continue to Phase IIa clinical trials for acute uncomplicated malaria [283]. The discovery and development of ozonides OZ277 and OZ439 highlight the potential of partnerships across academia, the pharmaceutical industry, and non-profit organizations to advance new therapeutics into the clinic.

Improving Access to Artemisinin Through Synthetic Biology

The complex chemical structure of artemisinin makes the compound particularly difficult to synthesize in an economical nature on the scale necessary to address the worldwide threat of malaria. Nonetheless, many synthetic chemists took up the challenge of developing a laboratory synthesis of artemisinin [284-296]. None of these have been scaled to production levels, although the strategies described in 2010 by Yadav [294] and in 2012 by Cook [296] deserve note as efforts specifically designed to reach that goal.

In the absence of an efficient chemical synthesis, Professor Jay Keasling spearheaded a program to utilize metabolic engineering and synthetic biology to increase the available supply of artemisinin (Fig. **27**). Using a synthetic biology approach, the complex architecture of the natural product can be assembled *via* heterologous expression of the biosynthetic pathway in a non-native host. As a sesquiterpene lactone, artemisinin's basic biosynthetic pathway is understood [297]. Farnesyl pyrophosphate is synthesized through the mevalonate or deoxyxylulose phosphate pathway and is transformed by various cyclase enzymes to more complex compounds. In the case of artemisinin, farnesyl pyrophosphate is cyclized to amorpha-4,11-diene. Selective biochemical oxidation by cytochrome P450 enzymes first produces artemisinic acid and further oxidation yields artemisinin. The enzymes that convert artemisinic acid to artemisinin by *A. annua* have not been identified, but chemical transformations of amorpha-4,11-diene [298, 299] and artemisinic acid [300-302] to artemisinin have been developed. The synthetic biology approach targets these advanced intermediates. Achieving a partial biosynthesis of artemisinin would solve many of the major challenges of the total chemical synthesis, including formation of all carbon-carbon bonds and stereocenters necessary to complete the synthesis. Furthermore, other than the engineered microbe, the inputs are cheap, readily available feedstocks such as ethanol or glucose. Fig. **27** summarizes the current state of the microbial production of artemisinin.

After initial work exploring the capability of *E. coli* to generate sesquiterpene compounds [303], the Keasling group disclosed the synthesis of amorpha-4,11-diene within an *E. coli* host [304]. The engineered microbe contained genetics from *Saccharomyces cerevisiae* to encode the mevalonate pathway for the production of farnesylpyrophosphate. Inserting the gene for amorphadiene synthase [305] into the host organism allows for the transformation of farnesylpyrophosphate to amorpha-4,11-diene. Subsequent work has led to improvements in the process for industrial production at sufficient concentration [306, 307]. In 2012, production of amorpha-4,11-diene was improved to 40 g/L within a *S. cerevisiae* host overexpressing all enzymes within the mevalonate pathway [299].

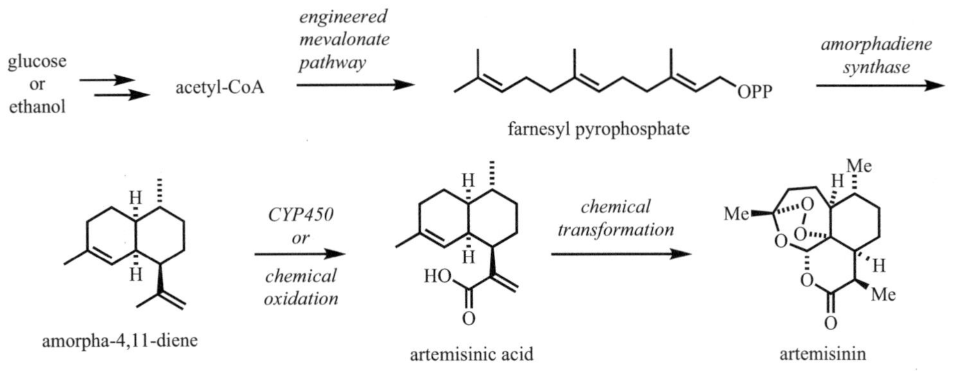

Fig. (27). Synthetic biology approach to artemisinin.

Keasling and coworkers have successfully identified the enzyme utilized by *A. annua* to carry out the oxidation of amorpha-4,11-diene to artemisinic acid, a cytochrome P450 encoded by the gene CYP71AV1 [308]. When the gene for the plant cytochrome P450 is expressed in *S. cerevisiae*, the more advanced artemisinic acid intermediate can be accessed from the microbial host.

CONCLUSIONS

Natural products and natural product inspired compounds comprise 75% of the FDA approved antibacterial and anti-viral agents over the past 30 years [3]. Even as antibiotic resistance to even the last lines of defense is emerging, industrial investment in antimicrobial development has been in significant decline. Factors including the cost and time to develop an approved agent and the low potential for return on investment have contributed to industry's decision to contract their antimicrobial discovery programs [309]. The emergence of MDR strains poses a potent global public health threat that requires renewed investment in the discovery of new and novel agents [310]. Since the evolution of resistance can fundamentally limit the utility of a drug, thereby minimizing the return on investment, the economics of resistance have contributed to the de-emphasis of antimicrobial drug development. Pharmaceutical companies must weigh the return on the investment of an antimicrobial agent that will typically be used in a short course or acute therapeutic regimen *versus* the development of maintenance drugs for lifestyle indications or chronic illness that are not subject to the same evolutionary pressures that lead to drug resistance [311]. Thus, while there is an unmet global need for a robust antimicrobial pipeline, the changing complexion of industrial discovery in this area has left the pipeline running nearly dry. In the wake of diminished private investment, more creative development strategies from a global perspective must be explored [310, 312]. This is especially true in the context of neglected diseases where public-private partnerships and the concept of "virtual drug discovery" are playing a critical role [313].

It is in this void that natural products can have a dramatic impact, providing potent, targeted, bioavailable therapies for infection and new technological developments can accelerate discovery. The golden era of antibiotic drug discovery from the 1950s–1980s preceded the genomic revolution. The availability of whole genome sequences and the development of molecular methods have improved both our functional knowledge of natural biosynthetic pathways and molecular targets for disease therapy. Though bacteria are the largest natural source of antibiotic agents, it is estimated that the vast majority of them are not culturable [314]. Analysis of the natural microbial diversity using culture free methods like ribosomal RNA analysis suggests that the number of unculturable microbes may exceed their culturable counterparts by 2-3 orders of magnitude [315, 316]. There is a vast untapped wealth of microbial diversity that could provide new antibiotic agents. Genomics has played a major role in identifying new sources of antibiotic agents from unculturable sources. Metagenomics is the analysis of environmental DNA isolated from naturally occurring microbial populations, obviating the challenges associated with culturing the organisms individually [317]. This technology is particularly attractive for natural product isolation because bacteria and fungi are the largest natural sources for anti-infectives. While an emerging field, there have already been amazing advancements to identify new and novel biosynthetic clusters for previously undiscovered natural antibiotics [318].

Another challenge for using natural products as lead compounds for anti-infectives is that of access. Synthetic biology may fill some of those gaps, allowing the cloning and heterologous expression of full biosynthetic clusters in surrogate hosts to improve production capabilities or to provide access to challenging synthetic transformations [298]. Functional bacterial genomics has also allowed access to new natural product-like scaffolds by the artificial expression of biosynthetic pathways with non-natural substrates [319]. Natural products themselves have also been studied as leads for medicinal chemistry efforts where the *de novo* or semisynthesis of the natural pharmacophore has been elaborated to yield synthetically tractable natural product-like therapeutic agents [320].

While there is no silver bullet in the path to decreasing cost and increasing efficiency in the process of anti-infective drug discovery, natural products are a privileged class in this space. There are clear unmet medical needs. The emergence of MDR organisms requires the development of new agents with a higher barrier to resistance or chemical agents that can evade resistance mechanisms. There has been more limited exploration of natural products in the context of viral or parasitic infection, areas where the requisite cell culture for screening may have limited their accessibility as primary bioactivity screens. Instead, the post-genomic era has delivered host and pathogen targets that have been used to develop HTS to identify new agents with known mechanistic activity. Natural products can be used to address these unmet needs by providing bioactive, bioavailable therapies for infection.

ABBREVIATIONS

ABSSSI = Acute Bacterial Skin and Skin Structure Infection

AIDS	= Acquired Immune Deficiency Syndrome
ALT	= Alanine Aminotransferase
API	= Active Pharmaceutical Ingredient
BARDA	= Biomedical Advanced Research Development Authority
CABP	= Community Acquired Bacterial Pneumonia
CAP	= Community Acquired Pneumonia
CBSSSI	= Complicated Bacterial Skin and Skin Structure Infection
CD	= *Clostridium Difficile*
CDC	= US Centers for Disease Control and Prevention
cIAI	= Complicated Intra-Abdominal Infection
CSSSI	= Complicated Skin and Skin Structure Infection
cUTI	= Complicated Urinary Tract Infection
DANA	= 2,3-Didehydro-*N*-Acetylneuraminic Acid
DNA	= Deoxyribonucleic Acid
EC_{50}	= 50% Effective Concentration
FASII	= Bacterial type II Fatty Acid Biosynthesis
FDA	= US Food and Drug Administration
HAART	= Highly Active Antiretroviral Therapy
HBeAg	= Hepatitis B e Antigen
HBV	= Hepatitis B Virus
HCV	= Hepatitis C Virus
HIV	= Human Immunodeficiency Virus
HTS	= High-Throughput Screening
IAI	= Intra-Abdominal Infection
IC_{50}	= 50% Inhibitory Concentration

IFN	=	Interferon
IV	=	Intravenous
MARVEL	=	Multinational Asian Clinical Research for Influenza Viral Extermination on Long-Acting Neuraminidase Inhibitor
MDR	=	Multi-Drug Resistant
mRNA	=	Messenger RNA
MRSA	=	Methicillin-Resistant *Staphylococcus aureus*
MSSA	=	Methicillin-Sensitive *Staphylococcus aureus*
NA	=	Neuraminidase
PDF	=	Peptide Deformylase
PBP	=	Penicillin Binding Protein
PI	=	Protease Inhibitor
PRSP	=	Pencillin-Resistant *Streptococcus pneumonia*
RESIST	=	Randomized Evaluation of Strategic Intervention In Multi-Drug Resistant
RNA	=	Ribonucleic Acid
rRNA	=	Ribosomal RNA
RTI	=	Respiratory Tract Infection
SCID-hu Thy/Liv	=	Severe-Combined Immunodeficient Mice with Human Thymus and Liver
SSSI	=	Skin and Skin Structure Infection
THF	=	Tetrahydrofuranyl
tRNA	=	Transfer RNA
VISA	=	Vancomycin Intermediate-Resistant *Staphylococcus aureus*
VRE	=	Vancomycin-Resistant *Enterococcus faecium*
VRSA	=	Vancomycin-Resistant *Staphylococcus aureus*.

ACKNOWLEDGEMENTS

This is communication number 8411 from CSIR-CDRI.

CONFLICT OF INTEREST

The authors confirm that this chapter content has no conflict of interest.

REFERENCES

[1] Mullin, R., Merck Cuts Sales Jobs, Halts Natural Products Research. *Chem. Eng. News* **2008**, *86* (19), 21.

[2] Lachance, H.; Wetzel, S.; Kumar, K.; Waldmann, H., Charting, Navigating, and Populating Natural Product Chemical Space for Drug Discovery. *J. Med. Chem.* **2012**, *55* (13), 5989-6001.

[3] Newman, D. J.; Cragg, G. M., Natural Products As Sources of New Drugs over the 30 Years from 1981 to 2010. *J. Nat. Prod.* **2012**, *75* (3), 311-335.

[4] Wright, G. D., Antibiotics: A New Hope. *Chem. Biol.* **2012**, *19* (1), 3-10.

[5] Cavalleri, B.; Pagani, H.; Volpe, G.; Selva, E.; Parenti, F., A-16686, A New Antibiotic From Actinoplanes .1. Fermentation, Isolation and Preliminary Physicochemical Characteristics. *J. Antibiot.* **1984**, *37* (4), 309-317.

[6] Ciabatti, R.; Kettenring, J. K.; Winters, G.; Tuan, G.; Zerilli, L.; Cavalleri, B., Ramoplanin (A-16686), A New Glycolipodepsipeptide Antibiotic .3. Structure Elucidation. *J. Antibiot.* **1989**, *42* (2), 254-267.

[7] Kettenring, J. K.; Ciabatti, R.; Winters, G.; Tamborini, G.; Cavalleri, B., Ramoplanin (A-16686), A New Glycolipodepsipeptide Antibiotic .4. Complete Sequence Determination By Homonuclear 2d Nmr-Spectroscopy. *J. Antibiot.* **1989**, *42* (2), 268-275.

[8] Pallanza, R.; Berti, M.; Scotti, R.; Randisi, E.; Arioli, V., A-16686, A New Antibiotic from Actinoplanes .2. Biological Properties. *J. Antibiot.* **1984**, *37* (4), 318-324.

[9] Skelton, N. J.; Harding, M. M.; Mortishiresmith, R. J.; Rahman, S. K.; Williams, D. H.; Rance, M. J.; Ruddock, J. C., Structure Elucidation and Solution Conformation of the Glycopeptide Antibiotic Ramoplanose (Uk-71,903) - A Cyclic Depsipeptide Containing an Antiparallel Beta-Sheet and a Beta-Bulge. *J. Am. Chem. Soc.* **1991**, *113* (20), 7522-7530.

[10] Reynolds, P. E.; Somner, E. A., Comparison of the Target Sites and Mechanisms of Action of Glycopeptide and Lipoglycodepsipeptide Antibiotics. *Drug Exp. Clin. Res* **1990**, *16* (8), 385-389.

[11] Nanotherapeutics Products: Ramoplanin. http://www.nanotherapeutics.com/products_pipeline_ramoplanin.php (accessed August 2012).

[12] de Lalla, F.; Nicolin, R.; Rinaldi, E.; Scarpellini, P.; Rigoli, R.; Manfrin, V.; Tramarin, A., Prospective-Study Of Oral Teicoplanin *Versus* Oral Vancomycin For Therapy Of Pseudomembranous Colitis And Clostridium-Difficile-Associated Diarrhea. *Antimicrob. Agents Chemother.* **1992**, *36* (10), 2192-2196.

[13] *Targocid Product Information*; Sanofi-Aventis: 2009.

[14] Bernareggi, A.; Borghi, A.; Borgonovi, M.; Cavenaghi, L.; Ferrari, P.; Vekey, K.; Zanol, M.; Zerilli, L. F., Teicoplanin Metabolism In Humans. *Antimicrob. Agents Chemother.* **1992**, *36* (8), 1744-1749.

[15] Birnbaum, J.; Kahan, F. M.; Kropp, H.; Macdonald, J. S., Carbapenems, A New Class Of Beta-Lactam Antibiotics. *Am. J. Med.* **1985**, *78* (6A), 3-21.

[16] Aldridge, K. E.; Morice, N.; Schiro, D. D., *In Vitro* Activity Of Biapenem (L-627), A New Carbapenem, Against Anaerobes. *Antimicrob. Agents Chemother.* **1994**, *38* (4), 889-893.

[17] Hikida, M.; Kawashima, K.; Nishiki, K.; Furukawa, Y.; Nishizawa, K.; Saito, I.; Kuwao, S., Renal Dehydropeptidase-I Stability Of Ljc 10,627, A New Carbapenem Antibiotic. *Antimicrob. Agents Chemother.* **1992**, *36* (2), 481-483.

[18] Zhanel, G. G.; Johanson, C.; Embil, J. M.; Noreddin, A. M.; Gin, A. S.; Vercaigne, L.; Hoban, D. J., Ertapenem: review of a new carbapenem. *Expert Rev. Anti-Infect. Ther.* **2005** *3*(1), 23-39.

[19] Castanheira, M.; Jones, R. N.; Livermore, D. M., Antimicrobial activities of doripenem and other carbapenems against Pseudomonas aeruginosa, other nonfermentative bacilli, and Aeromonas spp. *Diagn. Microbiol. Infect. Dis.* **2009**, *63* (4), 426-433.

[20] Sato, N.; Kijima, K.; Koresawa, T.; Mitomi, N.; Morita, J.; Suzuki, H.; Hayashi, H.; Shibasaki, S.; Kurosawa, T.; Totsuka, K., Population Pharmacokinetics of Tebipenem Pivoxil (ME1211), a Novel Oral Carbapenem Antibiotic, in Pediatric Patients with Otolaryngological Infection or Pneumonia. *Drug Metab. Pharmacokinet.* **2008**, *23* (6), 434-446.

[21] Kato, K.; Shirasaka, Y.; Kuraoka, E.; Kikuchi, A.; Iguchi, M.; Suzuki, H.; Shibasaki, S.; Kurosawa, T.; Tamai, I., Intestinal Absorption Mechanism of Tebipenem Pivoxil, a Novel Oral Carbapenem: Involvement of Human OATP Family in Apical Membrane Transport. *Mol. Pharm.* **2010**, *7* (5), 1747-1756.

[22] Zhanel, G. G.; Lam, A.; Schweizer, F.; Thomson, K.; Walkty, A.; Rubinstein, E.; Gin, A. S.; Hoban, D. J.; Noreddin, A. M.; Karlowsky, J. A., Ceftobiprole - A review of a broad-spectrum and anti-MRSA cephalosporin. *Am. J. Clin. Dermatol.* **2008**, *9* (4), 245-254.

[23] Bustos, C.; Pozo, J. L. D., Emerging agents to combat complicated and resistant infections: focus on ceftobiprole. *Infection Drug Resist.* **2010**, *3*, 5-14.

[24] Kontou, P.; Kuti, J. L.; Nicolau, D. R., Ceftobiprole - The first anti-MRSA cephalosporin antibiotic. *Formulary* **2008**, *43* (2), 66.

[25] *Ceftaroline*; Canadian Antimicrobial Resistance Alliance: 2010.

[26] Kanafani, Z. A.; Corey, G. R., Ceftaroline: a cephalosporin with expanded Gram-positive activity. *Future Microbiol.* **2009**, *4* (1), 25-33.

[27] Cubist Pharmaceuticals. Products and Pipeline: Gram-negative: CXA-201 (ceftolozane/tazobactam). http://www.cubist.com/products/cxa_201 (accessed August 2012).

[28] Ge, Y. G.; Whitehouse, M. J.; Friedland, I.; Talbot, G. H., Pharmacokinetics and Safety of CXA-101, a New Antipseudomonal Cephalosporin, in Healthy Adult Male and Female Subjects Receiving Single- and Multiple-Dose Intravenous Infusions. *Antimicrob. Agents Chemother.* **2010**, *54* (8), 3427-3431.

[29] Takeda, S.; Nakai, T.; Wakai, Y.; Ikeda, F.; Hatano, K., *In vitro* and *in vivo* activities of a new cephalosporin, FR264205, against Pseudomonas aeruginosa. *Antimicrob. Agents Chemother.* **2007**, *51* (3), 826-830.

[30] Toda, A.; Ohki, H.; Yamanaka, T.; Murano, K.; Okuda, S.; Kawabata, K.; Hatano, K.; Matsuda, K.; Misumi, K.; Itoh, K.; Satoh, K.; Inoue, S., Synthesis and SAR of novel parenteral anti-pseudomonal cephalosporins: Discovery of FR264205. *Bioorg. Med. Chem. Lett.* **2008**, *18* (17), 4849-4852.

[31] Choi, S.; Isaacs, A.; Clements, D.; Liu, D. H.; Kim, H.; Scott, R. W.; Winkler, J. D.; DeGrado, W. F., *De novo* design and *in vivo* activity of conformationally restrained antimicrobial arylamide foldamers. *Proc. Natl. Acad. Sci. U. S. A.* **2009**, *106* (17), 6968-6973.

[32] Liu, D. H.; Choi, S.; Chen, B.; Doerksen, R. J.; Clements, D. J.; Winkler, J. D.; Klein, M. L.; DeGrado, W. F., Nontoxic membrane-active antimicrobial arylamide oligomers. *Angew. Chem.-Int. Edit.* **2004**, *43* (9), 1158-1162.

[33] Scott, R. W., Defensin mimetics: nature knows best. *Am. Biotechnol. Lab.* **2009**, *27*, 16-19.

[34] Tew, G. N.; Scott, R. W.; Klein, M. L.; Degrado, W. F., *De Novo* Design of Antimicrobial Polymers, Foldamers, and Small Molecules: From Discovery to Practical Applications. *Acc. Chem. Res.* **2010**, *43* (1), 30-39.

[35] PolyMedix. PolyMedix Successfully Completes Phase 1 Exposure Escalation Safety Study With PMX-30063 Antibiotic. http://www.investors.polymedix.com/releasedetail.cfm?ReleaseID=600065 (accessed August 2012).

[36] PolyMedix. PMX-30063 Antibiotic Fact Sheet (March 2012) - PolyMedix. www.polymedix.com/uploads/files/Antibiotic-Fact-Sheet.pdf (accessed August 2012).

[37] Brilacidin (PMX-30063). http://www.polymedix.com/pipeline/Brilacidin (accessed August 2012).

[38] Harada, K.; Suzuki, M.; Kato, A.; Fujii, K.; Oka, H.; Ito, Y., Separation of WAP-8294A components, a novel anti-methicillin-resistant Staphylococcus aureus antibiotic, using high-speed counter-current chromatography. *J. Chromatogr. A* **2001**, *932* (1-2), 75-81.

[39] Kato, A.; Hirata, H.; Ohashi, Y.; Fujii, K.; Mori, K.; Harada, K., A new anti-MRSA antibiotic complex, WAP-8294A II. Structure characterization of minor components by ESI LCMS and MS/MS. *J. Antibiot.* **2011**, *64* (5), 373-379.

[40] Kato, A.; Nakaya, S.; Kokubo, N.; Aiba, Y.; Ohashi, Y.; Hirata, H.; Fujii, K.; Harada, K., A new anti-MRSA antibiotic complex, WAP-8294A - I. Taxonomy, isolation and biological activities. *J. Antibiot.* **1998**, *51* (10), 929-935.

[41] Kato, A.; Nakaya, S.; Ohashi, Y.; Hirata, H., WAP-8294A(2), a novel anti-MRSA antibiotic produced by Lysobacter sp. *J. Am. Chem. Soc.* **1997**, *119* (28), 6680-6681.

[42] Ohashi, Y.; Hirata, H.; Nakaya, S.; Katou, A.; Aiba, Y.; Kokubo, N.; Suzuki, N.; Maeda, M. Antibiotics WAP-8294A, Method for Preparing the Same and Antibacterial Compositions. U.S. Patent 5,648,455, 1997.

[43] Farrell, D. J.; Robbins, M.; Rhys-Williams, W.; Love, W. G., *In vitro* activity of XF-73, a novel antibacterial agent, against antibiotic-sensitive and -resistant Gram-positive and Gram-negative bacterial species. *Int. J. Antimicrob. Agents* **2010**, *35* (6), 531-536.

[44] Farrell, D. J.; Robbins, M.; Rhys-Williams, W.; Love, W. G., Investigation of the Potential for Mutational Resistance to XF-73, Retapamulin, Mupirocin, Fusidic Acid, Daptomycin, and Vancomycin in Methicillin-Resistant Staphylococcus aureus Isolates during a 55-Passage Study. *Antimicrob. Agents Chemother.* **2011**, *55* (3), 1177-1181.

[45] Maisch, T.; Bosl, C.; Szeimies, R. M.; Lehn, N.; Abels, C., Photodynamic effects of novel XF porphyrin derivatives on prokaryotic and eukaryotic cells. *Antimicrob. Agents Chemother.* **2005**, *49* (4), 1542-1552.

[46] Ooi, N.; Miller, K.; Hobbs, J.; Rhys-Williams, W.; Love, W.; Chopra, I., XF-73, a novel antistaphylococcal membrane-active agent with rapid bactericidal activity. *J. Antimicrob. Chemother.* **2009**, *64* (4), 735-740.

[47] Farrell, D.; Love, W.; Rhys-Williams, W., A new antimicrobial drug – comparison with mupirocin for the development of mutational resistance against MRSA in a 55-passage study. In *Abstracts of the Forty-eighth Interscience Conference on Antimicrobial Agents and Chemotherapy and the Forty-sixth Meeting of the Infectious Disease Society of America*, Washington, DC, 2008.

[48] Destiny Pharma Pipeline. http://antibacterials.co.uk/pipeline.shtml (accessed August 2012).

[49] Destiny Pharma News Archive. http://antibacterials.co.uk/news_archive.shtml (accessed August 2012).

[50] Destiny Pharma. Current News: September 2010: Destiny Pharma Destiny Pharma present clinical results at the 50th Annual ICAAC Meeting in Boston, USA. http://www.destinypharma.com/news_current.shtml (accessed August 2012).

[51] Higgins, D. L.; Chang, R.; Debabov, D. V.; Leung, J.; Wu, T.; Krause, K. A.; Sandvik, E.; Hubbard, J. M.; Kaniga, K.; Schmidt, D. E.; Gao, Q. F.; Cass, R. T.; Karr, D. E.; Benton, B. M.; Humphrey, P. P., Telavancin, a multifunctional lipoglycopeptide, disrupts both cell wall synthesis and cell membrane integrity in methicillin-resistant Staphylococcus aureus. *Antimicrob. Agents Chemother.* **2005**, *49* (3), 1127-1134.

[52] Leuthner, K. D.; Cheung, C. M.; Rybak, M. J., Comparative activity of the new lipoglycopeptide telavancin in the presence and absence of serum against 50 glycopeptide non-susceptible staphylococci and three vancomycin-resistant Staphylococcus aureus. *J. Antimicrob. Chemother.* **2006**, *58* (2), 338-343.

[53] Gotfried, M. H.; Shaw, J. P.; Benton, B. M.; Krause, K. M.; Goldberg, M. R.; Kitt, M. M.; Barriere, S. L., Intrapulmonary distribution of intravenous telavancin in healthy subjects and effect of pulmonary surfactant on *in vitro* activities of telavancin and other antibiotics. *Antimicrob. Agents Chemother.* **2008**, *52* (1), 92-97.

[54] Rubino, C. M.; Van Wart, S. A.; Bhavnani, S. M.; Ambrose, P. G.; McCollam, J. S.; Forrest, A., Oritavancin Population Pharmacokinetics in Healthy Subjects and Patients with Complicated Skin and Skin Structure Infections or Bacteremia. *Antimicrob. Agents Chemother.* **2009**, *53* (10), 4422-4428.

[55] Belley, A.; McKay, G. A.; Arhin, F. F.; Sarmiento, I.; Beaulieu, S.; Fadhil, I.; Parr, T. R.; Moeck, G., Oritavancin Disrupts Membrane Integrity of Staphylococcus aureus and Vancomycin-Resistant Enterococci To Effect Rapid Bacterial Killing. *Antimicrob. Agents Chemother.* **2010**, *54* (12), 5369-5371.

[56] Allen, N. E., From vancomycin to oritavancin: the discovery and development of a novel lipoglycopeptide antibiotic. *Antinfect. Agents Med. Chem.* **2010**, *9*, 23-47.

[57] Scheinfeld, N., Dalbavancin: A review. *Drugs Today* **2007**, *43* (5), 305-316.

[58] Chen, A. Y.; Zervos, M. J.; Vazquez, J. A., Dalbavancin: a novel antimicrobial. *Int. J. Clin. Pract.* **2007**, *61* (5), 853-863.

[59] Optimer Pharmaceuticals, Inc. Dificid, Full Prescribing Information. http://www.dificid.com/sites/default/files/prescribing.pdf (accessed August 2012).

[60] Hochlowski, J. E.; Swanson, S. J.; Ranfranz, L. M.; Whittern, D. N.; Buko, A. M.; McAlpine, J. B., Tiacumicins, A Novel Complex Of 18-Membered Macrolides .2. Isolation And Structure Determination. *J. Antibiot.* **1987**, *40* (5), 575-588.

[61] McAlpine, J. B.; Jackson, M.; Karwowski, J.; Theriault, R. J.; Hochlowski, J. Tiacumicin compounds. U.S. Patent 4,918,174, 1990.

[62] Theriault, R. J.; Karwowski, J. P.; Jackson, M.; Girolami, R. L.; Sunga, G. N.; Vojtko, C. M.; Coen, L. J., Tiacumicins, A Novel Complex of 18-Membered Macrolide Antibiotics .1. Taxonomy, Fermentation and Antibacterial Activity. *J. Antibiot.* **1987**, *40* (5), 567-574.

[63] Arnone, A.; Nasini, G.; Cavalleri, B., Structure Elucidation Of The Macrocyclic Antibiotic Lipiarmycin. *J. Chem. Soc.-Perkin Trans. 1* **1987**, (6), 1353-1359.

[64] Cavalleri, B.; Arnone, A.; Dimodugno, E.; Nasini, G.; Goldstein, B. P., Structure And Biological-Activity Of Lipiarmycin-B. *J. Antibiot.* **1988**, *41* (3), 308-315.

[65] Coronelli, C.; Parenti, F.; White, R.; Pagani, H. Lipiarmycin and its preparation. U.S. Patent 3,978,211, 1976.

[66] Coronelli, C.; White, R. J.; Lancini, G. C.; Parenti, F., Lipiarmycin, a new antibiotic from Actinoplanes. II. Isolation, chemical, biological, and biochemical characterization. *J. Antibiot.* **1975**, *28*, 253–259.

[67] Omura, S.; Imamura, N.; Oiwa, R.; Kuga, H.; Iwata, R.; Masuma, R.; Iwai, Y., Clostomicins, New Antibiotics Produced By Micromonospora-Echinospora Subsp Armeniaca Subsp Nov .1. Production, Isolation, and Physicochemical and Biological Properties. *J. Antibiot.* **1986**, *39* (10), 1407-1412.

[68] Parenti, F., Pagani, H. & Beretta, G. Lipiarmycin, a new antibiotic from Actinoplanes. I. Description of the producer strain and fermentation studies. *J. Antibiot.* **1975**, *28*, 247–252.

[69] Sergio, S.; Pirali, G.; White, R.; Parenti, F., Lipiarmycin, a new antibiotic from Actinoplanes. III. Mechanism of action. *J. Antibiot.* **1975**, *28*, 543–549.

[70] Talpaert, M.; Campagnari, F.; Clerici, L., Lipiarmycin: an antibiotic inhibiting nucleic acid polymerases. *Biochem. Biophys. Res. Commun.* **1975**, *63* (1), 328-334.

[71] Sonenshein, A. L.; Alexander, H. B.; Rothstein, D. M.; Fisher, S. H., Lipiarmycin-resistant ribonucleic acid polymerase mutants of Bacillus subtilis. *J. Bacteriol.* **1977**, *132* (1), 73-79.

[72] Sonenshein, A. L.; Alexander, H. B., Initiation of transcription *in vitro* is inhibited by lipiarmycin. *J. Mol. Biol.* **1979**, *127*, 55–72.

[73] Tupin, A.; Gualtieri, M.; Leonetti, J. P.; Brodolin, K., The transcription inhibitor lipiarmycin blocks DNA fitting into the RNA polymerase catalytic site. *EMBO J.* **2010**, *29* (15), 2527-2537.

[74] Optimer Pharmaceuticals. Optimer Pharmaceuticals Completes New Drug Application for Fidaxomicin and Requests Priority Review from FDA. http://investor.optimerpharma.com/releasedetail.cfm?ReleaseID=533687 (accessed August 2012).

[75] Optimer Pharmaceuticals. The New England Journal of Medicine Publishes Results of Fidaxomicin Phase 3 Trial Showing Significantly Lower Recurrence Rates and Improved Global Cure Rates Compared to Vancomycin in Patients with Clostridium difficile Infection (CDI). http://investor.optimerpharma.com/releasedetail.cfm?ReleaseID=547133 (accessed August 2012).

[76] TRIAL WATCH Phase III success for novel Clostridium difficile antibiotic. *Nat. Rev. Drug Discov.* **2010**, *9* (4).

[77] Louie, T.; Miller, M.; Donskey, C.; Mullane, K.; Goldstein, E. J. C., Clinical Outcomes, Safety, and Pharmacokinetics of OPT-80 in a Phase 2 Trial with Patients with Clostridium difficile Infection. *Antimicrob. Agents Chemother.* **2009**, *53* (1), 223-228.

[78] Kurabachew, M.; Lu, S. H. J.; Krastel, P.; Schmitt, E. K.; Suresh, B. L.; Goh, A.; Knox, J. E.; Ma, N. L.; Jiricek, J.; Beer, D.; Cynamon, M.; Petersen, F.; Dartois, V.; Keller, T.; Dick, T.; Sambandamurthy, V. K., Lipiarmycin targets RNA polymerase and has good activity against multidrug-resistant strains of Mycobacterium tuberculosis. *J. Antimicrob. Chemother.* **2008**, *62* (4), 713-719.

[79] Sum, P. E.; Petersen, P., Synthesis and structure-activity relationship of novel glycylcycline derivatives leading to the discovery of GAR-936. *Bioorg. Med. Chem. Lett.* **1999**, *9* (10), 1459-1462.

[80] Petersen, P. J.; Jacobus, N. V.; Weiss, W. J.; Sum, P. E.; Testa, R. T., *In vitro* and *in vivo* antibacterial activities of a novel glycylcycline, the 9-t-butylglycylamido derivative of minocycline (GAR-936). *Antimicrob. Agents Chemother.* **1999**, *43* (4), 738-744.

[81] Fluit, A. C.; Florijn, A.; Verhoef, J.; Milatovic, D., Presence of tetracycline resistance determinants and susceptibility to tigecycline and minocycline. *Antimicrob. Agents Chemother.* **2005**, *49* (4), 1636-1638.

[82] Bauer, G.; Berens, C.; Projan, S. J.; Hillen, W., Comparison of tetracycline and tigecycline binding to ribosomes mapped by dimethylsulphate and drug-directed Fe2+ cleavage of 16S rRNA. *J. Antimicrob. Chemother.* **2004**, *53* (4), 592-599.

[83] Breedt, J.; Teras, J.; Gardovskis, J.; Maritz, F. J.; Vaasna, T.; Ross, D. P.; Gioud-Paquet, M.; Dartois, N.; Ellis-Grosse, E. J.; Loh, E.; Tigecycline 305 c, S. S. G., Safety and efficacy of tigecycline in treatment of skin and skin structure infections: Results of a double-blind phase 3 comparison study with vancomycin-aztreonam. *Antimicrob. Agents Chemother.* **2005**, *49* (11), 4658-4666.

[84] Oliva, M. A. E.; Rekha, A.; Yellin, A.; Pasternak, J.; Campos, M.; Rose, G. M.; Babinchak, T.; Ellis-Grosse, E. J.; Loh, E.; Study, G., A multicenter trial of the efficacy and safety of tigecycline *versus* imipenem/cilastatin in patients with complicated intra-abdominal infections (Study ID Numbers: 3074A1-301-WW). *BMC Infect. Dis.* **2005**, *5*.

[85] Fomin, P.; Beuran, M.; Gradauskas, A.; Barauskas, G.; Datsenko, A.; Dartois, N.; Ellis-Grosse, E.; Loh, E., Tigecycline is efficacious in the treatment of complicated intra-abdominal infections. *Int. J. Surg.* **2005**, *3* (1), 35-47.

[86] Sacchidanand, S.; Penn, R. L.; Embil, J. M.; Campos, M. E.; Curcio, D.; Ellis-Grosse, E.; Loh, E.; Rose, G., Efficacy and safety of tigecycline monotherapy compared with vancomycin plus aztreonam in patients with complicated skin and skin structure infections: Results from a phase 3, randomized, double-blind trial. *Int. J. Infect. Dis.* **2005**, *9* (5), 251-261.

[87] Smith, K. L.; McCabe, S. M.; Awschlimann, J. R., Tigecycline - A novel glycylcycline antibiotic. *Formulary* **2005**, *40* (8), 245.

[88] Hunt, D., TP-434 is a novel broad-spectrum fluorocycline. In *Proceedings of the 50th Interscience Conference on Antimicrobial Agents and Chemotherapy Conference*, Boston, MA, 2010.

[89] U.S. National Institutes of Health. Study to Compare TP-434 and Ertapenem in CA Complicated Intra-abdominal Infections. http://clinicaltrials.gov/show/NCT01265784 (accessed June 2012).

[90] Jacobs, M. R., Retapamulin: a semisynthetic pleuromutilin compound for topical treatment of skin infections in adults and children. *Future Microbiol.* **2007**, *2* (6), 591-600.

[91] Yan, K.; Madden, L.; Choudhry, A. E.; Voigt, C. S.; Copeland, R. A.; Gontarek, R. R., Biochemical characterization of the interactions of the novel pleuromutilin derivative

retapamulin with bacterial ribosomes. *Antimicrob. Agents Chemother.* **2006**, *50* (11), 3875-3881.

[92] Woodford, N.; Afzal-Shah, M.; Warner, M.; Livermore, D. M., *In vitro* activity of retapamulin against Staphylococcus aureus isolates resistant to fusidic acid and mupirocin. *J. Antimicrob. Chemother.* **2008**, *62* (4), 766-768.

[93] U.S. National Institutes of Health. Study Comparing the Safety and Efficacy of Two Doses of BC-3781 *vs* Vancomycin in Patients with ABSSSI http://clinicaltrials.gov/ct2/show/results/NCT01119105 (accessed June 2012).

[94] Sader, H. S., Activity of BC-3781, a novel pleuromutilin compound, tested against clinical isolates of MRSA, including molecularly characterized community-acquired and hospital-associated strains. In *Proceedings of the 50th Interscience Conference on Antimicrobial Agents and Chemotherapy Conference*, Boston, MA, 2010.

[95] Wicha, W. W.; Ivezic-Schoenfeld, Z.; Novak, R., Efficacy of BC-3781 in murine pneumonia models. In *Proceedings of the 50th Interscience Conference on Antimicrobial Agents and Chemotherapy Conference*, Boston, MA, 2010.

[96] Nabriva Therapeutics Product Pipeline: Pleuromutilin. http://www.nabriva.com/programs/product-pipeline/ (accessed August 2012).

[97] Biedenbach, D. J.; Jones, R. N.; Ivezic-Schoenfeld, Z.; Paukner, S.; Novak, R., *In vitro* antibacterial spectrum of BC-7013, a novel pleuromutilin derivative for topical use in humans. In *Proceedings of the 49th Interscience Conference on Antimicrobial Agents and Chemotherapy*, San Francisco, CA, 2009.

[98] Craig, W. A.; Andes, D.; Ivezic-Schoenfeld, Z.; Wicha, W. W.; Novak, R., *In vivo* pharmacodynamic activity of BC-3205, a novel pleuromutilin derivative. In *Proceedings of the 49th Interscience Conference on Antimicrobial Agents and Chemotherapy*, San Francisco, CA, 2009.

[99] Maskell, J. P.; Williams, J. D., *In Vitro* Susceptibility of Oral Streptococci to Pristinamycin. *J. Antimicrob. Chemother.* **1987**, *19* (5), 585-590.

[100] Allington, D. R.; Rivey, M. P., Quinupristin/dalfopristin: A therapeutic review. *Clin. Ther.* **2001**, *23* (1), 24-44.

[101] Synercid I.V. (quinupristin and dalfopristin for injection). http://www.fda.gov/Safety/MedWatch/SafetyInformation/Safety-RelatedDrugLabelingChanges/ucm123454.htm (accessed August 2012).

[102] Sanders, W. E.; Sanders, C. C., Sisomicin: a review of eight years' experience. *Rev. Infect. Dis.* **1980**, *2* (2), 182–195.

[103] Aggen, J. B.; Armstrong, E. S.; Goldblum, A. A.; Dozzo, P.; Linsell, M. S.; Gliedt, M. J.; Hildebrandt, D. J.; Feeney, L. A.; Kubo, A.; Matias, R. D.; Lopez, S.; Gomez, M.; Wlasichuk, K. B.; Diokno, R.; Miller, G. H.; Moser, H. E., Synthesis and Spectrum of the Neoglycoside ACHN-490. *Antimicrob. Agents Chemother.* **2010**, *54* (11), 4636-4642.

[104] Armstrong, E. S.; Miller, G. H., Combating evolution with intelligent design: the neoglycoside ACHN-490. *Curr. Opin. Microbiol.* **2010**, *13* (5), 565-573.

[105] Endimiani, A.; Hujer, K. M.; Hujer, A. M.; Armstrong, E. S.; Choudhary, Y.; Aggen, J. B.; Bonomo, R. A., ACHN-490, a Neoglycoside with Potent *In Vitro* Activity against Multidrug-Resistant Klebsiella pneumoniae Isolates. *Antimicrob. Agents Chemother.* **2009**, *53* (10), 4504-4507.

[106] Scheinfeld, N., Telithromycin: a brief review of a new ketolide antibiotic. *J. Drugs Dermatol.* **2004**, *3* (4), 409-413.

[107] Ketek Prescribing Information. http://products.sanofi.us/ketek/ketek.html (accessed August 2012).

[108] Neuhauser, M. M.; Prause, J. L.; Danziger, L. H.; Pendland, S. L., *In vitro* bactericidal activities of ABT-773 against ermB strains of Streptococcus pneumoniae. *Antimicrob. Agents Chemother.* **2003**, *47* (3), 1132-1134.

[109] Cempra Pharmaceuticals: Solithromycin. http://www.cempra.com/products/Solithromycin-cem-101/ (accessed August 2012).

[110] Putnam, S. D.; Sader, H. S.; Farrell, D. J.; Biedenbach, D. J.; Castanheira, M., Antimicrobial characterisation of solithromycin (CEM-101), a novel fluoroketolide: activity against staphylococci and enterococci. *Int. J. Antimicrob. Agents* **2011**, *37* (1), 39-45.

[111] McGhee, P.; Clark, C.; Kosowska-Shick, K. M.; Nagai, K.; Dewasse, B.; Beachel, L.; Appelbaum, P. C., *In Vitro* Activity of CEM-101 against Streptococcus pneumoniae and Streptococcus pyogenes with Defined Macrolide Resistance Mechanisms. *Antimicrob. Agents Chemother.* **2010**, *54* (1), 230-238.

[112] Woosley, L. N.; Castanheira, M.; Jones, R. N., CEM-101 Activity against Gram-Positive Organisms. *Antimicrob. Agents Chemother.* **2010**, *54* (5), 2182-2187.

[113] Putnam, S. D.; Castanheira, M.; Moet, G. J.; Farrell, D. J.; Jones, R. N., CEM-101, a novel fluoroketolide: antimicrobial activity against a diverse collection of Gram-positive and Gram-negative bacteria. *Diagn. Microbiol. Infect. Dis.* **2010**, *66* (4), 393-401.

[114] Cempra Pharmaceuticals. Solithromycin. http://www.cempra.com/research/antibacterials/ (accessed August 2012).

[115] Bertrand, D.; Bertrand, S.; Neveu, E.; Fernandes, P., Molecular Characterization of Off-Target Activities of Telithromycin: a Potential Role for Nicotinic Acetylcholine Receptors. *Antimicrob. Agents Chemother.* **2010**, *54* (12), 5399-5402.

[116] U.S. National Institutes of Health. Efficacy and Safety Study of Oral CEM-101 Compared to Oral Levofloxacin in Treatment of Patients With Community-Acquired Bacterial Pneumonia. http://clinicaltrials.gov/show/NCT01168713 (accessed June 2012).

[117] Farrell, D. J.; Castanheira, M.; Sader, H. S.; Jones, R. N., The *in vitro* evaluation of solithromycin (CEM-101) against pathogens isolated in the United States and Europe (2009). *J. Infect.* **2010**, *61* (6), 476-483.

[118] Gordon, J. J.; Kelly, B. K.; Miller, G. A., Actinonin: an antibiotic substance produced by an actinomycete. *Nature* **1962**, *195*, 701-702.

[119] Gordon, J. J.; Devlin, J. P.; East, A. J.; Ollis, W. D.; Wright, D. E.; Ninet, L., Studies concerning the antibiotic actinonin. Part I. The constitution of actinonin. A natural hydroxamic acid with antibiotic activity. *J. Chem. Soc., Perkin Trans. 1 (1972-1999)* **1975**, (9), 819-825.

[120] Chen, D. Z.; Patel, D. V.; Hackbarth, C. J.; Wang, W.; Dreyer, G.; Young, D. C.; Margolis, P. S.; Wu, C.; Ni, Z. J.; Trias, J.; White, R. J.; Yuan, Z. Y., Actinonin, a naturally occurring antibacterial agent, is a potent deformylase inhibitor. *Biochemistry* **2000**, *39* (6), 1256-1262.

[121] Leeds, J. A.; Dean, C. R., Peptide deformylase as an antibacterial target: a critical assessment. *Curr. Opin. Pharmacol.* **2006**, *6* (5), 445-452.

[122] Clements, J. M.; Beckett, R. P.; Brown, A.; Catlin, G.; Lobell, M.; Palan, S.; Thomas, W.; Whittaker, M.; Wood, S.; Salama, S.; Baker, P. J.; Rodgers, H. F.; Barynin, V.; Rice, D.

W.; Hunter, M. G., Antibiotic activity and characterization of BB-3497, a novel peptide deformylase inhibitor. *Antimicrob. Agents Chemother.* **2001**, *45* (2), 563-570.

[123] Azoulay-Dupuis, E.; Mohler, J.; Bedos, J. P., Efficacy of BB-83698, a novel peptide deformylase inhibitor, in a mouse model of pneumococcal pneumonia. *Antimicrob. Agents Chemother.* **2004**, *48* (1), 80-85.

[124] Clements, J. M.; Ayscough, A. P.; Keavey, K.; East, S. P., Peptide deformylase inhibitors, potential for a new class of broad spectrum antibacterials. *Curr. Med. Chem. Anti-Infect. Agents* **2002**, *1*, 239-249.

[125] Bowker, K. E.; Noel, A. R.; MacGowan, A. P., *In vitro* activities of nine peptide deformylase inhibitors and five comparator agents against respiratory and skin pathogens. *Int. J. Antimicrob. Agents* **2003**, *22* (6), 557-561.

[126] Apfel, C. M.; Locher, H.; Evers, S.; Takacs, B.; Hubschwerlen, C.; Pirson, W.; Page, M. G. P.; Keck, W., Peptide deformylase as an antibacterial drug target: Target validation and resistance development. *Antimicrob. Agents Chemother.* **2001**, *45* (4), 1058-1064.

[127] Bouchillon, S. K.; Hackel, M.; Hoban, D. J.; Zalazain, M.; Butler, D., *In vitro* activity of GSK1322322, a novel peptide deformylase inhibitor, against 4,836 pathogens from skin and soft tissue infections and respiratory tract infections. In *Proceedings of the 50th Annual Interscience Conference on Antimicrobial Agents and Chemotherapy*, Boston, MA, 2010.

[128] Lewandowski, T.; Demarsh, P.; Peters, T.; Kulkarni, S., Potent activity of GSK1322322, a novel peptide deformylase inhibitor, after oral dosing in a murine multi-drug resistant Staphylococcus aureus infection model. In *Proceedings of the 50th Annual Interscience Conference on Antimicrobial Agents and Chemotherapy*, Boston, MA, 2010.

[129] U.S. National Institutes of Health. GSK1322322 *Versus* Linezolid in the Treatment of Acute Bacterial Skin and Skin Structure Infection. http://clinicaltrials.gov/ct2/show/record/NCT01209078 (accessed June 2012).

[130] Shiau, T. P.; Houchin, A.; Nair, S.; Xu, P.; Low, E.; Najafi, R.; Jain, R., Stieglitz rearrangement of N,N-dichloro-beta,beta-disubstituted taurines under mild aqueous conditions. *Bioorg. Med. Chem. Lett.* **2009**, *19* (4), 1110-1114.

[131] Francavilla, C.; Low, E.; Nair, S.; Kim, B.; Shiau, T. P.; Debabov, D.; Celeri, C.; Alvarez, N.; Houchin, A.; Xu, P.; Najafi, R.; Jain, R., Quaternary ammonium N,N-dichloroamines as topical, antimicrobial agents. *Bioorg. Med. Chem. Lett.* **2009**, *19* (10), 2731-2734.

[132] Wang, L.; Khosrovi, B.; Najafi, R., N-Chloro-2,2-dimethyltaurines: a new class of remarkably stable N-chlorotaurines. *Tetrahedron Lett.* **2008**, *49* (14), 2193-2195.

[133] Gottardi, W.; Nagl, M., N-chlorotaurine, a natural antiseptic with outstanding tolerability. *J. Antimicrob. Chemother.* **2010**, *65* (3), 399-409.

[134] Wang, L.; Belisle, B.; Bassiri, M.; Xu, P.; Debabov, D.; Celeri, C.; Alvarez, N.; Robson, M. C.; Payne, W. G.; Najafi, R.; Khosrovi, B., Chemical Characterization and Biological Properties of NVC-422, a Novel, Stable N-Chlorotaurine Analog. *Antimicrob. Agents Chemother.* **2011**, *55* (6), 2688-2692.

[135] Celeri, C.; Debabov, D.; Flagella, M., Biological characterization of N,N-dichloro-2,2-dimethyltaurine (NVC-422). In *Proceedings of the the American Society for Microbiology and the Infectious Diseases Society of America 48th Annual ICAAC/IDSA 46th Annual Meeting* Washington, DC, 2008.

[136] U.S. National Institutes of Health: Study to Evaluate NVC-422 for Urinary Catheter Blockage and Encrustation. http://clinicaltrials.gov/ct2/show/NCT01243125 (accessed August 2012).

[137] Page, M. G. P.; Dantier, C.; Desarbre, E., *In Vitro* Properties of BAL30072, a Novel Siderophore Sulfactam with Activity against Multiresistant Gram-Negative Bacilli. *Antimicrob. Agents Chemother.* **2010**, *54* (6), 2291-2302.

[138] Mushtaq, S.; Warner, M.; Livermore, D., Activity of the siderophore monobactam BAL30072 against multiresistant non-fermenters. *J. Antimicrob. Chemother.* **2010**, *65* (2), 266-270.

[139] Basilea Pharmaceutica. Basilea initiates phase I clinical program of its novel antibiotic BAL30072. http://www.basilea.com/News-and-Media/Basilea-initiates-phase-I-clinical-program-of-its-novel-antibiotic-BAL30072/381 (accessed August 2012).

[140] Heath, R. J.; White, S. W.; Rock, C. O., Lipid biosynthesis as a target for antibacterial agents. *Prog. Lipid Res.* **2001**, *40* (6), 467-497.

[141] Smith, S.; Witkowski, A.; Joshi, A. K., Structural and functional organization of the animal fatty acid synthase. *Prog. Lipid Res.* **2003**, *42* (4), 289-317.

[142] Young, K.; Jayasuriya, H.; Ondeyka, J. G.; Herath, K.; Zhang, C.; Kodali, S.; Galgoci, A.; Painter, R.; Brown-Driver, V.; Yamamoto, R.; Silver, L. L.; Zheng, Y.; Ventura, J. I.; Sigmund, J.; Ha, S.; Basilio, A.; Vicente, F.; Tormo, J. R.; Pelaez, F.; Youngman, P.; Cully, D.; Barrett, J. F.; Schmatz, D.; Singh, S. B.; Wang, J., Discovery of FabH/FabF Inhibitors from Natural Products. *Antimicrob. Agents Chemother.* **2006**, *50* (2), 519-526.

[143] Kodali, S.; Galgoci, A.; Young, K.; Painter, R.; Silver, L. L.; Herath, K. B.; Singh, S. B.; Cully, D.; Barrett, J. F.; Schmatz, D.; Wang, J., Determination of selectivity and efficacy of fatty acid synthesis inhibitors. *J. Biol. Chem.* **2005**, *280* (2), 1669-1677.

[144] Singh, S. B.; Jayasuriya, H.; Ondeyka, J. G.; Herath, K. B.; Zhang, C.; Zink, D. L.; Tsou, N. N.; Ball, R. G.; Basilio, A.; Genilloud, O.; Diez, M. T.; Vicente, F.; Pelaez, F.; Young, K.; Wang, J., Isolation, Structure, and Absolute Stereochemistry of Platensimycin, A Broad Spectrum Antibiotic Discovered Using an Antisense Differential Sensitivity Strategy. *J. Am. Chem. Soc.* **2006**, *128* (36), 11916-11920.

[145] Wang, J.; Soisson, S. M.; Young, K.; Shoop, W.; Kodali, S.; Galgoci, A.; Painter, R.; Parthasarathy, G.; Tang, Y. S.; Cummings, R.; Ha, S.; Dorso, K.; Motyl, M.; Jayasuriya, H.; Ondeyka, J.; Herath, K.; Zhang, C.; Hernandez, L.; Allocco, J.; Basilio, A.; Tormo, J. R.; Genilloud, O.; Vicente, F.; Pelaez, F.; Colwell, L.; Lee, S. H.; Michael, B.; Felcetto, T.; Gill, C.; Silver, L. L.; Hermes, J. D.; Bartizal, K.; Barrett, J.; Schmatz, D.; Becker, J. W.; Cully, D.; Singh, S. B., Platensimycin is a selective FabF inhibitor with potent antibiotic properties. *Nature* **2006**, *441* (7091), 358-361.

[146] Wang, J.; Kodali, S.; Lee, S. H.; Galgoci, A.; Painter, R.; Dorso, K.; Racine, F.; Motyl, M.; Hernandez, L.; Tinney, E.; Colletti, S. L.; Herath, K.; Cummings, R.; Salazar, O.; Gonzalez, I.; Basilio, A.; Vicente, F.; Genilloud, O.; Pelaez, F.; Jayasuriya, H.; Young, K.; Cully, D. F.; Singh, S. B., Discovery of platencin, a dual FabF and FabH inhibitor with *in vivo* antibiotic properties. *Proc. Natl. Acad. Sci. U. S. A.* **2007**, *104* (18), 7612-7616.

[147] Singh, S. B.; Ondeyka, J. G.; Herath, K. B.; Zhang, C.; Jayasuriya, H.; Zink, D. L.; Parthasarathy, G.; Becker, J. W.; Wang, J.; Soisson, S. M., Isolation, enzyme-bound structure and antibacterial activity of platencin A1 from Streptomyces platensis. *Bioorg. Med. Chem. Lett.* **2009**, *19* (16), 4756-4759.

[148] Singh, S. B.; Jayasuriya, H.; Herath, K. B.; Zhang, C.; Ondeyka, J. G.; Zink, D. L.; Ha, S.; Parthasarathy, G.; Becker, J. W.; Wang, J.; Soisson, S. M., Isolation, enzyme-bound structure, and activity of platensimycin A1 from Streptomyces platensis. *Tetrahedron Lett.* **2009**, *50* (37), 5182-5185.

[149] Zhang, C.; Ondeyka, J.; Dietrich, L.; Gailliot, F. P.; Hesse, M.; Lester, M.; Dorso, K.; Motyl, M.; Ha, S. N.; Wang, J.; Singh, S. B., Isolation, structure and biological activities of platencin A(2)-A(4) from Streptomyces platensis. *Bioorg. Med. Chem.* **2010**, *18* (7), 2602-2610.

[150] Zhang, C.; Ondeyka, J.; Herath, K.; Jayasuriya, H.; Guan, Z.; Zink, D. L.; Dietrich, L.; Burgess, B.; Ha, S. N.; Wang, J.; Singh, S. B., Platensimycin and Platencin Congeners from Streptomyces platensis. *J. Nat. Prod.* **2011**, *74* (3), 329-340.

[151] Zhang, C.; Ondeyka, J.; Guan, Z.; Dietrich, L.; Burgess, B.; Wang, J.; Singh, S. B., Isolation, structure and biological activities of platensimycin B4 from Streptomyces platensis. *J. Antibiot.* **2009**, *62* (12), 699-702.

[152] Zhang, C.; Ondeyka, J.; Zink, D. L.; Burgess, B.; Wang, J.; Singh, S. B., Isolation, structure and fatty acid synthesis inhibitory activities of platensimycin B1-B3 from Streptomyces platensis. *Chem. Commun.* **2008**, (40), 5034-5036.

[153] Herath, K. B.; Zhang, C.; Jayasuriya, H.; Ondeyka, J. G.; Zink, D. L.; Burgess, B.; Wang, J.; Singh, S. B., Structure and Semisynthesis of Platensimide A, Produced by Streptomyces platensis. *Org. Lett.* **2008**, *10* (9), 1699-1702.

[154] Jayasuriya, H.; Herath, K. B.; Ondeyka, J. G.; Zink, D. L.; Burgess, B.; Wang, J.; Singh, S. B., Structure of homoplatensimide A: a potential key biosynthetic intermediate of platensimycin isolated from Streptomyces platensis. *Tetrahedron Lett.* **2008**, *49* (22), 3648-3651.

[155] Martens, E.; Demain, A. L., Platensimycin and platencin: promising antibiotics for future application in human medicine. *J. Antibiot.* **2011**, *64* (11), 705-710.

[156] The first HIV protease inhibitors approved by the FDA:. *Antiviral Agents Bull.* 1995, pp 353-355.

[157] Sepkowitz, K. A., AIDS — The First 20 Years. *N. Engl. J. Med.* **2001**, *344* (23), 1764-1772.

[158] Le Douce, V.; Janossy, A.; Hallay, H.; Ali, S.; Riclet, R.; Rohr, O.; Schwartz, C., Achieving a cure for HIV infection: do we have reasons to be optimistic? *J. Antimicrob. Chemother.* **2012**, *67* (5), 1063-1074.

[159] Vella, S.; Palmisano, L., The global status of resistance to antiretroviral drugs. *Clin. Infect. Dis.* **2005**, *41 Suppl 4*, S239-246.

[160] Ghosh, A. K.; Chapsal, B. D.; Weber, I. T.; Mitsuya, H., Design of HIV protease inhibitors targeting protein backbone: an effective strategy for combating drug resistance. *Acc. Chem. Res.* **2008**, *41* (1), 78-86.

[161] Ghosh, A. K.; Kincaid, J. F.; Walters, D. E.; Chen, Y.; Chaudhuri, N. C.; Thompson, W. J.; Culberson, C.; Fitzgerald, P. M. D.; Lee, H. Y.; McKee, S. P.; Munson, P. M.; Duong, T. T.; Darke, P. L.; Zugay, J. A.; Schleif, W. A.; Axel, M. G.; Lin, J.; Huff, J. R., Nonpeptidal P2 Ligands for HIV Protease Inhibitors: Structure-Based Design, Synthesis, and Biological Evaluation. *J. Med. Chem.* **1996**, *39* (17), 3278-3290.

[162] Koh, Y.; Nakata, H.; Maeda, K.; Ogata, H.; Bilcer, G.; Devasamudram, T.; Kincaid, J. F.; Boross, P.; Wang, Y. F.; Tie, Y.; Volarath, P.; Gaddis, L.; Harrison, R. W.; Weber, I. T.; Ghosh, A. K.; Mitsuya, H., Novel bis-tetrahydrofuranylurethane-containing nonpeptidic protease inhibitor (PI) UIC-94017 (TMC114) with potent activity against multi-PI-resistant human immunodeficiency virus *in vitro*. *Antimicrob. Agents Chemother.* **2003**, *47* (10), 3123-3129.

[163] Ghosh, A. K.; Ramu Sridhar, P.; Kumaragurubaran, N.; Koh, Y.; Weber, I. T.; Mitsuya, H., Bis-Tetrahydrofuran: a Privileged Ligand for Darunavir and a New Generation of HIV Protease Inhibitors That Combat Drug Resistance. *ChemMedChem* **2006**, *1* (9), 939-950.

[164] De Meyer, S.; Azijn, H.; Surleraux, D.; Jochmans, D.; Tahri, A.; Pauwels, R.; Wigerinck, P.; de Bethune, M. P., TMC114, a novel human immunodeficiency virus type 1 protease inhibitor active against protease inhibitor-resistant viruses, including a broad range of clinical isolates. *Antimicrob. Agents Chemother.* **2005**, *49* (6), 2314-2321.

[165] Arasteh, K.; Yeni, P.; Pozniak, A.; Grinsztejn, B.; Jayaweera, D.; Roberts, A.; Hoy, J.; De Meyer, S.; Vangeneugden, T.; Tomaka, F., Efficacy and safety of darunavir/ritonavir in treatment-experienced HIV type-1 patients in the POWER 1, 2 and 3 trials at week 96. *Antivir. Ther.* **2009**, *14* (6), 859-864.

[166] Mills, A. M.; Nelson, M.; Jayaweera, D.; Ruxrungtham, K.; Cassetti, I.; Girard, P. M.; Workman, C.; Dierynck, I.; Sekar, V.; Abeele, C. V.; Lavreys, L., Once-daily darunavir/ritonavir *vs* lopinavir/ritonavir in treatment-naive, HIV-1-infected patients: 96-week analysis. *AIDS* **2009**, *23* (13), 1679-1688.

[167] Arribas, J. R.; Horban, A.; Gerstoft, J.; Fatkenheuer, G.; Nelson, M.; Clumeck, N.; Pulido, F.; Hill, A.; van Delft, Y.; Stark, T.; Moecklinghoff, C., The MONET trial: darunavir/ritonavir with or without nucleoside analogues, for patients with HIV RNA below 50 copies/ml. *AIDS* **2010**, *24* (2), 223-230.

[168] Klein, R.; Struble, K. Traditional approval of Prezista (darunavir), a new dosing regimen for treatment-naïve patients, new 400 mg tablets, and revised Pregnancy Category. http://www.fda.gov/ForConsumers/ByAudience/ForPatientAdvocates/HIVandAIDSActivities/ucm121607.htm (accessed September 22, 2012).

[169] Thaisrivongs, S.; Tomich, P. K.; Watenpaugh, K. D.; Chong, K.-T.; Howe, W. J.; Yang, C.-P.; Strohbach, J. W.; Turner, S. R.; McGrath, J. P., Structure-Based Design of HIV Protease Inhibitors: 4-Hydroxycoumarins and 4-Hydroxy-2-pyrones as Non-peptidic Inhibitors. *J. Med. Chem.* **1994**, *37* (20), 3200-3204.

[170] Bourinbaiar, A. S.; Tan, X.; Nagorny, R., Effect of the oral anticoagulant, warfarin, on HIV-1 replication and spread. *AIDS* **1993**, *7* (1), 129-130.

[171] Tummino, P. J.; Ferguson, D.; Hupe, D., Competitive inhibition of HIV-1 protease by warfarin derivatives. *Biochem. Biophys. Res. Commun.* **1994**, *201* (1), 290-294.

[172] Hirsh, J.; Dalen, J. E.; Deykin, D.; Poller, L., Oral anticoagulants. Mechanism of action, clinical effectiveness, and optimal therapeutic range. *Chest* **1992**, *102* (4 Suppl), 312S-326S.

[173] Skulnick, H. I.; Johnson, P. D.; Howe, W. J.; Tomich, P. K.; Chong, K. T.; Watenpaugh, K. D.; Janakiraman, M. N.; Dolak, L. A.; McGrath, J. P.; Lynn, J. C.; *et al.*, Structure-based design of sulfonamide-substituted non-peptidic HIV protease inhibitors. *J. Med. Chem.* **1995**, *38* (26), 4968-4971.

[174] Thaisrivongs, S.; Skulnick, H. I.; Turner, S. R.; Strohbach, J. W.; Tommasi, R. A.; Johnson, P. D.; Aristoff, P. A.; Judge, T. M.; Gammill, R. B.; Morris, J. K.; Romines, K. R.; Chrusciel, R. A.; Hinshaw, R. R.; Chong, K.-T.; Tarpley, W. G.; Poppe, S. M.; Slade, D. E.; Lynn, J. C.; Horng, M.-M.; Tomich, P. K.; Seest, E. P.; Dolak, L. A.; Howe, W. J.; Howard, G. M.; Schwende, F. J.; Toth, L. N.; Padbury, G. E.; Wilson, G. J.; Shiou, L.; Zipp, G. L.; Wilkinson, K. F.; Rush, B. D.; Ruwart, M. J.; Koeplinger, K. A.; Zhao, Z.; Cole, S.; Zaya, R. M.; Kakuk, T. J.; Janakiraman, M. N.; Watenpaugh, K. D., Structure-

Based Design of HIV Protease Inhibitors: Sulfonamide-Containing 5,6-Dihydro-4-hydroxy-2-pyrones as Non-Peptidic Inhibitors. *J. Med. Chem.* **1996**, *39* (22), 4349-4353.

[175] Turner, S. R.; Strohbach, J. W.; Tommasi, R. A.; Aristoff, P. A.; Johnson, P. D.; Skulnick, H. I.; Dolak, L. A.; Seest, E. P.; Tomich, P. K.; Bohanon, M. J.; Horng, M.-M.; Lynn, J. C.; Chong, K.-T.; Hinshaw, R. R.; Watenpaugh, K. D.; Janakiraman, M. N.; Thaisrivongs, S., Tipranavir (PNU-140690): A Potent, Orally Bioavailable Nonpeptidic HIV Protease Inhibitor of the 5,6-Dihydro-4-hydroxy-2-pyrone Sulfonamide Class. *J. Med. Chem.* **1998**, *41* (18), 3467-3476.

[176] Hicks, C. B.; Cahn, P.; Cooper, D. A.; Walmsley, S. L.; Katlama, C.; Clotet, B.; Lazzarin, A.; Johnson, M. A.; Neubacher, D.; Mayers, D.; Valdez, H., Durable efficacy of tipranavir-ritonavir in combination with an optimised background regimen of antiretroviral drugs for treatment-experienced HIV-1-infected patients at 48 weeks in the Randomized Evaluation of Strategic Intervention in multi-drug reSistant patients with Tipranavir (RESIST) studies: an analysis of combined data from two randomised open-label trials. *Lancet* **2006**, *368* (9534), 466-475.

[177] Klein, R.; Struble, K. FDA approval of Aptivus (tipranavir). http://www.fda.gov/ForConsumers/ByAudience/ForPatientAdvocates/HIVandAIDSActivities/ucm124850.htm (accessed October 20, 2012).

[178] Wainwright, A. New Aptivus® (tipranavir) Oral Solution Approved for Treatment-Experienced Pediatric and Adolescent HIV Patients http://www.boehringer-ingelheim.com/news/news_releases/press_releases/2008/24_june_2008.html (accessed October 20, 2012).

[179] Temesgen, Z.; Feinberg, J., Tipranavir: A new option for the treatment of drug-resistant HIV infection. *Clin. Infect. Dis.* **2007**, *45* (6), 761-769.

[180] Fujioka, T.; Kashiwada, Y.; Kilkuskie, R. E.; Cosentino, L. M.; Ballas, L. M.; Jiang, J. B.; Janzen, W. P.; Chen, I. S.; Lee, K. H., Anti-AIDS agents, 11. Betulinic acid and platanic acid as anti-HIV principles from Syzigium claviflorum, and the anti-HIV activity of structurally related triterpenoids. *J. Nat. Prod.* **1994**, *57* (2), 243-247.

[181] Kashiwada, Y.; Hashimoto, F.; Cosentino, L. M.; Chen, C.-H.; Garrett, P. E.; Lee, K.-H., Betulinic Acid and Dihydrobetulinic Acid Derivatives as Potent Anti-HIV Agents. *J. Med. Chem.* **1996**, *39* (5), 1016-1017.

[182] Li, F.; Goila-Gaur, R.; Salzwedel, K.; Kilgore, N. R.; Reddick, M.; Matallana, C.; Castillo, A.; Zoumplis, D.; Martin, D. E.; Orenstein, J. M.; Allaway, G. P.; Freed, E. O.; Wild, C. T., PA-457: A potent HIV inhibitor that disrupts core condensation by targeting a late step in Gag processing. *Proc. Natl. Acad. Sci. U. S. A.* **2003**, *100* (23), 13555-13560.

[183] Stoddart, C. A.; Joshi, P.; Sloan, B.; Bare, J. C.; Smith, P. C.; Allaway, G. P.; Wild, C. T.; Martin, D. E., Potent activity of the HIV-1 maturation inhibitor bevirimat in SCID-hu Thy/Liv mice. *PLoS One* **2007**, *2* (11), e1251.

[184] Martin, D. E.; Blum, R.; Wilton, J.; Doto, J.; Galbraith, H.; Burgess, G. L.; Smith, P. C.; Ballow, C., Safety and Pharmacokinetics of Bevirimat (PA-457), a Novel Inhibitor of Human Immunodeficiency Virus Maturation, in Healthy Volunteers. *Antimicrob. Agents Chemother.* **2007**, *51* (9), 3063-3066.

[185] Smith, P. F.; Ogundele, A.; Forrest, A.; Wilton, J.; Salzwedel, K.; Doto, J.; Allaway, G. P.; Martin, D. E., Phase I and II study of the safety, virologic effect, and pharmacokinetics/pharmacodynamics of single-dose 3-o-(3',3'-dimethylsuccinyl)betulinic

acid (bevirimat) against human immunodeficiency virus infection. *Antimicrob. Agents Chemother.* **2007**, *51* (10), 3574-3581.

[186] McCallister, S.; J., L.; G., R.; Thompson, M.; R., H.; D., M.; K., S.; Allaway, G. In *HIV-1 Gag Polymorphisms Determine Treatment Response to Bevirimat (PA-457)*, Antivir. Ther. Sitges, Spain, Sitges, Spain, 2008; p A10.

[187] Van Baelen, K.; Salzwedel, K.; Rondelez, E.; Van Eygen, V.; De Vos, S.; Verheyen, A.; Steegen, K.; Verlinden, Y.; Allaway, G. P.; Stuyver, L. J., Susceptibility of human immunodeficiency virus type 1 to the maturation inhibitor bevirimat is modulated by baseline polymorphisms in Gag spaccr peptide 1. *Antimicrob. Agents Chemother.* **2009**, *53* (5), 2185-2188.

[188] Heider, D.; Verheyen, J.; Hoffmann, D., Predicting Bevirimat resistance of HIV-1 from genotype. *BMC Bioinf.* **2010**, *11*, 37.

[189] Alcorn, K. Myriad halts HIV maturation inhibitor drug programme. http://www.aidsmap.com/Myriad-halts-HIV-maturation-inhibitor-drug-programme/page/1439004/ (accessed Nov. 23, 2012).

[190] Innaimo, S. F.; Seifer, M.; Bisacchi, G. S.; Standring, D. N.; Zahler, R.; Colonno, R. J., Identification of BMS-200475 as a potent and selective inhibitor of hepatitis B virus. *Antimicrob. Agents Chemother.* **1997**, *41* (7), 1444-1448.

[191] Price, P. M.; Banerjee, R.; Jeffrey, A. M.; Acs, G., The mechanism of inhibition of hepatitis B virus replication by the carbocyclic analog of 2'-deoxyguanosine. *Hepatology (Hoboken, NJ, U. S.)* **1992**, *16* (1), 8-12.

[192] Seifer, M.; Hamatake, R. K.; Colonno, R. J.; Standring, D. N., *In vitro* inhibition of hepadnavirus polymerases by the triphosphates of BMS-200475 and lobucavir. *Antimicrob. Agents Chemother.* **1998**, *42* (12), 3200-3208.

[193] de Man, R. A.; Wolters, L. M. M.; Nevens, F.; Chua, D.; Sherman, M.; Lai, C. L.; Gadano, A.; Lee, Y.; Mazzotta, F.; Thomas, N.; DeHertogh, D., Safety and efficacy of oral entecavir given for 28 days in patients with chronic hepatitis B virus infection. *Hepatology (Hoboken, NJ, U. S.)* **2001**, *34* (3), 578-582.

[194] Chang, T. T.; Gish, R. G.; Hadziyannis, S. J.; Cianciara, J.; Rizzetto, M.; Schiff, E. R.; Pastore, G.; Bacon, B. R.; Poynard, T.; Joshi, S.; Klesczewski, K. S.; Thiry, A.; Rose, R. E.; Colonno, R. J.; Hindes, R. G., A dose-ranging study of the efficacy and tolerability of entecavir in Lamivudine-refractory chronic hepatitis B patients. *Gastroenterology* **2005**, *129* (4), 1198-1209.

[195] Chang, T. T.; Gish, R. G.; de Man, R.; Gadano, A.; Sollano, J.; Chao, Y. C.; Lok, A. S.; Han, K. H.; Goodman, Z.; Zhu, J.; Cross, A.; DeHertogh, D.; Wilber, R.; Colonno, R.; Apelian, D., A comparison of entecavir and lamivudine for HBeAg-positive chronic hepatitis B. *N. Engl. J. Med.* **2006**, *354* (10), 1001-1010.

[196] Gish, R. G.; Chang, T. T.; de Man, R.; Gadano, A.; Sollano, J.; Han, K. H.; Lok, A. S.; Zhu, J.; Cross, A.; Brett-Smith, H.; Fernandes, L., Entecavir Results in Substantial Virologic and Biochemical Improvement and HBeAg Seroconversion Through 96 Weeks of Treatment in HBeAg Chronic Hepatitis B Patients (Study ETV-022). *Hepatology (Hoboken, NJ, U. S.)* **2005**, *Supplement 1*, A181.

[197] Klein, R.; Struble, K. Approval of Baraclude (entecavir) for Treatment of Chronic Hepatitis B Virus Infection. http://www.fda.gov/ForConsumers/ByAudience/ForPatientAdvocates/HIVandAIDSActivities/ucm124910.htm (accessed October 21, 2012).

[198] Zoulim, F., Antiviral therapy of chronic hepatitis B. *Antiviral Res.* **2006**, *71* (2–3), 206-215.

[199] Koklu, S.; Tuna, Y.; Gulsen, M. T.; Demir, M.; Koksal, A. S.; Kockar, M. C.; Aygun, C.; Coban, S.; Ozdil, K.; Ataseven, H.; Akin, E.; Purnak, T.; Yuksel, I.; Ataseven, H.; Ibis, M.; Yildirim, B.; Nadir, I.; Kucukazman, M.; Akbal, E.; Yuksel, O.; Basar, O., Long-Term Efficacy and Safety of Lamivudine, Entecavir, and Tenofovir for Treatment of HBV-Related Cirrhosis. *Clin. Gastroenterol. Hepatol.* **2012**, 88-94.

[200] Chang, T.-T.; Lai, C.-L.; Kew Yoon, S.; Lee, S. S.; Coelho, H. S. M.; Carrilho, F. J.; Poordad, F.; Halota, W.; Horsmans, Y.; Tsai, N.; Zhang, H.; Tenney, D. J.; Tamez, R.; Iloeje, U., Entecavir treatment for up to 5 years in patients with hepatitis B e antigen–positive chronic hepatitis B. *Hepatology (Hoboken, NJ, U. S.)* **2010**, *51* (2), 422-430.

[201] Bryant, M. L.; Bridges, E. G.; Placidi, L.; Faraj, A.; Loi, A. G.; Pierra, C.; Dukhan, D.; Gosselin, G.; Imbach, J. L.; Hernandez, B.; Juodawlkis, A.; Tennant, B.; Korba, B.; Cote, P.; Marion, P.; Cretton-Scott, E.; Schinazi, R. F.; Sommadossi, J. P., Antiviral L-nucleosides specific for hepatitis B virus infection. *Antimicrob. Agents Chemother.* **2001**, *45* (1), 229-235.

[202] Jones, R.; Nelson, M., Novel anti-hepatitis B agents: a focus on telbivudine. *Int. J. Clin. Prac.* **2006**, *60* (10), 1295-1299.

[203] Nelson, M. In *Telbivudine (L-dT) in phase III studies for chronic hepatitis B.*, HEP DART, Kuai, HI, Dec 14-18; Kuai, HI, 2003.

[204] Lai, C. L.; Leung, N.; Teo, E. K.; Tong, M.; Wong, F.; Hann, H. W.; Han, S.; Poynard, T.; Myers, M.; Chao, G.; Lloyd, D.; Brown, N. A., A 1-year trial of telbivudine, lamivudine, and the combination in patients with hepatitis B e antigen-positive chronic hepatitis B. *Gastroenterology* **2005**, *129* (2), 528-536.

[205] Lai, C.-L.; Gane, E.; Liaw, Y.-F.; Hsu, C.-W.; Thongsawat, S.; Wang, Y.; Chen, Y.; Heathcote, E. J.; Rasenack, J.; Bzowej, N.; Naoumov, N. V.; Di Bisceglie, A. M.; Zeuzem, S.; Moon, Y. M.; Goodman, Z.; Chao, G.; Constance, B. F.; Brown, N. A., Telbivudine *versus* Lamivudine in Patients with Chronic Hepatitis B. *N. Engl. J. Med.* **2007**, *357* (25), 2576-2588.

[206] Zeuzem, S.; Gane, E.; Liaw, Y. F.; Lim, S. G.; DiBisceglie, A.; Buti, M.; Chutaputti, A.; Rasenack, J.; Hou, J.; O'Brien, C.; Nguyen, T. T.; Jia, J. D.; Poynard, T.; Belanger, B.; Bao, W.; Naoumov, N. V., Baseline characteristics and early on-treatment response predict the outcomes of 2 years of telbivudine treatment of chronic hepatitis B. *J. Hepatol.* **2009**, *51* (1), 11-20.

[207] Chan, H. L. Y.; Heathcote, E. J.; Marcellin, P.; Lai, C.-L.; Cho, M.; Moon, Y. M.; Chao, Y.-C.; Myers, R. P.; Minuk, G. Y.; Jeffers, L.; Sievert, W.; Bzowej, N.; Harb, G.; Kaiser, R.; Qiao, X.-J.; Brown, N. A., Treatment of Hepatitis B e Antigen–Positive Chronic Hepatitis with Telbivudine or AdefovirA Randomized Trial. *Ann. Intern. Med.* **2007**, *147* (11), 745-754.

[208] Chu, C. K.; Ma, T. W.; Shanhmuganathan, K.; Wang, C. G.; Xiang, Y. J.; Pai, S. B.; Yao, G. Q.; Sommadossi, J. P.; Cheng, Y. C., USE OF 2'-FLUORO-5-METHYL-BETA-L-ARABINOFURANOSYLURACIL AS A NOVEL ANTIVIRAL AGENT FOR HEPATITIS-B VIRUS AND EPSTEIN-BARR-VIRUS. *Antimicrob. Agents Chemother.* **1995**, *39* (4), 979-981.

[209] Liu, S. H.; Grove, K. L.; Cheng, Y. C., Unique metabolism of a novel antiviral L-nucleoside analog, 2 '-fluoro-5-methyl-beta-L-arabinofuranosyluracil: a substrate for both

thymidine kinase and deoxycytidine kinase. *Antimicrob. Agents Chemother.* **1998**, *42* (4), 833-839.

[210] Pai, S. B.; Liu, S. H.; Zhu, Y. L.; Chu, C. K.; Cheng, Y. C., Inhibition of hepatitis B virus by a novel L-nucleoside, 2'-fluoro-5-methyl-beta-L-arabinofuranosyl uracil. *Antimicrob. Agents Chemother.* **1996**, *40* (2), 380-386.

[211] Yoo, B. C.; Kim, J. H.; Chung, Y. H.; Lee, K. S.; Paik, S. W.; Ryu, S. H.; Han, B. H.; Han, J. Y.; Byun, K. S.; Cho, M.; Lee, H. J.; Kim, T. H.; Cho, S. H.; Park, J. W.; Um, S. H.; Hwang, S. G.; Kim, Y. S.; Lee, Y. J.; Chon, C. Y.; Kim, B. L.; Lee, Y. S.; Yang, J. M.; Kim, H. C.; Hwang, J. S.; Choi, S. K.; Kweon, Y. O.; Jeong, S. H.; Lee, M. S.; Choi, J. Y.; Kim, D. G.; Lee, H. Y.; Yoo, K.; Yoo, H. W.; Lee, H. S., Twenty-four-week clevudine therapy showed potent and sustained antiviral activity in HBeAg-positive chronic hepatitis B. *Hepatology* **2007**, *45* (5), 1172-1178.

[212] Yoo, B. C.; Kim, J. H.; Kim, T. H.; Kohl, K. C.; Um, S. H.; Kim, Y. S.; Lee, K. S.; Hang, B. H.; Chon, C. Y.; Han, J. Y.; Ryu, S. H.; Kim, H. C.; Byun, K. S.; Hwang, S. G.; Kim, B. I.; Cho, M.; Yoo, K.; Lee, H. J.; Hwang, J. S.; Lee, Y. S.; Choi, S. K.; Lee, Y. J.; Yang, J. M.; Park, J. W.; Lee, M. S.; Kim, D. G.; Chung, Y. H.; Cho, S. H.; Choi, J. Y.; Kweon, Y. O.; Lee, H. Y.; Jeong, S. H.; Yoo, H. W.; Lee, H. S., Clevudine is highly efficacious in hepatitis B e antigen-negative chronic hepatitis B with durable off-therapy viral suppression. *Hepatology* **2007**, *46* (4), 1041-1048.

[213] Lau, G. K.; Leung, N., Forty-eight weeks treatment with clevudine 30 mg qd *versus* lamivudine 100 mg qd for chronic hepatitis B infection: a double-blind randomized study. *Korean J. Hepatol.* **2010**, *16* (3), 315-320.

[214] Kim, I. H.; Lee, S.; Kim, S. H.; Kim, S. W.; Lee, S. O.; Lee, S. T.; Kim, D. G.; Choi, C. S.; Kim, H. C., Treatment outcomes of clevudine *versus* lamivudine at week 48 in naïve patients with HBeAg positive chronic hepatitis B. *J. Korean Med. Sci.* **2010**, *25* (5), 738-745.

[215] Yang, H. W.; Lee, B. S.; Lee, T. H.; Lee, H. Y.; Nam, K. W.; Kang, Y. W.; Chae, H. B.; Kim, S. H.; Kim, S. B.; Lee, H.; Kim, A. N.; Song, I. H.; Lee, S. H.; Kim, H. S., Efficacy of initial treatment with clevudine in naive patients with chronic hepatitis B. *Korean J. Intern. Med.* **2010**, *25* (4), 372-376.

[216] Shin, S. R.; Yoo, B. C.; Choi, M. S.; Lee, D. H.; Song, S. M.; Lee, J. H.; Koh, K. C.; Paik, S. W., A comparison of 48-week treatment efficacy between clevudine and entecavir in treatment-naïve patients with chronic hepatitis B. *Hepatol. Int.* **2011**, *5* (2), 664-670.

[217] Seok, J. I.; Lee, D. K.; Lee, C. H.; Park, M. S.; Kim, S. Y.; Kim, H. S.; Jo, H. Y.; Kim, D. S., Long-Term Therapy with Clevudine for Chronic Hepatitis B Can Be Associated with Myopathy Characterized by Depletion of Mitochondrial DNA. *Hepatology* **2009**, *49* (6), 2080-2086.

[218] Kim, B. K.; Oh, J.; Kwon, S. Y.; Choe, W. H.; Ko, S. Y.; Rhee, K. H.; Seo, T. H.; Lim, S. D.; Lee, C. H., Clevudine myopathy in patients with chronic hepatitis B. *J. Hepatol.* **2009**, *51* (4), 829-834.

[219] Tak, W. Y.; Park, S. Y.; Cho, C. M.; Jung, M. K.; Jeon, S. W.; Kweon, Y. O.; Park, J. Y.; Sohn, Y. K., Clinical, biochemical, and pathological characteristics of clevudine-associated myopathy. *J. Hepatol.* **2010**, *53* (2), 261-266.

[220] Choung, B. S.; Kim, I. H.; Jeon, B. J.; Lee, S.; Kim, S. H.; Kim, S. W.; Lee, S. O.; Lee, S. T.; Kim, D. G., Long-Term Treatment Efficacy and Safety of Clevudine Therapy in Naive Patients with Chronic Hepatitis B. *Gut Liver* **2012**, *6* (4), 486-492.

[221] Pharmasset Voluntarily Halts Clinical Studies with Clevudine in Hepatitis B Infected Patients. http://www.fiercebiotech.com/press-releases/pharmasset-voluntarily-halts-clinical-studies-clevudine-hepatitis-b-infected-patien-0 (accessed August 2012).

[222] Hay, A. J.; Wolstenholme, A. J.; Skehel, J. J.; Smith, M. H., The molecular basis of the specific anti-influenza action of amantadine. *EMBO J.* **1985**, *4* (11), 3021-3024.

[223] Wang, C.; Takeuchi, K.; Pinto, L. H.; Lamb, R. A., Ion channel activity of influenza A virus M2 protein: characterization of the amantadine block. *J. Virol.* **1993**, *67* (9), 5585-5594.

[224] Bright, R. A.; Shay, D. K.; Shu, B.; Cox, N. J.; Klimov, A. I., Adamantane resistance among influenza A viruses isolated early during the 2005-2006 influenza season in the United States. *JAMA, J. Am. Med. Assoc.* **2006**, *295* (8), 891-894.

[225] Moscona, A., Neuraminidase Inhibitors for Influenza. *N. Engl. J. Med.* **2005**, *353* (13), 1363-1373.

[226] Hayden, F., Developing New Antiviral Agents for Influenza Treatment: What Does the Future Hold? *Clin. Infect. Dis.* **2009**, *48* (Supplement 1), S3-S13.

[227] von Itzstein, M.; Wu, W.-Y.; Kok, G. B.; Pegg, M. S.; Dyason, J. C.; Jin, B.; Phan, T. V.; Smythe, M. L.; White, H. F.; Oliver, S. W.; Colman, P. M.; Varghese, J. N.; Ryan, D. M.; Woods, J. M.; Bethell, R. C.; Hotham, V. J.; Cameron, J. M.; Penn, C. R., Rational design of potent sialidase-based inhibitors of influenza virus replication. *Nature* **1993**, *363* (6428), 418-423.

[228] Kim, C. U.; Lew, W.; Williams, M. A.; Liu, H.; Zhang, L.; Swaminathan, S.; Bischofberger, N.; Chen, M. S.; Mendel, D. B.; Tai, C. Y.; Laver, W. G.; Stevens, R. C., Influenza neuraminidase inhibitors possessing a novel hydrophobic interaction in the enzyme active site: design, synthesis, and structural analysis of carbocyclic sialic acid analogues with potent anti-influenza activity. *J. Am. Chem. Soc.* **1997**, *119* (4), 681-690.

[229] Meindl, P.; Bodo, G.; Palese, P.; Schulman, J.; Tuppy, H., Inhibition of neuraminidase activity by derivatives of 2-deoxy-2,3-dehydro-N-acetylneuraminic acid. *Virology* **1974**, *58* (2), 457-463.

[230] Gubareva, L. V., Molecular mechanisms of influenza virus resistance to neuraminidase inhibitors. *Virus Res.* **2004**, *103* (1–2), 199-203.

[231] Dharan, N. J.; Gubareva, L. V.; Meyer, J. J.; Okomo-Adhiambo, M.; McClinton, R. C.; Marshall, S. A.; St. George, K.; Epperson, S.; Brammer, L.; Klimov, A. I.; Bresee, J. S.; Fry, A. M., INfections with oseltamivir-resistant influenza a(h1n1) virus in the united states. *JAMA, J. Am. Med. Assoc.* **2009**, *301* (10), 1034-1041.

[232] Moss, R. B.; Davey, R. T.; Steigbigel, R. T.; Fang, F., Targeting pandemic influenza: a primer on influenza antivirals and drug resistance. *J. Antimicrob. Chemother.* **2010**, *65* (6), 1086-1093.

[233] Yamashita, M.; Tomozawa, T.; Kakuta, M.; Tokumitsu, A.; Nasu, H.; Kubo, S., CS-8958, a prodrug of the new neuraminidase inhibitor R-125489, shows long-acting anti-influenza virus activity. *Antimicrob. Agents Chemother.* **2009**, *53* (1), 186-192.

[234] Kubo, S.; Tomozawa, T.; Kakuta, M.; Tokumitsu, A.; Yamashita, M., Laninamivir Prodrug CS-8958, a Long-Acting Neuraminidase Inhibitor, Shows Superior Anti-Influenza Virus Activity after a Single Administration. *Antimicrob. Agents Chemother.* **2010**, *54* (3), 1256-1264.

[235] Kiso, M.; Kubo, S.; Ozawa, M.; Le, Q. M.; Nidom, C. A.; Yamashita, M.; Kawaoka, Y., Efficacy of the New Neuraminidase Inhibitor CS-8958 against H5N1 Influenza Viruses. *PLoS Pathog.* **2010**, *6* (2), e1000786.

[236] Itoh, Y.; Shinya, K.; Kiso, M.; Watanabe, T.; Sakoda, Y.; Hatta, M.; Muramoto, Y.; Tamura, D.; Sakai-Tagawa, Y.; Noda, T.; Sakabe, S.; Imai, M.; Hatta, Y.; Watanabe, S.; Li, C.; Yamada, S.; Fujii, K.; Murakami, S.; Imai, H.; Kakugawa, S.; Ito, M.; Takano, R.; Iwatsuki-Horimoto, K.; Shimojima, M.; Horimoto, T.; Goto, H.; Takahashi, K.; Makino, A.; Ishigaki, H.; Nakayama, M.; Okamatsu, M.; Takahashi, K.; Warshauer, D.; Shult, P. A.; Saito, R.; Suzuki, H.; Furuta, Y.; Yamashita, M.; Mitamura, K.; Nakano, K.; Nakamura, M.; Brockman-Schneider, R.; Mitamura, H.; Yamazaki, M.; Sugaya, N.; Suresh, M.; Ozawa, M.; Neumann, G.; Gern, J.; Kida, H.; Ogasawara, K.; Kawaoka, Y., *In vitro* and *in vivo* characterization of new swine-origin H1N1 influenza viruses. *Nature* **2009**, *460* (7258), 1021-1025.

[237] Koyama, K.; Takahashi, M.; Oitate, M.; Nakai, N.; Takakusa, H.; Miura, S.; Okazaki, O., CS-8958, a prodrug of the novel neuraminidase inhibitor R-125489, demonstrates a favorable long-retention profile in the mouse respiratory tract. *Antimicrob. Agents Chemother.* **2009**, *53* (11), 4845-4851.

[238] Ishizuka, H.; Yoshiba, S.; Okabe, H.; Yoshihara, K., Clinical pharmacokinetics of laninamivir, a novel long-acting neuraminidase inhibitor, after single and multiple inhaled doses of its prodrug, CS-8958, in healthy male volunteers. *J. Clin. Pharmacol.* **2010**, *50* (11), 1319-1329.

[239] Sugaya, N.; Ohashi, Y., Long-Acting Neuraminidase Inhibitor Laninamivir Octanoate (CS-8958) *versus* Oseltamivir as Treatment for Children with Influenza Virus Infection. *Antimicrob. Agents Chemother.* **2010**, *54* (6), 2575-2582.

[240] Watanabe, A.; Chang, S.-C.; Kim, M. J.; Chu, D. W.-s.; Ohashi, Y.; Group, f. t. M. S., Long-Acting Neuraminidase Inhibitor Laninamivir Octanoate *versus* Oseltamivir for Treatment of Influenza: A Double-Blind, Randomized, Noninferiority Clinical Trial. *Clin. Infect. Dis.* **2010**, *51* (10), 1167-1175.

[241] Yamashita, M., Laninamivir and its prodrug, CS-8958: long-acting neuraminidase inhibitors for the treatment of influenza. *Antivir. Chem. Chemother.* **2010**, *21* (2), 71-84.

[242] Biota wins BARDA contract to pursue clinical development of Laninamivir. http://www.biotapharma.com/ (accessed August 2012).

[243] Babu, Y. S.; Chand, P.; Bantia, S.; Kotian, P.; Dehghani, A.; El-Kattan, Y.; Lin, T. H.; Hutchison, T. L.; Elliott, A. J.; Parker, C. D.; Ananth, S. L.; Horn, L. L.; Laver, G. W.; Montgomery, J. A., BCX-1812 (RWJ-270201): discovery of a novel, highly potent, orally active, and selective influenza neuraminidase inhibitor through structure-based drug design. *J. Med. Chem.* **2000**, *43* (19), 3482-3486.

[244] Bantia, S.; Parker, C. D.; Ananth, S. L.; Horn, L. L.; Andries, K.; Chand, P.; Kotian, P. L.; Dehghani, A.; El-Kattan, Y.; Lin, T.; Hutchison, T. L.; Montgomery, J. A.; Kellog, D. L.; Babu, Y. S., Comparison of the anti-influenza virus activity of RWJ-270201 with those of oseltamivir and zanamivir. *Antimicrob. Agents Chemother.* **2001**, *45* (4), 1162-1167.

[245] Sidwell, R. W.; Smee, D. F.; Huffman, J. H.; Barnard, D. L.; Bailey, K. W.; Morrey, J. D.; Babu, Y. S., *In vivo* influenza virus-inhibitory effects of the cyclopentane neuraminidase inhibitor RJW-270201. *Antimicrob. Agents Chemother.* **2001**, *45* (3), 749-757.

[246] Kohno, S.; Kida, H.; Mizuguchi, M.; Shimada, J.; Group, f. t. S.-C. S., Efficacy and Safety of Intravenous Peramivir for Treatment of Seasonal Influenza Virus Infection. *Antimicrob. Agents Chemother.* **2010**, *54* (11), 4568-4574.

[247] Kohno, S.; Kida, H.; Mizuguchi, M.; Hirotsu, N.; Ishida, T.; Kadota, J.; Shimada, J., Intravenous peramivir for treatment of influenza A and B virus infection in high-risk patients. *Antimicrob. Agents Chemother.* **2011**, *55* (6), 2803-2812.

[248] Kohno, S.; Yen, M.-Y.; Cheong, H.-J.; Hirotsu, N.; Ishida, T.; Kadota, J.-i.; Mizuguchi, M.; Kida, H.; Shimada, J., Phase III Randomized, Double-Blind Study Comparing Single-Dose Intravenous Peramivir with Oral Oseltamivir in Patients with Seasonal Influenza Virus Infection. *Antimicrob. Agents Chemother.* **2011**, *55* (11), 5267-5276.

[249] Hikita, T.; Hikita, H.; Hikita, F.; Hikita, N.; Hikita, S., Clinical effectiveness of peramivir in comparison with other neuraminidase inhibitors in pediatric influenza patients. *Int. J. Pediatr.* **2012**, *2012*, e834181.

[250] Bennett, R. BioCryst Announces Outcome from the Peramivir Phase 3 Interim Analysis. http://www.businesswire.com/news/home/20121107006831/en/BioCryst-Announces-Outcome-Peramivir-Phase-3-Interim (accessed November 2012).

[251] Sidwell, R. W.; Huffman, J. H.; Khare, G. P.; Allen, L. B.; Witkowski, J. T.; Robins, R. K., Broad-spectrum antiviral activity of Virazole: 1-beta-D-ribofuranosyl-1,2,4-triazole-3-carboxamide. *Science* **1972**, *177* (4050), 705-706.

[252] Tam, R. C.; Lau, J. Y.; Hong, Z., Mechanisms of action of ribavirin in antiviral therapies. *Antivir. Chem. Chemother.* **2001**, *12* (5), 261-272.

[253] McHutchison, J. G.; Gordon, S. C.; Schiff, E. R.; Shiffman, M. L.; Lee, W. M.; Rustgi, V. K.; Goodman, Z. D.; Ling, M. H.; Cort, S.; Albrecht, J. K., Interferon alfa-2b alone or in combination with ribavirin as initial treatment for chronic hepatitis C. Hepatitis Interventional Therapy Group. *N. Engl. J. Med.* **1998**, *339* (21), 1485-1492.

[254] Reichard, O.; Norkrans, G.; Fryden, A.; Braconier, J. H.; Sonnerborg, A.; Weiland, O., Randomised, double-blind, placebo-controlled trial of interferon alpha-2b with and without ribavirin for chronic hepatitis C. The Swedish Study Group. *Lancet* **1998**, *351* (9096), 83-87.

[255] Fried, M. W.; Shiffman, M. L.; Reddy, K. R.; Smith, C.; Marinos, G.; Goncales, F. L., Jr.; Haussinger, D.; Diago, M.; Carosi, G.; Dhumeaux, D.; Craxi, A.; Lin, A.; Hoffman, J.; Yu, J., Peginterferon alfa-2a plus ribavirin for chronic hepatitis C virus infection. *N. Engl. J. Med.* **2002**, *347* (13), 975-982.

[256] Poynard, T.; Marcellin, P.; Lee, S. S.; Niederau, C.; Minuk, G. S.; Ideo, G.; Bain, V.; Heathcote, J.; Zeuzem, S.; Trepo, C.; Albrecht, J., Randomised trial of interferon alpha2b plus ribavirin for 48 weeks or for 24 weeks *versus* interferon alpha2b plus placebo for 48 weeks for treatment of chronic infection with hepatitis C virus. International Hepatitis Interventional Therapy Group (IHIT). *Lancet* **1998**, *352* (9138), 1426-1432.

[257] Lertora, J. J.; Rege, A. B.; Lacour, J. T.; Ferencz, N.; George, W. J.; VanDyke, R. B.; Agrawal, K. C.; Hyslop, N. E., Jr., Pharmacokinetics and long-term tolerance to ribavirin in asymptomatic patients infected with human immunodeficiency virus. *Clin. Pharmacol. Ther.* **1991**, *50* (4), 442-449.

[258] Roberts, S. S.; Miller, R. K.; Jones, J. K.; Lindsay, K. L.; Greene, M. F.; Maddrey, W. C.; Williams, I. T.; Liu, J.; Spiegel, R. J., The Ribavirin Pregnancy Registry: Findings after 5 years of enrollment, 2003-2009. *Birth Defects Res. A Clin. Mol. Teratol.* **2010**, *88* (7), 551-559.

[259] Witkowski, J. T.; Robins, R. K.; Khare, G. P.; Sidwell, R. W., Synthesis and antiviral activity of 1,2,4-triazole-3-thiocarboxamide and 1,2,4-triazole-3-carboxamidine ribonucleosides. *J. Med. Chem.* **1973**, *16* (8), 935-937.

[260] Wu, J. Z.; Walker, H.; Lau, J. Y. N.; Hong, Z., Activation and Deactivation of a Broad-Spectrum Antiviral Drug by a Single Enzyme: Adenosine Deaminase Catalyzes Two Consecutive Deamination Reactions. *Antimicrob. Agents Chemother.* **2003**, *47* (1), 426-431.

[261] Lin, C. C.; Yeh, L. T.; Vitarella, D.; Hong, Z., Viramidine, a prodrug of ribavirin, shows better liver-targeting properties and safety profiles than ribavirin in animals. *Antivir. Chem. Chemother.* **2003**, *14* (3), 145-152.

[262] Gish, R. G.; Arora, S.; Rajender Reddy, K.; Nelson, D. R.; O'Brien, C.; Xu, Y.; Murphy, B., Virological response and safety outcomes in therapy–naïve patients treated for chronic hepatitis C with taribavirin or ribavirin in combination with pegylated interferon alfa-2a: A randomized, phase 2 study. *J. Hepatol.* **2007**, *47* (1), 51-59.

[263] Benhamou, Y.; Afdhal, N. H.; Nelson, D. R.; Shiffman, M. L.; Halliman, D. G.; Heise, J.; Chun, E.; Pockros, P. J., A phase III study of the safety and efficacy of viramidine *versus* ribavirin in treatment-naïve patients with chronic hepatitis C: ViSER1 results. *Hepatology (Hoboken, NJ, U. S.)* **2009**, *50* (3), 717-726.

[264] Marcellin, P.; Gish, R. G.; Gitlin, N.; Heise, J.; Halliman, D. G.; Chun, E.; Rodriguez-Torres, M., Safety and efficacy of viramidine *versus* ribavirin in ViSER2: randomized, double-blind study in therapy-naive hepatitis C patients. *J. Hepatol.* **2010**, *52* (1), 32-38.

[265] Poordad, F.; Lawitz, E.; Shiffman, M. L.; Hassanein, T.; Muir, A. J.; Bacon, B. R.; Heise, J.; Halliman, D.; Chun, E.; Hammond, J., Virologic response rates of weight-based taribavirin *versus* ribavirin in treatment-naive patients with genotype 1 chronic hepatitis C. *Hepatology (Hoboken, NJ, U. S.)* **2010**, *52* (4), 1208-1215.

[266] Benz, F.; Knuesel, F.; Nuesch, J.; Treichler, H.; Voser, W.; Nyfeler, R.; Keller-Schierlein, W., Metabolic products of microorganisms. 143. Echinocandin B, a new polypeptide antibiotic from Aspergillus nidulans var echinulatus. Isolation and components. *Helv. Chim. Acta* **1974**, *57* (8), 2459-2477.

[267] Taft, C. S.; Stark, T.; Selitrennikoff, C. P., Cilofungin (LY121019) Inhibits Candida albicans (1-3)-beta-D-Glucan Synthase Activity. *Antimicrob. Agents Chemother.* **1988**, *32* (12), 1901-1903.

[268] Debono, M.; Gordee, R. S., Antibiotics That Inhibit Fungal Cell-Wall Development. *Annu. Rev. Microbiol.* **1994**, *48*, 471-497.

[269] Debono, M.; Abbott, B. J.; Fukuda, D. S.; Barnhart, M.; Willard, K. E.; Molloy, R. M.; Michel, K. H.; Turner, J. R.; Butler, T. F.; Hunt, A. H., Synthesis of New Analogs of Echinocandin-B by Enzymatic Deacylation and Chemical Reacylation of the Echinocandin-B Peptide - Synthesis of the Antifungal Agent Cilofungin (LY121019). *J. Antibiot.* **1989**, *42* (3), 389-397.

[270] Debono, M.; Turner, W. W.; Lagrandeur, L.; Burkhardt, F. J.; Nissen, J. S.; Nichols, K. K.; Rodriguez, M. J.; Zweifel, M. J.; Zeckner, D. J.; Gordee, R. S.; Tang, J.; Parr, T. R., Semisynthetic Chemical Modification of the Antifungal Lipopeptide Echinocandin-b (ECB) - Structure-Activity Studies of the Lipophilic and Geometric Parameters of Polyarylated Acyl Analogs of ECB. *J. Med. Chem.* **1995**, *38* (17), 3271-3281.

[271] Planche, V.; Ducroz, S.; Alanio, A.; Bougnoux, M. E.; Lortholary, O.; Dannaoui, E., *In Vitro* Combination of Anidulafungin and Voriconazole against Intrinsically Azole-

Susceptible and -Resistant Aspergillus spp. *Antimicrob. Agents Chemother.* **2012**, *56* (8), 4500-4503.

[272] Anidulafungin Plus Voriconazole *Versus* Voriconazole for the Treatment of Invasive Aspergillosis. http://clinicaltrials.gov/ct2/show/results/NCT00531479 (accessed August 2012).

[273] Posner, G. H.; Northrop, J.; Paik, I. H.; Borstnik, K.; Dolan, P.; Kensler, T. W.; Xie, S.; Shapiro, T. A., New chemical and biological aspects of artemisinin-derived trioxane dimers. *Bioorg. Med. Chem.* **2002**, *10* (1), 227-232.

[274] WHO *Guidelines for the Treatment of Malaria*; World Health Organization: Geneva, 2006.

[275] WHO *Global Report on Antimalarial Drug Efficacy and Drug Resistance: 2000–2010*; World Health Organization: Geneva, 2010.

[276] Tang, Y. Q.; Dong, Y. X.; Vennerstrom, J. L., Synthetic peroxides as antimalarials. *Med. Res. Rev.* **2004**, *24* (4), 425-448.

[277] Salako, L. A.; Guiguemde, R.; Mittelholzer, M. L.; Haller, L.; Sorenson, F.; Sturchler, D., Ro-42-1611 in the Treatment of Patients with Mild Malaria - A Clinical-Trial in Nigeria and Burkina-Faso. *Trop. Med. Parasitol.* **1994**, *45* (3), 284-287.

[278] Somomoyou, R.; Mittelholzer, M. L.; Sorenson, F.; Haller, L.; Sturchler, D., Efficacy of Ro-42-1611 (Arteflene) in the Treatment of Patients with Mild Malaria - A Clinical-Trial in Cameroon. *Trop. Med. Parasitol.* **1994**, *45* (3), 288-291.

[279] Vennerstrom, J. L.; Arbe-Barnes, S.; Brun, R.; Charman, S. A.; Chiu, F. C. K.; Chollet, J.; Dong, Y. X.; Dorn, A.; Hunziker, D.; Matile, H.; McIntosh, K.; Padmanilayam, M.; Tomas, J. S.; Scheurer, C.; Scorneaux, B.; Tang, Y. Q.; Urwyler, H.; Wittlin, S.; Charman, W. N., Identification of an antimalarial synthetic trioxolane drug development candidate. *Nature* **2004**, *430* (7002), 900-904.

[280] Valecha, N.; Looareesuwan, S.; Martensson, A.; Abdulla, S. M.; Krudsood, S.; Tangpukdee, N.; Mohanty, S.; Mishra, S. K.; Tyagi, P. K.; Sharma, S. K.; Moehrle, J.; Gautam, A.; Roy, A.; Paliwal, J. K.; Kothari, M.; Saha, N.; Dash, A. P.; Bjorkman, A., Arterolane, a New Synthetic Trioxolane for Treatment of Uncomplicated Plasmodium falciparum Malaria: A Phase II, Multicenter, Randomized, Dose-Finding Clinical Trial. *Clin. Infect. Dis.* **2010**, *51* (6), 684-691.

[281] Ranbaxy. Ranbaxy Commences Phase-Iii Clinical Trials For Its New Anti-Malarial Molecule. http://www.ranbaxy.com/news/newsdisp.aspx?cp=922 (accessed August 2012).

[282] Charman, S. A.; Arbe-Barnes, S.; Bathurst, I. C.; Brun, R.; Campbell, M.; Charman, W. N.; Chiu, F. C. K.; Chollet, J.; Craft, J. C.; Creek, D. J.; Dong, Y. X.; Matile, H.; Maurer, M.; Morizzi, J.; Nguyen, T.; Papastogiannidis, P.; Scheurer, C.; Shackleford, D. M.; Sriraghavan, K.; Stingelin, L.; Tang, Y. Q.; Urwyler, H.; Wang, X. F.; White, K. L.; Wittlin, S.; Zhou, L.; Vennerstrom, J. L., Synthetic ozonide drug candidate OZ439 offers new hope for a single-dose cure of uncomplicated malaria. *Proc. Natl. Acad. Sci. U. S. A.* **2011**, *108* (11), 4400-4405.

[283] Moehrle, J. J.; Duparc, S.; Siethoff, C.; van Giersbergen, P. L.; Craft, J. C.; Arbe-Barnes, S.; Charman, S. A.; Gutierrez, M.; Wittlin, S.; Vennerstrom, J. L., First-in-man safety and pharmacokinetics of synthetic ozonide OZ439 demonstrates an improved exposure profile relative to other peroxide antimalarials. *Br. J. Clin. Pharmacol.* **2012**.

[284] Liu, J.-M.; Ni, M.-Y.; Fan, J.-F.; Tu, Y.-Y.; Wu, Z.-H.; Wu, Y.-L.; Chou, W.-S., Structure and reaction of arteannuin. *Huaxue Xuebao* **1979**, *37* (2), 129-143.

[285] Schmid, G.; Hofheinz, W., Total Synthesis of Qinghaosu. *J. Am. Chem. Soc.* **1983**, *105* (3), 624-625.

[286] Xu, X. X.; Zhu, J.; Huang, D. Z.; Zhou, W. S., Total Synthesis of Arteannuin and Deoxyarteannuin. *Tetrahedron* **1986**, *42* (3), 819-828.

[287] Avery, M. A.; Jenningswhite, C.; Chong, W. K. M., The Total Synthesis of (+)-Artemisinin and (+)-9-Desmethylartemisinin. *Tetrahedron Lett.* **1987**, *28* (40), 4629-4632.

[288] Ravindranathan, T.; Kumar, M. A.; Menon, R. B.; Hiremath, S. V., Stereoselective Synthesis of Artemisinin. *Tetrahedron Lett.* **1990**, *31* (5), 755-758.

[289] Avery, M. A.; Chong, W. K. M.; Jenningswhite, C., Stereoselective Total Synthesis Of (+)-Artemisinin, The Antimalarial Constituent of Artemisia annua. *J. Am. Chem. Soc.* **1992**, *114* (3), 974-979.

[290] Liu, H. J.; Yeh, W. L.; Chew, S. Y., A Total Synthesis of the Antimalarial Natural Product (+)-Qinghaosu. *Tetrahedron Lett.* **1993**, *34* (28), 4435-4438.

[291] Constantino, M. G.; Beltrame, M.; daSilva, G. V. J., A novel asymmetric total synthesis of (+)-artemisinin. *Synth. Commun.* **1996**, *26* (2), 321-329.

[292] Liu, H. J.; Yeh, W. L., Total synthesis of (-)-qinghaosu IV (artemisinin D, arteannuin D). *Heterocycles* **1996**, *42* (2), 493-497.

[293] Yadav, J. S.; Babu, R. S.; Sabitha, G., Stereoselective total synthesis of (+)-artemisinin. *Tetrahedron Lett.* **2003**, *44* (2), 387-389.

[294] Yadav, J. S.; Thirupathaiah, B.; Srihari, P., A concise stereoselective total synthesis of (+)-artemisinin. *Tetrahedron* **2010**, *66* (11), 2005-2009.

[295] Hao, H. D.; Li, Y.; Han, W. B.; Wu, Y. K., A Hydrogen Peroxide Based Access to Qinghaosu (Artemisinin). *Org. Lett.* **2011**, *13* (16), 4212-4215.

[296] Zhu, C. Y.; Cook, S. P., A Concise Synthesis of (+)-Artemisinin. *J. Am. Chem. Soc.* **2012**, *134* (33), 13577-13579.

[297] Dewick, P. M., *Medicinal Natural Products - A Biosynthetic Approach*. John Wiley & Sons, LTD: Hoboken, NJ, 2001.

[298] Hale, V.; Keasling, J. D.; Renninger, N.; Diagana, T. T., Microbially derived artemisnin: A biotechnology solution to the global problem of access to affordable antimalarial drugs. *Am. J. Trop. Med. Hyg.* **2007**, *77* (6), 198-202.

[299] Westfall, P. J.; Pitera, D. J.; Lenihan, J. R.; Eng, D.; Woolard, F. X.; Regentin, R.; Horning, T.; Tsuruta, H.; Melis, D. J.; Owens, A.; Fickes, S.; Diola, D.; Benjamin, K. R.; Keasling, J. D.; Leavell, M. D.; McPhee, D. J.; Renninger, N. S.; Newman, J. D.; Paddon, C. J., Production of amorphadiene in yeast, and its conversion to dihydroartemisinic acid, precursor to the antimalarial agent artemisinin. *Proc. Natl. Acad. Sci. U. S. A.* **2012**, *109* (3), 111-118.

[300] Roth, R. J.; Acton, N., A Facile Semisynthesis of the Antimalarial Drug Qinghaosu. *J. Chem. Educ.* **1991**, *68* (7), 612-613.

[301] Vonwiller, S. C.; Warner, J. A.; Mann, S. T.; Haynes, R. K., Copper(II) Trifluoromethanesulfonate-Induced Cleavage Oxygenation of Allylic Hydroperoxides Derived from Qinghao Acid in the Synthesis of Qinghaosu Derivatives - Evidence for the Intermediacy of Enols. *J. Am. Chem. Soc.* **1995**, *117* (45), 11098-11105.

[302] Levesque, F.; Seeberger, P. H., Continuous-Flow Synthesis of the Anti-Malaria Drug Artemisinin. *Angew. Chem.-Int. Edit.* **2012**, *51* (7), 1706-1709.

[303] Martin, V. J. J.; Yoshikuni, Y.; Keasling, J. D., The *in vivo* synthesis of plant sesquiterpenes by Escherichia coli. *Biotechnol. Bioeng.* **2001**, *75* (5), 497-503.

[304] Martin, V. J. J.; Pitera, D. J.; Withers, S. T.; Newman, J. D.; Keasling, J. D., Engineering a mevalonate pathway in Escherichia coli for production of terpenoids. *Nat. Biotechnol.* **2003**, *21* (7), 796-802.

[305] Mercke, P.; Bengtsson, M.; Bouwmeester, H. J.; Posthumus, M. A.; Brodelius, P. E., Molecular cloning, expression, and characterization of amorpha-4,11-diene synthase, a key enzyme of artemisinin biosynthesis in Artemisia annua L. *Arch. Biochem. Biophys.* **2000**, *381* (2), 173-180.

[306] Tsuruta, H.; Paddon, C. J.; Eng, D.; Lenihan, J. R.; Horning, T.; Anthony, L. C.; Regentin, R.; Keasling, J. D.; Renninger, N. S.; Newman, J. D., High-Level Production of Amorpha-4,11-Diene, a Precursor of the Antimalarial Agent Artemisinin, in Escherichia coli. *PLoS One* **2009**, *4* (2).

[307] Anthony, J. R.; Anthony, L. C.; Nowroozi, F.; Kwon, G.; Newman, J. D.; Keasling, J. D., Optimization of the mevalonate-based isoprenoid biosynthetic pathway in Escherichia coli for production of the anti-malarial drug precursor amorpha-4,11-diene. *Metab. Eng.* **2009**, *11* (1), 13-19.

[308] Ro, D. K.; Paradise, E. M.; Ouellet, M.; Fisher, K. J.; Newman, K. L.; Ndungu, J. M.; Ho, K. A.; Eachus, R. A.; Ham, T. S.; Kirby, J.; Chang, M. C. Y.; Withers, S. T.; Shiba, Y.; Sarpong, R.; Keasling, J. D., Production of the antimalarial drug precursor artemisinic acid in engineered yeast. *Nature* **2006**, *440* (7086), 940-943.

[309] Wenzel, R. P., Business and medicine - The antibiotic pipeline - Challenges, costs, and values. *N. Engl. J. Med.* **2004**, *351* (6), 523-526.

[310] Theuretzbacher, U., Accelerating resistance, inadequate antibacterial drug pipelines and international responses. *Int. J. Antimicrob. Agents* **2012**, *39* (4), 295-299.

[311] White, A. R.; Need, B. W. P. U., Effective antibacterials: at what cost? The economics of antibacterial resistance and its control. *J. Antimicrob. Chemother.* **2011**, *66* (9), 1948-1953.

[312] Nathan, C.; Goldberg, F. M., The profit problem in antibiotic R&D. *Nat. Rev. Drug Discov.* **2005**, *4* (11), 887-891.

[313] Nwaka, S.; Ridley, R. G., Virtual drug discovery and development for neglected diseases through public-private partnerships. *Nat. Rev. Drug Discov.* **2003**, *2* (11), 919-928.

[314] Clardy, J.; Fischbach, M. A.; Walsh, C. T., New antibiotics from bacterial natural products. *Nat. Biotechnol.* **2006**, *24* (12), 1541-1550.

[315] Hugenholtz, P.; Goebel, B. M.; Pace, N. R., Impact of culture-independent studies on the emerging phylogenetic view of bacterial diversity. *J. Bacteriol.* **1998**, *180* (18), 4765-4774.

[316] Rappe, M. S.; Giovannoni, S. J., The uncultured microbial majority. *Annu. Rev. Microbiol.* **2003**, *57*, 369-394.

[317] Handelsman, J.; Rondon, M. R.; Brady, S. F.; Clardy, J.; Goodman, R. M., Molecular biological access to the chemistry of unknown soil microbes: A new frontier for natural products. *Chem. Biol.* **1998**, *5* (10), R245-R249.

[318] Banik, J. J.; Brady, S. F., Recent application of metagenomic approaches toward the discovery of antimicrobials and other bioactive small molecules. *Curr. Opin. Microbiol.* **2010**, *13* (5), 603-609.

[319] Bode, H. B.; Muller, R., The impact of bacterial genomics on natural product research. *Angew. Chem. Int. Edit.* **2005**, *44* (42), 6828-6846.

[320] von Nussbaum, F.; Brands, M.; Hinzen, B.; Weigand, S.; Habich, D., Antibacterial natural products in medicinal chemistry - Exodus or revival? *Angew. Chem. Int. Edit.* **2006**, *45* (31), 5072-5129.

Frontiers in Anti-Infective Drug Discovery, Vol. 2, 2014, 224-268

CHAPTER 4

Targeting the Molecular Basis of Resistance

Samar A.M. Salem[*] and Nehal M. Zuel-Fakkar

Dermatology, Venereology and Anderology Department, Faculty of Medicine, Ain Shams University, Cairo, Egypt

Abstract: Antimicrobial resistance is a type of drug resistance where a microorganism is able to survive exposure to the antimicrobial agent. While a spontaneous or induced genetic mutation in bacteria may confer resistance to antimicrobial drugs, genes that confer resistance can be transferred between bacteria in a horizontal fashion by conjugation, transduction or transformation. Resistance can be intrinsic as a naturally occurring trait arising from the biology of the organism, or acquired by mutation or by acquisition of new DNA. Many diseases are increasingly difficult to treat because of the emergence of drug-resistant organisms, including HIV and other viruses; bacteria such as *staphylococci*, *enterococci*, and *E. coli* which cause serious infections in hospitalized patients; bacteria that cause respiratory diseases such as pneumonia and tuberculosis; food-borne pathogens such as *Salmonella* and *Campylobacter*; sexually transmitted organisms such as *Neisseria gonorrhoeae*; *Candida* and other fungi; and parasites such as *Plasmodium falciparum*, the cause of malaria. The emergence of antimicrobial resistance is not a new or unexpected phenomenon. It is an inevitable result of the rapid replication and evolution of microbes. The main mechanisms by which microorganisms exhibit resistance to antimicrobials are: drug inactivation or modification, alteration of target site, alteration of metabolic pathway, and reduced drug accumulation by decreasing drug permeability and/or increasing active efflux (pumping out) of the drugs across the cell surface. Additionally, increased mutation rate as a stress response can occur. Factors contributing towards resistance include overuse of broad-spectrum antibiotics, incorrect diagnosis, unnecessary prescriptions, and improper use of antibiotics by patients. The molecular mechanisms of drug resistance provide the essential knowledge on new drug development and clinical use. These mechanisms include enzyme catalyzed antibiotic modifications, bypass of antibiotic targets and active efflux of drugs from the cell. Multidrug resistance can be reversed by a variety of pharmacological agents which promote drug accumulation. Monoclonal antibodies provide a potentially valuable alternative means of reversing multidrug resistance. Understanding the chemical rationale and underpinnings of resistance is an essential component of our response to this clinical challenge.

Keywords: Bacterial resistance, fungal resistance, mechanism of antimicrobial action, molecular mechanism of antimicrobial resistance, viral resistance.

***Address correspondence to Samar A.M. Salem:** Dermatology, Venereology and Anderology Department, Faculty of Medicine, Ain Shams University, Cairo, Egypt; Tel: 0020226830767; Fax: 0020226830767; E-mail: smousasalem@yahoo.com

Atta-ur-Rahman / M. Iqbal Choudhary (Eds.)

INTRODUCTION

The current worldwide increase in resistant bacteria and, simultaneously, the downward trend in the development of new antibiotics have serious health and economic implications [1]. Bacterial resistance often results in treatment failure, which can have serious consequences, especially in critically ill patients [2]. Risk groups include young children and the elderly with high susceptibility to infections and reduced immune response, people with compromised immune defences, such as cancer patients and HIV-positive people, for whom adequate antibiotic therapy to prevent and treat severe infections is necessary for their survival [1].

Resistance and the risk of inappropriate therapy increasingly limit therapeutic options [3]. In addition, antibiotic resistance endangers advanced medical procedures such as organ transplants and implants of prostheses, where antibiotics are vital for patient safety and to avoid complications [1].

Despite the relatively low overall prevalence of antifungal resistance, it still represents a management challenge for individual high-risk patients and those with persistent mycoses. Opportunistic fungal infections are widespread in immunosuppressed individuals [4]. The frequency of invasive fungal infections has risen with a striking increase in mortality due to invasive mycoses [5]. *Candida spp.* and *Aspergillus spp.* represent the most common life-threatening infections. The most common infecting species is *C. albicans*, which, when combined with *C. glabrata*, *C. parapsilosis*, *C. tropicalis* and *C. krusei* causes approximately 99% of all human cases [6]. The incidence of invasive mould infections has also risen in the past decade, especially those caused by *Aspergillus spp.* [7, 8], particularly *A. Fumigates* [8, 9]. In recent decades, there has also been an increase in rare mould infections, which are often resistant to antifungal drugs [10].

Drug resistance in particular has been a major concern for the fungistatic azole drugs and also more recently for echinocandins such as caspofungin [11-13]. In fact, drug resistance has been found for all known drug classes and poses a significant challenge in antifungal therapy [14, 15]. Even with the use of new, effective classes of antifungal drugs such as the azole voriconazole, and the candin micafungin, drug-resistant clinical isolates emerge [16]. Moreover, an additional threat has emerged due to the appearance of fungal strains with multi-drug resistance (MDR) [17].

A virus can change from copy to copy to make medicines less and less effective. Resistance means that the virus has changed in such a way that your medications are ineffective in preventing more copies from being made. In other words, resistance allows the virus to make more copies, even in the presence of medicines [18].

Anti-viral drugs including acyclovir, vidarabine, famciclovir, valacyclovir, pencyclovir are widely used in the treatment of HSV-1 infection. Nowadays, the occurrence of mutations in viral DNA polymerase and thymidine kinase has led to an increase in drug resistance to nucleoside analogs such as acyclovir [19].

Monogenic resistance to viruses has been demonstrated, generally involving mutations in receptors such as CCR5 for HIV1, erythrocyte P antigen for the parvovirus B19, or in genes controlling the receptor expression such as the fucosyltransferase (FUT2), which is required for the expression of norovirus ABH coreceptors. In fact, predisposition to viral diseases mirrors the resistance and contributes to the variability of their prevalence within populations [20].

PREDISPOSING FACTORS

Important predisposing factor for bacterial resistance include the global extensive overuse of antibiotics, *e.g.,* based on incorrect medical indications, mostly viral infections, as well as misuse by using the wrong agent, administration route, dose and treatment duration. At the same time, there is a lack of access to effective antibiotics in some developing countries [1].

Determining the relative risk of resistance development for any specific antibiotic is complicated. Factors as the antibacterial spectrum of the drug and its pharmacokinetics will influence the extent of impact on the body's normal bacterial flora [21]. Poor patient compliance with dosage regimens and the use of substandard antibiotics lead to sub-optimal concentrations that fail to control the infection and may promote growth of resistant bacterial populations. Thus, underuse may play as important a role in driving resistance as overuse [22].

Regarding fungal infections, several factors have contributed to their growing incidence. Besides the most commonly isolated *Candida* and *Aspergillus* species, emerging opportunistic fungi include *Mucor*, *Fusarium*, *Rhizomucor* and *Absidia* species, in addition to *Saccharomyces cerevisiae* [23]. Factors playing important roles in development of fungal resistance include advanced, invasive surgical techniques, induced immunosuppression resulting from transplantation protocols and chemotherapies, and disease conditions associated with human immunodeficiency virus infection. Such an increase in infection rates with the previously mentioned factors has necessitated additional and prolonged treatments with the available arsenal of antifungal drugs. This, in turn, has led to the emergence of drug-resistant strains of pathogenic fungi [24].

What adds to the problem is the difficulty of the early diagnosis of invasive fungal infections, as signs and symptoms are nonspecific, blood cultures are commonly negative, and patients are often unable to undergo invasive diagnostic procedures [25, 26]. For candidiasis, diagnosis is usually based on the isolation of *Candida spp.* from blood cultures or tissue biopsy specimens. However, in the early stages of infection, the sensitivity of blood cultures for diagnosis of systemic candidiasis is low and may require 2-5 days for growth. Clinical outcomes are improved with early start of treatment [27, 28], but empiric antifungal therapy increases selective pressure toward drug-resistant species [6, 12]. Broad use of prophylaxis, empiric and preemptive therapeutic approaches is usual for invasive mould infections as the diagnosis is often based on clinical and nonspecific radiographic findings [29, 30, 31]. Definitive diagnosis requires demonstration of hyphae in blood, respiratory specimens, or tissue. Yet, an evaluation of morphological features, reproductive structures, and biochemical properties may take days to weeks [4].

Genetic factors of resistance and predisposition to viral diseases explain a significant part of the clinical variability observed within host populations [19]. Such predispositions may concern multiple infections when the mutation induces a general immune defect: typical genetic predispositions to multiple infections are due to global primary immune deficiencies, which are generally rare and usually affect hematopoietic cells. On the contrary, a mutation may enhance the susceptibility to a single virus as in the well-studied example of the skin warts and cancer induced by HPV infection in individuals with a mutated cellular zinc regulator [20].

HOW DO ANTIMICROBIALS WORK?

Regarding antibacterial agents, most of them have 4 major modes of action according to which, they are classified. These are: (1) interference with cell wall synthesis, (2) inhibition of protein synthesis, (3) interference with nucleic acid synthesis, and (4) inhibition of a metabolic pathway. Disruption of bacterial membrane structure may be a fifth, although less well characterized, mechanism of action [32].

Antibacterial drugs that work by inhibiting bacterial cell wall synthesis include the beta-lactams, such as the penicillins, cephalosporins, carbapenems, and monobactams, and the glycopeptides, including vancomycin and teicoplanin [32, 33]. Beta-lactam agents inhibit synthesis of the bacterial cell wall by interfering with the enzymes required for the synthesis of the peptidoglycan layer, while Vancomycin and teicoplanin do so by binding to the terminal D-alanine residues of the nascent peptidoglycan chain, thereby preventing the cross-linking steps required for stable cell wall synthesis [33].

Macrolides, aminoglycosides, tetracyclines, chloramphenicol, streptogramins, and oxazolidinones act by inhibiting protein synthesis [32, 33]. Fluoroquinolones exert their antibacterial effects by disrupting DNA synthesis and causing lethal double-strand DNA breaks during DNA replication [34], whereas sulfonamides and trimethoprim [TMP] block the pathway for folic acid synthesis, which ultimately inhibits DNA synthesis [35, 36]. Polymyxins possibly exert their inhibitory effects by increasing bacterial membrane permeability, causing leakage of bacterial contents [37]. The cyclic lipopeptide daptomycin inserts its lipid tail into the bacterial cell membrane, causing membrane depolarization and bacterial death [38].

Gram-negative organisms have a poorly permeable outer membrane that hinders drug accumulation and express membrane transporters that actively pump antibiotics out of the cell [39]. Gram-positive bacteria, which lack the outer membrane, can resort only to the latter mechanism of protection [40]. Table **1** summarizes the mechanisms of action of antibacterial agents.

Table 1: Mechanisms of action of antibacterial agents [2].

● Interference with cell wall synthesis – Lactams: penicillins, cephalosporins, carbapenems, monobactams – Glycopeptides: vancomycin, teicoplanin
● Protein synthesis inhibition – Bind to 50S ribosomal subunit: macrolides, chloramphenicol, clindamycin, quinupristin-dalfopristin, linezolid – Bind to 30S ribosomal subunit: aminoglycosides, tetracyclines – Bind to bacterial isoleucyl-tRNA synthetase: mupirocin
● Interference with nucleic acid synthesis – Inhibit DNA synthesis: fluoroquinolones – Inhibit RNA synthesis: rifampin
● Inhibition of metabolic pathway: sulfonamides, folic acid analogues
● Disruption of bacterial membrane structure: polymyxins, daptomycin

tRNA = Transfer RNA.

Concerning the antifungals, the ideal antifungal agent should display high antifungal activity, broad antifungal spectrum, fungicidal action, reluctance to induce resistance, the ability to overcome multi-drug resistance and low animal toxicity. None of the available clinical antifungal agents fulfill all these requirements [17].

Currently available antifungal drugs belong to four major drug classes: polyenes (*e.g.*, amphotericin B), azoles (*e.g.*, fluconazole), echinocandins (*e.g.*, caspofungin), and pyrimidine analogs (*e.g.*, 5-fluorocytosine) [41-43]. These drug classes disrupt membrane integrity, ergosterol biosynthesis, cell wall function, and DNA synthesis respectively. The drugs within each class suffer from various limitations including toxicity (polyenes), resistance (azoles), narrow spectrum of activity (echinocandins), and lack of efficacy as a single agent (5-fluorocytosine) [44].

Polyenes are fungicidal agents used in short treatment regimens due to associated toxicity, which may account for the low incidence of resistance encountered. They act by binding to ergosterol, the fungal membrane sterol, which induces the formation of channels through which essential cellular components leak out, thereby causing cell death [45]. Consistent with this mode of action, amphotericin B-resistant *Candida* strains often have a marked decrease in ergosterol content [46]. Resistance in clinical isolates of *Cryptococcus neoformans* was also associated with a mutation preventing ergosterol biosynthesis at the C8-isomerization step [47].

Pyrimidine analogs include flucytosine, which inhibits cellular DNA and RNA synthesis, and is mainly used in combination therapy as *Candida* was observed to become resistant at high frequency. Flucytosine resistance occurs in *C. albicans* strains bearing molecular variants of cytosine deaminase, uracil phosphoribosyltransferase or uridine monophosphate pyrophosphorylase [48].

Azole antifungals include Triazole drugs (fluconazole, voriconazole, itraconazole and posaconazole) which interfere with ergosterol biosynthesis by blocking a key enzyme, lanosterol 14-alpha demethylase (Erg11p). The resulting ergosterol depletion and accumulation of 14 α -methylsterols (*e.g.,* lanosterol and 14α-methyl-3-6-diol) interfere with the functions of ergosterol as the predominant cellular membrane component [49]. Among the different categories of antifungal drugs, the development of azole resistance is the most relevant medical problem [50].

Voriconazole is a second generation triazole antifungal agent, exhibiting very high *in vitro* and *in vivo* activity against a wide variety of human pathogenic yeasts and moulds [51]. It is a drug of choice for the treatment of disseminated infections caused by filamentous fungi [52], and also exhibits a high activity against a number of human pathogenic yeasts [53], including *Candida albicans, Candida krusei* and *Candida glabrata* [54]. Very limited data are available on voriconazole action on multidrug-resistant (MDR) yeast. Voriconazole may be active against fluconazole-resistant *Candida* clinical isolates [54] and some other fluconazole-resistant fungi.

Echinocandins are new group of drugs (caspofungin, micafungin and anidulafungin) which are effective against a wide range of *Candida spp.*, including azole-resistant species [55-58]. They inhibit ß-1,3-D-glucan synthase, which disrupts the structure of the growing cell wall in susceptible yeast cells [57, 59]. Resistance is not a pervasive problem to the echinocandin drugs [60], although reports of echinocandin resistance with *Candida spp.* are more prevalent with expanding drug use [61, 62].

Of the other antifungal drugs currently used, terbinafine and amorolfine also target ergosterol biosynthesis. The former inhibits squalene epoxidase and the latter sterol C14-reductase and sterol Δ 8-7-isomerase. Resistance may be detected with more extensive use in different clinical situations and can be expected also for other antifungals [46].

MECHANISMS OF RESISTANCE TO ANTIMICROBIAL AGENTS

With better understanding of the molecular basis of resistance it can be envisaged that new diagnostic tools will be developed to allow rapid and appropriate changes in treatment [63]. For example, the key to the successful application of molecular diagnostic technology for antifungal resistance is a strong association between genetic mechanisms, *in vitro* reduced susceptibility, and clinical outcome [4].

Mechanisms of Resistance to Antibacterial Agents

Bacterial resistance can be defined either genotypically (the bacteria carry certain resistance elements); phenotypically (the bacteria can survive and grow above a certain level of antibiotic in the laboratory) or clinically (the bacteria are able to multiply in humans in the presence of drug concentrations achievable during therapy) [64].

Bacteria become resistant to antibiotics through several mechanisms [65]: (i) the production of enzymes that digest/metabolize the antibiotic; (ii) efflux pumps that eliminate the drug from the cell; (iii) modifications to the cellular target of the antibiotic that prevent binding; (iv) activation of an alternate pathway that bypasses drug action; and (v) particularly for gram-negative bacteria, down-regulation or elimination of transmembrane porins through which drugs enter the cell [66] (Fig. **1**).

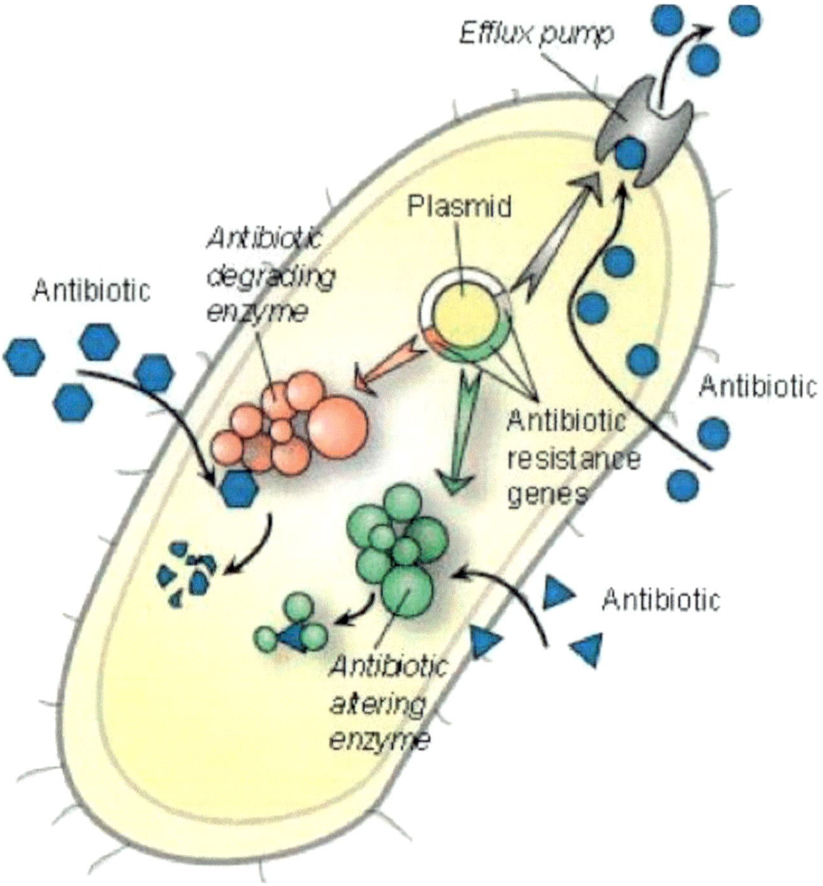

Figure 1: Mechanisms of resistance [1].

Thus, normally susceptible populations of bacteria may become resistant to antimicrobial agents through mutation and selection, or by acquiring from other bacteria the genetic information that encodes resistance. Through genetic exchange mechanisms, many bacteria have become resistant to multiple classes of antibacterial agents causing a serious concern. Strains of bacteria carrying resistance-conferring mutations are selected by antimicrobial use, which kills the susceptible strains but allows the newly resistant strains to survive and grow.

Acquired resistance that develops due to chromosomal mutation and selection is termed *vertical evolution* [2].

Bacteria also develop resistance *by horizontal evolution* through the acquisition of new genetic material from other resistant organisms. This may occur between strains of the same species or between different bacterial species or genera. Mechanisms of genetic exchange include conjugation, transduction, and transformation [33]. In each of these processes, transposons may facilitate the transfer and incorporation of the acquired resistance genes into the host's genome or into plasmids. During conjugation, a gram-negative bacterium transfers plasmid-containing resistance genes to an adjacent bacterium. During transduction, resistance genes are transferred from 1 bacterium to another *via* bacteriophage (bacterial viruses). Finally, transformation, the process whereby bacteria acquire and incorporate DNA segments from other bacteria that have released their DNA complement into the environment after cell lysis, can move resistance genes into previously susceptible strains [2, 33]. The introduction of new antibiotics has resulted in accumulation of genetic elements coding for resistance mechanisms that can be transferred between microbes and create clones with multiresistant properties [67, 68].

The important role played by small mutations in the evolution of resistance has also been demonstrated. For example, only 35 point-mutations distinguish a vancomycin-resistant strain of *S. aureus* from its sensitive counterpart [69].

Unfortunately, there are insufficient details in the annotation information commonly associated with genes deposited in public databases for representing the variety of resistance mechanisms. Thus, additional relevant meta-information is needed. Specifically, each resistance gene is associated with a resistance profile (set of antibiotics or classes of antibiotics targeted by the gene), yet this information is usually not available. Second, resistance often occurs by the cooperation of multiple genes, usually within a same operon (*e.g.,* vancomycin resistance VanA operon requires seven genes [70]), while most annotation information is targeted at individual genes. Finally, resistance frequently results from modifications to, or the disruption of an individual gene (*e.g.,* modifications of the drug target), information incompatible with standard annotation procedures.

Consequently, specialized resources are necessary for annotating and cataloging information related to antibiotic resistance [71]

Mechanisms of Resistance to Antifungal Agents

Resistant infections to antifungals can result from both primary resistance, which is observed as a shift toward colonization with inherently less susceptible organisms, and secondary resistance, which involves the emergence of cell-specific resistance mechanisms in normally susceptible strains [6, 72, 73].

It is known that there are at least four basic mechanisms conferring resistance to triazoles especially fluconazole: (i) overexpression of the *ERG11* gene encoding intracellular target for azole antifungals, 14α-lanosterol demethylase; (ii) alteration of the target structure; (iii) alterations in the ergosterol biosynthesis pathway, especially inactivation of the *ERG3* gene and (iv) an active efflux mediated by multidrug transporter proteins [74].

Mutations in the gene encoding the drug target Erg11 (yeasts) and Cyp51A (moulds) alter the apparent drug-binding domain [75, 76]. They are easily assessed with high throughput DNA sequencing [77], allele-specific realtime molecular probes [78], Light Cycler melt curve analysis [79] or DNA microarray technology [80]. Prominent efflux mediated triazole resistance arises from overexpression of the sterol pathway genes and upregulation of two principal families of efflux pumps, the ATP-binding cassette (ABC) *Candida* drug resistance (Cdr1, Cdr2) and the major facilitator superfamily (MFS) (Mdr1) [81]. The level of transcript for these genes provides a measure of relative resistance.

Multidrug resistance (MDR) has also been often correlated with the activity of energy dependent plasma membrane efflux transporters with low substrate specificity [82]. Constitutive overexpression of the ABC transporters CDR1 and CDR2, or the MFS transporter MDR1 was observed in *Candida spp.* with MDR phenotypes [83]. Yeast cells resistant to fluconazole because of the overexpression of *C. albicans* genes encoding multidrug transporter proteins demonstrate reduced sensitivity to voriconazole [84]. Another gene found to be upregulated in some *C. albicans* azole-resistant yeast clinical isolates is a multidrug transporter gene named *CaMDR1* (for *C. albicans* *m*ulti*d*rug *r*esistance 1, previously known as *BENr* for benomyl resistance) and belonging to the family of major facilitators. Transient upregulation of multidrug transporter genes, beside constitutive upregulation in azole-resistant clinical isolates, also occurs by the exposure of yeast or other fungal pathogens to different drugs [11]. In *C. albicans*, the ABC-transporter genes *CDR1* and *CDR 2* can be upregulated by short-term exposure to steroids, alternative antifungals (terbinafine and amorolfine) or other metabolic inhibitors [85]. Quantitative reverse transcription-PCR (RT-PCR) has replaced semiquantitative northern blot analysis to assess transcript levels [78, 86, 87]. Each gene linked to resistance is assessed relative to a constitutive, highly expressed normalization control gene. A multiplex approach now facilitates simultaneous expression profiling of many genes. The subjectivity of expression profiling when relating transcript levels to resistance phenotypes can be well eliminated by evaluating gain-of-function mutations in transcription factors that promote expression of specific drug resistance genes. These gain-of-function mutations can be directly targeted by microarray analysis, high-throughput sequencing, and multiplexed real-time PCR [4].

Triazole resistance in *A. fumigatus* is more limited than that in *Candida* species and predominantly involves mutations in Cyp51A (equivalent to Erg11). Drug pumps play an unclear role. Limited mutations in Cyp51A confer resistance to one or more triazole agents (voriconazole, itraconazole or posaconazole), and are ideally suited for molecular detection [62, 88].

Resistance to echinocandin drugs remains relatively low, but the more extensive use of echinocandins resulted in rising breakthrough infections involving high MIC strains [4].

A defect in sterol C5-desaturase (*erg3* mutants) was found to be linked with fluconazole resistant *S. cerevisiae* [89] was found to be genetically. This ergosterol biosynthetic enzyme is a non-haem oxygen requiring enzyme that introduces a double bond into the sterol B-ring. The mutants no longer make ergosterol, and also were found to accumulate different sterols under azole treatment [63].

A conserved gene of unknown function, *YER067W*, was found to be strongly induced in response to many stress conditions and repressed in drug resistant yeast strains. Gene expression patterns of *YER067W* suggest an involvement in energy metabolism. Yeast lacking *YER067W* display altered levels of reserve carbohydrates and a growth deficiency in media that requires acrobic metabolism. Impaired mitochondrial function and overall reduction of ergosterol content in the *YER067W* deleted strain could underly the observed increase in resistance to the drugs fluconazole and amphotericin B [90].

Mechanism of Resistance to Antiviral Agents

Antiviral drug resistance depends on the viral mutation frequency, intrinsic mutability of the antiviral target site, the selective pressure exerted by the drug, and the magnitude and rate of virus replication. Other factors include replication fitness and replication space. Resistance occur due to mutation and with this enormous daily virion production, errors of the replication process will inevitably occur. Viral reverse transcriptases (RTs), unlike DNA polymerases, do not encode for a proof reading or editing activity that can remove a misincorporated dNTP. In the absence of an intact immune system or other selection pressure, the faster replicating mutant would be expected to outgrow the slower viruses. The pattern and kinetics of viral resistance to antiviral agents can be understood in terms of a balance between replication fitness, replication space and selection pressure [18].

The Darwinian definition of fitness is the ability to produce offspring in the setting of natural selection. Clearly, there are differences in viral replication between mutant and wild-type which play an important role in the replacement of "the less fit viral species" in patients undergoing antiviral therapy [91].

Compensatory mutations that partly or wholly restore the level of viral fitness have been documented during therapy. Multiple polymerase mutations associated with significantly higher viral loads, increased resistance, as well as disease exacerbation. The swarm of genetic variants that can be found in any patient infected with a viral pathogen such as HBV tend to represent a mixture of viruses with varying replication fitnesses and selection advantages under the changing conditions of host-cell type, immune response or pressure from drug treatment [18].

Selection pressure; in clinical trials of drugs, most of the beneficial effect resulting from monotherapy is largely reversed weeks after initiation of treatment [92]. This reversal is directly associated with the emergence of drug-resistant mutants [93, 94]. These observations are also consistent with the existence of drug-resistant populations in patients before treatment [95] and similar populations of pre-existing resistant virus have been identified in drug-naive individuals [96]. Since these mutations are rarely without cost from the virological perspective [97], compromising mutations tend to survive under the pressure of selection by a second compensatory mutation that partially restores the original levels of viral replication. These findings have important clinical and pathogenesis implications, since the viral load in serum would be expected to drop significantly with drug therapy withdrawal [98].

Replication space is the number of cells that can be infected and the number of viral DNA in those cells (viral load) and continuation of replication depends upon growth of those infected cells and loss of viral DNA to other cells and according to the situation in this replication space the behavior of a mutant virus (the resistant virus) can be determined if it will overcome the original virus or not [99].

TRANSMISSION OF RESISTANT MICROBES

Once resistant clones are selected, their spread is endorsed by factors such as overcrowding and poor hygiene *e.g.,* the rapid dissemination of epidemic clones of methicillin-resistant *Staphylococcus aureus* (MRSA) in the hospital setting. Global spread of resistant clones is enhanced by increasing international trade, travelling and migration, ecosystem disturbances, urbanization and the increasing number of people with compromised immune systems [100]. The transmissibility of drug-resistant viral mutants has now emerged as a potentially important public health issue [18].

EXAMPLES OF RESISTANT MICRO-ORGANISMS

Streptococcus pneumoniae is the single most important cause of infections of the lower respiratory tract in adults and children. It is also the main cause of otitis media in children and causes severe meningitis in children and the elderly. A steady decrease of penicillin susceptibility has been reported worldwide, with increasing proportion of penicillin non-susceptible *Streptococcus pneumoniae* (PNSP). Many PNSP strains are also resistant to erythromycin [1].

Escherichia coli is the most common Gram-negative bacterium isolated from blood cultures in clinical settings. It is the most frequent cause of community and hospital acquired urinary tract infections; and is associated with peritonitis, synergistic wound infections; and food-borne infections. Broad-spectrum penicillins such as amoxicillin were the treatments of choice before resistance started to appear and make them ineffective [1].

Staphylococcus aureus is the leading cause of hospital and community acquired bone, joint and soft tissue infections. It also causes blood stream infections and endocarditis, and food poisoning. methicillin-resistant *Staphylococcus aureus* (MRSA) has now spread throughout the world [1], with some of them being susceptible only to vancomycin and other glycopeptides. However, decreased vancomycin susceptibility has now emerged within all pandemic MRSA lineages [101].

Enterococci are common causes of urinary tract and intra-abdominal infections. They cause endocarditis, and are opportunistic pathogens in immuno-compromised patients, where they cause septicaemia, meningitis and bone infections. As they have an exceptional ability to collect genetic elements coding for resistance mechanisms, *enterococci* were the first significant human pathogens to develop full resistance against third-line glycopeptide antibiotics (vancomycin and teicoplanin), Vancomycin-resistant *enterococci* (VRE) [102].

Mycobacterium tuberculosis shows the striking problems of multi-drug resistant (MDR) strains. Around 80% of these strains are resistant to three or four first-line drugs [103].

Resistant fungi include mainly *Candida spp.* especially *C. albicans* [6], and *Aspergillus spp.* [7, 8], particularly *A. Fumigates* [8, 9].

HOW TO COMBAT ANTIMICROBIAL RESISTANCE

National Programmes Control Strategies

National programme control strategies focus on surveillance of antibiotic use and resistance rates, optimizing antibiotic use with treatment guidelines and diagnostic testing, education of professionals and the public, prevention with infection control measures and immunization, industry involvement and drug development, regulatory issues with central prescribing restrictions and advertising restrictions, review with evaluation of interventions, audit of compliance and physician feedback, and international cooperation [104]. World health organization targeted six area of intervention to control bacterial resistance including reduction of the disease burden and spread of resistance, improvement of access to appropriate antibiotic therapy, improvement of antibiotic use, strengthening health-care systems and their surveillance capacities, enforcement of regulations and legislation, and the encouragement of the development of appropriate new antibiotics and vaccines [1].

Basic and applied research worked on several areas in this concern including expansion of the knowledge base on the molecular mechanisms behind resistance, functional genomics of antibiotic-producing organisms, new molecular targets for the development of drugs against pathogens causing severe resistance problems, novel approaches to address antimicrobial resistance through non-antimicrobial based therapies, the role of mobile genetic elements in the generation of antimicrobial resistance, improved understanding of ecological factors with impact on the genetic and molecular determinants of fitness and virulence of resistant bacterial pathogens, and management of lower respiratory tract infections [105].

Vaccines

There is no vaccine that specifically targets antibiotic resistant bacteria. However, the aim of immunization is to prevent common bacterial infections where resistance has emerged. This may help to reduce the burden of antibiotic resistance. In addition, by reducing the burden of bacterial infections with consequent lower antibiotic use, the likelihood of emerging resistance is reduced [1].

Bioinformatics programmes now exist to help predict which gene products are likely to be located on the surface of the bacterial cell from the analysis of genome sequences [106, 107]. This approach helped the identification of new vaccine *candidat*es against *S. pneumonia* [108], *N. Meningitides* [109, 110] and *M. Tuberculosis* [111].

The genomic technique has promoted the development of vaccines for bacterial infections. This genome-based approach is applied to streptococci, *Chlamydiae, staphylococci* and *Yersinia pestis* [112]. Vaccines against the bacteria most frequently associated with infections were developed, *e.g., S. aureus, E. coli* from urinary tract infections, *P. aeruginosa* and *enterococci*; as well as antibodies [113-116]. A bivalent polysaccharide vaccine against *Staphylococcus aureus* infections [114] is an important progress as it can limit the spread of resistant bacteria as MRSA. Successful CONJUGATE VACCINES have been introduced against *H. influenzae* SEROTYPEb [117], *Neisseria meningitides* [118], and *S. pneumonia* [119]. These vaccines are possibly expensive and indicated to prevent infections in selected high-risk patients [1].

Diagnostics

Diagnostics to Manage Antibacterial Resistance

Tests that differentiate viral from bacterial infection could likely reduce antibiotic consumption. Detection of antibiotic-resistant bacteria as MRSA in screening samples is important to identify and isolate the carriers. PCR-based tests are the main tests to identify antibiotic-resistant bacteria, but they must be performed on DNA extracts from pure bacterial cultures, which take approximately one day before the PCR can be performed [1]. A PCR based assay is a simple, sensitive, fast and feasible method for identification of enterococcal isolates at the genus level and detection of the type of vancomycin resistance genes harbored by those isolates [120]. Application of molecular methods for the detection of drug resistance in TB, for example novel mutations explaining the possible functional variation associated with INH resistance, is a rapid technique and appropriate therapy can be initiated [121]. Moreover, DNA microarray technique can be used in screening the type and composition of genetic elements carrying glycopeptides resistance genes in Enterococcus, and to investigate their correlation with the phenotype [122]. Microarray analyses can be also used to assess the molecular mechanisms involved in bacterial resistance against reactive oxygen species

[123]. Thus, improved diagnostic tools would be one of the most important steps to reduce unnecessary antibiotic use in viral infections and to limit the use of broad- spectrum antibiotics [1].

Specialized resources are necessary for annotating and cataloging information related to antibiotic resistance [71]. Several recent efforts have been made to partially unify this information but with limited functionality, such as Antibiotic Resistance Genes Online (ARGO) [124], MvirDB [125] and a compendium of TEM β-lactamase genes at the Lahey Clinic [126]. ARGO only contains part of β-lactamase, vancomycin and tetracycline resistance genes, and does not include rich annotation information such as resistance profile, mechanism of action, operon information or gene sequence. Furthermore, many of the links between ARGO and GenBank target incorrect records (*e.g.,* links to a genome instead of the relevant gene record). MvirDB is a broad repository of virulence-associated genes, including toxins, virulence factors and antibiotic resistance. The latter information is just a replicate of the ARGO database. The Lahey Clinic website is a comprehensive collection of TEM type β-lactamases, trying to standardize the nomenclature for these genes. In addition to these specialized resources, a more restricted way to get information on antibiotic resistance is through GenBank [127] and SwissProt [128], databases that lack many important relevant information in this domain.

A manually curated database (Antibiotic Resistance Genes Database [ARDB]) was developed unifying most of the publicly available genes and related information, and providing a reliable annotation service to researchers investigating the molecular basis of bacterial resistance. ARDB is supposed to be continually updated according to the diverse new continuously identified resistance genes [71].

Diagnostics to Manage Antifungal Resistance

Defining the MIC of an infecting organism, a presumptive measure for predicting clinical outcome and susceptibility, is important for management of high-risk patients. However, susceptibility testing is not routinely performed. Antifungal susceptibility testing usually come later, 48-72 h following identification, than the time needed to give a decision on patient management. More rapid tests are thus needed to be used in parallel with primary identification [4].

Molecular techniques provide a faster more accurate assessment of both primary and secondary resistance than classical methodologies. Nucleic acid-based diagnostics are the fastest growing component of many clinical laboratories. These applications are gradually replacing or complementing culture-based, biochemical and immunological assays for the detection of a wide range of microorganisms. The detection of ribosomal genes, or intervening noncoding regions, facilitates accurate detection of genera and species, and allows the detection of low microbial burdens (<10 colony forming units) in a primary specimen [129]. PCR and Nucleic Acid Sequence Based Amplification (NASBA)-based amplification detection platforms [130] can diagnose fungal infections at an early stage. Real-time PCR provides higher quality diagnostic information. While nucleic acid assays have been focused on the detection and identification of microbial pathogens, newer probing technologies provided allelic discrimination enabling parallel determinations of drug resistance [131].

Antifungal resistance is dominated by primary resistance to triazole drugs due to inherently less susceptible fungal species. Thus, knowing species-specific information guides treatment choices. For example, rapidly identifying organisms that show reduced triazole susceptibility like *C. glabrata* and *C. krusei* [132, 133] or polyene resistance like *A. terreus* [134] influences primary therapy with positive impact on clinical care. Also, appropriate therapy at an early stage (<12 h) following the first culture positive blood sample significantly improves outcome of *candida* infections [28]. Molecular diagnostic assays are ideal for rapid species determination. They can be used with primary specimens because of their sensitivity [4].

Molecular probing technology is perfect to evaluate secondary triazole resistance in *Candida*. It can be used to determine specific triazole resistance mechanisms that result from genetic changes in drug target site genes, chromosomal aneuploidy or genetic elements controlling expression of drug efflux transporters. Real-time PCR platforms that reliably distinguish single nucleotide changes [allele discrimination] are suitable for multiplexed assays [50, 135]. When combined with genus and/or species-specific probes, this approach can rapidly identify a specific fungal pathogen and determine whether a drug-resistant determinant is present [4].

The narrow range of resistance-associated mutations of *A. fumigatus* to triazole facilitated the application of real-time PCR with molecular beacon probes [88], pyrosequencing [136], and high-resolution melt curve analysis [137] for mutation profiling. Allele-specific molecular beacons could profile eight separate alleles in a single multiplexed PCR reaction [88]. Accordingly, this high-throughput evaluation of isolates classified them as susceptible or resistant. Moreover, a more comprehensive two-tiered molecular diagnostic assay for triazole drug resistance can detect resistance associated mutations [4].

Molecular diagnostic tools, as real-time PCR, highthroughput sequencing, and microarray technology, are also valuable in detecting the limited spectrum of fungal mutations conferring resistance to echinocandin [4].

Some researchers have chosen to avoid entirely the use of nutritional markers to manipulate the *C. albicans* genome, especially if the genes of interest are in pathways affected by nutritional status. Instead, drug resistance markers can be used. The use of drug makers also opens way for testing clinical isolates as is, without creating any auxotrophic mutations. This advantage heavily benefits the researchers that test *C. albicans* clinical isolates [138].

The *S. cerevisiae* genome project is undertaking the systematic disruption of all yeast genes, including approximately 200 transport genes, and from these strains comprehensive information on fungal drug transport can emerge [63].

Diagnostics to Manage Antiviral Resistance

There are three major methods for detecting and measuring antiviral drug-resistance: genotypic assays, phenotypic methods, and virtual phenotyping. Genotypic resistance assays use DNA sequencing methods to examine the polymerase region of the genome for recognizable resistance-associated mutations. This utilizes probes for previously identified subsets of resistance mutations known to occur [139]. Phenotypic assays typically use cell culture based methods for measuring the inhibitory concentration of an antiviral drug that reduces viral replication by at least fifty-percent. Usually a greater than ten-fold increase in IC50 is associated with "resistance" whilst a less than five-fold increase is regarded as "sensitive", and a five to tenfold increase represents partial resistance [140]. Virtual phenotyping in the matching of polymerase sequences from a HBV strain of interest to HBV strains that have both identical or near identical sequences and a known antiviral drug phenotype. A "virtual" phenotype for the test strain reported as the mean IC50 of all matches to the wild-type virus [141].

The relative replication fitness of viral mutants can be assessed using *in vitro* co-infection co competition assays. There are also *in vitro* assays that can describe the behaviour of mutants such as the kinetics of RNA- and DNA- polymerization [91], enzyme processivity [142], and enzyme fidelity and mutation frequencies [143]. The ability of the polymerase to catalyze the incorporation of nucleotides during synthesis of cDNA products before the enzyme dissociates from the template is described as processivity whilst the ability of the polymerase to correct base-pair the template during polymerization is defined as enzyme fidelity [18].

GENOMICS AS A TOOL TO COMBAT RESISTANCE

Identifying New Targets

In Bacteria

The genomic revolution has dramatically changed the approaches to drug development. The number of bacterial genomes continues to grow exponentially. The steadily growing collection of sequenced microbial genomes offers considerable opportunities to rapidly identify conserved and unique sequences that could serve as potential drug targets [1]. With this advent in genomics, the emphasis in drug-discovery programmes has changed from screening compound libraries to first seeking targets [3].

Some comparative genome analyses show that there might be fewer than 300 broad-spectrum essential potential target genes [144, 145]. Genome analysis can also be used to identify narrow-spectrum targets that might be of special concern in problem organisms such as *Mycobacterium tuberculosis*. Another possible use is to identify 'Achilles heels' that are associated with virulent or resistant isolates and are not shared by bacterial species in general. For example, MOLECULAR-TYPING studies on drug-resistant *S. pneumoniae* and *S. aureus* show a limited genetic diversity among these important pathogenic groups [146-149]. This lack of genetic diversity among successful clones implies the possible use of genomic analysis to identify targets that are specific to these problematic clones. Moreover, it is most likely that the old target sites have not been fully explored. Thus, new classes of antibiotics directed at the old targets could be found, such as cell wall biosynthesis, DNA replication, RNA synthesis, and protein synthesis [1].

In Fungi

Examination of the haploinsufficient phenotype, in which lowering the number of genes from two copies to one copy results in a heterozygote that is sensitized to any drug that acts on the product of this gene, ends in discovery of novel drug targets [150]. Pharmacogenetics represents a powerful tool to increase the likelihood of success of antifungal chemotherapy in seriously ill patients [23]. Following the isolation of the *C. albicans ERG24* gene and the sequential disruption of both alleles, it was indicated that an Erg24p inhibitor could be an effective antifungal compound [24].

The enzyme glucosamine-6-phosphate synthase, EC 2.6.1.16, has been identified as a novel target for antifungal agents. Highly selective irreversible potent inhibitors of the enzyme, glutamine analogs, have been obtained. Studies on molecular modelling of selectivity of the enzyme-inhibitor interaction [151] allowed the identification of the structural factors of glutamine analogs important for the high selectivity of inhibitor for glucosamine-6-phosphate synthase [152-154].

FMDP and EADP amino acid peptides exhibit broad antifungal spectrum and fungicidal action [155]. FMDP peptides also demonstrated *in vitro* activity against multi-drug resistant *S. cerervisiae*. Regarding transport characteristics, tripeptides are superior to dipeptides. In *C. albicans* they are taken up by two permeases: di-tripeptide and oligopeptide permeases, which ensures better uptake and slows down the development of resistance [156]. The portage transport concept was applied to eliminate the difficulty of inefficient transport of FMDP and EADP amino acid peptides to cells *via* highly specific amino acid permeases. Inhibitors built into oligopeptide structures were very well transported by peptide permeases and cleaved by intracellular peptidases, generating *in situ* the 'warhead' which cannot escape the cell and unable to be exported by specific amino acid permeases [17].

Validating and Prioritizing New Targets

Genomics based target validation is motivated by the ability to rapidly identify essential genes in which loss of function coincides with loss of viability or virulence attenuation. One form of target validation is to identify genes that are essential for bacterial growth under all conditions. So, high-density random TRANSPOSON MUTAGENESIS has been used to identify essential genes in particular species [157, 158]. Alternatively, mutagenesis can be targeted to a selected list of conserved genes. For example, in *S. pneumoniae*, 347 genes that are conserved in *Bacillus subtilis, Enterococcus faecalis, Escherichia coli* and *S. aureus* were designated as potential targets. Target-gene disruption was achieved by allelic exchange using PCR-generated DNA fragments from each target, which were cloned into a SUICIDE VECTOR. The resulting analysis identified 113 essential genes among the 347 *S. pneumoniae candida*tes [145]. A third method to identify essential genes is by expressing antisense RNA. Using this approach, ~150 essential *S. aureus* genes were identified by transformation with a plasmid library that contained staphylococcal DNA fragments behind a tetracycline-regulated promoter [159]. An alternative approach to choosing new drug targets is to identify gene products that are involved in virulence. The advantage of this approach is relatively narrow-spectrum targets identified that would reduce the probability of resistance emerging because they reduce the impact of antibiotic selection on the resident flora [160]. Techniques that are useful for this purpose identify genes that are specifically switched on during infection, and include *in vivo* expression technology (IVET) [161], differential fluorescence induction (DFI) [162] and signature-tagged mutagenesis (STM) [163, 164].

Another means by which genome-scale analysis might contribute to the selection of new targets is to analyse gene expression profiles during exposure to an antibiotic. In this approach, microarrays of DNA fragments that correspond to every open reading frame (ORF) in a genome are used to obtain the signature of a specific inhibitor. Potentially, this can identify a number of genes that are involved in the biosynthetic pathway that the inhibitor targets. An application for this is in the transcriptional response of *M. tuberculosis* to the antibiotic isoniazid [165] to identify a set of genes that are induced by isoniazid and to indicate a number of potential new targets for antimicrobial drugs. The understanding of the molecular basis for aminoglycoside resistance modification has been greatly enhanced by the availability of representative 3D-structures from the three classes of modifying enzymes: kinases, acetyltransferases and adenyltransferases [166]. Finally, an attractive approach is by the validation of prolyl-tRNA synthetase as an essential target. The advantage of this approach is that once the target, the peptide and the peptide binding site were validated by these methods, screening for small molecules that displaced the peptide was used as a direct way to get new drug leads [167].

In case of viral resistance gene therapy serves as an attractive alternative as it reconstitutes the immune system with resistant cells and could thereby provide a potential cure [168].

OPTIMIZING NEW ANTIBIOTICS

Traditionally, new antimicrobial agents have been identified from biological sources and from large collections of individual compounds that have been gathered from various laboratories. Classical biological sources are the actinomycetes and fungi, which are continuously used in the search for new antibiotics [169]. A successful antibiotic should be able to cross bacterial cell membranes, avoid bacterial efflux pumps, not be a target for bacterial modifying or hydrolyzing enzymes that could inactivate it, reach its target at a sufficiently high concentration, have a broad spectrum of antibacterial activity, reach inhibitory concentrations at the site of infection, have little or no toxicity and have minimal side effects in humans [3].

The details of a new phosphorylation-dependent signal transduction system that controls cephalosporin resistance in *enterococci* are partially unravelled. Deeper understanding of the mechanism underlying cephalosporin resistance in *E. faecalis* may enable the development of new therapeutics designed to reduce the incidence of hospital-acquired enterococcal infections [170].

COMBINATORIAL CHEMISTRY APPROACH

Combinatorial chemistry facilitates the rapid synthesis of a large number of distinct compounds that can then be assayed for antimicrobial activity [171]. Modern industrial pharmacology relies on high-throughput screening of biological libraries for inhibitors of new drug targets. However, with the need to develop new classes of antibiotics with potentially greater ability to withstand resistance, approaches where the primary goal is not to kill the bacteria but to reduce their virulence and reproduction and thereby limit their possibilities to harm the affected host are also needed [1]. The most commonly applied chemical approach to generate variation in small molecules is referred to as 'target-orientated synthesis', in which the targets are specific drug *candida*tes. An exciting alternative approach is 'diversity-orientated synthesis' [172] which aims to synthesize collections of structurally diverse and complex small molecules. These would then be screened for biological activity, leading eventually to the identification of therapeutic protein targets that are capable of being modulated by small molecules [3].

Knowledge about pathogenesis and bacterial/host interactions help to develop drug targets related to the pathogenic process such as bacterial virulence factors rather than an integral function of the microorganism itself [1].

OPTIMIZING KNOWN INHIBITORS

In Bacteria

In addition to generating completely new compounds, combinatorial chemistry can still be frequently used to build new diversity that is based on antibiotics in clinical use, including tetracyclines [173], macrolides [174] and oxadolidinones [175]. An alternative approach is to re-investigate old hits that were never developed for reasons such as narrow spectrum of activity, toxicity, weak ligand binding, and so on [3].

In Fungi

One of the ways to overcome drug resistance is by administering combination therapy, which has the additional advantages of reducing the doses and toxicity, increasing spectrum of activity, and converting a fungistatic to a fungicidal drug, thus facilitating clearance of the pathogen and decreasing the resistance development [176, 177]. However, to develop an effective drug combination regimen, it is important to understand the molecular mechanism behind the combined drug effect. This will help in developing chemical probes for exploring biological pathways targeted by the drug combination. Investigating the mechanism of action of antifungal synergies will definitely result in great progress in the development of optimal and safe combination therapies for the treatment of drug-resistant fungal infections [44]. Making use of chemogenomic profiling, a technology in which the cellular response to inhibitory compounds is measured by evaluating the fitness of a library of genome-wide deletion mutant strains, a bioinformatics-driven approach that predicts synergy between antifungal drug combinations was developed. Strains with reduced fitness in the presence of a compound are identified, and the genes deleted in those strains provide information on cellular pathways targeted by the compound as well as pathways that are required for conferring sensitivity to that compound [178]. Chemogenomic profiling and genetic interaction studies are thus considered very important technologies in investigating the molecular and genetic basis of synergistic drug relationships [44] (Fig. **2**).

New face of an old drug is a strategy was based on the recognition of the molecular basis of very poor selective toxicity of polyene macrolide antibiotics (PMA) otherwise exhibiting excellent properties and removal of this discriminating feature upon rational modification [17].

Because of their unique properties among antifungal agents, PMA are of particular interest despite the high animal toxicity and water insolubility. These

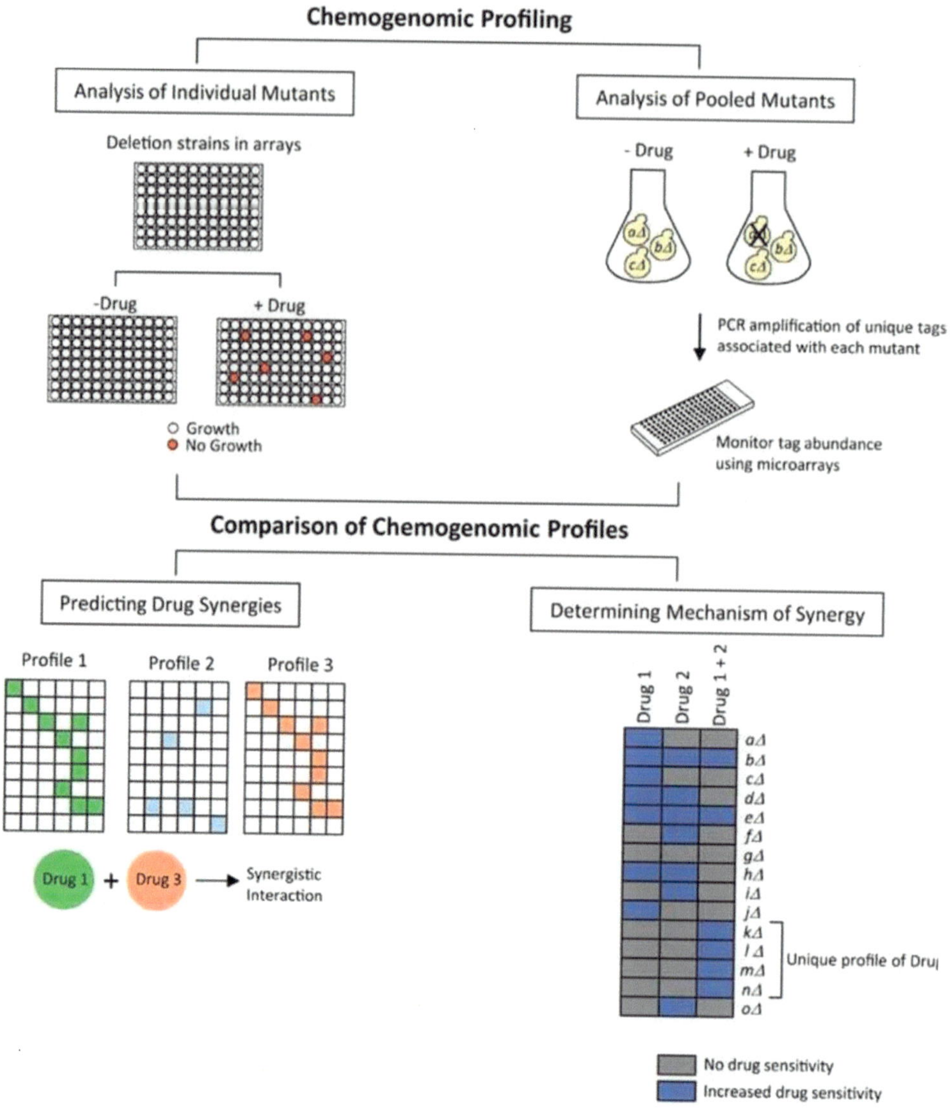

Figure 2: Predicting drug synergies and determining synergy mechanisms. Chemogenomic profiling is conducted by screening drugs against collections of yeast deletion mutants. For analyzing individual mutants, the collection is arrayed in microplates, and the growth of each strain is examined in the presence or absence of the drug. For analyzing pooled mutants, the collection is grown in a single culture, with or without drug, and growth is measured by monitoring the abundance of unique tags associated with each mutant, using DNA microarrays consisting of tag complements. Two drugs with similar chemogenomic profiles would be predicted to exhibit a synergistic interaction (for simplicity, exactly matching profiles are depicted). If the combination of two synergizing drugs generates a unique chemogenomic profile of sensitive mutants, then genes deleted in those mutants provide information on the drug synergy mechanism [44].

drugs have very high antifungal activity; a very broad antifungal fungicidal spectrum; and a reluctance to induce resistance. In order to lower the toxicity and to improve the water solubility of PMA, new delivery systems were developed with partial success. However, the most suitable approach to achieve this aim seems to be the rational chemical modification of PMA. Amphotericin B (AmB) was selected, on the basis of its characteristics, as an optimal *candida*te from the PMA group for the rational modification [17].

In Viruses

Increasing the antiviral effectiveness of therapy is accompanied by an increasing probability that drug resistant mutants will be selected, but only up to a point. At high levels of antiviral activity, suppressing virus replication reduces the likelihood that resistance mutations will be selected because replication is the process responsible for the emergence of the mutations [179]. This key relationship can be described as a bell-shaped curve and leads to the inevitable conclusion that no replication (NR) equates to no resistance (NR), or put another way: NR=NR [92, 180]. Virological suppression remains the primary goal of treatment. This goal should be pursued in all cases, where clinically feasible, by selecting active drugs for salvage therapy using a resistance assay [168].

RATIONAL DRUG DESIGN

When a new biological target has been well defined structurally and functionally its rational design can be used to characterize an inhibitor structure [181]. Combinatorial chemistry can then be used to explore this structure space and identify lead compounds for optimization. In this way, the new class of antibiotics that are active *in vivo, new* PEPTIDE DEFORMYLASE inhibitors, has been identified, and was the first to be discovered using mechanism-based drug design and combinatorial chemistry [182, 183].

Another target for rational drug design is the protein PBP2A, an important determinant of broad-spectrum beta-lactam resistance in MRSA, whose structure was determined recently at high resolution [184]. The structural information shows in detail how to design new classes of drug to overcome MRSA beta-lactam resistance [3].

COMBINATORIAL BIOLOGY

The principle of combinatorial biology is to use the enzymes from antibiotic biosynthetic pathways to create new chemical structures [185, 186]. Of the antibiotics in clinical use, those with the most complex chemical structures are all based on secondary metabolites of microorganisms. The goal of combinatorial biology is to exploit and direct the evolution of complex biosynthetic pathways to expand the range of secondary metabolites, such as antibiotics [186]. A limitation with this approach is that it provides derivatives of known antibiotics, such as erythromycin [187] and vancomycin [188], rather than new classes of antibiotic.

DEVELOPING RESISTANCE INHIBITORS

Beta-Lactamase Inhibitors

Traditionally, new antibiotics with a greater potency or broader spectrum have been derived from antibiotics that are already successful. An example is the development of beta-lactam antibiotics into second and third generation cephalosporins with better resistance to beta-lactamases. Alternatively, secondary inhibitors may be used to counteract the resistance mechanism [189]. Inhibitors extend the effective spectrum of a beta-lactam antibiotic by conferring potency against beta-lactamase producing pathogens. A combination of the beta-lactamase enzyme inhibitor clavulanic acid with the beta-lactam antibiotic amoxicillin is effectively and successfully used. However, it is necessary to develop a second generation of beta-lactamase inhibitor molecule to combat the continued evolution of beta-lactamases [3].

Efflux Inhibitors

Potential applications of the substantial research on the mechanistics of MDR pumps include the design of transport inhibitors that block these efflux pumps. Clinically useful pump inhibitors could allow the return of drugs rendered outdated by efflux in both prokaryotic and eukaryotic systems [190].

In Bacteria

The intrinsic resistance of Gram negative bacteria to many antibiotics requires constitutively expressed pumps of the resistance nodulation- division (RND) type, as well as the outer membrane barrier [191]. Inactivation of the pumps of *P. aeruginosa*, or *E. coli* thus makes these bacteria susceptible to many antibiotics against which they are normally resistant [3]. Active efflux of macrolide antibiotics is an important way of resistance in Gram-positive pathogens. *e.g.,* in *Staphylococcus epidermidis* [40]. Also, genes of tetracycline efflux transporters have been shown to exist in Gram-negative bacteria [192]. Moreover, multidrug resistance in bacteria is often caused by the overexpression of MULTIDRUG EFFLUX systems [193].

Although increased efflux alone might not be sufficient to create a clinically relevant level of resistance, it can enhance survival until further changes resulting in high-level resistance occur. Consequently, the design of drugs that are less efficiently pumped out is important [3] *e.g.,* tetracyline derivatives that have a higher affinity for the ribosomal binding site and that are not subject to efflux, as Glycyclines, have been synthesized to combat tetracycline resistant strains [194]. An alternative is to find inhibitors of efflux pumps *e.g.,* the development of tetracycline analogs inhibiting efflux transporters to be used in combination with tetracyclines [195]. The aims are to restore antibiotic susceptibility to resistant mutants, and to make intrinsically resistant species susceptible to a broader range of antibiotics. The screening of small-molecule compound libraries has led to the identification of inhibitors of several multidrug transport systems in *S. aureus* [196-198] and *E. coli* [195]. A broad-spectrum efflux-pump inhibitor, active against all three Mex pumps in *P. aeruginosa* and against the AcrAB-TolC pump in *E. coli* [199] are developed. Self-organizing maps, a type of non supervised learning algorithms, were chosen to implement a virtual screening protocol for identification of new inhibitors of P-glycoprotein which is an ATP-driven efflux pump. These protein homology models now may serve as tools for subsequent molecular dynamics simulations and studies, which will guide the target-based development of new efflux- pump inhibitors [200].

In Fungi

Effective efflux inhibition in fungi, as in bacteria, can be done by targeting the actual transporter/drug complex; by preventing the correct assembly of drug transporter complexes, necessitating detailed structural information on all of the components in such complexes; by targeting the transcriptional regulators that modulate expression of efflux systems [190]; by managing the repressors/activators that can control the level of efflux expression [201]; by abolishing transcription of the transporter genes; or by targeting signal transduction systems that control certain multidrug pumps [202, 203].

Previously, attempts to find MDR reversal agents have mainly focused on the screening of chemical libraries for inhibitors. Inhibitors were identified largely from studies monitoring the accumulation of radiolabeled drugs; drugs that display changes in fluorescence upon entering the cell; changes in rates of ATP hydrolysis; or, in the case of microbes, a reduction in the minimal inhibitory concentration of specific antimicrobial pump substrates [190].

Seeking for inhibitors of P-gp-mediated MDR has been intensive as it is a significant problem [204-206]. Three generations of chemical modulators can inhibit the action of P-gp. First generation inhibitors are pharmaceuticals that are already in use for other treatments, and include calcium channel blockers, such as verapamil; immunosuppresants, such as cyclosporine A; anti-hypertensives, such as reserpine, quinidine and yohimbine; and anti-estrogens, such as tamoxifen and toremifena. However, the clinical efficacy of these compounds is limited by their toxicity. Second generation P-gp modulators have the MDR reversal properties of the first generation modulators, with significantly less toxicity, but with deleterious effects *in vivo*. They can result in the toxic accumulation of co-administered anticancer drugs in blood plasma or in organs such as the liver, kidney, or intestine [207]. Several third generation modulators that are highly potent, selective inhibitors of P-gp are now developed [208].

ALTERNATIVE STRATEGIES

Optimizing Antibiotic Use

An approach to reduce the prevalence of resistant bacteria is to limit the antibiotic consumption. However, this will probably have limited success. The availability of rapid molecular diagnostic methods would allow the use narrow-spectrum drugs with safety reducing the selective pressure for the spread of resistance (passive approach) and is beneficial for increasing the efficacy of dosing with traditional BROADSPECTRUM ANTIBIOTICS. A successful diagnostic test needs to combine rapidity, sensitivity, specificity, and ubiquity [209], and would probably be based on nucleic acid amplification [210].

Antibiotic combination therapy and the use of MUTANT-PREVENTIVE CONCENTRATIONS (MPCs) of antibiotics are more proactive approaches to be used. In combination therapy, the more effective action antibiotic will reduce the probability of selecting resistance among surviving bacteria in a treated population [211]. This approach is particularly relevant in treatment of multidrug-resistant *M. tuberculosis* [212].

In viral infections, one management option in multidrug-experienced patients with limited or no drug options available, might be to continue the failing therapy if the virus has low replication capacity/fitness. Patients with a virus of high replication capacity/fitness who fail therapy may benefit from treatment change, even if there are few available options, in order to attempt to select for a virus with lower fitness [168]. The chances of drug resistance can sometimes be minimized by using multiple drugs simultaneously. This works because individual mutations can be independent and may tackle only one drug at a time; if the individuals are still killed by the other drugs, then the mutations cannot persist. However, cross resistance where mutations confer resistance to two or more treatments can be problematic [213].

Non-Antimicrobial Strategies

The use of BACTERIOPHAGE as an antibacterial therapy is of interest in dealing with antibiotic resistance [214, 215]. The rationale is that bacteriophage that targets and kills specific bacterial pathogens *in vitro* might also be able to achieve this *in vivo*. For example, bacteriophages, can selectively kill pathogenic streptococci, including antibiotic-resistant strains, without affecting the normal flora [216, 217]. The problems encountered with this approach are narrow host range, the emergence of bacterial resistance, and a failure to achieve high phage concentrations at the site of infection [3].

Synthetic antibiotic fusion products are a promising approach and are currently being developed for hybrid molecules, which combine an antibacterial activity with an effector molecule of the innate immune system. Other therapies such as immunomodulators, resistance inhibitors, and gene therapy with anti-sense inhibitors are also alternatives to antibacterial drugs [1]. Prebiotic, probiotic and synbiotic based approaches have been used to develop new therapies utilizing the bacterial colonization phenomenon. As an example, vaginal capsules with lactobacilli have been used to prevent recurrent urinary tract infections [218]. Such probiotics could be used to prevent infections and reduce the ecological pressure due to antibiotics [1].

CONCLUDING REMARKS

The development of microbial resistance is an issue of global concern nowadays. The hazardous consequences of this resistance should be evaded by avoiding the predisposing factors, early and proper diagnosis of infections, studying the molecular basis of resistance, and the development of new technologies to expand the therapeutic modalities available.

ACKNOWLEDGEMENTS

None declared.

CONFLICT OF INTEREST

The authors confirm that this chapter content has no conflict of interest.

REFERENCES

[1] Nordberg P, Monnet DL, Cars O. Antibacterial drug resistance. Background document for the WHO project: Priority Medicines for Europe and the World "A Public Health Approach to Innovation." Available from: http://soapimg.icecube.snowfall.se/stopresistance/Priority_Medicine_Antibacterial_background_docs_final.pdf [cited: 7th November 2012] [cited: 15th July 2012].

[2] Tenover FC. Mechanisms of Antimicrobial Resistance in Bacteria. Am J Med 2006; 119 (6A): S3-S10.

[3] Hughes D. Exploiting genomics, genetics and chemistry to combat antibiotic resistance. Nature reviews | Genetics 2003; 4: 432-41.

[4] Perlin DS. Antifungal drug resistance: do molecular methods provide a way forward? Curr Opin Infect Dis 2009; 22: 568-73.

[5] Rapp RP. Changing strategies for the management of invasive fungal infections. Pharmacotherapy 2004; 24: 4S-28S; quiz 29S-32S.

[6] Pfaller MA, Diekema DJ. Epidemiology of invasive candidiasis: a persistent public health problem. Clin Microbiol Rev 2007; 20: 133-63.

[7] Bhatti Z, Shaukat A, Almyroudis NG, Segal BH. Review of epidemiology, diagnosis, and treatment of invasive mould infections in allogeneic hematopoietic stem cell transplant recipients. Mycopathologia 2006; 162:1-15.

[8] Maschmeyer G, Haas A, Cornely OA. Invasive aspergillosis: epidemiology, diagnosis and management in immunocompromised patients. Drugs 2007; 67:1567-1601.

[9] Marr KA. Fungal infections in hematopoietic stem cell transplant recipients. Med Mycol 2008; 46:293-302.

[10] Malani AN, Kauffman CA. Changing epidemiology of rare mould infections: implications for therapy. Drugs 2007; 67:1803-1812.

[11] Sanglard D. Resistance of human fungal pathogens to antifungal drugs. Curr Opin Microbiol 2002; 5: 379-85.

[12] Maertens J. Evaluating prophylaxis of invasive fungal infections in patients with haematologic malignancies. Eur J Haematol 2007; 78: 275-82.

[13] Perlin DS. Resistance to echinocandin-class antifungal drugs. Drug Resist Updat 2007; 10: 121-30.

[14] Pemán J, Cantón E, Espinel-Ingroff A. Antifungal drug resistance mechanisms. Expert Rev Anti Infect Ther 2009; 7: 453-60.

[15] Mukherjee PK, Wang M. Antifungal drug resistance: significance and mechanisms. In: Ghannoum MA, Perfect JR, Eds. Antifungal Therapy. New York: Informa Healthcare; 2010; pp. 63-86.

[16] Tanabe K, Niimi K, Niimi M. What's new in the molecular basis of antifungal drug resistance in pathogenic yeasts. Nihon Rinsho 2008; 66(12): 2273-8.

[17] Borowski E. Novel approaches in the rational design of antifungal agents of low toxicity. Farmaco 2000; 55(3): 206-8.

[18] Richman DD. The impact of drug resistance on the effectiveness of chemotherapy for chronic hepatitis B. Hepatology 2000; 32: 866-7.

[19] Khania S, Motamedifara M, Golmoghaddamb H, Hosseinic HM, Hashemizadeha Z. *In vitro* study of the effect of a probiotic bacterium Lactobacillus rhamnosus against herpes simplex virus type 1. Braz J Infect Dis 2012; 16(2): 129-35.

[20] Verrier ER, Langevin C, Tohry C, *et al.* Genetic Resistance to Rhabdovirus Infection in Teleost Fish Is Paralleled to the Derived Cell Resistance Status. PLoS ONE 2012; 7(4): e33935.

[21] Sullivan A, Edlund C, Nord CE. Effect of antimicrobial agents on the ecological balance of human microflora. Lancet Infect Dis 2001; 1: 101-14.

[22] World Health Organization. WHO Global Strategy for Containment of Antimicrobial Resistance.Geneva:WHO,2001.Availablefrom:http://www.who.int/csr/resources/publications/drugresist/en/EGlobal_Strat.pdf [cited 7th November 2012].

[23] Lupetti A, Danesi R, Campa M, Del Tacca M, Kelly S. Molecular basis of resistance to azole antifungals. Trends Mol Med 2002; 8 (2): 76-81.

[24] Jia N, Arthington-Skaggs B, Lee W, *et al.* *Candida albicans* Sterol C-14 Reductase, Encoded by the *ERG24* Gene, as a Potential Antifungal Target Site. Antimicrob Agents Chemother 2002; 46(4): 947-57.

[25] Stevens DA. Diagnosis of fungal infections: current status. J Antimicrob Chemother 2002; 49 (Suppl 1): 11-19.

[26] Chamilos G, Kontoyiannis DP. Defining the diagnosis of invasive aspergillosis. Med Mycol 2006; 44 (Suppl): 163-72.

[27] Garey KW, Rege M, Pai MP, *et al.* Time to initiation of fluconazole therapy impacts mortality in patients with candidemia: a multiinstitutional study. Clin Infect Dis 2006; 43: 25-31.

[28] Morrell M, Fraser VJ, Kollef MH. Delaying the empiric treatment of *Candida* bloodstream infection until positive blood culture results are obtained: a potential risk factor for hospital mortality. Antimicrob Agents Chemother 2005; 49: 3640-45.

[29] Ruping MJ, Vehreschild JJ, Cornely OA. Antifungal treatment strategies in high risk patients. Mycoses 2008; 51 (Suppl 2): 46-51.

[30] Thursky KA, Playford EG, Seymour JF, Sorrell TC, Ellis DH, Guy SD, Gilroy N, Chu J, Shaw DR. Recommendations for the treatment of established fungal infections. Intern Med J 2008; 38: 496-520.

[31] Walsh TJ, Anaissie EJ, Denning DW, *et al.* Treatment of aspergillosis: clinical practice guidelines of the Infectious Diseases Society of America. Clin Infect Dis 2008; 46: 327-60.

[32] Neu HC. The crisis in antibiotic resistance. *Science* 1992; 257: 1064-73.

[33] McManus MC. Mechanisms of bacterial resistance to antimicrobial agents. *Am J Health Syst Pharm* 1997; 54: 1420 -33.

[34] Drlica K, Zhao X. DNA gyrase, topoisomerase IV, and the 4-quinolones. *Microbiol Mol Biol Rev* 1997; 61: 377-92.

[35] Yao J, Moellering RJ. Antibacterial agents. In: Murray PR, Baron EJ, Jorgensen JH, Pfaller MA, Yolken RH, Eds. Manual of Clinical Microbiology. 8th ed. Washington, DC: ASM Press 2003; pp. 1039 -73.

[36] Petri WAJ. Antimicrobial agents: sulfonamides, trimethoprim-sulfamethoxazole, quinolones, and agents for urinary tract infections. In: Brunton LL, Lazo JS, Parker KL, Eds. Goodman & Gilman's The Pharmacological Basis of Therapeutics. 11th ed. New York: McGraw- Hill 2006; pp. 1111-26.

[37] Storm DR, Rosenthal KS, Swanson PE. Polymyxin and related peptide antibiotics. Annu Rev Biochem 1977; 46: 723-63.

[38] Carpenter CF, Chambers HF. Daptomycin: another novel agent for treating infections due to drug-resistant gram-positive pathogens. Clin Infect Dis 2004; 38: 994 -1000.

[39] Poole K. Multidrug resistance in Gram-negative bacteria. Curr Opin Microbiol 2001; 4: 500-508.

[40] Markham PN, Neyfakh AA. Efflux-mediated drug resistance in Gram-positive bacteria. Curr Opin Microbiol 2001; 4: 509-14.

[41] Petrikkos G, Skiada A. Recent advances in antifungal chemotherapy. Int J Antimicrob Agents 2007; 30: 108-17.

[42] Pasqualotto AC, Denning DW. New and emerging treatments for fungal infections. J Antimicrob Chemother 2008; 61(Suppl. 1): i19-i30.

[43] Denning DW, Hope WW. Therapy for fungal diseases: opportunities and priorities. Trends Microbiol 2010; 18(5): 195-204.

[44] Agarwal AK, Tripathi SK, Xu T, Jacob MR, Li X-C, Clark AM. Exploring the Molecular Basis of Antifungal Synergies Using Genome-Wide Approaches. Front Microbiol 2012; 3: 115.

[45] Brajtburg J, Powderley WG, Kobayashi GS, Medoff G. Amphotericin B: current understanding of mechanism of action. Antimicrob Agents Chemother 1990; 34: 183-88.

[46] White TC, Marr KA, Bowden RA. Clinical, cellular, and molecular factors that contribute to antifungal drug resistance. Clin Microbiol Rev 1998; 11: 382-402.

[47] Kelly SL, Lamb DC, Taylor M, Corran AJ, Baldwin BC, Powderly WG. Resistance to amphotericin B associated with defective sterol delta 8-7 isomerase in a *Cryptococcus neoformans* strain from an AIDS patient. FEMS Microbiol Lett 1994; 122: 39-42.

[48] Fasoli MO, Kerridge D, Morris PG, Torosantucci A. 19F nuclear magnetic resonance study of fluoropyrimidine metabolism in strains of *Candida glabrata* with specific defects in pyrimidine metabolism. Antimicrob Agents Chemother 1990; 34: 1996-2006.

[49] Kelly SL, Lamb DC, Kelly DE, *et al.* Resistance to fluconazole and cross-resistance to amphotericin B in *Candida albicans* from AIDS patients caused by defective sterol delta 5,6-desaturation. FEBS Lett 1997; 400: 80-82.

[50] Perlin DS. Application of real-time PCR to the diagnosis of invasive fungal infections. In: Logan J, Edwards K, Saunders N, Eds. Real-time PCR: current technology and applications. Norfolk, UK: Caister Academic Press; 2009; pp. 221-34.

[51] Johnson LB, Kauffman CA. Voriconazole: a new triazole antifungal agent. Clin Infect Dis 2003; 36: 630-7.

[52] Linares MJ, Charriel G, Solis F, Rodriguez F, Ibarra A, Casal M. Susceptibility of filamentous fungi to voriconazole tested by two microdilution methods. J Clin Microbiol 2005; 43: 250-3.

[53] Swinne D, Watelle M, Nolard N. *In vitro* activity of voriconazole, fluconazole, itraconazole and amphotericin B against non *Candida* albicans yeast isolates. Rev Iberoam Micol 2005; 22: 24-8.

[54] Nguyen MH, Yu CY. Voriconazole against fluconazole-susceptible and resistant *Candida* isolates: *in vitro* efficacy compared with that of itraconazole and ketoconazole. J Antimicrob Chemother 1998; 42: 253-6.

[55] Kartsonis NA, Nielsen J, Douglas CM. Caspofungin: the first in a new class of antifungal agents. Drug Resist Updat 2003; 6: 197-218.

[56] Denning DW. Echinocandin antifungal drugs. Lancet 2003; 362:1142-51.

[57] Wiederhold NP, Lewis RE. The echinocandin antifungals: an overview of the pharmacology, spectrum and clinical efficacy. Expert Opin Investig Drugs 2003; 12:1313-33.

[58] Morris MI, Villmann M. Echinocandins in the management of invasive fungal infections, part 1. Am J Health Syst Pharm 2006; 63:1693-1703.

[59] Bowman JC, Hicks PS, Kurtz MB, *et al.* The antifungal echinocandin caspofungin acetate kills growing cells of Aspergillus fumigatus *in vitro*. Antimicrob Agents Chemother 2002; 46: 3001-12.

[60] Pfaller MA, Boyken L, Hollis RJ, *et al. In vitro* susceptibility of invasive isolates of *Candida spp.* to anidulafungin, caspofungin, and micafungin: six years of global surveillance. J Clin Microbiol 2008; 46: 150-56.

[61] Cleary JD, Garcia-Effron G, Chapman SW, Perlin DS. Reduced *Candida* glabrata susceptibility secondary to an FKS1 mutation developed during candidemia treatment. Antimicrob Agents Chemother 2008; 52: 2263-65.

[62] Garcia-Effron G, Dilger A, Alcazar-Fuoli L, Park S, Mellado E, Perlin DS. Rapid detection of triazole antifungal resistance in Aspergillus fumigatus. J Clin Microbiol 2008; 46: 1200-6.

[63] Lamb D, Kelly D, Kelly S. Molecular aspects of azole antifungal action and resistance. Drug Resist Updat 1999; 2: 390-402.

[64] Andersson D. The ways in which bacteria resist antibiotics (background document) Seminar on the Global Threat of Antibiotic Resistance - Exploring Roads Towards Concerted Action, Uppsala, Sweden, 5-7 May 2004. Available from: http:// www.reactgroup.org [cited: 15th July 2012]

[65] Alekshun MN, Levy SB. Molecular mechanisms of antibacterial multidrug resistance. Cell 2007; 128: 1037-50.

[66] Vila J, Marti S, Sanchez-Cespedes J. Porins. Efflux pumps and multidrug resistance in *Acinetobacter baumannii*. J Antimicrob Chemother 2007; 59:1210-15.

[67] Livermore DM. Bacterial resistance: origins, epidemiology, and impact. Clin Infect Dis 2003; 36(Suppl 1): S11-23.

[68] Livermore D. Can better prescribing turn the tide of resistance? Nat Rev Microbiol 2004; 2: 73-8.

[69] Mwangi MM, Wu SW, Zhou Y, *et al.* Tracking the *in vivo* evolution of multidrug resistance in *Staphylococcus aureus* by whole-genome sequencing. Proc Natl Acad Sci USA 2007; 104: 9451-6.

[70] Courvalin P. Vancomycin resistance in gram-positive cocci. Clin Infect Dis 2006; 42(Suppl. 1): S25-S34.

[71] Liu B, Pop M. ARDB—Antibiotic Resistance Genes Database. Nucleic Acids Res 2009; 37(Database issue): D443-D447.

[72] Marr KA. Invasive *Candida* infections: the changing epidemiology. Oncology (Huntingt) 2004; 18: 9-14.

[73] Pfaller MA, Diekema DJ, Gibbs DL, *et al.* Results from the ARTEMIS DISK Global Antifungal Surveillance study, 1997 to 2005: an 8.5-year analysis of susceptibilities of *Candida* species and other yeast species to fluconazole and voriconazole determined by CLSI standardized disk diffusion testing. J Clin Microbiol 2007; 45: 1735-45.

[74] Sanglard D, Bille J. Current understanding of the modes of action of and resistance mechanisms to conventional and emerging antifungal agents for treatment of *Candida* infections. In: Calderone RA, ed. *Candida* and Candidiasis. Washington, DC: ASM Press 2002; pp. 349-83.

[75] Marichal P, Koymans L, Willemsens S, *et al.* Contribution of mutations in the cytochrome P450 14alpha-demethylase (Erg11p, Cyp51p) to azole resistance in *Candida* albicans. Microbiology 1999; 145 (Pt 10): 2701-13.

[76] Sanglard D, Ischer F, Parkinson T, Falconer D, Bille J. *Candida* albicans mutations in the ergosterol biosynthetic pathway and resistance to several antifungal agents. Antimicrob Agents Chemother 2003; 47: 2404-12.

[77] Wiederhold NP, Grabinski JL, Garcia-Effron G, Perlin DS, Lee SA. Pyrosequencing to detect mutations in FKS1 that confer reduced echinocandin susceptibility in *Candida* albicans. Antimicrob Agents Chemother 2008; 52: 4145-8.

[78] Park S, Perlin DS. Establishing surrogate markers for fluconazole resistance in *Candida* albicans. Microb Drug Resist 2005; 11: 232-8.
[79] Loeffler J, Hagmeyer L, Hebart H, Henke N, Schumacher U, Einsele H. Rapid detection of point mutations by fluorescence resonance energy transfer and probe melting curves in *Candida* species. Clin Chem 2000; 46: 631-5.
[80] Yan L, Zhang J, Li M, *et al.* DNA microarray analysis of fluconazole resistance in a laboratory *Candida* albicans strain. Acta Biochim Biophys Sin 2008; 40: 1048-60.
[81] White TC, Holleman S, Dy F, Mirels LF, Stevens DA. Resistance mechanisms in clinical isolates of *Candida* albicans. Antimicrob Agents Chemother 2002; 46: 1704-13.
[82] Kretschmer M, Leroch M, Mosbach A, *et al.* Fungicide-Driven Evolution and Molecular Basis of Multidrug Resistance in Field Populations of the Grey Mould Fungus *Botrytis cinerea.* PLoS Pathog 2009; 5(12): e1000696.
[83] Morschhäuser J, Barker KS, Liu TT, Blaß-Warmuth J, Homayouni R, Rogers PD. The transcription factor Mrr1p controls expression of the MDR1 efflux pump and mediates multidrug resistance in *Candida albicans*. PLoS Pathog 2007; 3: e164.
[84] Wakieć R, Prasad R, Morschhäuser J, Barchiesi F, Borowski E, Milewski S. Voriconazole and multidrug resistance in *Candida albicans*. Mycoses 2007; 50: 109-115.
[85] de Micheli M, Bille J, Schueller C, Sanglard D. A common drug-responsive element mediates the upregulation of the *Candida albicans* ABC transporters *CDR1* and *CDR2*, two genes involved in antifungal drug resistance. Mol Microbiol 2002, 43: 1197-1214.
[86] Kofla G, Ruhnke M. Development of a new real-time TaqMan PCR assay for quantitative analyses of *Candida* albicans resistance genes expression. J Microbiol Methods 2007; 68: 178-83.
[87] Gygax SE, Vermitsky JP, Chadwick SG, *et al.* Antifungal resistance of *Candida* glabrata vaginal isolates and development of a quantitative reverse transcription-PCR-based azole susceptibility assay. Antimicrob Agents Chemother 2008; 52: 3424-6.
[88] Balashov SV, Gardiner R, Park S, Perlin DS. Rapid, high-throughput, multiplex, real-time PCR for identification of mutations in the cyp51A gene of Aspergillus fumigatus that confer resistance to itraconazole. J Clin Microbiol 2005; 43: 214-22.
[89] Watson PF, Rose ME, King DJ, Ellis SW, England H, Kelly SL. Defective sterol C5-6 desaturation and azole resistance:A new hypothesis on the mode of action of azole antifungals. Biochem Biophys Res Commun 1989; 164: 1170-5.
[90] Domitrovic T, Kozlov G, Freire JCG, *et al.* Structural and Functional Study of Yer067w, a New Protein Involved in Yeast Metabolism Control and Drug Resistance. PLoS One 2010; 5(6): e11163.
[91] Reardon JE. Human immunodeficiency virus reverse transcriptase. A kinetic analysis of RNAdependent and DNA-dependent DNA polymerization. J Biol Chem 1993; 268: 8743-51.
[92] Locarnini S, Birch C. Antiviral chemotherapy for chronic hepatitis B infection: Lessons learned from treating HIV infected patients. J Hepatol 1999; 30: 536-50.
[93] Schuurman R, Nijhuis M, van Leeuwen R, *et al.* Rapid changes in human immunodeficiency virus type 1 RNA load and appearance of drug-resistant virus populations in persons treated with lamivudine (3TC). J Infect Dis 1995; 171:1411-9.
[94] Wainberg MA, Salomon H, Gu Z, *et al.* Development of HIV-1 resistance to (-)2'-deoxy-3'-thiacytidine in patients with AIDS or advanced AIDS-related complex. AIDS 1995; 9: 351-7.

[95] Najera I, Holguin A, Quinones-Mateu ME, *et al.* Pol gene quasispecies of human immunodeficiency virus: mutations associated with drug resistance in virus from patients undergoing no drug therapy. J Virol 1995; 69: 23-31.

[96] Kobayashi S, Ide T, Sata M. Detection of YMDD motif mutations in some lamivudine-untreated asymptomatic hepatitis B virus carriers. J Hepatol 2001; 34: 584-6.

[97] Coffin JM. HIV population dynamics *in vivo*: implications for genetic variation, pathogenesis, and therapy. Science 1995; 267: 483-9.

[98] Tillmann HL, Trautwein C, Bock T, *et al.* Mutational pattern of hepatitis B virus on sequential therapy with famciclovir and lamivudine in patients with hepatitis B virus reinfection occurring under HBIg immunoglobulin after liver transplantation. Hepatology 1999; 30: 244-56.

[99] Zhang YY, Summers J. Low dynamic state of viral competition in a chronic avian hepadnavirus infection. J Virol 2000; 74: 5257-65.

[100] Smith RD, Beaglehole R, Woodward D, Drager N, Eds. Global public goods for health: health economics and public health perspective. Oxford: Oxford University Press 2003.

[101] Howe RA, Monk A, Wootton M, Walsh TR, Enright MC. Vancomycin susceptibility within methicillin-resistant Staphylococcus aureus lineages. Emerg Infect Dis 2004; 10: 855-7.

[102] Cohen ML. Epidemiology of drug resistance: implications for a post-antimicrobial era. Science 1992; 257: 1050-5.

[103] Global Tuberculosis Control: Surveillance, Planning Financing. Geneva: World Health Organization; 2004. Available from: http://www.who.int/tb/publications/global_report/2004/en/full.pdf

[104] Carbon C, Cars O, Christiansen K. Moving from recommendation to implementation and audit: part 1. Current recommendations and programs: a critical commentary. Clin Microbiol Infect 2002; 8(Suppl 2): 92-106.

[105] European Commission. Sixth EU Framework Programme for Research and Technological Development. Latest information on LifeSciHealth calls. Available from: http://fp6.cordis.lu/lifescihealth/calls.cfm [Accessed 29 July 2004].

[106] Fraser CM, Eisen J, Fleischmann RD, Ketchum KA, Peterson S. Comparative genomics and understanding of microbial biology. Emerg Infect Dis 2000; 6: 505-12.

[107] Moxon ER, Hood DW, Saunders NJ, Schweda EK, Richards JC. Functional genomics of pathogenic bacteria. Philos Trans R Soc Lond B Biol Sci 2002; 357: 109-16.

[108] Wizemann TM, Heinrichs JH, Adamou JE, *et al.* Use of a whole genome approach to identify vaccine molecules affording protection against *Streptococcus pneumoniae* infection. Infect Immun 2001; 69: 1593-8.

[109] Pizza M, Scarlato V, Masignani V, *et al.* Identification of vaccine *candida*tes against serogroup B meningococcus by whole-genome sequencing. Science 2000; 287: 1816-20.

[110] Comanducci M, Bambini S, Brunelli B, *et al.* NadA, a novel vaccine *candida*te of *Neisseria meningitidis*. J Exp Med *2002*; 195: 1445-54.

[111] Cockle PJ, Gordon SV, Lalvani A, Buddle BM, Hewinson RG, Vordermeier HM. Identification of novel *Mycobacterium tuberculosis* antigens with potential as diagnostic reagents or subunit vaccine *candida*tes by comparative genomics. Infect Immun 2002; 70: 6996-7003.

[112] Rappuoli R, Covacci A. Reverse vaccinology and genomics. Science 2003; 302(5645): 602.

[113] Shlaes DM. The abandonment of antibacteials: why and wherefore? Curr Opin Pharmacol 2003; 3: 470-3.
[114] Fattom AI, Horwith G, Fuller S, Propst M, Naso R. Development of StaphVAX, a polysaccharide conjugate vaccine against S. aureus infection: from the lab bench to phase III clinical trials. Vaccine 2004; 22: 880-7.
[115] Koch S, Hufnagel M, Theilacker C, Huebner J. Enterococcal infections: host response, therapeutic, and prophylactic possibilities. Vaccine 2004; 22: 822-30.
[116] Roberts JA, Kaack MB, Baskin G, *et al.* Antibody responses and protection from pyelonephritis following vaccination with purified Escherichia coli PapDG protein. J Urol 2004; 171: 1682-5.
[117] Heath PT, McVernon J. The UK Hib vaccine experience. Arch Dis Child 2002; 86: 396-9.
[118] Ramsay ME, Andrews N, Kaczmarski EB, Miller E. Efficacy of meningococcal serogroup C conjugate vaccine in teenagers and toddlers in England. Lancet 2001; 357: 195-6.
[119] Obaro SK. The new pneumococcal vaccine. Clin Microbiol Infect 2002; 8: 623-33.
[120] Pe´rez-Herna´ndez X, Me´ndez-A´ lvarez S, Claverie-Martı´n F. A PCR assay for rapid detection of vancomycin-resistant *enterococci*. Diagn Microbiol Infect Dis 2002; 42: 273-7.
[121] Ramasubban G, Therese K L, Vetrivel U, *et al.* Detection of novel coupled mutations in the katG gene (His276Met, Gln295His and Ser315Thr) in a multidrug-resistant Mycobacterium tuberculosis strain from Chennai, India, and insight into the molecular mechanism of isoniazid resistance using structural bioinformatics approaches. Int J Antimicrob Agents 2011; 37(4): 368-72.
[122] Cassone M, Del Grosso M, Pantosti A, Giordano A, Pozzi G. Detection of genetic elements carrying glycopeptide resistance clusters in Enterococcus by DNA microarrays. Mol Cell Probes 2008; 22(3): 162-7.
[123] Peeters E, Sass A, Mahenthiralingam E, Nelis H, Coenye T. Transcriptional response of *Burkholderia cenocepacia* J2315 sessile cells to treatments with high doses of hydrogen peroxide and sodium hypochlorite. BMC Genomics 2010; 11: 90.
[124] Scaria J, Chandramouli U, Verma SK. Antibiotic Resistance Genes Online (ARGO): a Database on vancomycin and beta-lactam resistance genes. Bioinformation 2005; 1: 5-7.
[125] Zhou CE, Smith J, Lam M, Zemla A, Dyer MD, Slezak T. MvirDB—a microbial database of protein toxins, virulence factors and antibiotic resistance genes for bio-defence applications. Nucleic Acids Res 2007; 35: D391-4.
[126] ß-Lactamase Classification and Amino Acid Sequences for TEM, SHV and OXA Extended-Spectrum and Inhibitor Resistant Enzymes. Lahay Clinc. Available from: http://www.lahey.org/Studies/ [cited 7th November 2012].
[127] Benson DA, Karsch-Mizrachi I, Lipman DJ, Ostell J, Wheeler DL. GenBank. Nucleic Acids Res 2008; 36: D25-D30.
[128] UniProt Consortium The universal protein resource (UniProt) Nucleic Acids Res 2008; 36: D190-5.
[129] Perlin DS, Zhao Y. Molecular diagnostic platforms for detecting Aspergillus. Med Mycol 2009; 47 Suppl 1: S223-32.
[130] De Marco D, Perotti M, Ossi CM, Burioni R, Clementi M, Mancini N. Development and validation of a molecular method for the diagnosis of medically important fungal infections. New Microbiol 2007; 30: 308-12.
[131] Weile J, Knabbe C. Current applications and future trends of molecular diagnostics in clinical bacteriology. Anal Bioanal Chem 2009; 394: 731-42.

[132] Pfaller MA, Diekema DJ, Jones RN, *et al.* International surveillance of bloodstream infections due to *Candida* species: frequency of occurrence and *in vitro* susceptibilities to fluconazole, ravuconazole, and voriconazole of isolates collected from 1997 through 1999 in the SENTRY antimicrobial surveillance program. J Clin Microbiol 2001; 39: 3254-9.

[133] Pfaller MA, Diekema DJ, International Fungal Surveillance Participant Group. Twelve years of fluconazole in clinical practice: global trends in species distribution andfluconazole susceptibility of bloodstream isolates of *Candida*. Clin Microbiol Infect 2004; 10 Suppl 1: 11-23.

[134] Steinbach WJ, Perfect JR, Schell WA, Walsh TJ, Benjamin DK Jr. *In vitro* analyses, animal models, and 60 clinical cases of invasive Aspergillus terreus infection. Antimicrob Agents Chemother 2004; 48: 3217-25.

[135] Perlin DS, Balashov S, Park S. Multiplex detection of mutations. Methods Mol Biol 2008; 429: 23-31.

[136] Trama JP, Mordechai E, Adelson ME. Detection of Aspergillus fumigatus and a mutation that confers reduced susceptibility to itraconazole and posaconazole by real-time PCR and pyrosequencing. J Clin Microbiol 2005; 43:906-8.

[137] Tuohy MJ, Reja V, Park S, *et al.* Use of a high-resolution melt assay to characterize codon 54 of the cyp51A gene of Aspergillus fumigatus on a Rotor-Gene 6000 instrument. Antimicrob Agents Chemother 2010; 54(5): 2248-51.

[138] Samaranayake DP, Hanes SD. Milestones in *Candida* albicans gene manipulation. Fungal Genet Biol 2011; 48(9): 858-65.

[139] Stuyver L, Van Geyt C, De Gendt S, *et al.* Line probe assay for monitoring drug resistance in hepatitis B virus-infected patients during antiviral therapy. J Clin Microbiol 2000; 38: 702-7.

[140] Chin R, Shaw T, Torresi J, *et al. In vitro* susceptibilities of wild-type or drug-resistant hepatitis B virus to (-)-beta-D-2,6-diaminopurine dioxolane and 2'-fluoro-5-methyl- beta-L-arabinofuranosyluracil. Antimicrob Agents Chemother 2001; 45: 2495-2501.

[141] Harrigan PR, Salim M, Stammers DK, *et al.* A Mutation in the 3' Region of the Human Immunodeficiency Virus Type 1 Reverse Transcriptase (Y318F) Associated with Nonnucleoside Reverse Transcriptase Inhibitor Resistance. J Virol 2002; 76: 6836-40.

[142] Back N, Nijhuis M, Keulen W, *et al.* Reduced replication of 3TC-resistant HIV-1 variants in primary cells due to a processivity defect of the transverse transcriptase enzyme. EMBO J 1996; 15(15): 4040-9.

[143] Kim CM, Koike K, Saito I, Miyamura T, Jay G. HBx gene of hepatitis B virus induces liver cancer in transgenic mice. Nature 1991; 351: 317-20.

[144] Chalker AF, Lunsford RD. Rational identification of new antibacterial drug targets that are essential for viability using a genomics-based approach. Pharmacol Ther 2002; 95:1-20.

[145] Thanassi JA, Hartman-Neumann SL, Dougherty TJ, Dougherty BA, Pucci MJ. Identification of 113 conserved essential genes using a high-throughput gene disruption system in *Streptococcus pneumoniae*. Nucleic Acids Res 2002; 30: 3152-62.

[146] Feikin DR, Klugman KP. Historical changes in pneumococcal serogroup distribution: implications for the era of pneumococcal conjugate vaccines. Clin Infect Dis 2002; 35: 547-55.

[147] Oliveira DC, Tomasz A, de Lencastre H. Secrets of success of a human pathogen: molecular evolution of pandemic clones of meticillin-resistant *Staphylococcus aureus*. Lancet Infect Dis 2002; 2: 180-89.

[148] Sa-Leao R, Tomasz A, Santos Sanches I, de Lencastre H. Pilot study of the genetic diversity of the pneumococcal nasopharyngeal flora among children attending day care centers. J Clin Microbiol 2002; 40: 3577-85.

[149] Sa-Leao R, Vilhelmsson SE, de Lencastre H, Kristinsson KG, Tomasz A. Diversity of penicillinnonsusceptible *Streptococcus pneumoniae* circulating in Iceland after the introduction of penicillin-resistant clone Spain(6B)-2. J Infect Dis 2002; 186: 966-75.

[150] Giaever G, Shoemaker DD, Jones TW, *et al.* Genomic profiling of drug sensitivities *via* induced haploinsufficiency. Nat Genet 1999; 21: 278-83.

[151] Wojciechowski M, Mazerski J, Borowski E. Constrained search of conformational hyperspace of inactivators of glucosamine-6-phosphate synthase. J Enzyme Inhib1995; 10: 17-26.

[152] Milewski S, Chmara R, Andruszkiewicz R, Borowski E. Synthetic derivatives of N3-fumaroyl-L-2,3-diaminopropanoic acid inactivate glucosamine synthetase from *Candida* albicans. Biochim Biophys Acta 1985; 828: 247-54.

[153] Andruszkiewicz R, Chmara R, Milewski S, Borowski E. Synthesis of N3-fumaramoyl-L-2,3-diaminopropanoic acid analogues, the irreversible inhibitors of glucosamine synthetase. Int J Peptide Protein Res 1986; 27: 449-53.

[154] Andruszkiewicz R, Milewski S, Borowski E. Amide and ester derivatives of N3-trans-epoxysuccinoyl-L-2,3-diaminopropanoic acid: inhibitors of glucosamine-6-phosphate synthase. J Enzyme Inhib 1995; 9: 123-33.

[155] Andruszkiewicz R, Zieniawa T, Chmara H, Kasprzak L, Borowski E. Synthesis and anti*candida*l activities of optimized analogs of antibiotic Sch 37137. J Antbiot 1994; 47: 715-23.

[156] Milewski S, Andruszkiewicz R, Borowski E. Substrate specificity of peptide permeases in *Candida albicans*. FEMS Microbiol Lett 1988; 50: 73-78.

[157] Gerdes SY, Scholle MD, D'Souza M, *et al.* From genetic footprinting to antimicrobial drug targets: examples in cofactor biosynthetic pathways. J Bacteriol 2002; 184: 4555-72.

[158] Akerley BJ, Rubin EJ, Novick VL, Amaya K, Judson N, Mekalanos JJ. A genome-scale analysis for identification of genes required for growth or survival of *Haemophilus influenzae*. Proc Natl Acad Sci USA 2002; 99: 966-71.

[159] Ji Y, Zhang B, Van SF, *et al.* Identification of critical staphylococcal genes using conditional phenotypes generated by antisense RNA. Science 2001; 293: 2266-9.

[160] Knowles DJ. New strategies for antibacterial drug design. Trends Microbiol 1997; 5: 379-83.

[161] Merrell DS, Camilli A. Detection and analysis of gene expression during infection by *in vivo* expression technology. Philos Trans R Soc Lond B Biol Sci 2000; 355: 587-99.

[162] Valdivia RH, Falkow S. Fluorescence-based isolation of bacterial genes expressed within host cells. Science 1997; 277: 2007-11.

[163] Hensel M, Shea JE, Gleeson C, Jones MD, Dalton E, Holden DW. Simultaneous identification of bacterial virulence genes by negative selection. Science 1995; 269: 400-3.

[164] Mecsas J. Use of signature-tagged mutagenesis in pathogenesis studies. Curr Opin Microbiol 2002; 5: 33-7.

[165] Wilson M, DeRisi J, Kristensen HH, *et al.* Exploring drug-induced alterations in gene expression in Mycobacterium tuberculosis by microarray hybridization. Proc Natl Acad Sci USA 1999; 96: 12833-8.

[166] Jana S, Deb JK. Molecular targets for design of novel inhibitors to circumvent aminoglycoside resistance. Curr Drug Targets 2005; 6(3): 353-61.
[167] Tao J, Wendler P, Connelly G, *et al.* Drug target validation: lethal infection blocked by inducible peptide. Proc Natl Acad Sci USA 2000; 97: 783-6.
[168] De Luca A. The impact of resistance on viral fitness and its clinical implications. In: Geretti AM, Ed. Antiretroviral Resistance in Clinical Practice. London: Mediscript 2006; Chapter 12.
[169] Donadio S, Monciardini P, Alduina R, *et al.* Microbial technologies for the discovery of novel bioactive metabolites. J Biotechnol 2002; 99: 187-98.
[170] Kristich CJ, Little JL, Hall CL, Hoff JS. Reciprocal Regulation of Cephalosporin Resistance in *Enterococcus faecalis*. mBio 2011; 2(6): e00199-11.
[171] Blondelle SE, Perez-Paya E, Houghten RA. Synthetic combinatorial libraries: novel discovery strategy for identification of antimicrobial agents. Antimicrob Agents Chemother 1996; 40: 1067-71.
[172] Schreiber SL. Target-oriented and diversity-oriented organic synthesis in drug discovery. Science 2000; 287: 1964-9.
[173] Koza DJ. Synthesis of 7-substituted tetracycline derivatives. Org Lett 2000; 2: 815-7.
[174] Akritopoulou-Zanze I, Sowin TJ. Solid-phase synthesis of macrolide analogues. J Comb Chem 2001; 3: 301-11.
[175] Gordeev MF. Combinatorial lead discovery and optimization of antimicrobial oxazolidinones. Curr Opin Drug Discov Devel 2001; 4: 450-61.
[176] Johnson MD, Macdougall C, Ostrosky-Zeichner L, Perfect JR, Rex JH. Combination antifungal therapy. Antimicrob Agents Chemother 2004; 48: 693-715.
[177] Mukherjee PK, Sheehan DJ, Hitchcock CA, Ghannoum MA. Combination treatment of invasive fungal infections. Clin Microbiol Rev 2005; 18: 163-94.
[178] Jansen G, Lee AY, Epp E, *et al.* Chemogenomic profiling predicts antifungal synergies. Mol Syst Biol 2009; 5: 338.
[179] Condra JH, Emini EA. Preventing HIV-1 Drug Resistance. Science and Medicine 1997; 4: 2-11.
[180] Richman D, Ed. Antiviral drug resistance: issues and challenges. Chichester(UK): John Wiley & Sons 1996.
[181] Klebe G. Recent developments in structure-based drug design. J Mol Med 2000; 78: 269-81.
[182] Clements JM, Beckett RP, Brown A, *et al.* Antibiotic activity and characterization of BB-3497, a novel peptide deformylase inhibitor. Antimicrob Agents Chemother 2001; 45: 563-70.
[183] Hackbarth CJ, Chen DZ, Lewis JG, *et al.* N-alkyl urea hydroxamic acids as a new class of peptide deformylase inhibitors with antibacterial activity. Antimicrob Agents Chemother 2002; 46: 2752-64.
[184] Lim D, Strynadka NC. Structural basis for the β -lactam resistance of PBP2a from methicillin-resistant *Staphylococcus aureus*. Nature Struct Biol 2002; 9: 870-6.
[185] Rodriguez E, McDaniel R. Combinatorial biosynthesis of antimicrobials and other natural products. Curr Opin Microbiol 2001; 4: 526-34.
[186] Baltz R. In: Hughes D, Andersson DI, Eds. Antibiotic Development and Resistance. Taylor and Francis, London, New York 2001; pp. 233-257.

[187] McDaniel R, Thamchaipenet A, Gustafsson C, Fu H, Betlach M, Ashley G. Multiple genetic modifications of the erythromycin polyketide synthase to produce a library of novel 'unnatural' natural products. Proc Natl Acad Sci USA 1999; 96: 1846-51.

[188] Losey HC, Jiang J, Biggins JB, *et al.* Incorporation of glucose analogs by GtfE and GtfD from the vancomycin biosynthetic pathway to generate variant glycopeptides. Chem Biol 2002; 9: 1305-14.

[189] Miller LA, Ratnam K., Payne DJ. β-lactamase-inhibitor combinations in the 21st century: current agents and new developments. Curr Opin Pharmacol 2001; 1: 451-8.

[190] McKeegan KS, Borges-Walmsley MI, Walmsley AR. Structural understanding of efflux-mediated drug resistance: potential routes to efflux inhibition. Curr Opin Pharmacol 2004; 4(5): 479-86.

[191] Nikaido H. Multiple antibiotic resistance and efflux. Curr Opin Microbiol 1998; 1: 516-23.

[192] McMurry LM, Levy SB. Tetracycline resistance in Gram-positive bacteria. In: Fischetti VA, Novick RP, Ferretti JJ, Portnoy DA, Rood JI, Eds. Gram-positive Pathogens. Washington, DC: ASM Press 2000; pp. 660-77.

[193] Alekshun MN, Levy SB. Regulation of chromosomally mediated multiple antibiotic resistance: the mar regulon. Antimicrob Agents Chemother 1997; 41: 2067-75.

[194] Someya Y, Yamaguchi A, Sawai T. A novel glycycline, 9-(N,N-dimethylglycylamido)-6-deoxytetracycline, is neither transported nor recognized by the transposon Tn10-encoded metal-tetracycline/H+ antiporter. Antimicrob Agents Chemother 1995; 39(1): 247-9.

[195] Nelson ML, Levy SB. Reversal of tetracycline resistance mediated by different bacterial tetracycline resistance determinants by an inhibitor of the Tet(B) antiport protein. Antimicrob Agents Chemother 1999; 43: 1719-24.

[196] Markham PN, Westhaus E, Klyachko K, Johnson ME, Neyfakh AA. Multiple novel inhibitors of the NorA multidrug transporter of *Staphylococcus aureus*. Antimicrob Agents Chemother 1999; 43: 2404-8.

[197] Gibbons S, Oluwatuyi M, Kaatz GW. A novel inhibitor of multidrug efflux pumps in *Staphylococcus aureus*. J Antimicrob Chemother 2003; 51: 13-7.

[198] Kaatz GW, Moudgal VV, Seo SM, Kristiansen JE. Phenothiazines and thioxanthenes inhibit multidrug efflux pump activity in *Staphylococcus aureus*. Antimicrob Agents Chemother 2003; 47: 719-26.

[199] Renau TE, Léger R, Flamme EM, *et al.* Inhibitors of efflux pumps in Pseudomonas aeruginosa potentiate the activity of the fluoroquinolone antibacterial levofloxacin. J Med Chem 1999; 42: 4928-31.

[200] Pleban K, Kaiser D, Kopp S, Peer M, Chiba P, Ecker GF. Targeting drug-efflux pumps — a pharmacoinformatic approach. Acta Biochjmjca Polonica 2005; 52 (3): 737-40.

[201] Grkovic S, Brown MH, Skurray RA. Regulation of bacterial drug export systems. Microbiol Mol Biol Rev 2002; 66: 671-701.

[202] Maseda H, Sawada I, Saito K, Uchiyama H, Nakae T, Nomura N. Enhancement of the mexAB-OprM efflux expression by the quorum sensing autoinducer an its cancellation by a regulator MexT, of the mexEF-OprN efflux pump operon of Pseudomonas aeruginosa. Antimicrob Agents Chemother 2004; 48: 1320-8.

[203] Rahmati S, Yang S, Davidson AL, Zechiedrich EL. Control of the AcrAB multidrug efflux pump by quorum-sensing regulator SdiA. Mol Microbiol 2002; 43: 677-85.

[204] Thomas H, Coley HM. Overcoming multidrug resistance in cancer: an update on the clinical strategy of inhibiting P-glycoprotein. Cancer Control 2003; 10:159-65.

[205] Robert J, Jarry C. Multidrug resistance reversal agents. J Med Chem 2003; 46: 4805-17.

[206] Varma MVS, Ashokraj Y, Dey CS, Panchagnula R. P-glycoprotein inhibitors and their screening: a perspective from bioavailability enhancement. Pharmacol Res 2003; 48: 347-59.

[207] Krishna R, Mayer LD. Multidrug resistance (MDR) in cancer. Mechanisms, reversal using modulators of MDR and the roles of MDR modulators in influencing the pharmacokinetics of anticancer drugs. Eur J Pharm Sci 2000; 11: 265-83.

[208] Dantzig AH, Alwis DP, Burgess M. Considerations in the design and development of transport inhibitors as adjuncts to drug therapy. Adv Drug Deliv Rev 2003; 55: 133-50.

[209] Boissinot M, Bergeron MG. Toward rapid real-time molecular diagnostic to guide smart use of antimicrobials. Curr Opin Microbiol 2002; 5: 478-82.

[210] Schweitzer B, Kingsmore S. Combining nucleic acid amplification and detection. Curr Opin Biotechnol 2001; 12: 21-7.

[211] Grohs P, Kitzis MD, Gutmann L. *In vitro* bactericidal activities of linezolid in combination with vancomycin, gentamicin, ciprofloxacin, fusidic acid, and rifampin against *Staphylococcus aureus*. Antimicrob Agents Chemother 2003; 47: 418-20.

[212] Fattorini L, Tan D, Iona E, Mattei M, Giannoni F, Brunori L, Recchia S, Orefici G. Activities of moxifloxacin alone and in combination with other antimicrobial agents against multidrug-resistant *Mycobacterium tuberculosis* infection in BALB/c mice. Antimicrob Agents Chemother 2003; 47: 360-2.

[213] Gale M, Kwieciszewski B, Dossett M, Nakao H, Katze MG. Antiapoptotic and Oncogenic Potentials of Hepatitis C Virus Are Linked to Interferon Resistance by Viral Repression of the PKR Protein Kinase. J Virol. 1999; 73(8): 6506-16.

[214] Sulakvelidze A, Alavidze Z, Morris JG. Bacteriophage therapy. Antimicrob Agents Chemother 2001; 45: 649-59.

[215] Bull JJ, Levin BR, DeRouin T, Walker N, Bloch CA. Dynamics of success and failure in phage and antibiotic therapy in experimental infections. BMC Microbiol 2002; 2: 35.

[216] Loeffler JM, Nelson D, Fischetti VA. Rapid killing of Streptococcus pneumoniae with a bacteriophage cell wall hydrolase. Science 2001; 294: 2170-2.

[217] Nelson D, Loomis L, Fischetti VA. Prevention and elimination of upper respiratory colonization of mice by group A streptococci by using a bacteriophage lytic enzyme. Proc Natl Acad Sci USA 2001; 98: 4107-12.

[218] Reid G, Bruce AW. Urogenital infections in women: can probiotics help? Postgrad Med J 2003; 79: 428-32.

Send Orders for Reprints to reprints@benthamscience.net

Frontiers in Anti-Infective Drug Discovery, Vol. 2, 2014, 269-397

CHAPTER 5

Anti-Malaria Chemotherapy: State-of-the-Art in Prevention and Treatment and Novel Leads for Drug Development

Ana Maria Madeira M. Faísca Phillips*

Department of Chemistry, Faculty of Sciences and Technology, Universidade Nova de Lisboa, Campus de Caparica, Quinta da Torre, 2829-516 Caparica, Portugal

Abstract: Malaria is an infectious disease endemic to 106 countries of the tropical and subtropical regions of the world. According to the World Health Organization there were 216 million cases of malaria in 2010 that resulted in 655000 deaths. Children under the age of 5 are the most vulnerable, but approximately half of the world's population is at risk. Malaria is a febrile illness caused by parasitic protozoa of the genus *Plasmodium*, and transmitted exclusively by Anopheles mosquitoes. Control involves both prevention, through the use of indoor insecticide spraying with pyrethroids, insecticide treated bed nets, drug treatment of populations at high risk of infection and disease treatment. Malaria can be cured, but the development of resistance by *Plasmodium* is recurrent. Due to its high mortality and morbidity, the eradication of this disease has high priority in the UN 2000 Millennium Development Goals. As a result of renewed efforts, malaria related mortality decreased by 26% in the period 2000-2010, but control tools are limited. Presently there are no vaccines registered for this disease. The most deadly variant, caused by *Plasmodium falciparum*, is treated with artemisinin-based combination therapy with a 4-aminoquinoline or an amino alcohol. Recent reports of mosquito resistance to pyrethroid insecticides and of *Plasmodium* to artemisinin are serious causes for concern. The development of novel drugs remains a big challenge. This chapter highlights the state-of-the-art in malaria prevention and treatment. The literature published since 2000 on the development of new leads for chemotherapy is also reviewed.

Keywords: Malaria, antimalarial, *Plasmodium*, protozoa, *Anopheles*, infectious disease, pharmacology, artemisinin combination therapy, quinine, erythrocytes, antibiotics, aminoquinolines.

INTRODUCTION

Malaria is an infectious disease caused by parasitic protozoa of the genus *Plasmodium*, transmitted exclusively by the female *Anopheles* mosquito. It is

***Address correspondence to Ana Maria Madeira M. Faísca Phillips:** Department of Chemistry, Faculty of Sciences and Technology, Universidade Nova de Lisboa, Campus de Caparica, Quinta da Torre, 2829-516 Caparica, Portugal; Tel: (+351) 212948300, Ext. 10983; Fax: (+351) 212948550; E-mail: amfp@fct.unl.pt

Atta-ur-Rahman / M. Iqbal Choudhary (Eds)

endemic to 106 countries of the tropical and subtropical regions of the World. According to the World Health Organization, nearly 3.3 billion people were at risk of malaria in 2010, and in that year alone there were 216 million cases of which 655,000 resulted in death [1]. Due to its high mortality and morbidity, malaria is a disease of major importance. Although the figures for 2010 are staggering, they already represent a substantial improvement over the year 2000, when eradication of malaria was considered one of the priorities of the Millennium by the United Nations Organization, in its Millennium Development Goals. As a result of renewed interest, efforts and increased human and material resources for the fight against this disease, the number of reported cases of confirmed malaria decreased by more than 50% in 43 of the 99 countries with ongoing transmission during the period 2000 to 2010, and by 25 to 50% in another 8 countries [1]. It is estimated that during the same period the incidence of malaria decreased globally by 17%, and the mortality rate by 26% [1, 2].

Malaria is curable and controllable. When the parasite is inoculated into a human host by a feeding mosquito, it travels *via* the blood stream to the liver where it multiplies, returning afterwards to the blood stream where it infects the erythrocytes. The symptoms of malaria are initially similar to those of a minor systemic viral illness: headache, lassitude, fatigue, abdominal discomfort, muscle and joint aches, usually followed by fever, chills, perspiration, anorexia, vomiting and worsening malaise [3]. Appropriate diagnostic means are also important initially, to identify the disease correctly. If the disease is not controlled initially by effective medicines or if there is a delay in treatment, it may develop into severe malaria, especially when *P. falciparum* is the causal agent. Severe malaria may have the following symptoms: coma (cerebral malaria), metabolic acidosis, severe anaemia, hypoglycaemia, acute renal failure or acute pulmonary edema and ultimately it may result in death if not treated [3]. This progress can be very rapid and can take place within hours or days. Normally the main objective is to prevent death, then to prevent disabilities and recrudescence [4]. Young children under 5 are usually the most susceptible to the disease, and indeed 86% of malaria deaths occur in children under 5 years of age. In areas where populations are exposed to a high rate of malarial inoculations, partial immunity to the clinical disease and its severe symptoms is acquired. Nevertheless, immunity changes during pregnancy. Travellers moving to endemic areas are also at high risk.

THE MALARIA PARASITES

There are five species of *Plasmodium* parasites (of the *Apicomplexa* phylum) that affect humans: *P. falciparum*, *P. vivax*, *P. ovale*, *P. malariae* and *P. knowlesi* [2]. Nowadays *P. vivax* and *P. falciparum* are the most prevalent parasites. *Plasmodium falciparum* is the most dangerous. Malaria caused by this *Plasmodium* species often results in severe and life threatening conditions [5] and *P. falciparum* is responsible for approximately 90% of the deaths from malaria. In tropical countries *P. falciparum* is the most prevalent malaria parasite. *Plasmodium vivax* is more widely distributed and accounts for about 40% of the world malaria cases, but it is far less dangerous; it is also the dominant species outside Africa [3]. The other three species are less common. Although *P. vivax* and *P. ovale* very rarely cause fatal symptoms [3], these two species can form hypnozoites that stay dormant in the liver for long periods of time and can cause multiple relapses long after the first infection. Infection caused by *P. malariae* is often called "quartan" due to the periodic acute fevers it causes every four days, while with *P. vivax* and *P. ovale* this happens every third day; malaria caused by *P. vivax* is also known as "tertian". In *P. falciparum* malaria, the acute fevers occur at subtertian periods. *Plasmodium ovale* is the least distributed species, and is found only in sub-Saharan Africa, New Guinea and in the Philippines. *Plasmodium knowlesi* is a species that principally infects monkeys, but it has been causing an increasing number of human malaria cases in South-East Asia in recent years [3]. Parasitic *Plasmodium* species also infect birds, reptiles, chimpanzees and rodents.

THE LIFE CYCLE OF THE MALARIA PARASITE

Malaria is carried and transmitted to men by the female *Anopheles* mosquito only, when it bites to get a blood meal. The male mosquito only feeds on plant nectar and does not transmit the disease. The life cycle of the parasite [6], illustrated in Fig. (**1**), includes two stages: an exogeneous sexual phase (sporogony) with multiplication in the mosquito and an endogenous asexual phase (schizogony) with multiplication in the vertebrate host. The asexual phase includes two stages: a phase in the parenchyma cells of the liver, where pre-erythrocytic schizogony occurs, and another in the red blood cells, the erythrocytic schizogony. While sucking blood, the mosquito transfers saliva containing the *Plasmodium* parasite into the blood stream of the host. At this stage *Plasmodium* is in a highly infective sporozoite form. About 15 to 20 sporozoites are transferred. The parasite goes rapidly to the liver without being detected by the host's immune system and here starts the asexual liver stage in the life cycle of *Plasmodium*. The sporozoites invade the parenchyma cells of the liver where, by increasing their size and repeatedly replicating their nuclei and other organelles, they develop into tissue schizonts. In *P. vivax* and *P. ovale*, the sporozoites may remain in a dormant stage, the hypnozoites or develop into tissue schizonts. The hypnozoites can remain dormant in the liver for long periods of time, even years, and reactivate. In *P. falciparum* and *P. malariae* only schizonts form. The multinucleated schizonts subdivide into 10,000-30,000 identical daughter cells, consisting of a single nucleus and a narrow cytoplasmic ring, the merozoites. After one to two weeks the schizonts rupture releasing the merozoites into the blood stream. This starts the asexual erythrocytic phase of the parasite's life cycle.

Some merozoites invade the red blood cells, the erythrocytes, where they grow, absorbing the haemoglobin, and develop into trophozoites, or ring forms. Their nuclei divide 3 to 5 times into a variable number of small nuclei, then the cytoplasm divides, and as a result of this segmentation the blood schizonts are produced. The schizonts grow and subdivide into merozoites. After some time that varies from one *Plasmodium* species to another, the erythrocyte ruptures and releases 16-32 new merozoites into the blood stream. These new merozoites may also invade the erythrocytes and start a new erythrocyclic life cycle. This cycle, from erythrocyte invasion to schizont rupture lasts 48 h with *P. falciparum, P. vivax* and P. *ovale* and 72 h with *P. malariae*. After a number of asexual life cycles, some merozoites develop into sexual forms, the gametocytes, which are transferred to a mosquito during a blood meal. In the mosquito mid-gut the gametocytes reproduce sexually developing from diploid zygotes into motile ookinetes that attach themselves to the outer gut membrane, differentiating into oocysts. The oocysts divide many times producing thousands of infective sporozoites, which migrate to the salivary glands of the mosquito, ready to be transmitted to humans again, thus starting a new cycle.

Antimalarials usually act on different stages of the parasite's life cycle, and this distinction is commonly used to classify them. Table **1** shows the classification used. To treat someone suffering from malaria, a blood schizontocide and a gametocide are needed if the protozoan is *P. falciparum*. If the protozoa causing the disease are *P. vivax* or *P. ovale*, a tissue schizontocide is also needed.

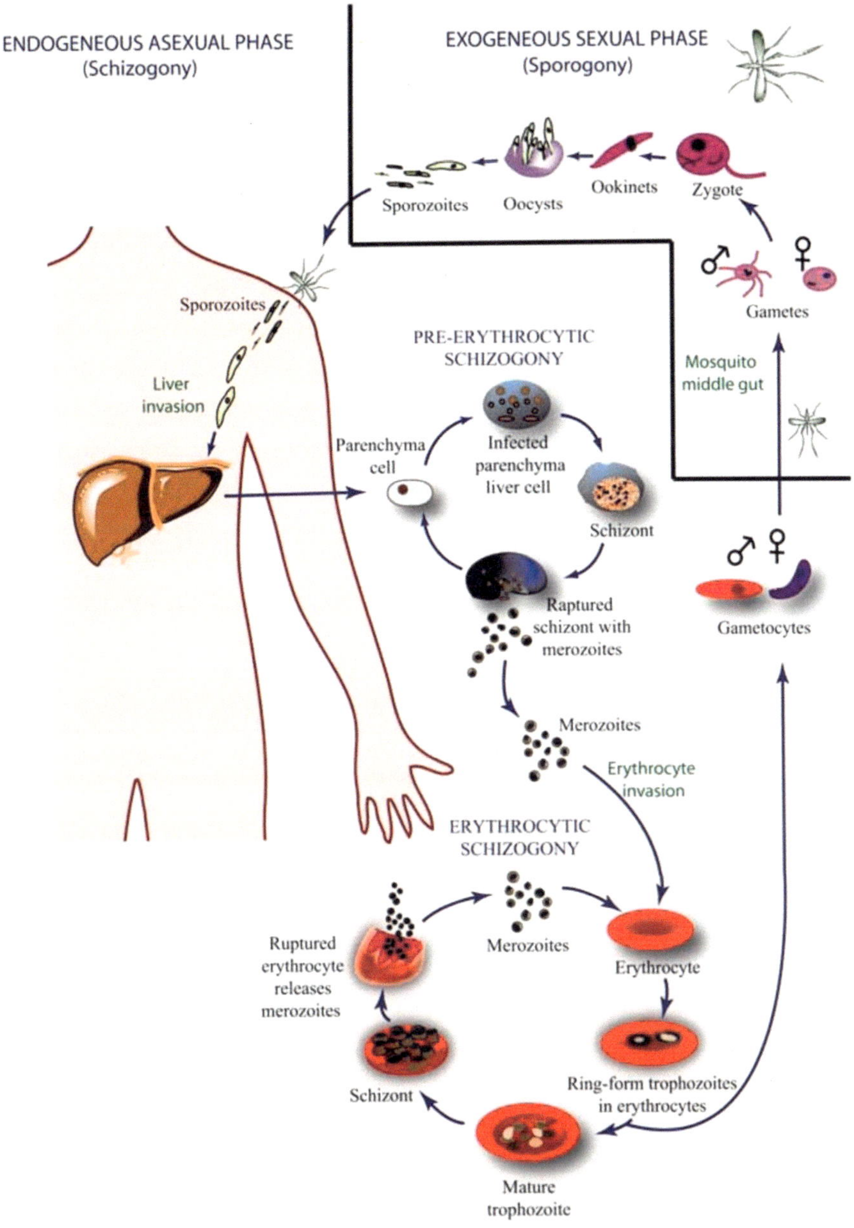

Figure 1: The life cycle of *P. falciparum*, with an exogeneous sexual phase (sporogony) with multiplication in certain *Anopheles* mosquitoes and an endogenous asexual phase (schizogony) with a liver stage and an erythrocytic stage of multiplication in man.

MALARIA CONTROL

Control involves both prevention, through the use of indoor insecticide spraying (mostly with pyrethroids), insecticide treated bed nets, drug treatment of populations at high risk of infection and disease treatment. Malaria can be cured. To maximize the effectiveness of the treatment and to prevent the development of resistance, combinations of drugs are recommended nowadays. Severe malaria, caused by *P. falciparum*, is often treated with artemisinin-based combination therapy (ACTs) with a 4-aminoquinoline or with an amino alcohol like quinine. Presently there are no vaccines registered for this disease, although attempts to develop one are underway. Recent reports of mosquito resistance to pyrethroid insecticides and of *Plasmodium* to artemisinin are serious causes for concern [1, 2]. Indeed, the development of resistance by *Plasmodium* is a continuous problem [8], and hence the development of novel drugs, to improve or substitute existing ones, is a continuous challenge. Affordability is yet another issue, since ACTs are nearly 10 times as expensive as the previous first-line drugs [9].

Table 1: **Classification of Antimalarial Drugs According to the Stage of the Parasite's Life Cycle on Which they Act**

Type of Drug	Drug Activity
Tissue Schizonticides	**They act on the liver forms of the parasite. When the primary exoerythrocytic stage is blocked, schizont development is impeded, and red blood cell invasion is prevented.** **These drugs are used for causal prophylaxis. *P. falciparum* is the most susceptible species.**
Blood Schizonticides	**They act on blood schizonts and related erythrocytic asexual forms of the parasite. These are the stages that are associated with acute disease, although sometimes there are only a few symptoms.** **They produce clinical cure.** **They also act on sexual erythrocytic forms of *P. vivax, P. ovale* and *P. malariae.* They don't act directly on the mature gametocytes of *P. falciparum.***
Gametocides	**They destroy the sexual forms of the parasite in the blood, the gametes. This prevents transmission of the infection to the mosquito.**
Sporontocides	**They prevent the development of oocysts and sporozoites in the mosquito. This prevents further transmission of malaria to humans.**
Hypnozoites	**Tissue schizonticides that act on the latent forms of the parasite that develop in the liver with *P. vivax* and *P. ovale.* They are used as anti-relapse drugs, preventing reactivation of the disease. These types of drugs are needed with these two species of *Plasmodium* to achieve radical cure of malaria.**

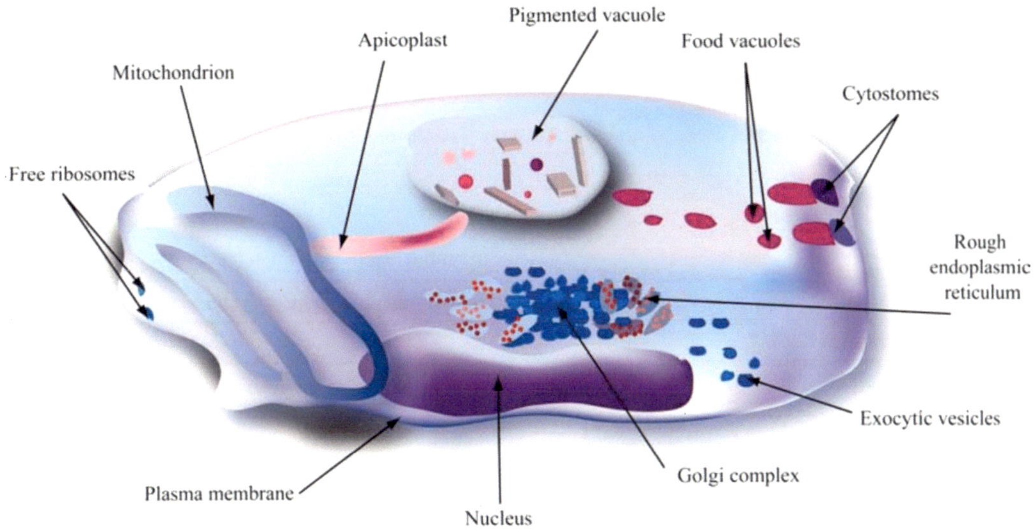

Figure 2: Schematic representation of the Mid-Trophozoite stage of *Plasmodium falciparum*, with its characteristic irregular outline [8].

Since an understanding of cell biology can lead to the development of better drugs, or to the exploitation of new drug targets, this is another area of intense research. The genome of *P. falciparum* has now been unveiled, and many present day studies focus on the development of molecular markers to identify genetic mutations related to antimalarial drug resistance [8]. A discussion of this subject is, however, beyond the scope of the present review. Nevertheless, to guide the reader through some of the aspects focused herein, Fig. (**2**) shows a schematic representation of the ultra-structure of *P. falciparum* in the mid trophozoite state. In this chapter, the state-of-the-art in malaria prevention and treatment is highlighted, as well as the pipeline of prospective drugs at several stages of clinical development. It ends with a brief overview of possible areas for future intervention.

CURRENTLY AVAILABLE ANTIMALARIAL DRUGS

The World Health Organization (WHO) recommends a number of drugs for the treatment and prophylaxis of malaria (Table **2**) [3, 7]. In this section, a brief look at their historical development, chemical and pharmaceutical properties, and the recommendations for their use, is presented. The pharmacokinetic parameters indicated aim to be representative. In many cases more than one study was published.

Table 2: Main Drugs Currently Available for Malaria Treatment According to WHO [7]

Chemical Class	Drug
Amino-alcohols	Quinine, quinidine, mefloquine, halofantrine, lumefantrine
4-Aminoquinolines	Chloroquine, amodiaquine, piperaquine
8-Aminoquinoline	Primaquine
Sulfonamides and sulfones	Sulfadoxine, sulfalene, dapsone
Diaminopyrimidine	Pyrimethamine
Biguanides	Proguanil, chlorproguanil
Naphthoquinone	Atovaquone
Sesquiterpene lactones	Artemisinin, arteether, artemether, artesunate, dihydroartemisinin
Antibiotics	Azythromycin, clindamycin, doxycycline, tetracycline

THE CINCHONA ALKALOIDS: QUININE AND QUINIDINE

Quinine

Quinine (QN) is the oldest antimalarial known [10]. A quinoline with a (8*S*,9*R*) quinuclidine methanol group, it is usually extracted from the bark of various species of the *Cinchona* tree, indigenous to Peru, where it is present in up to 13% of the dry matter. The medicinal properties of the bark were discovered by the Peruvian Quechua long ago. The plant was brought to Europe by the Jesuits in the 17th century, and it was already then used as an antimalarial drug. The powdered bark contains quinine and its diastereoisomer quinidine, both plasmodicidal alkaloids (Fig. **3**). A crude mixture of crystalline alkaloids was extracted from the cinchona bark by B. Gomes, in Portugal, in 1810 [11]. Quinine and cinchonine were later isolated by P. J. Pelletier and J. B. Caventou in Paris in 1820, and have been used as such since then. The first total synthesis was accomplished by R. B. Woodward and W. E. Dooring in 1944, and although a few more methods of total synthesis were developed since then, none is as economically viable as the extraction of the substance from the *Cinchona* tree bark. Quinine was the antimalarial drug of choice until the 1940s, but because of its side effects, other drugs started to be used. Quinine is a highly effective blood schizonticide against all forms of human malaria, hence it is effective for the clinical cure of malaria [12]. Radical cure is possible with *P. falciparum*. It has no effect on the exo-erythrocytic phase or the gametocytic phase. It is however an effective gametocytocide for *vivax*, *ovale* and *malariae* malaria [12]. It is inactive against latent erythrocytic stages. Long experience with this drug proves its value. Quinine has its own characteristic side effects, like giddiness, ringing in the ears, tremors and blurred vision, which occur while the drug is being administered [3]. These symptoms subside when the administration of the drug is stopped. Given intravenously it lowers blood pressure. More serious effects may occur, but they are rare. Nowadays quinine is still a drug of choice for the immediate relief of the symptoms of severe *P. falciparum* malaria, and it is recommended by WHO as a first line alternative to artesunate or artemether. It is also the drug of choice for pregnant women [7]. After an initial emergency parenteral antimalarial treatment, and once the patient can take oral medicines, one of the possibilities for follow-up treatment, besides an ACT, is quinine plus an antibiotic like clindamycin or doxycycline [3]. In a study in Thailand, after standard treatment for severe falciparum malaria the mean parasite clearance time was 76 h [13]. QN with an antibiotic is also recommended as second-line option for the treatment of uncomplicated falciparum malaria [3], and this was the subject of a recent review [14]. It is usually active against most strains that are resistant to chloroquine. IC_{50} values measured against laboratory strains and clinical isolates of *P. falciparum* varied between 96 and 380 nM and between 136 and 286 nM respectively [6].

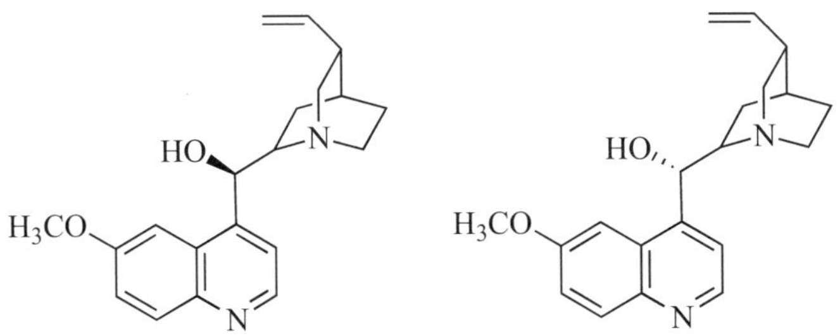

(-)-Quinine **1** (+)-Quinidine **2**

Figure 3: The first antimalarials, quinine and quinidine.

The mechanism of action of quinine is thought to involve inhibition of plasmodial haem polymerase [15-19]. In order to grow, the parasite breaks down the host's haemoglobin to obtain amino acids for its own protein synthesis (Fig. **4**). This takes place inside a lysosome-like organelle, the food vacuole. Ferriprotoporphyrin IX, *i.e.,* free haem, is obtained as a by-product. Free haem is toxic to the parasite, and as part of the detoxification process free haem is converted into hemozoin, the malaria pigment crystals, by the parasite's haem polymerase. When the action of haem polymerase is blocked by the antimalarial, there is a build up of free haem that eventually leads to parasite death. In addition, QN can also block DNA transcription in the parasite, since it can become intercalated in the parasite's DNA.

Pharmacology of Quinine

Quinine is rapidly absorbed from the gastrointestinal tract. It is extensively metabolised *via* the cytochrome P450 enzyme CYP3A4 in the liver [3]. The initial metabolite is 3-hydroxyquinine (3-OH-QN) that has about 10% of the antimalarial activity. QN has a half-life of 10 hours [12] and its bioavailability is about 80% [20]. A mean plasma concentration of 2-5 mg L^{-1} is probably necessary to reduce parasitaemia in acute *P. vivax* malaria, and 5 mg L^{-1} to eliminate asexual parasites from the blood stream [12]. Slightly higher amounts are needed with *P. falciparum*, which vary with the strains. It is generally given as a 7-day course followed by an antibiotic like tetracycline, pyrimethamine-sulphadoxine (Fansidar), doxycycline or clindamycin. In a study of its pharmacokinetics on healthy individuals, a single oral dose of 600 mg quinine sulphate produced a maximum concentration in the blood of 11.2 mg L^{-1} after 2.8 h, and mean $AUC_{0\rightarrow\infty}$ 12 h mg L^{-1} [21]. The major metabolite 3-OH-QN reached a mean maximum concentration in the blood of 1.35 mg L^{-1} after 62.8 h [21]. These values are higher in patients with uncomplicated *P. falciparum* malaria. In areas of multi-drug resistant strains, 7-day regimens of quinine and tetracycline provide cure rates over 90% in patients with uncomplicated falciparum malaria [22]. The pharmacokinetics of quinine was determined recently on adult patients in Thailand. Patients were treated with the standard oral treatment of quinine (quinine sulphate, 10 mg kg^{-1} b.w. thrice daily for 7 days). It was found that a maximum concentration of 11.4 μg mL^{-1} of quinine was reached in the blood after 1.5 days. The active metabolite 3-OH-QN reached C_{max} after 2.5 days. The $AUC_{0\rightarrow 7}$ was 10 fold higher for quinine than for its metabolite, and it was a mean of 51.7 d μg mL^{-1}. The mean parasite clearance time was 73 h. Some patients took rifampicin at the same time, but in those cases the parasite clearance time (PCT) was the same, an indication that rifampicin did not contribute to kill the parasite. The maximum concentration of 3-OH-QN in the blood was 1.26 μg mL^{-1} [22]. The authors concluded that for cure a continuous concentration of 6 μg mL^{-1} is required for 7 days. The pharmacokinetics of quinine is not altered significantly during pregnancy [23, 24]. The pharmacokinetics of quinine is not affected when taken in combination with the antibiotics doxycycline [20] and clindamycin.

THE 4-AMINOQUINOLINES: CHLOROQUINE, PIPERAQUINE AND AMODIAQUINE

The fact that the availability of quinine depended on supplies of bark from Cinchona plantations led to a further search for synthetic analogues (Fig. **5**). Chloroquine (CQ) was discovered in this way [25-27]. Later the development of resistance and the desire to have antimalarials with improved properties and fewer side effects but which still retained the useful properties of CQ became additional driving forces for research in this area. The strategies adopted in which the 4-aminoquinoline ring is kept have been 1) to link two aminoquinoline moieties by linkers of various lengths and nature, 2) to modify the side chain by elongation or shortening, 3) to introduce lipophilic aromatic moieties into the side chain, and more recently 4) the synthesis of hybrid 4-aminoquinolines, that is drug hybrids containing both an aminoquinoline moiety, and a synthetic mimic of another current antimalarial molecule [28]. Following some of these approaches two important drugs widely used nowadays in the treatment of malaria were developed: piperaquine and amodiaquine. Although the precise mode of action of the 4-aminoquinolines is not yet completely understood, it is known that they accumulate in the food vacuole [11], and it is thought that like quinine, they target the processes that take place inside the digestive food vacuole related to the metabolism of haemoglobin and detoxification (Fig. **4**) [16].

Chloroquine

Chloroquine (CQ), initially named resochin, was developed by German scientist H. Andersag at Bayer AG as a substitute for quinine [25]. It is a totally synthetic

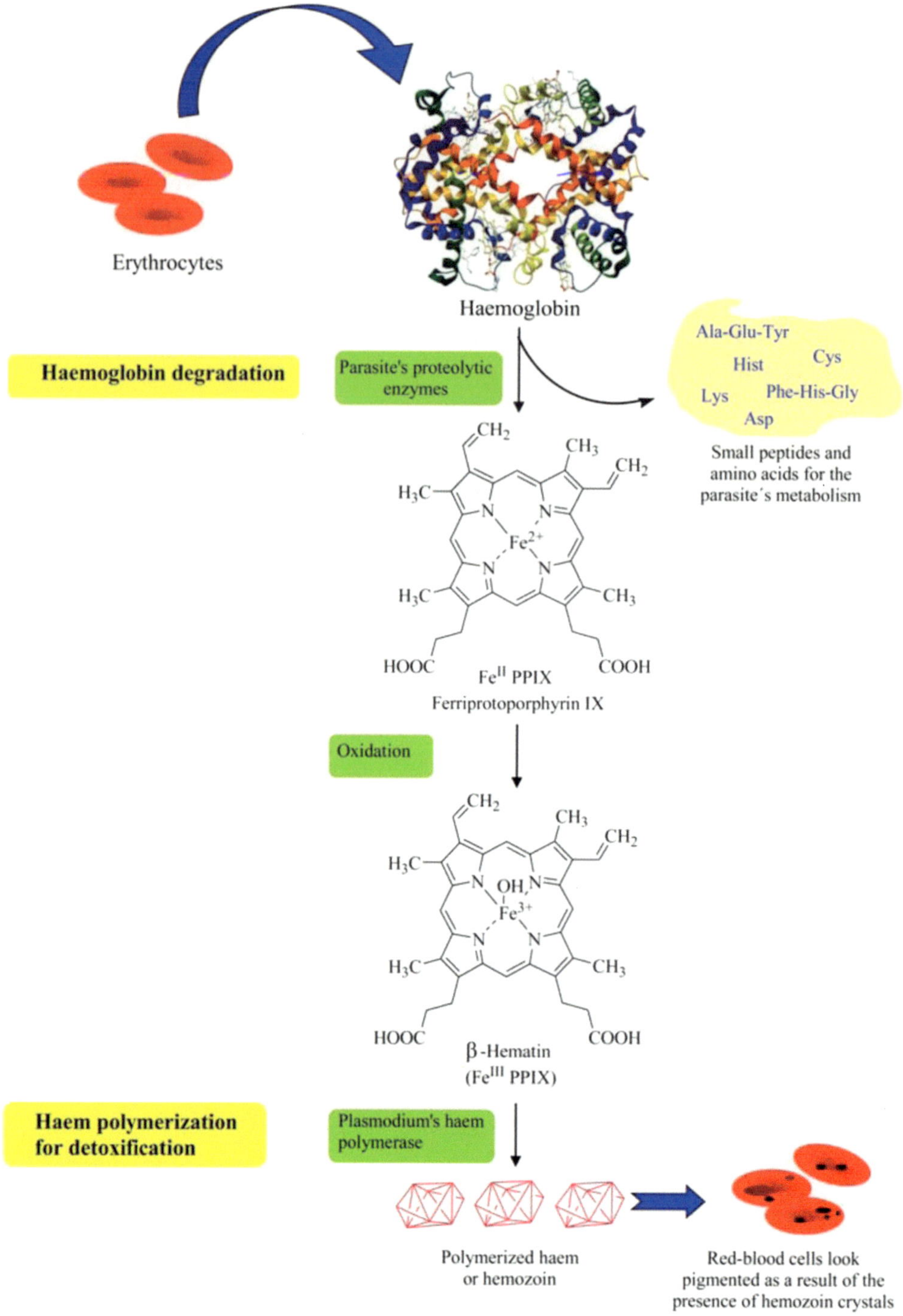

Figure 4: Haemoglobin digestion by *P. falciparum*.

drug, a 7-chloroquinoline with a flexible pentadiaminoalkane side chain at position 4 (**3**, Fig. **5**). Due to its high effectiveness, fast action, low toxicity and low cost, it became the most successful antimalarial drug ever used. It was the drug recommended by WHO for its Global Malaria Eradication Programme launched in 1955 [6]. Together with DDT spraying, landscaping measures and surveillance in national programmes, thousands of lives were saved and the final result was the eradication of malaria from areas with temperate climates and seasonal malaria transmission. In 1975 WHO declared that Europe was free of malaria. However, due to the extensive use of this drug, *Plasmodium falciparum* started to develop resistance in the 1960s independently in four different regions of the world, and nowadays resistance has spread to almost the entire malaria endangered area. More than 80% of wild isolates are resistant to CQ [6]. Nevertheless, CQ is still being used as a first line option in countries where strains are sensitive. It remains effective against most strains of *P. vivax*, *P. ovale* and *P. malariae*, but resistance to *P. vivax* is increasing. It is the drug recommended by WHO for the treatment of vivax malaria in areas where this drug is effective [7]. The treatment should be followed with a 14-day course of primaquine, to eradicate the persistent liver stages and hence prevent relapse [1]. It is still also the drug of choice to prevent malaria, used for prophylaxis by travellers going to sensitive areas. In addition, it is also recommended for the treatment of malariae and ovale malaria [1].

CQ is a very potent schizonticidal drug effective against erythrocytic stages of all *Plasmodium* species [12]. It has no effect on sporozoites or hypnozoites. It is gametocytocidal against *P. vivax, P. ovale*, and *P. malariae* and it is also effective against immature gametocytes of *P. falciparum*. However, it is ineffective against the mature ones [12]. The way it acts is not entirely clear, but like other aminoquinolines and also quinine, it targets metabolic processes that take place inside the food vacuole. CQ concentrates in the food vacuole, and an accumulation of undigested haemoglobin may be observed [11]. Hence it seems that it inhibits the process of haemoglobin degradation. Like quinine, it also intercalates with DNA and it fragments parasitic RNA. It can kill plasmodia at a concentration three orders of magnitude lower than the concentration at which it is toxic to mammalian cells [11]. When *P. falciparum* infection is safely excluded, chloroquine remains the standard of care for *P. malariae*, *P. ovale* and for *P. vivax* malaria [29].

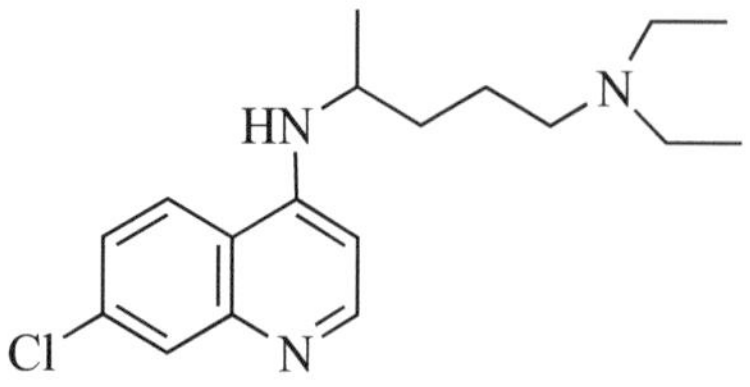

Chloroquine **3**

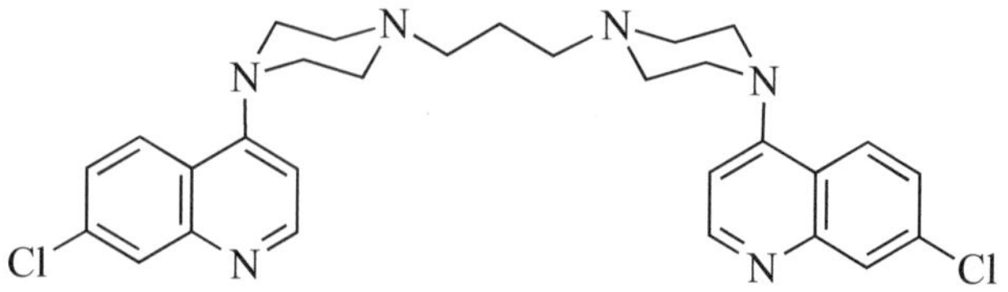

Piperaquine **4**

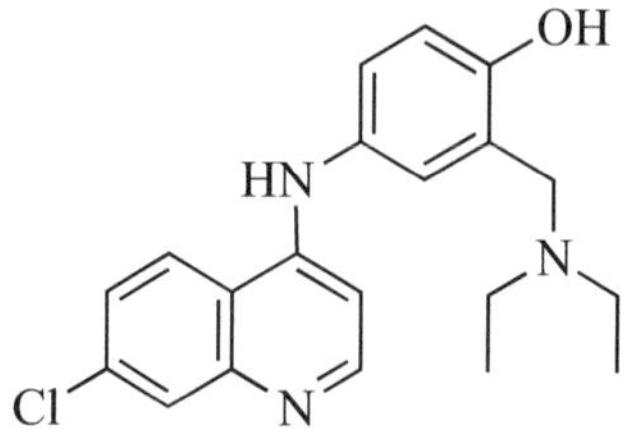

Amodiaquine **5**

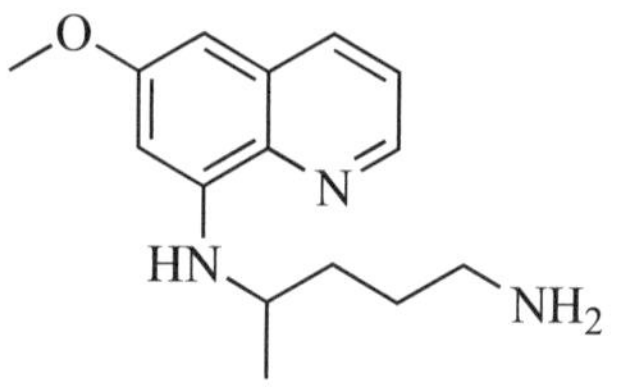

Primaquine **6**

Figure 5: The aminoquinolines.

Pharmacology of Chloroquine

CQ is rapidly absorbed from the gastrointestinal tract after oral administration, and it has a high bioavailability of between 80 and 90% [30]. Only about 50% is metabolized, predominantly to desethylchloroquine, which has similar antimalarial activity against *P. falciparum*. Bisdesethylchloroquine and 7-chlor-4-aminoquinoline are minor metabolites. The half-life is estimated at 1-2 months [3]. Recently there was a study on the pharmacokinetics of chloroquine in healthy volunteers [31], who received the standard WHO three-day CQ regimen: 1,000 mg CQ (600 mg base) on days 1 and 2, and 500 mg (300 mg base) on day 3. It was found that a maximum concentration of CQ of 16.5 kg μg mL^{-1} was present in the plasma after 6.6 h, and $AUC_{0\rightarrow\infty}$ was 1,690 kg h μg mL^{-1}. The pharmacokinetics of the metabolite desethylchloroquine was as follows: a maximum concentration of 4.99 kg μg mL^{-1} was present in the plasma after 13.2 h, and $AUC_{0\rightarrow\infty}$ was 761 kg h μg mL^{-1}. In this study the authors also determined the pharmacokinetics of chloroquine in the presence of azithromycin. However, although it has been observed by others that the effectiveness of these compounds increases when they are administered together [32], this study did not reveal a pharmacokinetic interaction between the two drugs. The therapeutic dose is 10 mg kg^{-1} b.w. At 20 mg kg^{-1} CQ causes serious side effects, 30 mg kg^{-1} is potentially lethal. In long-term prophylaxis, it may cause serious and irreversible side effects, such as neuromyopathy, retinopathy, erythema multiform and bone-marrow toxicity, but this is rare [6]. The effective concentration against *P. vivax* is 15 ng mL^{-1} in plasma and 30 ng mL^{-1} in serum [7]. Since the concentrations in whole blood are usually several times higher than those in plasma or serum, and the metabolite monodesethylchloroquine can also act against *P. vivax*, as it does against *P. falciparum*, whole-blood concentrations of 70-90 ng mL^{-1} of chloroquine and its metabolite should be adequate to suppress *P. vivax* [7].

Parasite clearance in the blood stream occurs within 48-72 h. CQ is well tolerated by pregnant women and children. In a study with pregnant and non-pregnant women with acute *P. vivax* malaria, the pharmacokinetics was found to be similar in both groups [33]. When 25 mg CQ base/kg were administered over 3 days to pregnant women, a peak plasma concentration of 960.5 ng mL^{-1} was observed after 3 h, with $AUC_{0-\infty}$ 122,216 h ng mL^{-1}. The half-life was 180.4 h. These values were similar to those obtained with non-pregnant women. At day 28 there was 100% cure, but by day 42 this value had dropped to 83% for the first group, 69% for the second.

Piperaquine

Piperaquine (PPQ) is a totally synthetic bis(quinolyl)piperazine (**4**, Fig. **5**) developed independently in the 1960s by researchers in China, at the Shanghai Research Institute of Pharmaceutical Industry, and at Rhone Poulenc in France. It was used extensively for twenty years, particularly in China, for prophylaxis and treatment of falciparum and vivax malaria [34]. It is active against exoerythrocytic forms of the parasite and it is also is a fast-acting blood schizonticide. It is thought to act by a mechanism similar to that of chloroquine and other aminoquinolines, accumulating in the lysosomal food vacuole, where it interferes with the haem metabolism. Its activity against resistant parasites is thought to be due to its large steric bulk, which prevents it from fitting into the binding site of the *trans*-membrane protein *Pf*CRT (*P. falciparum* chloroquine resistance transporter), a membrane transporter protein that, as a result of a genetic modification by a gene which underwent a mutation, *pfcrt*, is thought to be responsible for resistance [6]. The transporter protein reduces the concentration of these drugs in the food vacuole, preventing them from exerting their antiparasitic action. The effectiveness of piperaquine may also be due to the fact that it is more effectively trapped inside the acidic food vacuole as a result of its four negative charges [6]. However, nowadays widespread resistance to piperaquine has also developed. There are also reports of cross-resistance with chloroquine [6]. Cross-resistance occurs when two drugs have similar mechanisms of resistance, and the parasite being resistant to one, is also resistant to the other. There are also reports that cross-resistance between PPQ and dihydroartemisinin can be induced *in vitro*. In Africa, where piperaquine has not been introduced for treatment, wild isolates of *P. falciparum* are still sensitive to this drug, with IC_{50} values of 40 nM [35]. Piperaquine is well tolerated and its most important side-effect is an increase in blood pressure [6].

Pharmacology of Piperaquine

Piperaquine is highly lipophilic and basic, poorly soluble in water [37]. It has a long half-life, of 20 to 30 days [38]. Five metabolites of piperaquine have been identified recently in the urine of 2 healthy individuals, after administration of tablets containing PPQ and DHA together with a fatty meal (PPQ 120 mg, DHA 960 mg), but only two were present in blood and plasma and appear to be the main metabolites: piperaquine N-oxide and 3-[4-(7-choro-quinolin-4-yl)-piperazin-1-yl]-propionic acid [38].

The pharmacokinetics has been determined in a study with healthy Vietnamese adults [39]. Single doses of 500 mg of piperaquine were administered, and the maximum concentration of the drug was found to be 69.6 ng mL^{-1} after 4 hours, with $AUC_{0-\infty}$ 4,484 ng mL kg^{-1}, and a half-life of 483 h. A single dose of 1000 mg, gave similar parameters, with a peak blood plasma concentration of 195.5 ng mL^{-1} being observed after 4 hours, $AUC_{0-\infty}$ 13,370 ng mL kg^{-1} and a half-life of 494 h. When used to treat falciparum malaria, PPQ is conventionally given as four equal doses of between 2.8 and 10.8 mg base kg^{-1} [40].

The pharmacokinetic profile of this highly lipid-soluble drug with slow absorption, good bioavailability, long elimination half-life, large volume of distribution and its low cost, make it a promising partner for combination therapies with artemisinins for example. A fixed combination with dihydroartemisinin is now one of the ACTs recommended by WHO for malaria treatment [3]. Although the drug was used extensively in China, only a few publications are available in the English literature on its pharmacokinetics in individuals with malaria, and the studies were carried out using the PPQ-DHA fixed combination antimalarials. For further details see under Artemisinin-Based Combination Therapies).

Amodiaquine

Structure-activity relationship studies have shown that antimalarial activity is retained when the side chain of chloroquine is shortened or lengthened. Some of these modifications led to the development of amodiaquine (AQ) (**5**, Fig. **5**), a drug with higher lipophilicity as a result of the incorporation of an aromatic ring in the side chain, a 4-aminophenol group [28]. Its potential for malaria treatment was discovered in 1946, and it is thought to function as a blood schizonticide by a mechanism similar to that of chloroquine. It produces clinical cure of all types of human malaria and radical cure of falciparum and malariae infections [12]. It is an excellent suppressive agent. It is also a gametocytocidal agent against *P. vivax*, *P. ovale* and *P. malariae*, and it is effective against immature gametocytes of *P. falciparum*. Over the years resistance has developed against this antimalarial [41], and there is even cross-resistance with chloroquine [42]. However, in areas where CQ resistance has been identified, amodiaquine is still more effective, and hence it remains an important drug. Nowadays it is used in several countries as a first-line drug, particularly in combination therapies [7]. The minimum concentration of amodiaquine required to inhibit, *in vitro*, the maturation of blood schizonts of a sensitive strain of *P. falciparum* (*e.g.*, strain Uganda 1) is 50 μg salt L^{-1} of blood [12]. For a CQ-resistant Vietnam (Marks) strain, it is 100 μg salt L^{-1} of blood [12].

Amodiaquine causes some side effects. Hepatoxicity may occur after prophylatic use for a period of 3 weeks to 10 months, but the chances of this occurring are 1 in 15,500. Another pathology which has been associated with long term use is agranulocytosis, a severe condition characterized by low white blood cell counts and hence a higher susceptibility to infections as a result of a suppressed immune system. The incidence is also low, 1 in 2,100, but for these reasons amodiaquine is not recommended nowadays for long-term treatments or prophylaxis [27]. It is assumed to be safe when used in short therapeutic regimes [27]. Although some studies suggest that amodiaquine at standard doses is not teratogenic, there is yet not enough data on its safety and pharmacokinetics in pregnancy [43]. Artesunate plus amodiaquine is nowadays an ACT recommended for malaria therapy by WHO (see under Artemisinin-Based Combination Therapies).

Pharmacology of Amodiaquine

Amodiaquine has low bioavailability. However, it is considered to be a prodrug of desethylamodiaquine (DAQ), the main metabolite that forms rapidly in the liver, and a potent antimalarial with a plasma concentration 6- to 7-fold higher than the parent drug. DEA has a long elimination half-life of more than 100 h. The use of AQ to treat uncomplicated falciparum malaria has been recently reviewed [41]. In a study in which amodiaquine hydrochloride (3 mg base kg^{-1}) was given by constant rate intravenous injection over 10 minutes to healthy male volunteers, and over 4 h by constant rate infusion to adults with falciparum malaria (10 mg base kg^{-1}), a peak plasma concentration of 415 ng mL^{-1} and of 322 ng mL^{-1} was found in healthy volunteers and patients respectively [44]. The data obtained in this study suggested that parenteral amodiaquine should be given by constant rate intravenous infusion and that an effective dose would be the administration of 5 mg base kg^{-1} every 8 hours to a total of 25 mg kg^{-1}. Amodiaquine (25-30 mg base kg^{-1} body weight given over 3 days) has been used effectively for the treatment of chloroquine-resistant vivax malaria [3]. Primaquine must be added for radical cure.

The pharmacokinetics was studied in patients with uncomplicated falciparum malaria in Zambia [45]. Two different oral dose regimens were followed: either 10 mg kg^{-1} AQ on day 1, and 5 mg at 6 h, 24 h, and 48 h later or 10 mg kg^{-1} on day 1 and 24 h later, and 5 mg 48 h later. For AQ, the maximum concentration in the plasma was 21 ng mL^{-1} after 2.0 h, $AUC_{0\rightarrow 36}$ was 77 h ng mL^{-1}, and the half-life 3.7 h. DAQ had a maximum concentration in the plasma after 3.9 h of

161 ng mL^{-1}, $AUC_{0\rightarrow6}$ was 621 h ng mL^{-1}. The profiles in malaria patients are similar to those in healthy individuals, although the time to reach the maximum concentration in the plasma was three times higher in malaria patients.

Primaquine

Primaquine (PQ) is an 8-aminoquinoline (**6**, Fig. **5**). It has a chiral centre, but the commercially available preparations are all racemic [46]. It was introduced as an antimalarial in the United States of America by Elderfield and co-workers in 1946, after an intensive search for a drug to prevent relapse of malaria in American troops during the war in the Pacific [47]. Pamaquine was used then, but it was too toxic. PQ is active against all exoerythrocytic forms of the parasite [48]. Asexual stages of *P. falciparum* are not susceptible to primaquine, but those of *P. vivax* are [3]. PQ is gametocytocidal against *P. falciparum*, including multidrug-resistant *P. falciparum* and has significant blood stage activity against *P. vivax*. It is also active against gametocytes of other species that cause human malaria. In fact PQ is the only drug known to act on mature gametocytes, *i.e.,* those present in the blood stream when malaria symptoms are observable [3]. It is also highly effective on hypnozoites that can persist in the liver for long periods of time and cause relapses [3]. Although PQ is active against asexual blood stages, its activity is low, and it is normally used with another antimalarial, a schizonticide, in the case of acute attacks [48].

The mechanism of action of primaquine is still unclear [6]. It has been suggested that it may have an antagonistic effect on ubiquinone, with subsequent inhibition of electron transport in mitochondrial respiration [6]. Another possibility is that reactive metabolites create oxidative stress in the parasite's cells [49]. Primaquine is generally well tolerated, but in patients with glucose phosphate dehydrogenase (G6PD) deficiency it can cause haemolytic anaemia, which may be severe and life threatening [3]. Qualitative screening tests can be used to identify individuals who are G6PD deficient, prior to prescription of the drug [50]. There are however a few exceptions: those who have one of the milder G6PD deficient variants and recent haemolysis and some women who are heterozygous for the gene and also have mild deficiency. This side effect is known to be due to intra-erythrocytic oxidative stress mediated by redox-active metabolites [48]. Methemoglobinemia may also occur. In addition, primaquine should not be given to pregnant women and to nursing women. It is recommended for children, but not to infants. Anti-relapse treatment with PQ should only be used when there is confirmation that vivax malaria occurs [3].

So far there is no unambiguous evidence of the development of resistance against primaquine [7], although variations in the sensitivity of hypnozoites to the drug may be observed from region to region. This lack of resistance development is difficult to understand, and besides the drug's physical and chemical properties, it is thought that this may be related to its low half-life or its ability to sterilise the parasite's gametocytes [51]. The anti-relapse effect of primaquine is a function of the total dose rather than the duration of the treatment [7]. It is recommended that a lack of optimum response should be compensated for through the use of different regimens [7].

Nowadays, six decades after its introduction as an antimalarial, PQ is still the only transmission-blocking antimalarial available. It is recommended by WHO as an antigametocyte medicine to be used as a single dose in combination with an ACT for the treatment of uncomplicated falciparum malaria [3]. It is also used for primary prophylaxis against all species of malaria and for anti-relapse therapy in persons exposed to *P. vivax* and *P. ovale* [48]. Primaquine is recommended by WHO as first line drug for the treatment of *P. vivax* and *P. ovale* malaria in combination with chloroquine with the indication that the usual dose should be lowered when there is mild mild-to-moderate G6PD deficiency, but it is contra-indicated in severe G6PD deficiency [3]. It produces radical cure.

Although primaquine has always been used as a racemate, a few studies have shown that there is a difference in the metabolic rate as well as the hepatotoxicity of the two enantiomers, which could have implications for treatment and if explored, it could lead to future improvements of this valuable antimalarial [52].

Pharmacology of Primaquine

Primaquine is absorbed rapidly and almost completely from the gastrointestinal tract. The maximum concentration in the body is reached within 1 to 4 h. It is metabolised in the liver primarily to carboxyprimaquine, which has much lower activity [53], and other unidentified minor metabolites. The half-life is variable, ranging from 1 to 16 h, in patients and healthy volunteers [20]. It has a bioavailability of 96% [54]. The pharmacokinetics has been studied in healthy volunteers in Thailand. After an oral dose of 15 mg, a mean peak plasma concentration of primaquine of 65 ng mL^{-1} was achieved after 2 h, and the mean AUC was 468 h ng mL^{-1}. The mean elimination half-life was 4.4 h. Almost identical results were obtained in the mean plasma concentration-time profile of the drug after the volunteers had a chronic dose (15 mg daily for 14 days) [55]. Nevertheless, there were marked interindividual differences in the pharmacokinetics observed after the chronic therapy.

The recommended dose of primaquine is 15 mg for 14 days to prevent relapses. This dose may be increased to eliminate hypnozoites fully with some *P. vivax* strains. For radical cure a blood schizonticide is usually given at the same time [12].

THE AMINO ALCOHOLS: MEFLOQUINE, HALOFANTRINE AND LUMEFANTRINE

These antimalarial compounds have in common an aryl amino alcohol unit, which is also found in quinine and quinidine, but for historical reasons they are described separately in this review (Fig. **6**). They exert their toxicity on the erythrocytic stages of the *Plasmodium*'s life cycle [10]. It is thought that their mechanisms of action involve the metabolic processes that take place inside the food vacuole, like the cinchona alkaloids and the 4-aminoquinolines [11].

Mefloquine

Mefloquine (MQ), the most widely used drug of this class of antimalarials, is a quinoline methanol derivative developed at the Water Reed Army Research Institute, United States of America (**7**, Fig. **6**). This totally synthetic drug was selected from about 300 analogues of quinine synthesized in the 1970s, and it started to be used for therapy in 1985 as Lariam [6]. Mefloquine is effective against all forms of malaria, and it is used for treatment and prevention [56]. In

2000 it was the most widely used drug for the treatment of multidrug resistant falciparum malaria [57]. It has high activity against most chloroquine-resistant *Plasmodium* strains, *e.g.*, IC_{50} = 8.4 nM (CQ-sensitive laboratory strain D6), IC_{50} = 3.4 nM (CQ-resistant strain W2) and IC_{50} = 6.2-10.7 nM (CQ-resistant isolates from Cameroon) [6]. Mefloquine has been widely used in Asia. Over the years considerable resistance has developed. Since it is highly effective against CQ-resistant vivax malaria, it was recommended as a monotherapy for treatment, for example in Cambodia - Greater Mekong sub-region, from 1993 to 2000 [7]. As resistance gradually build-up throughout the country, the first line treatment policy was changed to a three-day course of artesunate plus mefloquine. When it adopted this policy, Cambodia became the first country to have an ACT for first line treatment as national policy [7].

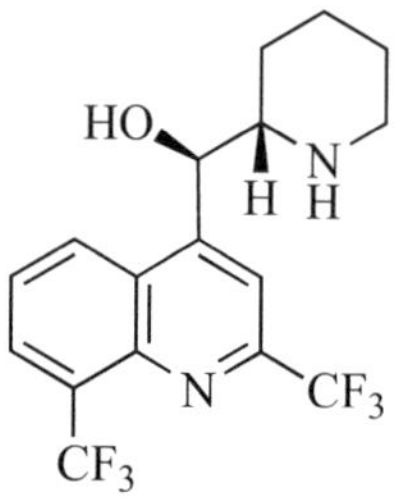

(+)-(11*R*,12*S*)-Mefloquine **7**

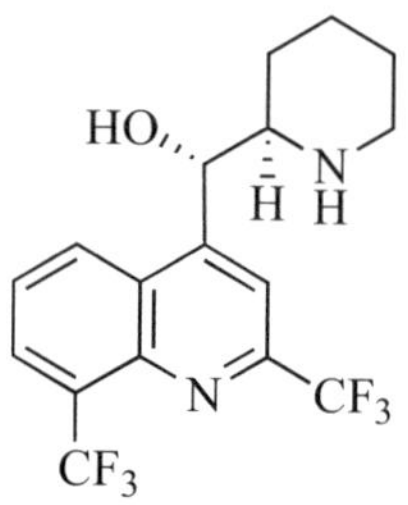

(-)-(11*S*,12*R*)-Mefloquine **8**

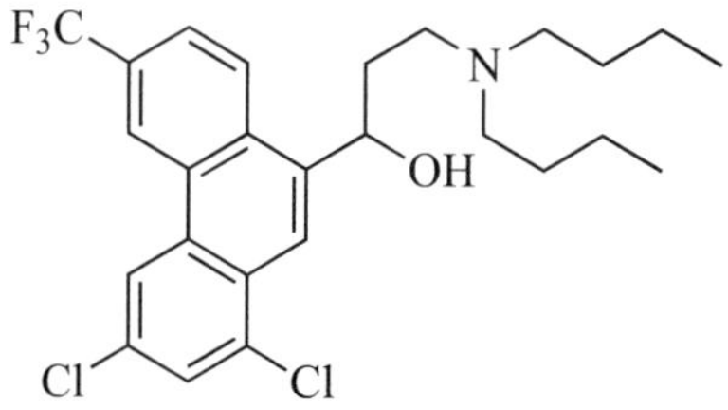

Halofantrine **9**

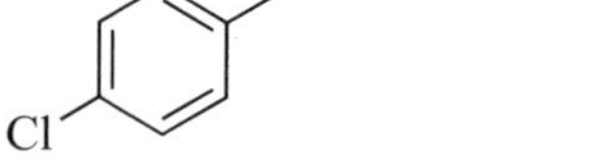

Lumefantrine **10**

Figure 6: The erythro optical isomers of mefloquine and other aminoalcohols currently in use to treat malaria.

Mefloquine is a blood schizonticide, effective against erythrocytic stages of the parasites. It has no effect on the exo-erythrocytic phase or on gametocytes in *P. falciparum*. Its mode of action is different from that of the 4-aminoquinolines, although it also targets the food vacuole. It is known that it makes it swell. It is thought that mefloquine inhibits vesicular docking indirectly or that, due to its high affinity for phospholipids on the membrane, it causes an antagonistic effect on vesicular docking [58].

Mefloquine may cause minor side effects, such as nausea, vomiting, abdominal pain, anorexia, diarrhoea, headache, dizziness, loss of balance, dysphoria, somnolence and sleep disorders, notably insomnia and abnormal dreams [3]. Since prophylatic use of mefloquine has been associated with neuropsychiatric side effects such as insomnia, depression and panic attacks in 5-29% of all those using it, prophylatic use is forbidden for people who require unimpeded abilities such as air-crew members [6]. Mefloquine is safe to use on children and has been used in pregnancy, but it was associated with an increase in stillbirths in Thailand, and it became less favoured for this purpose since then [59, 60].

Mefloquine is used in malaria therapy as the erythro racemate, but there has been interest in studying if one of the enantiomers could be more efficient to treat malaria or to have fewer undesirable side effects. *In vitro* the (+) enantiomers have higher IC_{50} values than the (-)-enantiomers by a factor of 1.6-1.8 on some strains of *P. falciparum* (D6 and W2) [61]. Recent research shows that the pharmacokinetics of the two enantiomers is different [62, 63], and in young children the differences are higher [64]. The (-)-enantiomer is present in plasma in higher concentrations and it has a longer half-life. There is also evidence that the (+)-enantiomer is more effective to treat malaria [65]. In addition it has been shown that the (-)-enantiomer binds to adenosine receptors in the central nervous system, which may explain some of the psychotropic effects associated with this antimalarial [66]. It has been suggested that the better *in vitro* antimalarial activity of the (+)-enantiomer could be accounted for by a stereoselective specific transport in the food vacuole of the parasite through the Pgh-1 transporter [67]. Recent data however suggests that although there is a difference in the safety and tolerability profiles between the (+)-enantiomer and racemic mefloquine, the overall difference does not appear to suggest that a replacement is necessary [68]. Nowadays mefloquine is recommended as an ACT in combination with artesunate for malaria therapy (See under Artemisinin-Based Combination Therapies).

Pharmacology of Mefloquine

Mefloquine is well absorbed from the gastrointestinal tract. It is converted by hepatic microsomal enzymes into its carboxy metabolite, a process probably mediated by CYP3A4 [20]. This metabolite is inactive against *P. falciparum*. MQ has a long elimination half-life of 21 days, which decreases to 14 days in malaria patients [3]. In the treatment of multidrug-resistant falciparum malaria, it has been used in doses ranging from 15 to 25 mg of base/kg of body weight [12]. The time taken for a maximum plasma concentration to be reached varies from individual to individual. The pharmacokinetics of MQ was studied in Thai male patients with acute, uncomplicated falciparum malaria [69]. An initial dose of 750 mg MQ was used, followed by 500 mg 6 h later. A mean maximum concentration of 2,212 ng mL^{-1} was reached after 20.3 h. The mean AUC was 17.2 d μg mL^{-1}, and the half-life 12 days. The mean parasite clearance time was 82.3 h. Some patients were treated concurrently with artesunate and mefloquine, and in those, the parasite clearance time was shorter, 47.5 h.

The concentration of mefloquine that gives a 95% protective level in areas with chloroquine-resistant *Plasmodium falciparum* is 620 ng mL^{-1} [60]. A single oral dose of 1.0 g of mefloquine was found to clear chloroquine-resistant *P. falciparum* parasites in 103.1 ± 18.0 h in semi-immune patients [70]. As for chloroquine-resistant vivax malaria, a single dose of 15 mg base kg^{-1} body weight given over three days has been found to be highly effective for treatment, giving 100% cure [71].

Halofantrine

Halofantrine (HF) is another synthetic quinine analogue, an amino alcohol (**9**, Fig. **6**) belonging to the class of 9-phenantrenmethanols, developed at the Water Reed Army Research Institute, United States of America in 1972. It was introduced for therapy in 1988, and marketed as Halfan. It was thought that since this class of compounds had not yet been used for malaria treatment, the risk of cross-resistance was minimal. HF is a highly lipophilic drug, insoluble in water. It is administered as a racemate, and its (+) and (-) enantiomers do not show a difference in activity *in vitro* [72]. It is a blood schizonticidal effective against asexual forms of *P. falciparum* and *P. vivax*. It has no action on sporozoites, gametocytes or hypnozoites in the liver [73]. Halofantrine is active against chloroquine-resistant *Plasmodium* strains, with a mean IC_{50} of 1.2 nM (Cameroon wild isolates); against chloroquine-sensitive isolates, mean IC_{50} values of 1.5 nM were observed [6]. Its mechanism of action is thought to be similar to that of mefloquine [6]. Halofantrine is effective against vivax malaria [12] and multidrug-resistant (including mefloquine) *P. falciparum* malaria [58], but nowadays it has been withdrawn from the market in a few countries [74], for safety, due to its cardiotoxicity. It can cause significant prolongation of the QT_c interval and hence cardiac arrhythmias [12], which could result in death. It is contraindicated in patients with a history of irregular heartbeat.

Pharmacology of Halofantrine

Halofantrine is poorly absorbed after oral administration, and its bioavailability is variable, <36 %, making it difficult to determine precisely its pharmacokinetics. Bioavailability increases with high-fat meals, but it is contra-indicated with food, because of the increased risk of cardiotoxicity. The maximum plasma concentration is usually reached within 6 h [73]. The elimination half-life is 1-2 days, and that of its main metabolite, N-desbutylhalofantrine, which is also an effective antimalarial, is 3-5 days. A typical dose that has been used for the treatment of malaria is 3 × 500 mg at 6 h intervals [73]. Healthy volunteers who were given this regime of halofantrine hydrochloride, and fed 2 hours before the second and third doses, showed three to five-fold increases in absorption. A mean maximum plasma concentration of 3200 ng mL^{-1} was attained 9 to 17 hours after this multiple dose [6].

Data pooled for 1474 patients who were given the same oral multiple dose of halofantrine, showed that in the case of acute uncomplicated *P. falciparum* infections, the mean parasite clearance time was 57.9 h, and 57.3 h in the case of *P. vivax* infections [73]. A 24 mg base kg^{-1} b.w. dose divided into three portions taken over a period of 12 hours has been shown to be efficient to treat vivax malaria [12].

Lumefantrine

Lumefantrine (LU) also known as benflumetol (**10**, Fig. **6**), is another aryl amino alcohol, a fluorine derivative, used in medicine as a racemate. It was developed in the 1970s in the Academy of Military Medical Sciences in Beijing, China. Lumefantrine is a blood schizonticide, effective against erythrocytic stages of *P. falciparum* [58]. It has a lower antimalarial activity than halofantrine. IC_{50} = 34-44 nM (laboratory strains) and 11.9 nM (Cameroon parasites) [6]. It is very effective against chloroquine resistant *P. falciparum* strains. The possibility of the enantiomers of lumefantrine differing in their activity against *Plasmodium* parasites has been investigated. However, (+)-lumefantrine, (-)-lumefantrine and racemic lumefantrine were found to be highly active, potent inhibitors of schizont maturation in fresh, natural isolates of *P. falciparum* but with similar potencies *i.e.,* the mean EC-50 values are 8.87, 9.71 and 12.44 nmol L^{-1} blood-medium-mixture, respectively [75]. Although lumefantrine is structurally similar to halofantrine, it does not have the dangerous cardiac side effects, and also no other significant toxicity [6]. It is very well tolerated, and only minor side effects such as nausea, abdominal discomfort, headache or dizziness have been reported, which are also characteristic symptoms of malaria [6]. Lumefantrine is not available as a monotherapy, and it has never been used alone for the treatment of malaria [6]. Presently it is available as combination therapy with artemether, marketed as Riamet or Coartem. It was registered first in China as an ACT in 1992, and it is nowadays one of the ACTs recommended by WHO for malaria therapy. At present it is used in 56 countries as first- or second-line treatment [3]. Other characteristics of this ACT are discussed under Artemisinin-Based Combination Therapies. Lumefantrine is thought to function by a mechanism similar to that of quinine, mefloquine and halofantrine, targeting the parasite's food vacuole.

Pharmacology of Lumefantrine

Data on the pharmacokinetics of lumefantrine is not readily accessible, since most of the preclinical research was done in China, without being published [20]. Recent reports concentrate on the properties of combination therapies. It is also known that lumefantrine is extensively metabolized in the liver primarily by cytochrome P450 3A4 [58]. The major metabolite is desbutyl-lumefantrine (DBL). So far there has not been much supportive pharmacokinetic data to show the effect of this metabolite in treatment [76]. Recent data shows that DBL is a more potent antimalarial than the parent compound, with an IC_{50} value of 9.0 nM *versus* 55.5 nM for LU against chloroquine-sensitive and resistant laboratory strains of *P. falciparum*. Also a mild synergy with dihydroartemisinin was observed, an indication that this metabolite could be useful for ACT combination therapies [76].

The Sulfonamides and Sulfones: Sulfadoxine, Sulfalene and Dapsone

The sulphur-based drugs belong to a large family of synthetic compounds of which many have antimicrobial properties. When some antibiotics were screened for their ability to treat other infectious diseases, including malaria, the sulfonamides sulfadoxine **11** and sulfalene **12** and the sulfone dapsone **13** were discovered (Fig. **7**). They all have a common mechanism of action: they target the parasite's folic acid biosynthetic pathway [77]. Folic acid is essential for the survival and growth of *Plasmodium* parasites (Fig. **8**) [78]. It consists of a pteridine ring, para-aminobenzoic acid and one molecule of L-glutamate [79]. One of its derivatives, tetrahydrofolic acid, plays a key role in the biosynthesis of the nucleotides thymine and purine, needed for the synthesis of DNA, RNA, and several amino acids (Met, Gly, Ser, Glu, and His). Humans biosynthesize tetrahydrofolic acid from pre-formed dihydrofolic acid which they obtain from their diet, but malaria parasites, like many bacteria, are unable to utilize dietary dihydrofolic acid, and synthesize the folic acids they need using p-aminobenzoic acid as a substrate. Nevertheless, some recent evidence suggests they may be able to use pre-formed folate [79]. Although the importance of this pathway seems to be minimal, with the *de novo* synthesis being the more efficient one, it appears that the possibility of this exogenous acquisition of folate from the host is related to the ability of the microorganism to become drug resistant [80]. The sulphur-based drugs are analogues of p-aminobenzoic acid, which is used by the enzyme dihydropteroate synthase (DHPS) to synthesize dihydrofolate, an early step in folic acid biosynthesis, and therefore they can compete with it and block the action of DHPS (Fig. **8**). By blocking folic acid biosynthesis, antifolates inhibit indirectly parasite DNA synthesis and cell growth. Since the malaria parasite has a high rate of replication, it is particularly sensitive to antifolate drugs. DHPS inhibitors are named class I antifolates. DHPS is completely absent in humans.

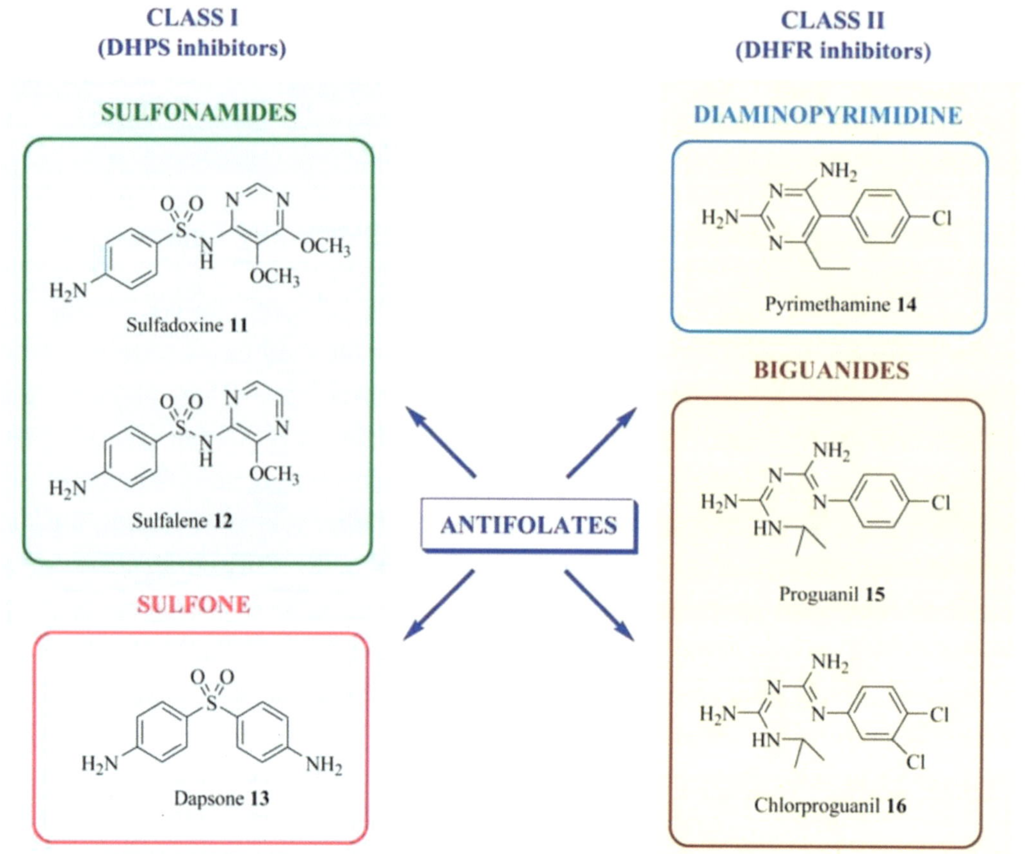

Figure 7: Antimalarial drugs that target the folic acid metabolic pathway.

These drugs have long half-lives, of between 60 and 200 h [81] and as a result they do not need to be administered several times to be effective. However, they are not very efficient in treating malaria, and for this reason they are usually used in fixed-combinations with other drugs, usually pyrimethamine or chloroguanil, which also have as target the folic acid metabolism, but inhibit a different enzyme, dihydrofolate reductase (DHFR). DHFR controls the reduction of the dihydrofolate to tetrahydrofolate, a step occurring later in the same biosynthetic route to folic acid (Fig. **8**). DHFR inhibitors are named class II antifolates. Parasitic DHFR is sufficiently different from the human enzyme to allow the development of antimalarials targeting this biosynthetic step. The sulphur drugs and the DHFR inhibitors have a synergistic effect, that is, the combined effect of their action is greater than the sum of the effect of each compound working individually. As a result, they can be used in lower amounts, which helps to reduce the side effects of some of the sulphur drugs and the fact that they are used in combinations brings the additional benefit of reducing the probability of resistance developing.

Sulfadoxine

This is a long-acting sulfonamide (**11**, Fig. **7**), usually used in combination with other drugs to treat infectious diseases [58]. Sulfadoxine (SDX) was first used to treat malaria in combination with the antifolates pyrimethamine (PYM) **14** and proguanil (PG) **15** in the late 1950s, to increase their efficacy, and to forestall or prevent the development of resistance (Fig. 7). The combination pyrimethamine-sulfadoxine (SP) became, like chloroquine, one of the antimalarial drugs most widely used ever [82]. Sulfadoxine and pyrimethamine are used in a fixed-dose combination of 20 parts to 1, administered orally or intramuscularly, with the trade name Fansidar. Although Fansidar is used as a co-formulation of two substances, the resulting product is considered a monotherapy because the two drugs act on the same biosynthetic pathway of the parasite, the folic acid biosynthetic pathway [3]. Their effect is synergistic.

Sulfadoxine is a class I antifolate. It is an analogue of *p*-aminobenzoic acid and a competitive inhibitor of the enzyme dihydropteroate synthetase (DHPS). Pyrimethamine inhibits dihydrofolate reductase (DHFR). SP is highly effective against asexual blood forms of *P. falciparum* and produces clinical cure [3]. It is also a suppressive agent. The combination is inactive against sporozoites and the latent exoerythrocytic stage, and it does not produce a radical cure or suppressive cure of *P. vivax*. It actually enhances gametocytogenesis, but the resulting gametocytes are unable to infect mosquitoes, so it reduces the transmission of malaria. This combination has been widely used to treat chloroquine-resistant malaria. It is also effective against wild type *P. vivax* [1]. Because of its long half-life, 4-9 days for sulfadoxine, and 4 days for pyrimethamine [3], and its low cost and safety in pregnant women and children, sulfadoxine-pyrimethamine is also used for intermittent preventive treatment of malaria in infants, children and pregnant women living in areas of high transmission. Despite widespread development of resistance, it remains effective nowadays in areas of moderate resistance [1]. Its *in vitro* activity against *P. falciparum* has varied in time: IC_{50} (SPX, Mozambique isolates) = 0.91 μM [83]; IC_{50} (SDX, Bangladesh strains) = 40.5 μM; IC_{50} (PYM, Bangladesh strains) = 1.7 μM [84]; IC_{50} (PYM, PYM-susceptible African isolates) = 15.4 nM [85].

Malaria treatment with sulfadoxine-pyrimethamine is regarded as sufficiently safe. However, in administration for prolonged periods as in prophylaxis, the toxicity of the sulfonamide combination partner may become significant, resulting in an increased risk of agranulocytosis and toxic epidermal necrolysis (the Steven-Johnson syndrome). For these reasons prophylatic use of this combination was discontinued in some countries a few years ago [6]. Nowadays there is also the problem of resistance, and thus the more recent tendencies are to use SP in combination with artemisinins. Artesunate plus sulfadoxine-pyrimethamine is one of the currently recommended ACTs for malaria treatment as discussed later (see under Artemisinin-Based Combination Therapies) [1]. Nevertheless, the treatment failure rate of SP remained low by 2007; around 162 efficacy studies conducted in 45 countries in the period 2000-2007 showed a low failure rate of 4.7% and 5% only in South America and in the Middle East and central Asia, respectively. In Africa the situation was worse, varying from 18.7% to 52.8% from the Western to the Eastern regions [7].

Pharmacology of Sulfadoxine

Currently, sulfadoxine-pyrimethamine is the only available antimalarial effective when given as a single dose [86]. The bioavailability of sulfadoxine is 70-100%, and that of pyrimethamine 100% [20]. After oral administration, about 5% of sulfadoxine appears in the plasma as acetylated metabolite, and about 2 to 3% as the glucuronide. Pyrimethamine is transformed to several unidentified metabolites. The pharmacokinetics of Fansidar has been reviewed recently [87]. In a study with adult patients with acute falciparum malaria, who received a single dose of Fansidar (1.36 mg kg^{-1} PYM, 27.3 mg kg^{-1} SDX), a maximum concentration of sulfadoxine in the plasma of 63.2 μg mL^{-1} was reached after 24 h and the AUC was 816 d μg mL^{-1}. The half-life was 7.8 d. A maximum concentration of pyrimethamine of 278.5 ng mL^{-1} was present after 9.3 h, and the

AUC was 1,602 d ng mL^{-1}. The half-life was 3.27 d. In addition, the authors of this work recommended a revision of the doses used presently for the treatment of malaria in children, suggesting an update to the same doses as those of adults based on data obtained in this study. In a different study with children infected with *Plasmodium falciparum* and treated with SP (SDX = 25 mg kg^{-1}, PYM = 1.25 mg kg^{-1} bw), parasite clearance was achieved in 1.85 days [83].

Sulfalene

Sulfalene **12**, also known as sulfametopyrazine or sulfamethoxypyrazine, is another important synthetic sulfonamide available for antimalaria therapy. It is also an antibacterial, which is used currently for the treatment of chronic bronchitis and urinary tract infections. Sulfalene is normally used in a fixed combination with pyrimethamine, in a 20 to 1 ratio, with the trade name Metakelfin (SLP). Its efficacy is similar to that of Fansidar, but Fansidar has been much more widely used [77]. Its metabolites are not active against malaria. Like sulfadoxine, it is a class I antifolate, a competitive DHPS inhibitor. It is also used in combination with trimethoprim. It is a blood schizonticide, active against all species of *Plasmodium* but more effective against *P. falciparum.* If administered in correct doses it is well tolerated, but like all sulfonamides, it may produce side effects in certain individuals [12]. The combination of artesunate plus sulfalene-pyrimethamine is an ACT recommended by WHO as an alternative to artesunate plus sulfadoxine-pyrimethamine for the treatment of uncomplicated and severe falciparum malaria [3] (see under Artemisinin-Based Combination Therapies).

Pharmacology of Sulfalene

Sulfalene is readily absorbed, and it oral bioavailability is 70-100% [20]. Peak plasma concentrations are reached after 4-6 h [12]. The drug has a high liposolubility, and a long terminal half-life of 65 h [12]. In a trial in rural Nigeria, it was found that a single dose of SLP cleared *Plasmodium falciparum* infections in 7 days. After 3 days 95% of the patients already showed no asexual forms of *P. falciparum* in the peripheral blood [88]. Lower doses used for children (patients < 10 yrs old) had a similar effect. In a more recent trial in Northeast India, it was found to be effective treating patients with chloroquine-resistant *P. falciparum* malaria, but resistance to this drug has already been reported in parts of India too [89].

Dapsone

Dapsone (DDS) **13** is the sulfone most widely used for the treatment of malaria (Fig. **7**). It is also active against a wide range of bacteria, but it is mainly well known as a drug for the treatment of leprosy, and as second-line treatment and prophylaxis against *Pneumocyctis carinii* pneumonia in HIV patients. It was synthesized for the first time by Fromm and Wittmann in 1908, as a result of a search for azo-dyes [77]. Its antimalarial activity was discovered in the 1930s, but it was thought to be too toxic for use due to the large amounts tried at the time. By 1949 it was discovered that it treated malaria at much smaller doses (100-200 mgs), but it proved to be unreliable in the treatment of acute falciparum malaria, and of limited efficacy. It was later introduced in synergic combinations with other antifolates for malaria prevention and chemotherapy. Dapsone is a class I antifolate, a competitive inhibitor of DHPS like sulfoxidine and sulfalene. In formulations, the most common drug partners are pyrimethamine or chlorproguanil. It is used in an 8:1 combination with pyrimethamine for prophylaxis [3], marketed as Maloprim, and in a 8:10 combination (CD) with chlorproguanil (CPG) **16**, a biguanide, for the treatment of chloroquine-resistant falciparum malaria. The latter combination, marketed as LapDap, only became available for clinical use in 2003, so it is still in post-marketing surveillance [90], but by 2006 it was already available in many African countries [77]. It is a rational alternative to sulfadoxine-pyrimethamine, particularly in areas where resistance to this antimalarial prevails, such as East Africa [20]. LapDap is however inactive against strains harbouring a quadruple mutant, abundant in Asia and South America [6]. IC_{50} values measured against a K39 strain, a PY-resistant strain of *P. falciparum* were found to be: chlorcycloguanil alone = 4.8 nM; dapsone alone = 51 μM [91].

Dapsone is highly active against the asexual blood forms of *P. falciparum.* It produces clinical cure, but it is used in combination with the other antifolates because it acts slowly. It is inactive against sporozoites and the primary exoerythrocytic stage of the parasite. It has the same effect as the sulfonamides in increasing gametocyte production, but the resulting gametes do not infect the mosquitoes [12]. It is inactive on the latent exoerythrocytic stages and hence it does not produce a radical or suppressive cure of vivax malaria. Dapsone has two important metabolites: monoacetyldapsone, which has no activity [92], and dapsone hydroxylamine. Monoacetyldapsone can be deacetylated to give dapsone too. Dapsone hydroxylamine is probably responsible for the two most commonly reported side effects of dapsone: methemoglobinemia and haemolysis, which may occur when high doses of more than 200 mg are taken. Haemolysis can be particularly serious in patients deficient in glycose-6-phosphate (G6PD), if more than 50 mg are taken daily [3]. Another side effect that has been reported following prophylaxis with dapsone-pyrimethamine, if taken twice a week, is the development of agranulocytosis [11]. Medications with dapsone are also not recommended for lactating women, because relatively large amounts of dapsone are excreted in breast milk (14% of the adult dose) [3].

By 2004 SP was still the first choice drug for the treatment of uncomplicated falciparum malaria in most of Africa [93], although cases of resistance had been reported. A large study involving 1850 children from 5 African countries was carried out with the aim of showing the possibility of using CD as an alternative treatment in case of SP failure and to compare the efficacy of SP and CD. The results showed that the efficacy of CD was slightly better (95% to 89%, CD to SP). Haematological adverse effects were more common with CD than with SP but they were reversible [93].

Pharmacology of Dapsone

Dapsone is slowly and completely absorbed from the gastrointestinal tract. Its bioavailability following oral administration is > 90% [20]. Dapsone is eliminated quickly in comparison with sulfadoxine, with a mean half-life of about 26 h, although there is large interindividual variability. The pharmacokinetics of Maloprim (100 mg DDS + 12.5 mg PYR) was studied in healthy individuals, after weekly administration of Maloprim [94]. The studies showed that after the last dose a mean maximum plasma concentration of dapsone of 1,134 ng mL^{-1} was reached after 1.7 h, and the mean AUC was 35.0 h μ mL^{-1}. The mean elimination

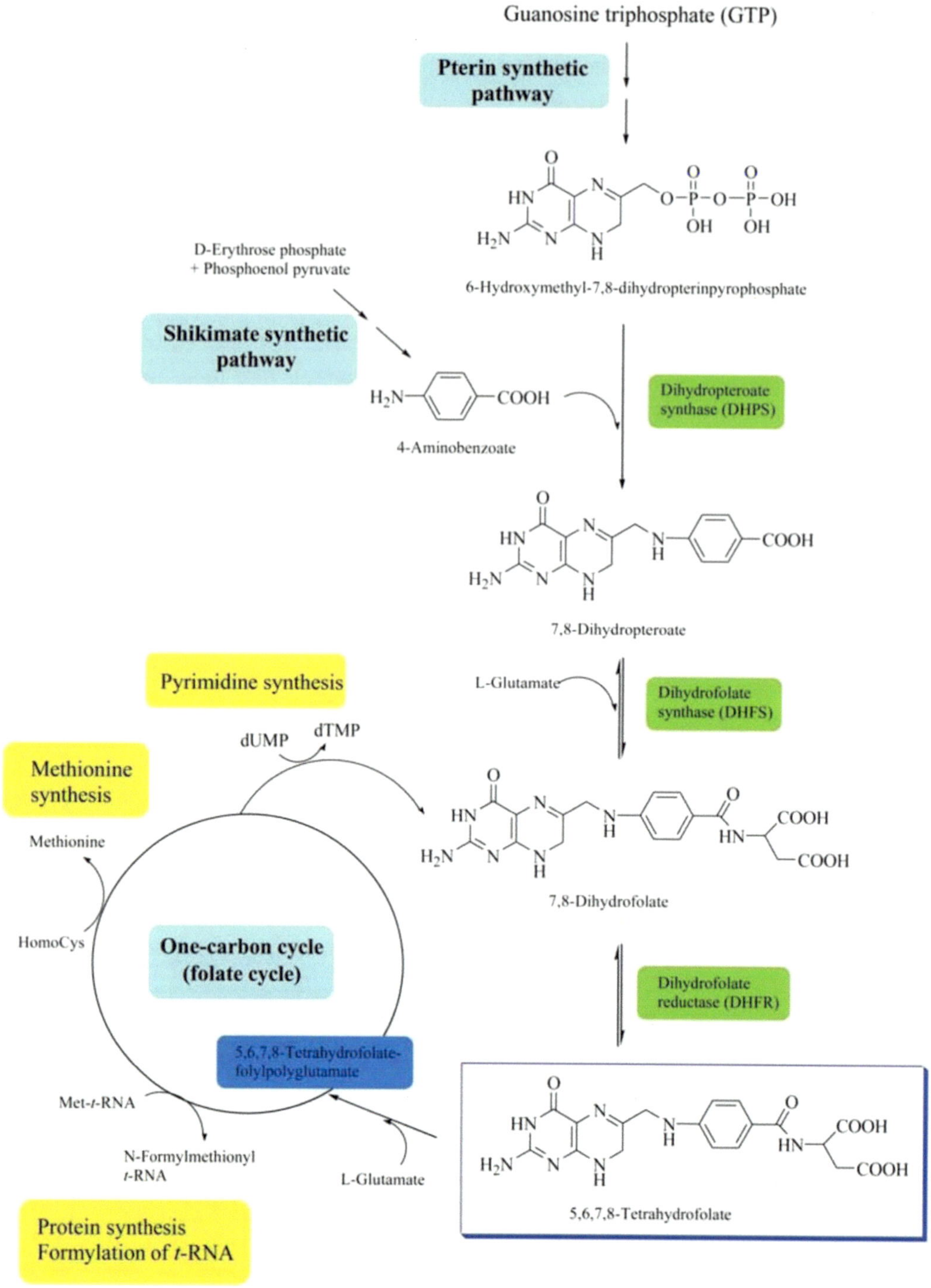

Figure 8: Folate synthesis in *Plasmodium* [78].

half-life of DDS was 22.6 h and that of PYR 104.9 h. The half-life of the major metabolite of dapsone, monoacetyldapsone, was similar, 22 h. In the case of pyrimethamine, a peak plasma concentration of 116 ng mL^{-1} was reached after 41.5 h, and the mean AUC was 104.9 h μg mL^{-1} [94].

The pharmacokinetics of the combination dapsone-proguanil (DDS+PROG) was studied after administration of a 1:20 daily dose to healthy volunteers [95]. In the case of DDS, after the last dose, the maximum concentration in the plasma was 285 ng mL^{-1}, and the elimination half-life 23.3 h. For PROG C_{max} was 151 ng mL^{-1} and $t_{½}$ was 18.3 h. The peak plasma concentration of the active metabolite of proguanil, cycloguanil was 56 ng mL^{-1} and $t_{½}$ 15.0 h. The pharmacokinetics of CD in healthy adults is similar to those in malaria patients. However, peak plasma concentrations in children are reached in half of the time needed by adults [96]. In a study with patients infected with pyrimethamine-sulfadoxine resistant falciparum malaria [97], in Tanzania, it was found that a 3-day dose regimen of chlorproguanil plus dapsone (2:2.5 mg kg^{-1} body weight) administered once a day, was enough to provide parasite clearance in 93% of all patients, suggesting that this drug combination could be a useful alternative for the treatment of malaria in areas where resistance to pyrimethamine-sulfadoxine prevails.

DIAMINOPYRIMIDINES: PYRIMETHAMINE

Nowadays pyrimethamine **14** is the only pyrimidine included in the WHO's list of currently available drugs for the treatment of malaria [7]. It was selected during the 1950's after a study made on a large number of pyrimidines and analogues to investigate the relationship between chemical structure and their participation as precursors and modifiers of nucleic acid biosynthesis [98]. Trimethoprim, another pyrimidine, has also been used in the past for malaria therapy, particularly in combination with sulfamethoxazole. It is less active than pyrimethamine or cycloguanil against *Pf*DHFR. Nowadays its use is more confined to the treatment of bacterial infections.

Pyrimethamine

Pyrimethamine (PYR) is a 2,4-diaminopyrimidine. It was synthesized in 1951 by an American and British team during searches for analogues of folic acid for the treatment of tumours [99]. It was found to be highly active against human malaria and it was used as a monotherapy with the trade name Daraprim in the 1950s. PYR is a class II antifolate, a highly active inhibitor of *P. falciparum* dihydrofolate reductase (DHFR) with a $K_i = 2.6$ nM [6], hence it blocks indirectly the synthesis of nucleic acids in the parasite (Fig. **8**). It has a higher binding affinity for DHFR than for the human enzyme and hence a good therapeutic index. It inhibits the plasmodial enzyme at a concentration 3500 times lower than the human enzyme [98]. In addition to inhibiting DHFR, PYR also appears to inhibit nuclear division in the parasite. It is also active against the other 3 human malaria parasites [3]. Comparing doses, pyrimethamine is one of the most powerful suppressive agents known against *P. falciparum* and sometimes against *P. vivax* [12]. It is active against asexual blood stages of the parasite and it produces clinical and radical cure in most cases of malaria [12]. It is not active against sporozoites, although it may have some effect on exoerythrocytic stages. In addition, although it appears to have no effect on gametocytes, it inhibits subsequent sporozoite development in the mosquito vector. PYR is inactive on latent erythrocytic stages, therefore it cannot be used for radical treatment of vivax malaria. The IC_{50} value of PYR against a wild-type *P. falciparum* strain (TM4) was found recently to be 58 nM [100].

Initially PYR was used as a monotherapy on its own, and one weekly dose could provide a completely suppressive cure of malaria. It was not recommended on its own for the treatment of acute attacks of malaria, because of its slow action. It was extensively used as a monotherapy on its own in some Asian and South American countries. Resistance appeared soon after and it is no longer used alone, but in synergistic combinations with class I antifolates, more commonly with the sulfonamides sulfoxidine or sulfalene or with the sulfone dapsone, as highlighted in their respective sections. On its own pyrimethamine is also used for the treatment of toxoplasmosis and isosporiasis and as prophylaxis against *Pneumocystis carinii* pneumonia [3]. PYR is generally a well-tolerated drug. After prolonged treatment depression of the haematopoiesis may occur due to interference with folic acid metabolism. It may also cause occasional skin rashes and hypersensitivity [3]. However, it is safe to be taken during pregnancy. In combination with sulfoxidine it became one of the most successful antimalarials ever used [82] (see under Sulfadoxine too).

Pharmacology of Pyrimethamine

PYR is almost completely absorbed from the gastrointestinal tract and peak plasma concentrations are reached within 2-6 h after oral doses. Its bioavailability is 100% [101]. It has a half-life of 4 days. The effective concentration to inhibit blood schizogony of *P. falciparum* is 10-100 μg mL^{-1}, which can be achieved with a single 25 mg dose [12]. PYR is nowadays available in oral and parental formulations with the sulfonamides for treatment of malaria or with dapsone for prophylaxis. Its pharmacokinetics upon administration in combination with sulfadoxine is described under Pharmacology of Sulfadoxine. In addition, sulfadoxine-pyrimethamine combined with artesunate is nowadays one of the ACTs recommended by WHO for malaria treatment (see under Artemisinin-Based Combination Therapies).

THE BIGUANIDES: PROGUANIL AND CHLORPROGUANIL

These drugs inhibit the action of dihydrofolate reductase, in the folic acid biosynthetic pathway. They are therefore class II antifolates. However, the original biguanides have almost no activity themselves, but they act as prodrugs. They are metabolized in the body to their triazine forms, cycloguanil (**17**) and chlorcycloguanil (**18**) respectively, the true DHFR inhibitors, *via* the polymorphic cytochrome P450 enzyme CYP2C19 (Fig. **9**). They have been used both for prophylaxis and treatment, either on their own or in combination with other antimalarials, often antifolates. Proguanil has been used with chloroquine, dapsone and nowadays with atovaquone, and chlorproguanil with dapsone [77].

Proguanil

Proguanil (PG) was the first biguanide described as an antimalarial and also the first antimalarial known to act on the folic acid biosynthetic pathway. It was discovered in 1945 at Imperial Chemical Industries (ICI), United Kingdom, as part of an intensive research program to search for synthetic antimalarials [77]. After oral administration proguanil is rapidly metabolized in the liver, *via* oxidative ring closure to form the triazine cycloguanil (CPG). Cycloguanil is a class II antifolate, a highly active inhibitor of DHFR, with K_i = 1.5 nM [6]. The parent compound has weak intrinsic antimalarial activity [3]. CPG also inhibits human dihydrofolate reductase, but its affinity for the parasitic enzyme is much higher, and hence it can be successfully used for therapy. Some populational groups are "poor metabolizers" of this drug, which may account for its inefficiency at times. The incidence in Caucasian and African populations is only 3%, but among Orientals it is as high as 20% [3].

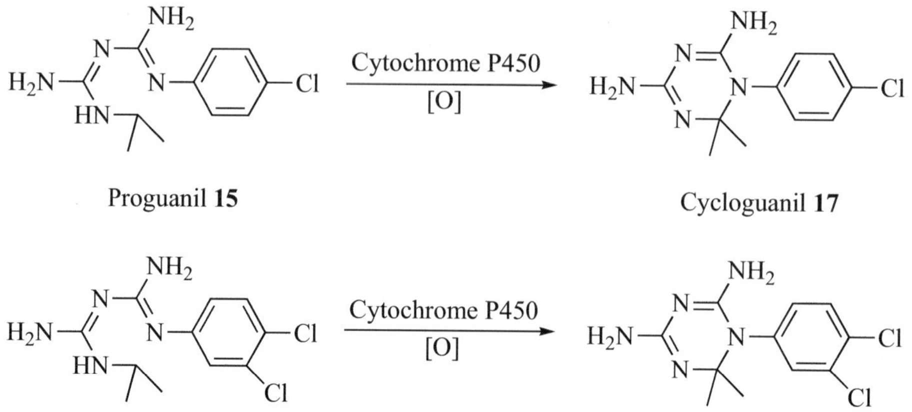

Figure 9: Proguanil and chlorproguanil have almost no antimalarial activity on their own. They act as prodrugs for cycloguanil and chlorcycloproguanil, respectively, metabolites formed by metabolic oxidative ring closure by the action of cytochrome P450. The metabolites are highly active antimalarial compounds.

Proguanil is highly active against the primary active exoerythrocytic forms of *P. falciparum* and *P. vivax* and also against the asexual blood stages of all species of human malaria parasites. PG is probably inactive against sporozoites and it has no effect on gametocytes, but when taken in appropriate doses it inhibits the development of sporogenic forms in the mosquito vector [12]. Sporogony in *P. vivax* is affected in a similar manner. PG is probably inactive on latent exoerythrocytic stages of the parasites, and hence it is not effective for radical cure of vivax malaria. The mean active plasma levels of proguanil in man are 10-20 μg L^{-1} for *P. vivax* and > 100 μg L^{-1} for a Costa strain of *P. falciparum* [3]. Against a drug-sensitive African strain, cycloguanil was found to be fully active *in vitro* at 5 μg L^{-1}, and at 250 μg L^{-1} against a drug-resistant strain from S. E. Asia [3].

Proguanil was introduced on the market in the 1950s as Palundrine®. It is highly active as a causal prophylatic in falciparum malaria, and it is also a good general suppressive against *P. falciparum* and *P. vivax* malaria. PG has a marked inhibitory effect on transmission. However, it acts too slowly to treat acute attacks of malaria in nonimmune persons. It has been widely used for many years as a prophylatic, alone or with chloroquine, marketed as Savarin® [20, 77], as a result of its outstanding properties: low toxicity, wide range of action and low cost [12]. As a result of the development of resistance, its popularity for use alone has decreased.

Proguanil has few adverse effects: mild gastric intolerance, diarrhoea, occasional aphthous ulceration and hair loss. In patients with renal impairment doses should be reduced because haematological changes occur [3]. The biotransformation to cycloguanil is also reduced during pregnancy and in women taking oral contraceptives [3]. In recent years a new fixed-ratio combination has been developed, atovaquone-proguanil 2.5:1, marketed as Malorone® [102]. It is useful for the treatment and prophylaxis of multidrug resistant falciparum malaria, but because of its high cost, it is not widely used in malaria endemic countries, and it remains more for prophylaxis of those travelling to these areas [7]. The high cost of this medication is related to the complexity of the synthetic route to obtain atovaquone [60]. This combination is also regarded as a monotherapy, because the two drugs act in synergy. Atovaquone (ATO) inhibits the parasite mitochondrial electron transport. The atovaquone-proguanil combination is currently the most potent prophylatic agent known [103]. This combination is recommended by WHO as a first-line option drug for the treatment of uncomplicated falciparum malaria in travellers returning to non-endemic countries, including those in special risk groups [3].

Pharmacology of Proguanil

Proguanil is absorbed from the gastrointestinal tract rapidly after oral administration. Peak plasma concentrations occur after approximately 4 h, and those of its active metabolite, cycloguanil, about 1 h after the peak plasma concentration of the parent drug [3]. They are eliminated slowly, and the half-life of both is approximately 20 h. The bioavailability of both is approximately 100% [20]. Proguanil must be taken daily for causal prophylaxis or suppression, and very low doses are effective. For treatment doses > 1000 mg daily are needed, but the drug is no longer used for treatment alone [12]. Cycloguanil has also been administered in the past by intramuscular injection, in the form of an embolate [3]. The use of PG in combination with dapsone is described under Pharmacology of Dapsone.

The pharmacokinetics of atovaquone-proguanil has been studied in healthy adult volunteers [104]. After a daily dose of the combination (400 mg PG, 1000 mg ATO) for 3 days, a peak plasma concentration of 509 ng mL^{-1} was found for PG after 3 h, and $AUC_{0-\infty}$ was 5,998 h ng mL^{-1}. The half-life of PG was 14.5 h. For CPG, C_{max} was 79.2 ng mL^{-1} after 6 h, and $AUC_{0-\infty}$ was 1,203 h ng mL^{-1}. The half-life was 11.8 h. In volunteers who took proguanil alone, a daily dose of 400 mg for 3 days, a peak plasma concentration of 547 ng mL^{-1} was reached after 3 h, and $AUC_{0-\infty}$ was 6,437 h ng mL^{-1}. The half-life was 13.7 h. The pharmacokinetic parameters of the metabolite were found to be C_{max} = 82.1 ng mL^{-1} after 6 h, $AUC_{0-\infty}$ = 1,355 h ng mL^{-1}, and the half-life 11.1 h. This study showed that the pharmacokinetics of proguanil is similar when it is taken alone or in combination with atovaquone. In studies with more than 500 patients showing symptoms of acute uncomplicated falciparum malaria, it was found that when the recommended dose of 4 tablets of Malarone was taken daily for 3 days, parasite clearance was achieved in 44-72 h and more than 98% of the patients were cured [105].

Chlorproguanil

The discovery of the antimalarial properties of proguanil led to the search of analogues that could have even better properties. Chlorination of the aromatic ring gave chlorproguanil (CPG), a compound with even higher antiplasmodial activity. Like proguanil, it also undergoes metabolic oxidative ring closure, catalyzed by cytochrome P450 to the triazine chlorcycloguanil, and it is the metabolite that has the high antimalarial activity. It is also a class II antifolate, acting as a DHFR inhibitor

[20]. Chlorproguanil is highly active against primary exoerythrocytic forms of *P. falciparum* and it is active against the asexual blood stages of all species of human malaria parasites [12, 20]. CPG has no apparent effect on gametocytes, but in appropriate doses it inhibits the sporogenic forms in the mosquito. The sporogony of *P. vivax* is affected in a similar manner. It has no effect on latent exoerythrocytic forms, therefore it is not effective for radical cure of vivax malaria [12].

Chloproguanil was initially marketed as Lapudrine®, and it was used for prophylaxis. Since it is more potent than proguanil, and it is retained in the body longer, it was recommended at lower doses. However it was not used as much as proguanil. The side effects that have been seen in the past are the same as those observed with proguanil [106]. In recent years it attracted attention for use as a combination partner. It was introduced in 2003 in combination with the sulfone dapsone and marketed as LapDap® [106]. By 2006 chlorproguanil was only available in combination with dapsone [106]. This antifolate combination was also regarded as a monotherapy, it was cheap and because chlorproguanil has a shorter half-life than pyrimethamine, it was thought that it had less selection pressure for resistance [20]. However it was used only for a few years, and in 2008 it was withdrawn [107] due to toxicity associated with dapsone [108].

Pharmacology of Chlorproguanil

Chlorproguanil has similar properties to proguanil. After oral administration it is metabolized in the liver to chlorocycloguanil and the maximum plasma concentration is reached within 4 h. It has a half-life ranging from 17 to 30 h. The pharmacokinetics of CPG was determined after a single oral dose of Lapudrine (320 mg) [109]. The mean maximum plasma concentration was found to be 36.7 ng mL^{-1} after 3.8 h. The elimination half-life was 17.5 h.

Naphthoquinones: Atovaquone

The antimicrobial properties of naphthoquinones have been known for more than 50 years [110]. The Fieser's research group had already prepared more than 300 naphthoquinone derivatives as potential antimalarials [6]. Atovaquone **19** was however the only naphthoquinone that eventually became approved for human

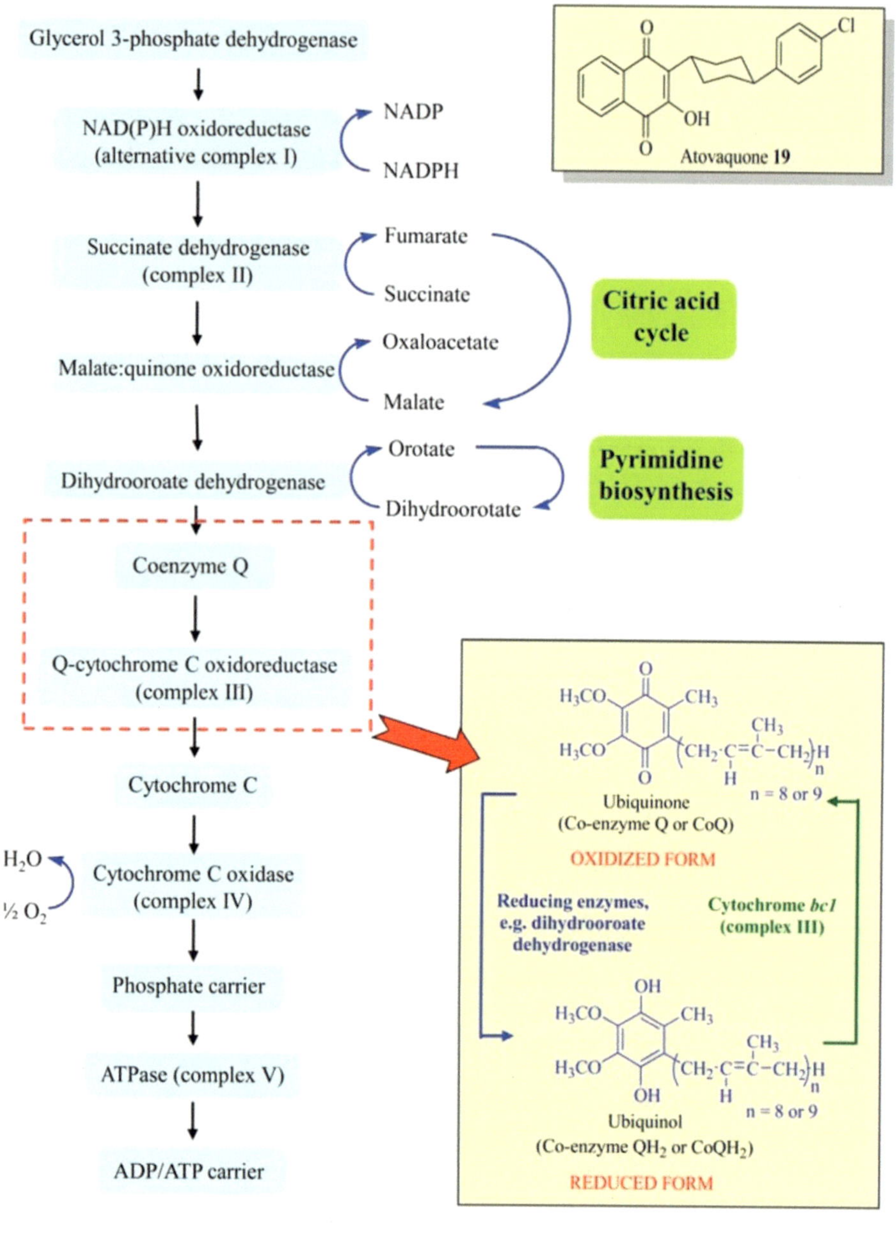

Figure 10: The mitochondrial respiratory chain in *P. falciparum* [112-116]. The glycerol 3-phosphate shuttle is illustrated. Complexes I, III and IV use the energy from electron transfer to pump electrons into the membrane space and create an electrochemical gradient. The energy is used by the ATPase complex (complex V) to produce ATP. The parasite does not depend on oxidative phosphorylation for its ATP but when Coenzyme Q is blocked, by the action of atovaquone and similar mitochondial electron transport inhibitors, pyrimidine synthesis and hence DNA synthesis are blocked. Other enzymes which transfer electrons to CoQ are also blocked.

treatment, because other options were only effective in very high doses. Nevertheless, it was only during the 1990s that atovaquone was approved by the FDA after the clinical trials undertaken in those years. The combination atovaquone-proguanil was registered throughout Europe in 1999 [111].

Atovaquone

Atovaquone (ATO) is a synthetic naphthalene derivative, a hydroxynaphthoquinone, and an analogue of ubiquinone (coenzyme Q), the electron carrier in the electron transport chain. ATO was developed by GlaxoWellcome Inc., in 1992. It is a potent selective inhibitor of mitochondrial electron transport in *Plasmodium* species, acting on the cytochrome bc_1 complex (Fig. **10**). The passage of electrons from ubiquinone to cytochrome bc_1 (complex III) requires the binding of ubiquinone to this complex. When atovaquone is present, it binds irreversible to the cytochrome *bc1* complex, preventing any further reactions and as a result the mitochondrial membrane potential drops. This inhibits any transport process across the mitochondrial membrane, it inhibits many parasitic enzymes linked to the electron transport system, including the synthesis of pyrimidine required for DNA synthesis, and eventually it results in the death of the parasite [112-116]. The mammalian cytochrome complex is up to 1000 times less sensitive than the parasite's complex [6], hence this drug can be used successfully as an antiplasmodial. ATO is active against all *Plasmodium* species [3, 117]. It inhibits pre-erythrocytic development in the liver [3], it is active on both the asexual and the sexual stages of *P. falciparum* [118] and it also inhibits oocyst development in the mosquito vector [3]. Some IC_{50} values that have been recorded are: 0.56-4.53 nM (laboratory strains) [119] and 1.1 [120], 3.56 [121] and 6.2 nM [122] (field isolates). When atovaquone is used on its own there is rapid development of resistance, due to a mutation at the mitochondrial gene that encodes cytochrome b. This causes an approximately 1000-fold increase in IC_{50} values [7]. For this reason atovaquone is not used on its own, but a combination with proguanil has been developed, which prevents the rapid development of resistance [103, 123, 124]. Marketed as Malarone, it acts in a synergic manner and hence it is considered a monotherapy. This drug has been used for treatment and prophylaxis of multidrug-resistant falciparum malaria since the mid 1990s, but it has not found widespread use due to its high cost [3]. For prophylaxis, the activity of atovaquone-proguanil against the liver stages of the parasite is particularly important, because the parasites are killed before erythrocyte infection starts. Presently it is the most potent prophylatic agent known [77]. It is suitable for use by air crews [20]. Atovaquone is generally well tolerated and the more common side effects have been skin rashes, headache, fever, insomnia, nausea, diarrhoea, vomiting, raised liver enzymes, hyponatraemia and, very rarely, haematological disturbances, such as anaemia and neutropenia [3]. Atovaquone is licensed in many countries for the treatment of the AIDS associated disease *Pneumocyctis carinii* pneumonia and it is active against toxoplasmosis. Atovaquone-proguanil is recommended by WHO as a first-line option drug for the treatment of uncomplicated falciparum malaria in travellers returning to non-endemic countries, including those in special risk groups [3].

Pharmacology of Atovaquone

Atovaquone is poorly absorbed from the gastrointestinal tract, and it is excreted almost exclusively in an unchanged form. It is a highly lipophilic drug that has a relatively poor bioavailability of approximately 23% [20]. This value can increase to about 47% when ATO is taken concurrently with a fatty meal [58]. The bioavailability is reduced in AIDS patients and in late pregnancy [3]. ATO has a half-life of 50-70 h due to enterohepatic recycling [3]. The first peak plasma concentration occurs between 1 and 8 h, and the second at 24-96 h [58]. The pharmacokinetics of atovaquone has been studied in healthy adult individuals after 1000 mg were taken once daily for three days [104]. It was found that a maximum concentration of ATO in the plasma of 10.52 μg mL^{-1} was reached after 3 h, with the $AUC_{0\rightarrow\infty}$ being 549 h μg mL^{-1}. The mean half-life of ATO in this study was 57.1 h. Similar results were obtained when the volunteers took Malarone (ATO 1000 mg, PG 400 mg) for a similar period. This is the recommended dose for treatment of acute falciparum malaria. In this case a maximum concentration of atovaquone of 11.54 μg mL^{-1} was found in the plasma after 3 h, $AUC_{0-\infty}$ was 510 h μg mL^{-1} and the half-life was 59.0 h. The same dose of Malarone given in Thailand to patients with acute falciparum malaria once a day for 3 days, produced parasite clearance in 65 h, and 100% cure rate [110].

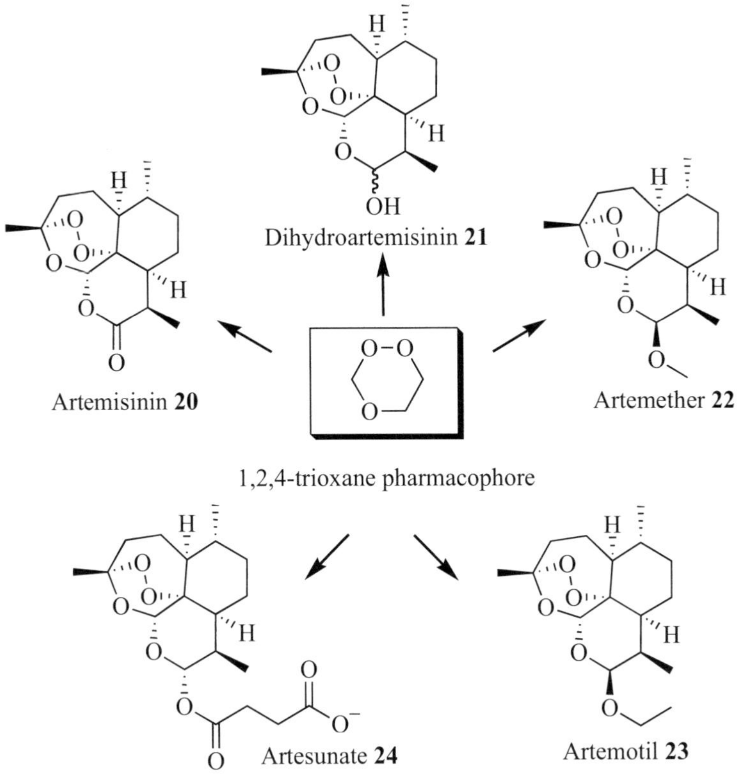

Figure 11: Artemisinin and derivatives presently in use to treat malaria. The common peroxide bridge within the 1,2,4-trioxane system is believed to be responsible for their bioactivity. It has been shown that artemisinins lacking a peroxidic oxygen atom are devoid of activity.

THE ARTEMISININS

Artemisia annua, the annual wormwood, has been used for more than 1000 years in Chinese traditional medicine for the treatment of fever [3]. In 1971, working in an army program to find a treatment for malaria, Tu Youyou [125] of China's Academy of Chinese Medical Sciences, Beijing, isolated the active ingredient from the leaves of *Artemisia annua,* and named it *qinghaosu* or artemisinin. Artemisinin (ART) **20** is a sesquiterpene lactone with a 1,2,4-trioxane substructure, the endoperoxide, which is responsible for its antimalarial activity [126]. Since artemisinin is only poorly soluble in water and in oil, there has been since then a search for derivatives that could have better physical properties and greater potency. A number of semi-synthetic derivatives are nowadays also used for therapy, resulting from modifications at the C10 position, all of which contain the endoperoxide bridge (Fig. **11**). The most commonly used are artenimol or β-dihydroartemisinin (DHA) **21**, artemether (AM) **22**, artemotil (AE) (previously known as arteether) **23** and artesunate (AS) **24**, all of which are more potent than artemisinin [126-130]. They are used to treat uncomplicated and severe malaria in both adults and children. In fact, besides the cinchona alkaloids quinine and quinidine, the artemisinins are the only class of compounds useful to manage severe malaria [127]. The artemisinins are presently the most active and rapid-acting antimalarial drugs known [6]. Nevertheless, although they produce rapid clearance of parasites, they have a short half-life. If used as a monotherapy, a seven-day course of therapy is required to prevent recrudescence. Hence, usually they are not used as monotherapies, but in combination with longer-acting blood schizonticidal drugs. This strategy is also recommended by WHO to prevent the development of resistance.

Artemisinin and its derivatives act very efficiently against asexual erythrocytic forms of *P. falciparum* [126], and in contrast to other antimalarials, they also act against the early ring stages present in the erythrocytes a few hours after infection. Artemisinin and artemether do not act on trophozoites, however dihydroartemisinin acts very fast on all three asexual stages. The artemisinins are also active against *P. vivax*. They are inactive against extra-erythrocytic forms (sporozoites, liver schizonts, merozoites) [126], and thus are not useful for causal prophylaxis. They are also less active against gametocytes, but in areas where they are used, a decrease in the transmission of malaria has been observed, suggesting that there is some inhibitory effect [126]. In *P. falciparum* malaria, artemisinin kills stage 4 gametocytes, which are otherwise sensitive only to primaquine [4].

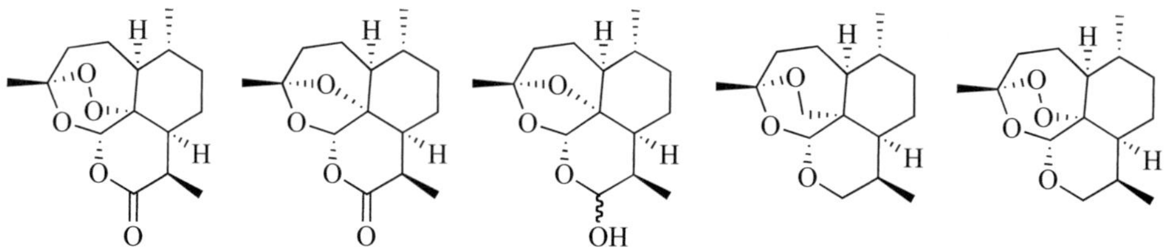

Artemisinin **20** **26** **27** **28** **29**

Figure 12: Artemisinin and analogues. Compounds **26-28** have no antimalarial activity, which suggests that the peroxide bridge is essential for bioactivity. In contrast compound **29** is more active than artemisinin [132].

The exact mechanism of action of the artemisinins is not known [131-133]. It has been shown that the peroxide structure is essential for the antimalarial activity (Fig. **12**), since related compounds lacking this unit are devoid of activity [134-136]. The artemisinins concentrate mainly in the food vacuole [137, 138].

Fe(II) is thought to be the main species responsible for bioactivation and this has been the subject of several studies [132]. Sincc the degradation of haemoglobin by the parasite produces large quantities of soluble haem in the Fe^{2+} form, haem iron is abundant. Initially it was proposed that Fe(II) cleaves the endoperoxide bridge, generating toxic oxygen radicals [141]. It was later proposed that the oxygen centred radicals generated rearrange to form carbon centred radicals [142, 143], which alkylate haem. A reductive scission model was proposed as a probable mechanism for this process (Fig. **13**) [132, 139-141] Alkylation can take place at positions α, β, γ or δ. Experiments showed that ferrous haem (not exogenous Fe^{2+}) bound to the artemisinins and promoted this process. It has also been shown by electron paramagnetic resonance spin trapping techniques [144-146] that carbon radicals alkylate haem. In a different model of haem activation, the open peroxide model [147-149], it was proposed that Fe acts as a Lewis acid, facilitating ionic rather than radical bioactivation of the artemisinins (Fig. **14**). Reaction with a water molecule leads to the formation of an unsaturated hydroxide species capable of modifying proteins irreversibly by direct oxidation. Other reactive oxygen species can also be produced in this manner, which can oxidize amino acids and this could be an important means of antimalarial action of these drugs. The alkylation of proteins by artemisinins is indeed a well established process [132].

Although intracellular iron (II) also exists in the food vacuole in equilibrium with iron (III), experiments comparing different redox forms of haem, ferrous iron, and deoxygenated and oxygenated haemoglobin under similar *in vitro* conditions showed that haem was the species that reacted with artemisinin more efficiently [150]. In humans the most abundant form of iron is oxyhaemoglobin, to which peroxide antimalarials are stable, which explains the selectivity of these drugs towards infected but not healthy erythrocytes.

Other potential targets for the artemisinins have been pointed out, such as inhibition of *Pf*ATP6, the parasite membranes and the mitochondria. It has been found that artemisinin is a highly selective inhibitor of a Ca^{2+} transporting ATP-ase (SERCA *i.e.,* sarco/endoplasmic reticulum membrane calcium ATP-ase). The role of this protein is to reduce cytosolic free calcium concentrations by concentrating Ca^{2+} into the membranes, an activity crucial for parasite survival [132]. However, *Pf*ATP6 resides in the sarcoplasmic endoplasmic reticulum, not in the food vacuole. The new mechanism was proposed [150], which assumes that endoperoxide cleavage takes place not in the food vacuole but in the cytoplasm, catalyzed by a cytoplasmic Fe (II) source, and that the radicals formed inhibit the parasite's calcium ATPase, *Pf*ATPase 6 (SERCA). A few studies have since been undertaken to test this hypothesis [132]. Parasite membrane damage by artemisinins has also been shown to occur [151], but so far there is no evidence of loss of mitochondrial functions as an initial stage of antimalarial activity with these drugs [132]. Presumably the antimalarial activity of these compounds results from more than one mechanism of action.

Artemisinin and its derivatives are active against all four species of malaria parasites that infect humans [3]. They are very well tolerated and show excellent human safety. There have been reports of mild gastrointestinal disturbances, dizziness and tinnitus [3]. The only potentially serious adverse effect reported is type 1 hypersensitivity reactions in approximately 1 in 3000 patients. Since there has yet been no evaluation of their tolerance during pregnancy, it is recommended that they should be avoided in the first trimester, because although fetotoxicity has not been reported in humans, it has been observed in animal experiments [3]. Neurotoxicity has also been observed in animals only. These adverse effects are associated with dihydroartemisinin, the main metabolite of all artemisinin semi-synthetic drugs.

Artemisinin and its derivatives are highly active antimalarial agents. In a review published in 2001, *in vitro* IC_{50} values against chloroquine-resistant *P. falciparum* strains were reported for artemisinin and derivatives as follows: 10-100 nM (artemisinin), 0.36-7.00 nM (dihydroartemisinin), 1.66-2.18 nM (artesunate), 0.57-6.10 nM (artemether), and 1.74-3.44 nM (arteether) [129].

Resistance to artemisinin has developed recently, appearing initially in the Cambodia-Thailand border area [7]. There is also early evidence of artemisinin resistance in Myanmar and Vietnam [1], which has led to greater efforts by WHO to press against the use of monotherapies for malaria treatment. In 2011 the *Global Plan for Artemisinin Resistance Containment* (GPARC) was published by WHO with recommendations for the successful management of artemisinin resistance, which include a call for increased monitoring and surveillance, improved access to diagnostics and treatment with artemisinin-based combination therapy (ACTs), and investment in research. The ACTs recommended nowadays for malaria treatment are described in the next section in this chapter.

Artemisinins pose the problem that although they are inexpensive by international standards, the derivatives are significantly more expensive than traditional antimalarials such as chloroquine and sulphadoxine/pyrimethamine [82]. A sufficient supply of artemisinin is also needed as raw material. The main cultivation areas are in China and Vietnam and the maximum yields are approximately 0.6%. Although synthetic routes do exist, production on a large-scale is not economically viable. The cost is a reflection of the complexity of the *de novo* synthetic procedures needed to obtain the unusual endoperoxide trioxane moiety.

Pharmacology of Artemisinin and its Derivatives

Artemisinin **20** is a potent antimalarial. It is converted to inactive metabolites *via* the cytochrome P450 enzyme CYP2B6 and other enzymes [3]. The derivatives artemether, artemotil and artesunate have antimalarial activity of their own, but the main therapeutic effect is due to the primary metabolite dihydroartemisinin, which forms rapidly after administration. DHA is then converted into inactive metabolites *via* hepatic cytochrome P-450 and other enzyme systems [127]. EC_{50} values depend on the compound and lie usually around or below 10 nM [126]. Recommended doses for the treatment of uncomplicated falciparum malaria in humans are 10 mg kg^{-1} day^{-1} for artemisinin and 2-5 mg kg^{-1} day^{-1} for artemisinin derivatives [126].

Artemisinin

Artemisinin **20** is a potent inducer of its own metabolism [3]. The pharmacokinetics of artemisinin has been studied a few times. For example, in two different studies [152, 153], after administration of a single oral dose of 500 mg ART to healthy individuals, a mean peak plasma concentration of 450 and 443 ng mL^{-1} was reached within 2.3 and 1.8 h respectively, and the half-life was determined to be 2 h in the first study and 0.97 h in the second. Multiple dose pharmacokinetics have also been investigated [154]. A study in Tanzania with uncomplicated falciparum malaria patients showed that when 500 mg of artemisinin are administered on the first day of treatment, followed by 2 doses of 250 mg taken daily for 4 days, and another dose of 500 mg on the last day of treatment, the mean time to parasite clearance was 31 h. On the first day a maximum mean concentration of antimalarial in the plasma of 588 ng mL^{-1} was reached after 2.4 h. On day 6, the maximum concentration was only 116 ng mL^{-1}, which was reached after 3.1 h. This decrease suggests that the metabolic capacity increases as a result of pronounced autoinduction. The area under the plasma concentration-time curve ($AUC_{0\rightarrow\infty}$) changed from 2,601 to 432 h ng mL^{-1} from day 1 to day 6. The half-life was 2.3 and 2.2 h respectively.

Dihydroartemisinin

Dihydroartemisinin **21** is the main active metabolite of the artemisinin derivatives, but it can also be used on its own. DHA has an hemiacetal substructure, obtained *via* reduction of the lactone substructure of artemisinin. It is relatively insoluble in water. When administered orally, peak plasma concentrations occur after 2.5 h, and after 4 h *via* the rectal route [3]. It is converted to inactive metabolites by the hepatic cytochrome P-450 and other enzyme systems. DHA has an elimination half-life of about 45 minutes [127]. The cure rates are similar to those of oral artesunate [3]. The pharmacokinetics of dihydroartemisinin was studied in patients with acute falciparum malaria [155], after administration of 200 mg of oral dihydroartemisinin. They were also administered 200 mg of artesunate 24 h later. A maximum mean concentration of 4,028 nmol L^{-1} of antimalarial in the blood plasma was reached after 2.63 h. $AUC_{0\rightarrow\infty}$ was 14,804 h nmol L^{-1} and the half-life 1.09 h. The treatment was completed with an additional 4 mg of artesunate and 25 mg of mefloquine per kg body weight

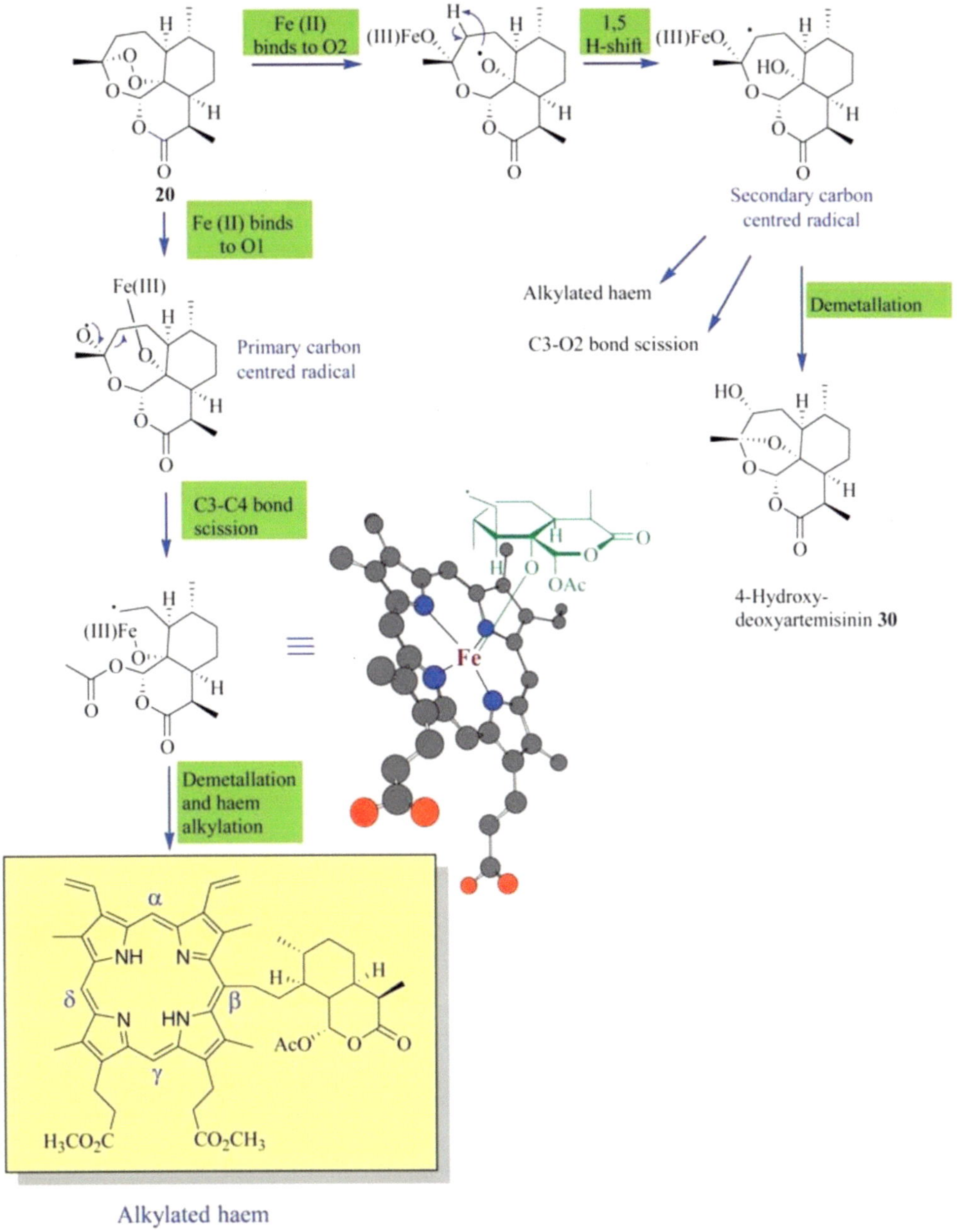

Figure 13: Haem alkylation, a probable mechanism of action of artemisinin and other peroxide antimalarials. This may prevent haem polymerization and detoxification as hemazoin. Since the peroxide bridge is unsymmetrical, more than one radical intermediate can be produced in the presence of Fe(II) ions. Both primary and secondary radicals have been spin-trapped by electron magnetic resonance spin trapping techniques. The reductive scission model is illustrated [132, 139-141].

administered after 48 h, and still 10 mg kg^{-1} of mefloquine 24 h after this. Dihydroartemisinin plus piperaquine is an ACT recommended by WHO as a first-line option treatment of uncomplicated *P. falciparum* malaria worldwide [12].

Artemether

Artemether **22** results from methylation of the hemiacetal substructure of dihydroartemisinin. It is insoluble in water, and it is more lipid-soluble than artemisinin or artesunate [3]. The peak plasma concentration occurs 2-3 h after oral administration but after intramuscular injection absorption is slow and erratic, and the peak plasma concentration occurs only 6-18 h later [3]. It has a half-life of 1 h. The pharmacokinetics of artemether was studied in patients with acute uncomplicated *P. falciparum* malaria, after oral or intramuscular administration of a 2 mg kg^{-1} body weight dose of AM [156]. A second dose was given 24 h later by the alternative route. Patient treatment was eventually concluded with the administration of 15 mg kg^{-1} body weight of mefloquine on the third day. Measurements were done by bioassays, which do not distinguish between the parent drug and the active metabolite DHA [157], and hence the values obtained and described here refer to DHA equivalents. After oral administration, a maximum concentration of 1,905 nmol L^{-1} was measured in the blood plasma after 1.0 h, with $AUC_{0\rightarrow\infty}$ = 6,045 h nmol L^{-1} and a half-life of 1.34 h. When the drug was administered intramuscularly, peak concentrations were reached in a median of 8 h, but they were only 121 nmol L^{-1}. The median $AUC_{0\rightarrow\infty}$ was then only 2,718 h nmol L^{-1}. The relative bioavailability of oral artemether during the first 24 h, clinically the most important period, was over three times that of intramuscular artemether. Artemether is recommended by WHO as a first-line option for the initial emergency 24 treatment of severe malaria, as an option to artesunate or quinine, for adults or for children. Artemether-lumefantrine is one of the first line options for the treatment of uncomplicated falciparum malaria in travellers returning to non-endemic countries [3].

Artemotil

Artemotil, also known as β-arteether **23**, is another semi-synthetic derivative of artemisinin. It is obtained by ethylation of the hemiacetal substructure of

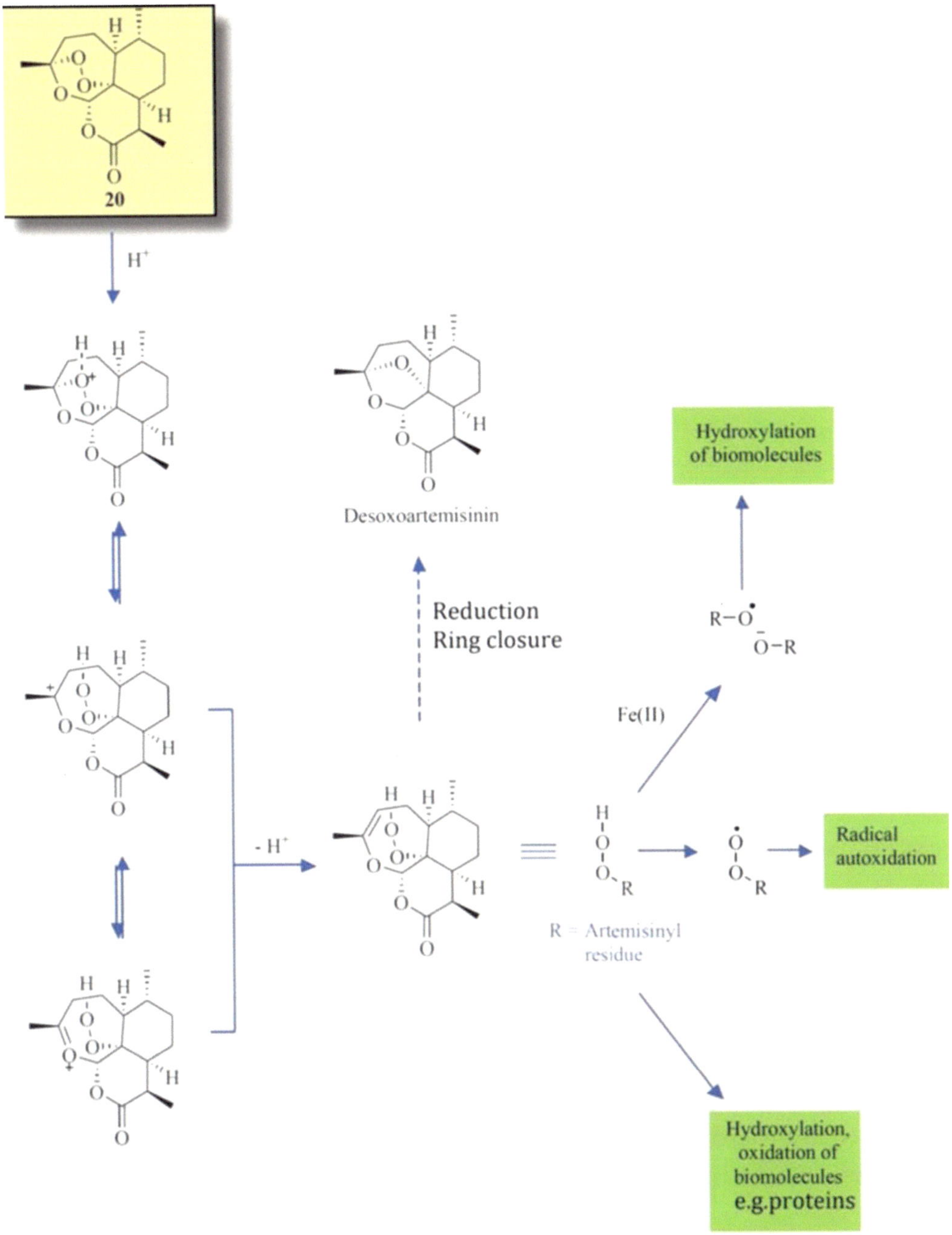

Figure 14: The open-peroxide model. The figure shows a proposal for peroxide ring opening to generate hydroperoxides, and the subsequent possibilities for decomposition. Instead of a proton, a Lewis acid like Fe(II) could activate the endoperoxide for ring opening [147, 149]. The species formed can oxidize amino acids, proteins.

dihydroartemisinin. It is water-insoluble, and it is administered by intramuscular injection only [3]. AE is absorbed slowly and more erratically than artemether, and can be detected in the plasma until more than 24 h after administration [3]. It is a fast-acting blood schizonticide specifically indicated for the treatment of chloroquine-resistant *P. falciparum* malaria and cerebral malaria [126]. The pharmacokinetics of arteether was studied on Thai patients with acute uncomplicated falciparum malaria after intramuscular administration of different doses of antimalarial to determine effective dose regimens [158]. From this study they concluded that the best regimen was one equivalent of the standard regimen used with artemether, *i.e.,* 3.2 mg kg^{-1} body weight of artemotil on the first day of treatment, followed by administration of 1 dose of 1.6 mg per kg body weight taken daily for 4 days thereafter. The pharmacokinetics after administration of the last dose were as follows: the mean peak plasma concentration was found to be 105.8 ng mL^{-1}, AUC (96,120 h) equal to 1,956 h ng mL^{-1}, and the half-life 22.4 h. Parasite clearance was achieved in a mean of 25.5 h.

Artesunate

Artesunate (AS) **24** is also obtained *via* modification of dihydroartemisinin. The hemiacetal hydroxyl group is acylated with succinic acid, and AS is used as the sodium salt. It is water-soluble and it can be administered orally, by intravenous or by intramuscular injection, or as suppositories [3]. It is absorbed rapidly, and the peak plasma concentration occurs 1.5 h after oral administration, 0.5 h after intramuscular administration and 2 h after rectal administration. It is eliminated rapidly and it has a half-life of 45 min [3]. The water solubility is important since it means that it can be administered intravenously which may be critical in cases of severe malaria when the patients are too ill and due to their condition administration *via* another route is not possible. The absolute bioavailability after a single dose of oral artesunate in adults with uncomplicated falciparum malaria is about 60% [159]. After intramuscular administration, DHA bioavailability is greater than 80% [160]. The pharmacokinetics of artesunate has been reviewed [161]. It was studied in patients with acute falciparum malaria [162], after administration of 200 mg of oral artesunate. They were also administered 200 mg of dihydroartemisinin 24 h later. Measurements were done by bioassays, which do not distinguish between the parent drug and the active metabolite DHA [157], and hence the values obtained and described here refer to

DHA equivalents. A maximum mean concentration of 3,889 nmol/L^{-1} of antimalarial in the plasma was reached after 1.55 h. $AUC_{0\rightarrow\infty}$ was 12,664 h nmol L^{-1} and the half-life 1.17 h. The treatment was completed with an additional 4 mg of artesunate and 25 mg of mefloquine per kg body weight administered after 48 h, and still 10 mg kg^{-1} of mefloquine 24 h after this. These results were similar to some obtained in a different study with Vietnamese patients [163]. The results highlighted here were obtained in the study referred to above in which the pharmacokinetics of dihydroartemisinin was also determined. A comparison of the data obtained for the two antimalarials led the authors of the study to conclude that since the pharmacokinetics of the two drugs are similar, and DHA is potentially cheaper and easier to manufacture than artesunate, that DHA could be a satisfactory alternative to artesunate in combination therapies to treat uncomplicated falciparum malaria. The big advantage of artesunate is its water-solubility, which allows for intravenous use. A few studies have been carried out on the pharmacokinetics of artesunate administered intravenously [161]. The AS concentration is initially high. Artesunate metabolises rapidly through esterase-catalyzed hydrolysis to dihydroartemisinin. The average AS half-life is less than 5 minutes. For example, administration of 120 mg artesunate over 2 min, leads to peak plasma concentrations ranging from 13,685 to 16,530 ng mL^{-1}. AUC values ranging from 846-1,269 h ng mL^{-1} were obtained. In all studies, T_{max} of DHA following intravenous administration was less than 25 min. The maximum concentration of DHA in the plasma was in the range 2,192 to 2,758 ng mL^{-1}. AUC ranged from 1,845 to 3,298 h ng mL^{-1}.

Artesunate is the first line antimalarial recommended by WHO for the treatment of severe malaria, for adults or children. Artemether or quinine are alternatives if artesunate is not available [3]. After the initial emergency 24 h treatment, artesunate plus clindamycin or doxycycline is one of the alternatives recommended for follow-up treatment.

ANTIBIOTICS: TETRACYCLINE, DOXYCYCLINE, CLINDAMYCIN AND AZITHROMYCIN

After the discovery of penicillin by Fleming in 1928, many antibiotics were isolated from fungal broths and characterized. By the 1950's some were already known to have antiplasmodial activity [164], including the tetracyclines, used nowadays in malaria therapy and chemoprophylaxis. Besides tetracycline and its derivative doxycycline, clindamycin and azithromycin are other non-sulfur antibiotics included in the WHO's list of principle antimalarial drugs available nowadays (Fig. **15**) [7].

All these antibiotics are thought to have a similar mode of action. They are translation inhibitors in prokaryotic synthesis and they are thought to inhibit protein synthesis inside the mitochondrion and the bacterial apicoplast [6]. The apicoplast is a non-photosynthetic plastid organelle, probably a remnant of endosymbiotic red algae, unique to parasites of the phylum Apicomplexa that includes protozoa like *Plasmodium* [165]. Many metabolic functions take place in the apicoplast [166], including fatty acid and haem biosynthesis [167] and hence this organelle is essential to the life of the parasite. The apicoplast has its own genome and it expresses about 30 genes, although the vast majority of the proteome is encoded in the nuclear genome [168]. Antibiotics disrupt translation during the first replication cycle of the parasite [169]. The apicoplasts metabolic functions are not disrupted in this first cycle, especially since many are catalyzed by nuclear-encoded proteins, and the parasite continues to grow normally in this first cycle [170]. However, during the second cycle, when the progeny of antibiotic-treated parasites invade a new host cell, the apicoplast cannot perform its normal functions and the new schizonts will not mature properly, erythrocyte rupture does not take place, leading to parasite death. This effect is called "the delayed-death effect" and as a result of this phenomenon even when antibiotics have potent antimalarial effects, they are slow to act.

Antibiotics have been used alone for the treatment of malaria, *e.g.,* clindamycin [81], but usually they are used in combination with other antimalarials. In fact the use of quinine or artesunate with an antibiotic is recommended as a first line treatment in severe malaria after the initial 24 h emergency treatment, and as second-line combination for the treatment of uncomplicated falciparum malaria [3]. Antibiotics are also used for chemoprophylaxis, as for instance doxycycline [3]. The use of antibiotics is important not only because of their antimalarial action, but also because septicaemia and severe malaria are associated and there is a diagnostic overlap, particularly in children [4]. Complications may also arise in malaria from bacterial infections.

The concept of antibiotic-based combination therapy (ABC) was introduced in 2009 [171], suggesting that a standardized (possibly co-formulated) combination of an antibiotic with antimalarial activity with a traditional antimalarial like quinine or artesunate should become standard treatment for severe malaria in the same way that ACTs are recommended for the treatment of malaria. Although the use of antibiotics in the treatment of malaria may give rise to fears that resistance could develop against this class of drugs which are used for the treatment of other illnesses, it has been suggested that the well-controlled environment in which intravenous therapy takes place, for example in severe malaria, in which patients are likely to receive the full course of treatment, would make this less probable to happen. Tetracyclines are one of the cheapest classes of antibiotics available [172].

Tetracycline

Tetracycline (TC) **32** was discovered in 1953 [172]. It consists of a linear system of four fused rings to which a variety of functional groups are attached (Fig. **15**). Originally it was obtained from certain species of *Streptomyces* bacteria, namely *S. aureofaciens*, *S. rimosus* and *S. viridofaciens* [172], but nowadays it is produced mainly synthetically. TC is amphoteric, with low solubility. It is used in therapy as the hydrochloride or phosphate salts, which are soluble in water. However, the intravenous preparations are stable for a few hours only [12]. Tetracycline is a broad-spectrum antibiotic, effective against Gram-positive and Gram-negative bacteria. In fact, besides the penicillins, the tetracyclines are the most widely prescribed antibiotics [173]. In malaria, TC is effective against primary erythrocytic forms of *P. falciparum* [12]. It is a blood schizonticide, which is also active against chloroquine-resistant strains and those resistant to dehydrofolate reductase inhibitors. It has no effect on gametocytes, and it is also not effective for radical cure of vivax malaria, since it has no effect on exoerythrocytic forms of the parasite. The effect on sporozoites is unknown [12]. In 2001 IC_{50} values measured against 5 strains of *P. falciparum* from Africa, Indochina, Uganda, Gambia and Brazil were found to vary from 33.8 to 88.9 μM [174].

When tetracycline is used alone for the treatment of malaria, parasite and fever clearance are slow. Hence tetracycline is usually used together with another antimalarial like quinine. In the USA, for example, tetracycline is recommended for the treatment of *P. falciparum* or *P. vivax* malaria from chloroquine-resistant areas in combination with quinine or quinidine [175]. There are no major side effects from tetracycline use, although a few adverse reactions have been reported such as nausea, vomiting, diarrhoea, and sometimes there are adverse effects on the skin, mucous membranes and the gastrointestinal tract. Tetracycline complexes may deposit in teeth and bones, so it should not be given to women after the fourth month of pregnancy or to infants and young children.

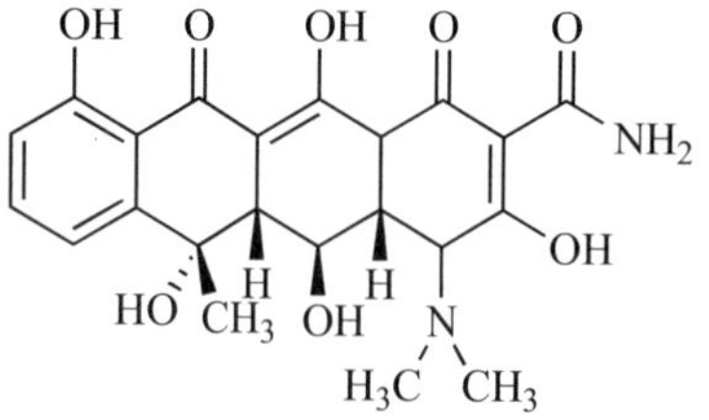

Tetracycline **32**

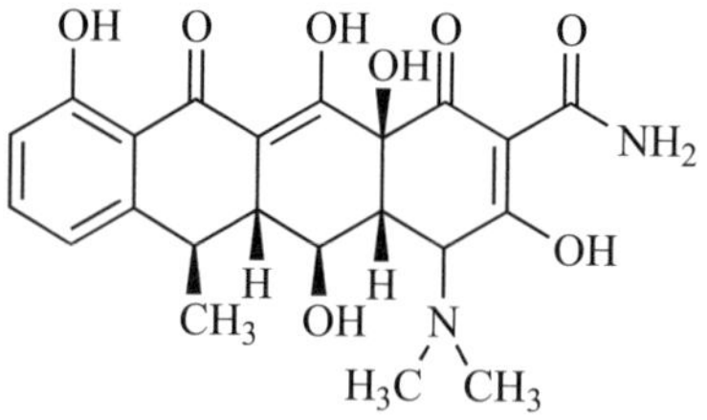

Doxycycline **33**

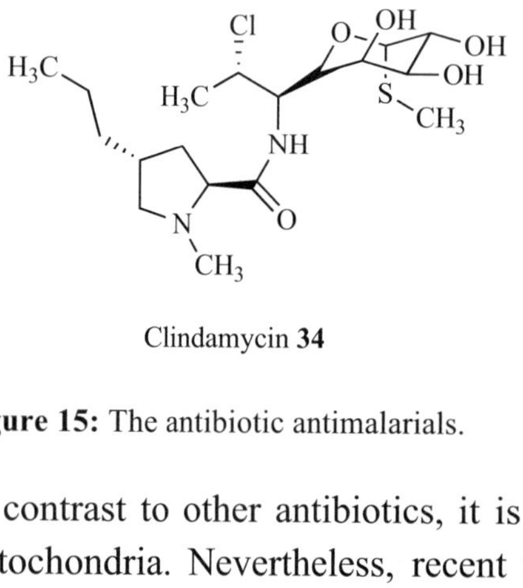

Clindamycin **34**

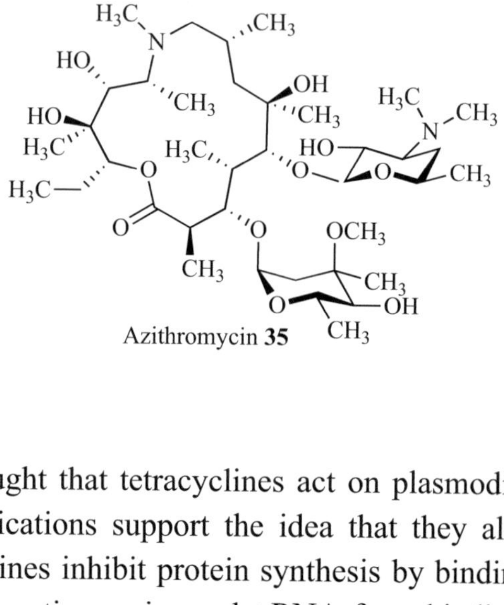

Azithromycin **35**

Figure 15: The antibiotic antimalarials.

In contrast to other antibiotics, it is thought that tetracyclines act on plasmodial mitochondria. Nevertheless, recent publications support the idea that they also target the apicoplast [176]. The tetracyclines inhibit protein synthesis by binding to the 30S subunit of ribosomes and preventing aminoacyl-*t*-RNA from binding. As a result, amino acid addition to the growing protein chain is impeded. Protein release is also inhibited [173].

Pharmacology of Tetracycline

Tetracycline is absorbed from the gastrointestinal tract following oral administration. About 5% of tetracycline is metabolised and excreted as

D-epitetracycline [177]. In a study on the pharmacokinetics in healthy volunteers [178], it was found that after oral intake of 500 mg of tetracycline by fasted subjects, a maximum concentration of 4.1 μg mL^{-1} was reached in the plasma after 4.2 h, and the mean $AUC_{0\rightarrow\infty}$ was 74.7 h μg mL^{-1}. The mean elimination half-life was 8.1 h. With meals the serum levels are reduced by about 50%, and the elimination half-life also decreases [178].

A study was carried out in Thailand, a country in which P. falciparum malaria is resistant to many antimalarials, to see the effectiveness of oral quinine plus tetracycline in treating patients with acute uncomplicated falciparum malaria [179]. Patients were administered quinine (600 mg quinine sulphate at 8 h intervals) and tetracycline (250 mg at 6 h intervals) for a period of 7 days. The mean PCT was 73.2 h and the cure rate was 100%. At the same time in other patients to whom oral artesunate was administered, the parasite clearance took place in half the time, with a similar cure success rate. Studies undertaken between 2002 and 2007 in six countries showed that quinine-tetracycline was 100% effective in Pakistan and in Cambodia [7], another area where resistance to antimalarials is high. In Cambodia, 4 patients out of 60 treated at the same time with artesunate showed falciparum resistance to this drug.

Doxycycline

Besides tetracycline, there are other naturally produced compounds with a basic tetracycline skeleton that have useful antibiotic properties. Chlortetracycline and oxytetracycline are examples. However, soon after their discovery, there were attempts to produce synthetic or semi-synthetic derivatives with better properties, such as improved water solubility or greater oral absorption. Structure-activity studies showed that the linearly fused tetracycline ring system should be kept to preserve activity, as well as the stereochemical configuration at the 4a, 12a (A-B ring junction) and the 4 (dimethylamino group) positions, and the keto-enol system (positions 11, 12, and 12a) near the phenolic ring D [172]. Doxycycline (DX) **33** was invented and developed for medicinal applications by Pfizer Inc. in the 1960s, as a semi-synthetic derivative of oxytetracycline. It was marketed as Vibramycin. The first report of its effectiveness to treat malaria dates back to 1971 [180]. DX has the advantage over tetracycline of having a longer half-life, which implies that it needs fewer administrations to be effective. It is relatively water insoluble, but highly lipophilic. It is a broad spectrum antibiotic, also used to treat anthrax infections and acne. It also active against certain species of *Plasmodium*. DX is active against primary exo-erythrocytic forms of *Plasmodium falciparum* so it can be used for malaria chemoprophylaxis. In chemoprophylaxis, destruction of the pre-erythrocytic forms, the tissue schizonts, prevents the development of merozoites and parasite release into the blood stream, which leads to the clinical symptoms of malaria that are observed. Nowadays doxycycline is a first line drug for chemoprophylaxis of malaria [181, 182]. It is the drug of choice in cases in which mefloquine cannot be administered because of its neuropsychiatric side effects, for example for aircrews and divers. It is also a blood schizonticide [182] and it can be used for the treatment of various types of malaria, *i.e.,* uncomplicated *P. falciparum, P. vivax and P. ovale* malaria, but because it acts slowly, it is used only in conjunction with fast acting blood schizonticidals like quinine. In the case of the last two, primaquine must also be administered. It is not recommended for pregnant women after the first trimester and for children under 8 years of age [3]. In the case of severe malaria, as a first line option treatment, doxycycline or clindamycin used in conjunction with quinine or artesunate are recommended as a follow-up on the initial emergency 24 h treatment with artesunate, quinine or artemether, as alternatives to ACTs [3]. The side effects of DX are similar to those of tetracycline [3], but it has fewer gastrointestinal effects. It may be used on patients with renal impairment, in which the use of tetracycline is not recommended, because it may accumulate and lead to renal failure [3].

IC_{50} values of doxycycline were measured against three *P. falciparum* strains, including a multi-drug resistant strain, and the mean values observed were in the range 2.7-4.4 μM [183]. Against 71 isolates in Senegal, the mean values were 11.3 μM, with no significant differences in activity between CQ-susceptible and CQ-resistant isolates [184]. IC_{50} values measured against 5 strains of *P. falciparum* from Africa, Indochina, Uganda, Gambia and Brazil were found to vary from 7.7 to 14.9 μM [174]. There have been no confirmed reports of resistance against doxycycline [6]. Studies undertaken during 2000-2007 showed that quinine-doxycycline was 100% effective in the treatment of uncomplicated falciparum malaria in Pakistan and Cambodia [7].

Pharmacology of Doxycycline

After oral administration doxycycline is quickly absorbed, mostly from the duodenum, and its bioavailability is 95% [185]. Like other tetracyclines, it is relatively metabolically inert, except for minor amounts of 4-epidoxycycline that have been detected in faeces and urine [186]. In a study on the pharmacokinetics in healthy volunteers [178], it was found that after oral intake of 200 mg of doxycycline by fasted subjects, a maximum concentration of 5.4 μg mL^{-1} was reached in the blood plasma after 4.3 h, and the mean $AUC_{0\rightarrow\infty}$ was 108.4 h μg mL^{-1}. The mean elimination half-life was 8.8 h. With meals the serum levels are reduced by about 20%, and the elimination half-life increases [178].

The pharmacokinetics of doxycycline was studied recently on patients recovering from severe falciparum malaria and receiving combination treatment [177]. After an initial treatment with intravenous artesunate, when the patients could take oral treatment, doxycycline was administered in combination with artesunate or quinine sulphate. The doxycycline treatment taken concurrently with the other drugs lasted for seven days, at a dose of 200 mg every 24 h. On day zero, after 200 mg of doxycycline intake, a maximum concentration of 3.17 μg mL^{-1} was found in the blood plasma after 2 h, and $AUC_{0\rightarrow\infty}$ was 49.6 h μg mL^{-1} [187]. The elimination half-life was 10.5 h. On day 7, the pharmacokinetics determined on the convalescent group was as follows: the peak plasma concentration was 4.44 μg mL^{-1}, reached after 3 h, and $AUC_{0\rightarrow\infty}$ was 73.0 h μg mL^{-1}. The elimination half-life was 11.6 h. From this study the authors concluded that the recommended dose of doxycycline of 3.5 mg kg^{-1} body weight may not be optimal for treatment. Doxycycline is known to have no effects on the pharmacokinetics of quinine [20].

For prophylaxis, doxycycline is taken once a day beginning 1-2 days before travel, while in malarious areas, and for 4 weeks after leaving. The daily dose for adults is 100 mg and for children 8 years of age is 2.2 mg kg^{-1} [182]. Adherence to the recommended doses for the periods stated is vital for its effectiveness [182]. For example, in a multinational military deployment in East Timor, consisting of

11,000 people who were present in this malaria endemic country from September 1999 to February 2000, it was found that in troops taking mefloquine there were no cases of malaria, but in the case of doxycycline, there were 11 cases per 1000 [188]. This was attributed to lack of compliance to the prescribed dose by some troops, since in the Italian Defence Forces there were no cases of malaria. Doxycycline has been reported to be as effective as mefloquine for malaria prophylaxis in the surrounding areas [188]. Since resistance to doxycycline in malaria has not been documented yet, DX can be used by travellers to all malaria-endemic countries [182].

Clindamycin

Clindamycin (CL) **34** is a lincosamide antibiotic, a derivative of lincomycin, which was first isolated from the actinomycete *Streptomyces lincolnensis* in a soil sample from Lincoln, Nebraska. Lincosamides have the carbohydrate 6-amino-6,8-dideoxy-D-erythro-D-galacto-octose as basic structural unit. Lincomycin is nowadays produced in fermentations of *Streptomyces lincolnensis*, and clindamycin is a chlorinated semi-synthetic derivative of lincomycin that exhibits better antibacterial activity and is also active against protozoa [189]. It is used as the phosphate ester, and it is very soluble in water. CL was introduced as an antibiotic in 1960. It is often used to treat infections with anaerobic bacteria, methicillin-resistant *Staphylococcus aureus* (MRSA) infections, and also as a topical treatment for acne. It has virtually no activity against aerobic Gram-negative bacteria, but excellent activity against both Gram-positive cocci and Gram-positive or -negative anaerobes [190]. The antimalarial properties of clindamycin have been known for a while. In one study, the IC_{50} mean values measured against three *P. falciparum* strains, including a multi-drug resistant one, were in the range 18-28 $\mu g\ mL^{-1}$ [183]. It was also observed that in the presence of the newer antibiotic fosmidomycin, there was good synergy and the IC_{50} values dropped considerably. CL also increases the activity of quinine. CL is effective not only against *P. falciparum* but also *P. vivax* [3]. It is not active against the exo-erythrocytic stages of the parasites [189].

The first report of the successful treatment of falciparum malaria with clindamycin alone dates back to 1975 [191]. Clindamycin is effective as a monotherapy for the treatment of malaria, as long as it is administered for at least 5 days, twice daily [192]. However, parasite clearance is slow, taking about 4-6 days, and hence it is not recommended for use as a monotherapy, but only in conjunction with a faster acting antimalarial [192], like quinine or chloroquine. CL is well tolerated. The adverse side effects are mild [192], and include gastrointestinal side effects like diarrhoea and perioral rashes. However, in some patients pseudomembranous colitis may develop during or after treatment, which can be fatal [3].

An advantage of clindamycin over the tetracyclines is that it may be used by pregnant women safely [193] and also by children [192]. The pharmacokinetic properties remain unchanged during pregnancy [194]. Small amounts are secreted in human milk.

The lincosamides block protein synthesis in bacteria by inhibiting the peptidyl transferase reaction on the 50S ribosomal subunit [195, 196]. Clindamycin inhibits bacterial protein synthesis and acts specifically on the 50S subunit of the bacterial ribosome, probably interfering with the process of peptide chain initiation [189]. It may also stimulate dissociation of peptidyl-tRNA from ribosomes [195, 196]. In *Plasmodium* it disrupts the apicoplast translation machinery during the first replication cycle, in the same way as the tetracyclines and the macrolides, provoking a "delayed-death effect" [168, 197]. Clindamycin is recommended as second-line treatment in combination with artesunate or quinine for the treatment of uncomplicated falciparum malaria. CL is recommended as the first choice of treatment together with quinine or artesunate throughout pregnancy. In the case of severe malaria, as first-line treatment options, antibiotics like clindamycin or doxycycline in conjunction with quinine or artesunate are recommended as a follow-up on the initial emergency 24 h treatment with artesunate, quinine or artemether, as alternatives to ACTs [3].

Pharmacology of Clindamycin

After intramuscular or intravenous administration, clindamycin phosphate is rapidly hydrolyzed in plasma to active clindamycin. The ester is not active. When administered orally, the hydrochloride is rapidly absorbed from the gastrointestinal tract. Clindamycin is metabolized into three major, biologically active derivatives (clindamycin sulfoxide, de-*N*-methyl clindamycin, and de-N-methyl clindamycin sulfoxide) and is excreted mainly into the bile, and about 20% is excreted by the kidneys [192].

The pharmacokinetics studied in a group of healthy volunteers, after oral administration of 600 mg of clindamycin hydrochloride, were as follows [198]: the mean absolute bioavailability F was 0.53, a peak plasma concentration of 5.3 mg L^{-1} was reached after 0.76 h, $AUC_{0\rightarrow\infty}$ was 16.9 h mg L^{-1}, and the mean half life was 2.4 h.

Several studies have been carried out on the use of quinine-clindamycin to treat uncomplicated falciparum malaria [199]. A study in Thailand on adult patients with multi-drug resistant falciparum malaria [200] showed that quinine in combination with clindamycin was 100% effective in treating the disease. Patients were treated with an oral dose of quinine sulphate (10 mg salt/bw thrice daily) plus clindamycin (5 mg base kg^{-1} body weight 4 x daily) for a total of 7 days, and parasite clearance was achieved after a mean of 78 h.

Azithromycin

Azithromycin (AZ) **35** belongs to the macrolide family of antibiotics, which have as characteristic structural feature a macrocyclic 12-, 14-, or 16-membered lactone ring to which sugar molecules are attached [201]. The widely used antibiotic erythromycin is also a member of this family. It is produced from a strain of the actinomycete *Streptomyces erythreus*, later reclassified as *Saccharopolyspora erythrea.* Azithromycin is a semi-synthetic derivative of erythromycin with an extra atom in the ring, a methyl-substituted nitrogen atom, and it is therefore a 15-membered azalide. It has 10 asymmetric centres in the macrocyclic ring, which make it difficult to produce synthetically. AZ was discovered in 1980 by a team of researchers working at the Croatian pharmaceutical company Pliva [202, 203]. The presence of the extra nitrogen atom in the ring causes increased bioavailability, increased tissue penetration and longer elimination half-life in comparison with erythromycin [204]. Nowadays it is one of the world's best selling antibiotics, with a broad spectrum of activity. It is often used to treat middle ear infections, strep throat, pneumonia, typhoid, sinusitis and certain sexually transmitted infections. Its antimalarial potential was discovered at the Walter Reed Army Institute of Research, USA [205-207]. The *in vitro* activity against multidrug-resistant *P. falciparum* K1 strain was determined by measuring the ^{3}H-hypoxanthine incorporation, and it was found to inhibit parasite growth with IC_{50} value of 8.4±1.2 μM [208].

The macrolides have a similar mechanism of action to that of the lincosamides, despite the fact that their chemical structures are very different [189]. Against bacteria, AZ acts by binding reversibly to the 50S ribosomal subunit, thus interfering with microbial protein synthesis [209]. Nucleic acid synthesis is not affected. It has been shown that in plasmodia, the antimalarial properties of AZ are a result of its binding to the apicoplast 50S ribosomal subunit and inhibiting protein synthesis in the apicoplast [209].

Azithromycin is active against pre-erythrocytic forms of *Plasmodium* [210], but it also causes the "delayed-death effect" since it does not prevent maturation of liver-stage merozoites, but these are incapable of causing the subsequent blood-stage infection. It is therefore slow to act [211], but it has been combined with other drugs like quinine or chloroquine for effective treatment [168]. Clinical trials have shown that azithromycin is a good chemoprophylatic agent, less effective than doxycycline against falciparum malaria [212, 213], but as effective as doxycycline against vivax malaria [213]. It has no apparent effect on *P. vivax* hypnozoites [214]. AZ is also active against blood schizonts [215, 216], but it is a weak antimalarial with a slow parasite clearance rate, and it was concluded in a recent review, that it offers no equivalence or superiority either as monotherapy or combination therapy for the treatment of *P. falciparum*- or *P. vivax*-induced malaria, compared with other existing antimalarials [214].

AZ is well tolerated. Reported adverse effects are nausea, vomiting, diarrhoea, pruritis and dizziness, but they usually disappeared when drug intake stopped [217]. Some studies show that it is safe for use in children and pregnant women [207, 218]. Presently azithromycin is not one of the drugs recommended by WHO for the treatment or prophylaxis of malaria [3], although it is already listed as an available antimalarial in the recent "Global report on antimalarial drug efficacy and drug resistance: 2000-2010" [7].

Pharmacology of Azithromycin

After oral administration, azithromycin is rapidly adsorbed from the gastrointestinal tract. AZ is eliminated mostly as an unchanged drug *via* biliary excretion [219]. The absolute oral bioavailability is approximately 34-52% with single doses of 500 mg to 1.2 g, probably due to incomplete absorption [219]. The standard dose to treat bacterial infections in adults is 250 to 500 mg orally every six hours or 0.5 to 1 g every 12 hours for seven days or more [214]. The half-life of azithromycin is approximately 68 h [220]. There have been a few studies of the pharmacokinetics of AZ as highlighted in a recent review [214]. In healthy Bangladeshi individuals, a single 500 mg tablet was administered under fasting conditions followed by a period of 3 weeks in which no drug was taken. The following data were determined: a maximum plasma concentration of 382.4 ng mL^{-1} was reached after 4.83 h, $AUC_{0\rightarrow\infty}$ was 6.307.5 h ng mL^{-1} and the mean half-life was 41.44 h [221].

A study carried out in India showed that when AZ was used alone in adults with acute uncomplicated falciparum malaria, clearance of parasites was incomplete [32]. In a study in Bangladesh, azithromycin-artesunate administered once daily for 3 days (30 mg kg^{-1} per day of AZ plus 4 mg kg^{-1} per day of ART) to patients with uncomplicated falciparum malaria, parasite clearance was obtained in a mean of 25.1 h [216].

ARTEMISININ-BASED COMBINATION THERAPIES (ACTs)

The appealing properties of artemisinin and its derivatives, *i.e.,* strong and fast initial activity, favourable pharmacokinetics and apparently excellent human safety and tolerability [220, 222] have made them become favourites for the treatment of malaria. During the 1990s WHO promoted a series of trials in different countries through its Roll Back Malaria Programme to test the efficacy of artemisinins in combination with other antimalarials to treat uncomplicated falciparum malaria [223, 224]. These combinations became known as artemisinin-based combination therapy (ACT). One of the reasons to try them as combinations was to prevent the development of resistance. The fact that artemisinins have very short half-lives of 2 to 5 h implies that they have to be administered for more than 5 days to be fully effective, which led to high failure rates. When they are combined with other antimalarials with longer half-lives, preferably of more than 24 h, they can be used for shorter periods, and the replicating parasites are not exposed to sub-therapeutical drug levels that favour the development of resistant parasites [223]. The three-day course recommended nowadays by WHO gives 90% reduction of parasites, which are then completely eliminated by the longer-acting drug partner, normally a schizonticide, leading to radical cure. In addition, the gametocytocidal activity of the artemisinins helps to reduce transmission. There are nowadays 5 ACTs recommended for use [1], and even formulations as syrups, powders, and granules to make them appealing to children [223]:

- artemether plus lumefantrine,
- artesunate plus amodiaquine,
- artesunate plus mefloquine,
- artesunate plus sulfadoxine-pyrimethamine, and
- dihydroartemisinin plus piperaquine.

The choice of ACT to use will depend on the resistance patterns in the area or country of intended use. All these drugs are now available as fixed-combinations except for artesunate-sulfadoxine-pyrimethamine [223]. One advantage of fixed-dose combination formulations is that they promote adherence to the treatment. WHO started to recommend the use of combination therapy in 2003, after the first signs of resistance to mefloquine-artesunate were observed in the Pailin province in Cambodia in 2002, particularly for areas where resistance to many antimalarials is common [225, 226]. The Thailand-Cambodia border has been historically the centre of emergence of resistance. However, by 2011 resistance had spread to other areas in East Asia. WHO launched then its Global Plan for Artemisinin Resistance Containment (GPARC) [7], a high-level plan to protect ACTs as an effective treatment for *P. falciparum* malaria. Nowadays ACTs are recommended by WHO as first line options for malaria treatment [3]. Nevertheless their use is not as widespread as it could be, due to cost and poor access, which are still enormous obstacles [227].

The dose and frequency of administration of the antimalarial drug have to be adequate so as to provide drug concentrations sufficiently high for a certain period of time to kill all the parasites [228]. The drug-concentration time profile is determined from the pharmacokinetics. The pharmacokinetic parameters of the drugs when administered alone may differ from those observed when they are used in a combination. Optimal designs for population pharmacokinetics are being developed [228] to optimize sampling schedules that can become very tiresome for weakened malaria patients, and also to make economical use of resources [228]. Experience has shown that the ACTs are more effective than the individual drugs when administered alone. In the last decade the pharmacokinetic parameters of most ACTs were determined, but the data is still incomplete especially for particularly vulnerable groups such as pregnant women and children. The spread of resistance may also create the need for dose readjustment [57]. Table **3** summarises the pharmacokinetic data obtained in some studies on the five ACTs presently recommended by WHO for the treatment of malaria. The data presented is illustrative, not exhaustive.

The pharmacokinetics of AS and DHA, administered singly or as a combination therapy, have been reviewed recently [160]. For the artesunate-amodiaquine (1:2.5) combination, pharmacokinetics has been studied in healthy volunteers [230]. It was found that the total drug exposure of both drugs was reduced considerably when they were administered as ACTs. AUC for the main active metabolites, DHA and DSA, decreased considerably, from 2044 to 1410 h ng mL^{-1} and from 12,041 to 8,437 h ng mL^{-1}, respectively. AUC is the key parameter for parasite killing and it is a useful predictor of therapeutic response. Since it is known that the ACT is more effective clearing parasitaemia and preventing recrudescence than AQ alone [231], it appears that the effectiveness is related to an additive or possibly synergistic effect. However, this decrease in AUC may become important in areas of high resistance, resulting in reduced parasite killing.

Table 3: Pharmacokinetic Parameters of the ACTs Currently Approved for Malaria Treatment[a]

Antimalarial	Dosage	Drug	C_{max}, ng mL^{-1}	T_{max}, h	AUC, h ng mL^{-1}	$T_{½}$, h	PCT, h	Ref.
Artesunate plus Amodiaquine	AQ 10 mg kg^{-1}, AS: 4 mg kg^{-1}; single dose (healthy volunteers)	AS	141.6	0.86	183.3	NA	72[b]	[229, 230]
		DHA	446.2	2.08	1410.5	2.20		
		AQ	22.7	2.18	108.5	3.9		
		DSA	301.4	2.18	8437	137		
	Artesunate alone: 4 mg kg^{-1} (healthy vol.)	AS	231.8	0.62	206.4	NA		
		DHA	844.5	1.10	2044.4	1.5		
	Amodiaquine alone: 10 mg kg^{-1} (healthy vol.)	AQ	29.2	2.32	162.4	5.3		
		DSA	268.7	3.68	12,041	241		
Artesunate plus Mefloquine	Standard dose: AS: 4 mg^{-1}/kg for 3 d, MQ: 15 mg kg^{-1} on day 1, 10 mg kg^{-1} on day 2 (in malaria)	MQ	3,239	70.9	1095,421	322	40	[232]
		AS	451	0.93	NA	NA		
		DHA	2,043	1.4	3,745	0.8		
	Artesunate: 4 mg kg^{-1} for 3 d; after the 3rd day, MQ administered (in malaria)	AS^1	201	0.50	237	0.58	48	[233]
		AS^2	316	1.00	338	0.29	72	
		DHA^1	1088	1.01	2701	0.85		[235]
		DHA^2	1452	1.50	3766	0.77		
	Alternative: 200 mg AS, 750, 500 mg MQ, 6 and 12 h later (in malaria)	MQ	1623	15.0	12.8*	264	47.5	[236]
	MQ alone: 750 mg, 500 mg 6 h later (in malaria)	MQ	2212	20.3	17.2*	288	82.3	[236]
Artesunate plus Sulphadoxinea and Pyrime-thamine	400 mg AS plus 1500 mg SDX, 75 mg PYR, on day 1, then 100 mg AS once a day for 4 d. (healthy volunteers)	SDX	98900	8.0	18876,700	180	72[c]	[237,238]
		PYR	790	3.0	112,000	177		
	SP alone: 1500 mg SDX, 75 mg PYR (healthy volunteers)	SDX	92900	10.0	15840,500	165		
		PYR	860	4.0	124,600	158		
Artmether plus Lumefantrine	20 mg AM, 120 mg LU, twice daily for 3 d Coartem® (in malaria)	AM	66.2	2	211,000	2.2	29	[241]
		DHA	205	2-3	604,000	1.6		[241]
		LU	9000	3-4	561,000	72-96		[242]
	80 mg AM, 480 mg LU at 0, 8, 24, 48 h; (in malaria) Co-artemether	AM	133	2.13	2035	0.86	30	[243]
		DHA	137	2.44	3135	1.06		
	80 mg AM at 0, 8, 24, 48 h (in malaria)	AM	157	1.73	1834	1.16	30	
		DHA	161	1.86	2926	0.95		

(Table 3) contd.....

Antimalarial	Dosage	Drug	C_{max}, ng mL^{-1}	T_{max}, h	AUC, h ng mL^{-1}	$T_{½}$, h	PCT, h	Ref.
Dihydroarte-misinin plus Piperaquine	DHA alone: 2 mg kg^{-1} bw (±50 kg bw); Single dose (healthy vol.)	DHA	181	1.5	377	0.96		[247]
	640 mg PPQ phosphate, 80 mg DHA, Artekin® Single dose (healthy vol.)	PPQ	586.9	2.1	46419	303		[248]
		DHA	244	1.6	450	1.25		[249]
	960 mg PPQ phosphate, 120 mg DHA Single dose (healthy vol.)	DHA	159	1.5	370	1.01	28[d]	[250,251]
	PPQ alone: 640 mg; Single dose (healthy vol.)	PPQ	578.5	2.3	44293	317		[248]
	Dihydroartemisinin alone: 120 mg (healthy vol.)	DHA	442	2.5	858	1.02		[252]

[a]units are µg d mL^{-1}; [b]three-day course in uncomplicated falciparum malaria; [c]AS (4 mg kg^{-1} d^{-1}) for 3 days + SP (25 mg kg^{-1} SDX+1.25 mg kg^{-1}) single dose on day 1, in uncomplicated falciparum malaria; [d]DHA (2.4 mg kg^{-1} d^{-1}) + PPQ (19.2 mg kg^{-1} d^{-1}) together for 3 days in uncomplicated falciparum malaria.

The standard dose prescribed for the artesunate-mefloquine combination is 4 mg kg^{-1} AS per day, with a total MQ dose of 25 mg kg^{-1} split into 2 days [232]. This ACT was introduced as an inexpensive combination therapy directed especially at Sub-Saharan Africa [233], and has now been adopted by many countries in Africa, *i.e.,* Burundi, Liberia, Sudan and Sierra Leone as the first-line therapy, and it has also been recommended for use in Central Angola, for example, where high levels of chloroquine resistance were found to occur [234].

Pharmacokinetic studies in malaria patients treated with the artesunate-mefloquine combination showed significant interactions between the two drugs. Parameters for the standard dose of 4 mg kg^{-1} bw of artesunate were obtained in two locations: Wang Pha in Thailand and Pailin in Cambodia. They were found to be similar, although the areas under the concentration-time curve were slightly greater in Pailin [235]. However, here parasite clearance took an average of 72 h, markedly slower than in Wang Pha, where this was achieved in 48 h. The difference between the two sites corresponds to the development of some resistance by *P. falciparum* to artesunate in Cambodia. In a different study, in which the same dose of artesunate was administered at the same time as mefloquine, it was found that the pharmacokinetics were similar to those observed in Wang Pha, the area where greater sensitivity to artesunate is observed [232], showing that the presence of mefloquine does not affect the artesunate or dihydroartemisinin disposition kinetics. However, the opposite is not true. The presence of artesunate causes significant changes in mefloquine pharmacokinetics. Mefloquine concentrations are lowered, with C_{max} being reached faster and changing from 2,212 ng mL^{-1} to 1,623 ng mL^{-1} [236]. Consequently AUC also drops. A larger volume of distribution and faster clearance was also observed in patients receiving the combination treatment. Despite these differences, the time for parasite clearance is nearly halved when combination therapy is used.

The artesunate-sulfadoxine-pyrimethamine combination was also studied in healthy volunteers [237]. It was found that artesunate had no effect on the pharmacokinetics of SP, although it has been observed in the past that the combination is more effective to treat malaria than the individual component drugs when administered alone [228]. In malaria, the repeated administration of AS causes a drastic reduction in parasitaemia, which is assisted by a continuous inhibition of folic acid biosynthesis in the parasite for more than 14 days by SP [238]. Cure rates improve, transmission decreases, and the development of resistance is delayed with the ACT. This ACT is being used nowadays in parts of South America, the Middle East, and South Asia where SP susceptibility is still high [227].

The artemether-lumefantrine (1:6) combination is referred to as co-artemether. It was originally developed in China, and in 2007 it was the only ACT registered internationally [239]. Presently it is the only ACT registered in Europe [127]. Lumefantrine is active against all human malaria parasites [227]. The two components have been shown to be synergistic in their action against *P. falciparum in vitro* [240]. The pharmacokinetics of the two drugs given in combination is not much different from those used when they are administered individually [20]. T_{max} of artemether and DHA increase by almost 0.5 h when artemether is used in combination with lumefantrine, but this is not statistically significant [241-243]. There is also a slight delay in absorption and the absorption time also increases, but the total AUC does not change [239, 244, 245]. Since lumefantrine is highly lipophilic, the bioavailability of this antimalarial increases up to 2-fold when it is administered together with food, which is therefore recommended [239]. Recent research has shown that desbutyl-lumefantrine (DBL), a metabolite of lumefantrine, is a more potent antimalarial than the parent compound with which it acts in synergy against *P. falciparum* and *P. vivax* [246]. It is also synergistic with DHA.

The pharmacokinetics of the dihydroartemisinin-piperaquine (1:8) combination studied in healthy volunteers showed that when a single dose of piperaquine (640 mg) was administered in the presence of artesunate there was no effect on piperaquine pharmacokinetics [247, 248]. Administration of dihydroartemisinin (2 mg kg^{-1} body weight) to volunteers with an average body weight of 50 kg had the same effect as when the drug was administered in combination with piperaquine [249]. However it was found that when twice this amount was administered, C_{max} doubled and AUC was 2.4 times higher. In a different study [250-252] a significant difference was found between single and combined administration of dihydroartemisinin. The oral bioavailability of piperaquine is also increased when it is administered with fat. A fixed-dose combination is now commercially available in many countries in Asia, and also more recently in Africa [227].

THE PIPELINE OF ANTIMALARIALS IN DEVELOPMENT

In the past 40 years antimalarial drug resistance has been increasing in frequency and intensity and it has also been spreading [253]. As a result, the efficacy of some of the more commonly used antimalarials has dropped in the affected areas. Resistance is one of the major obstacles in the fight against malaria. It develops mainly as a result of the extensive use of some antimalarial drugs. It can develop during treatment, when the concentration of a drug falls below subtherapeutic levels, before all the parasites are completely eliminated. It causes selection. It allows the few parasites present that were less susceptible to the drug to be transmitted to the vector and multiply in the next life cycle [254]. Since the concentration of the drug in the body at a given time depends on the pharmacokinetics of the drug, pharmacokinetics is the one of the most important aspects influencing the onset of resistance [255]. If the drug has a short half-life it has to be administered more frequently. Lack of compliance implies that plasma concentrations drop below the values required to eliminate the parasites. If the drug has a long half-life, problems may arise during prolonged periods at which the concentration of the drug has fallen to low levels. Combinations of drugs with suitable pharmacokinetics can help to solve this problem. Genetic mutations that confer resistance can also occur spontaneously, but they are rare [7, 256]. Point mutations in the genes encoding for a drug target in the parasite will result in less affinity of the target for the drug, and hence the drug will be less effective [7]. Various aspects related to resistance are focused in a few recent reviews [257, 258].

Resistance has been reported to occur with *P. falciparum, P. vivax* and *P. malariae.* The resistance of *P. falciparum* to two of the most widely used antimalarial drugs, chloroquine and sulfadoxine-pyrimethamine occurs now on a global scale [82], but resistance has also been reported to almost all other antimalarials being currently used, *e.g.,* amodiaquine, mefloquine, quinine, although it varies considerably from region to region [3]. Recently there have also been reports of resistance to the artemisinins in a number of countries in South-East Asia, particularly on the Cambodia-Thailand border, Myanmar and Vietnam [1]. *P. vivax* shows resistance to sulfadoxine-pyrimethamine in many areas, and also to chloroquine, but in this case it is confined largely to Indonesia, East Timor, Papua New Guinea and other parts of Oceania [6]. It has also been reported in Brazil and Peru. Immunity is reduced in pregnancy and also when individuals move out of the transmission areas. The increase in the numbers of international travellers has also contributed to an increase in imported malaria [259].

Resistance can be prevented or at least be delayed by combining drugs or through the use of antimalarials with different modes of action. The chance of the parasite developing resistance against both simultaneously is much lower. The use of combinations of drugs is common practice in the treatment of other diseases such as tuberculosis, most HIV and cancer [253]. In malaria the situation can also be complicated by cross-resistance, which can occur among drugs that belong to the same chemical family or which have similar modes of action [3]. Multidrug resistance also occurs, which implies that the parasite is resistant to more than two antimalarial compounds of different chemical classes and modes of action. Table **4** summarizes the main target molecules or processes aimed at by antimalarials presently in use or under development [260-262].

Table 4: Main Drug Targets for Malaria Chemotherapy [260-262]

Target Location	Pathway/Mechanism	Target Molecule or Process	Examples
Cytosol	Folate metabolism	Dihydrofolate reductase	**Pyrimethamine, proguanil, cycloguanil, chlorproguanil, trimethoprim, P218**
		Dihydropteroate synthase	**Sulfadoxine, sulfalene, dapsone**
	Purine biosynthesis (Salvage pathway)	Purine nucleoside phosphorylase	**BCX4945**
	Pyrimidine biosynthesis	Dihydrooroate dehydrogenase	**DSM265**
Parasite membrane	Phospholipid metabolism		**Albitiazolium**
	Membrane transport	*Pf*CRT	**Piperaquine**
Food vacuole	Haemoglobin metabolism	Hemozoin formation	**Chloroquine, quinine, quinidine, amodiaquine, halofantrine, lumefantrine, mefloquine, 8-aminoquinolines, ferroquine**
		Haem iron as activator of protein alkylation	**Artemisinins**
		Free radical generation	**Artemisinins**
Mitochondrion	Electron transport	Ubiquinol-cytochrome C oxidoreductase	**Atovaquone**
Apicoplast	Translation		**Tetracyclines, clindamycin, azythromycin, spiroindole**
	Isoprenoid biosynthesis	DOXP reductoisomerase	**Fosmidomycin**
Endoplasmic reticulum	**Ca^{2+} level regulation (ATP-dependant Ca^{2+} pump)**	**ATPase 6 (SERCA)**	**Artemisinins**

Resistance is the main factor determining the life span of a drug [253]. It is therefore clear that there is a basic need for sustainable development and discovery of new drugs for the future, to fill in any gaps that may arise. This also applies to the need to develop new insecticides, for use in nets, since insecticide resistance to the pyrethroids, the agents that are most commonly used for this purpose, has already been reported in 27 countries in Africa and 41 countries worldwide [1]. New research and development in this area is needed for improved antimalarial drugs, vector control tools, diagnostics and vaccines. Ideally new antimalarials should be cheap, well tolerated, require the administration of fewer doses, and be useful for many types of malaria [253, 263].

Although antimalarials are needed in many parts of the world, the market is small in terms of profit, and by 1999 the pipeline for new antimalarials was almost empty [259]. The United Nations resolution to eradicate malaria from the planet, implied in one of its Goals for the Millennium, brought a new impetus to research in this area.

Nowadays there are a few international organizations committed to the fight against malaria [264]:

- Foundation for Innovative New Diagnostics (FIND)
- Global Fund to Fight AIDS, Tuberculosis and Malaria
- Medicines for Malaria Venture (MMV)
- Multilateral Initiative on Malaria (MIM)
- PATH Malaria Vaccine Initiative (MVI)
- Roll Back Malaria
- Special Programme for Research and Training in Tropical Diseases (TDR)

The global malaria medicine pipeline is now more extensive than in the past [265]. Many of the products being developed have the support of the Medicines for Malaria Venture, an organization created in 1999. Built on experiences from the Special Program for Research and Training in Tropical Diseases [82], it operates in concert with the Roll Back Malaria Program of the WHO, bringing together teams of scientists from the academia and industry, through suitable finance mechanisms, to develop projects leading to the development of novel antimalarial products. Nowadays it has partnerships with more than 260 research institutions and countries across the world.

Fig. (**16**) shows the pipeline of antimalarial drugs being developed worldwide at the first quarter of 2012, according to the Medicines for Malaria Venture [266]. It includes medicines that have been already approved and are now in Phase IV of development, *i.e.,* they are undergoing post-marketing real world surveillance studies, as opposed to those previously carried out in a controlled environment [267]. The properties of these antimalarials have been discussed previously in this chapter. Table **5** shows endoperoxide ring nomenclature. Tables **6** and **7** summarize some of the properties of the prospective antimalarials.

Drugs Waiting Registration (See Table 6)

An ACT, in the form of one tablet consisting of a fixed-dose combination of artesunate **23** and mefloquine **7** is one of the new options awaiting registration. The artesunate-mefloquine combination is already recommended by WHO for the treatment of uncomplicated and severe *P. falciparum* and also for *P. vivax* malaria, but it has been administered so far as a combination of two separate tablets of mefloquine and artesunate. At this stage is also a new formulation of artesunate for the treatment of acute malaria, in the form of suppositories.

Drugs in Phases IIB and III (See Table 6)

Two new antibiotic combinations are being developed. One is a fixed-dose of the antibiotic azithromycin **35** in combination with chloroquine **3**, being developed as intermittent preventive treatment in pregnant women, as an alternative to sulphadoxine-pyrimethamine, against which resistance has developed in some parts of the world. The other is Co-trimoxazole, a combination of trimethoprim **37** and sulphamethoxazole **38**. This combination is already recommended as part of the standard treatment for people infected with the human immunodeficiency virus (HIV) and those with acquired immunodeficiency syndrome, and also for integrated management of childhood illness in Africa [268]. In malaria Co-trimoxazole acts as an antifolate, and it is another possible successor to sulphadoxine-pyrimethamine.

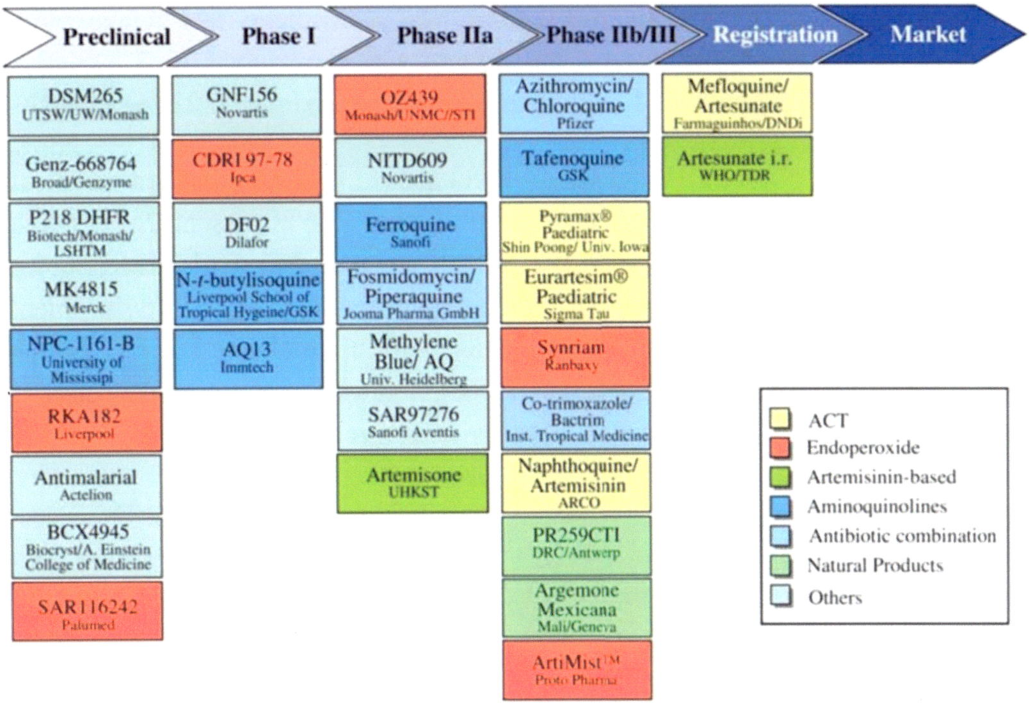

Figure 16: The world pipeline of antimalarials in development according to the Medicines for Malaria Venture [266].

ACTs in this stage of development include Eurartesim® Paediatric, a child friendly dispersible formulation consisting of a fixed dose of dihydroartemisinin **21** and piperaquine **4**, already available as tablets for adults and recommended by WHO for the treatment of uncomplicated falciparum malaria. Pyramax® Paediatric is an ACT consisting of a fixed combination of pyronaridine **39** and artesunate **23**, which is being developed as a fixed combination for children. Pyronaridine is a blood schizonticide, a Mannich base which instead of the usual quinoline heterocycle possesses an azaacridine ring system. It is effective against *P. falciparum* and *P. vivax* malaria. The tablet formulation received a positive scientific opinion from the European Medicines Agency. A fixed-dose combination of artemisinin **20** and naphthoquine **40** is also being developed as an alternative for the treatment of all forms of malaria.

A completely new fixed-dose combination is Synriam, already launched in India as an alternative for the treatment of *P. falciparum* malaria. This non-artemisinin based combination therapy (NACT) combines a synthetic fast-acting blood schizonticide, arterolane **41**, with a half-life of approximately 1 to 3 h, with a longer acting one, piperaquine **4**, with a half-life of approximately 23 days [242].

Monotherapies in phases IIB and III of development include tafenoquine **42**, an alternative to primaquine **6**. PQ is the only drug available at present that is active against hypnozoites of the relapsing parasites *P. vivax* and *P. ovale*. Tafenoquine is the only molecule in the pipeline with activity against *P. vivax* hypnozoites. ArTiMist, a sublingual spray formulation of artemether **22** is another monotherapy being developed to treat uncomplicated *P. falciparum* malaria in young children and infants. It is also effective in severe malaria.

Included in this group are also two herbal medicines. One is *Argemone mexicana*, a weed found in many tropical areas, used by traditional healers in Mali as a decoction for the treatment of malaria. IC_{50} values of the aqueous decoction and methanol extracts of the aerial parts of the plant, against *P. falciparum* (chloroquine-resistant K1 strain) were found to be 5.89 and 1.00 μg mL^{-1} respectively [270]. In a trial conducted in Mali, its performance was compared with that of artesunate-amodiaquine ACT [271]. Both treatments were well-tolerated. Second-line treatment was not required for 89% of patients treated with *Argemone mexicana versus* 95% treated with the ACT. In cases of severe malaria it was found to perform as well as the artesunate-amodiaquine treatment.

The other antimalarial herbal medicine is PR259 CTI, a quantified 80% ethanol extract from the stem bark of *Nauclea pobeguinii*, containing strictosamide **43** as the major alkaloid [272]. It has moderate *in vitro* activity against *P. falciparum*, with IC_{50} values in the range 32-44 μg mL^{-1}.

Drugs in Phase IIA (see Table 6)

There are two NACTs in this stage of development: fosmidomycin **44**-piperaquine **4** and methylene blue **45**-amodiaquine **5**. Fosmidomycin (FOS) is an antibiotic that has potent activity against Gram-negative bacteria. Initially it was isolated from cultures of *Streptomyces lavendulae*, but nowadays it is produced synthetically. It is also active against *Plasmodium* parasites, being at present the most potent and rapid acting antibiotic against malaria [167]. It targets isoprenoid biosynthesis in the apicoplast of the parasite, more particularly the action of 1-deoxy-D-xylulose 5-phosphate (DOXP) reductoisomerase, the second enzyme of the pathway [273]. Since in mammals isoprenoids are derived from an alternative pathway, the mevalonate pathway, FOS can be used safely to treat malaria. It is a blood schizonticide, but in contrast to other antibiotics with antimalarial properties it does not exert a delayed death effect [274], and hence it acts more rapidly. The combination dihydroartemisinin-piperaquine is an ACT currently recommended by WHO for the treatment of malaria. A synergic effect has been observed *in vitro* against *P. falciparum* drug-sensitive 3D7 and CQ-resistant K1 strains when fosmidomycin was added to piperaquine, which led to the identification of these drugs as therapeutic partners [275]. Phase II trials started at the end of 2011 in Thailand.

The second NACT in this stage of development is a combination of the first compound ever used to treat malaria, methylene blue (MB) and amodiaquine. Methylene blue as a monotherapy is not recommended for malaria treatment nowadays. It is however used in medicine as a component of a drug prescribed frequently, Prosed®, which is a urinary analgesic/anti-infective/anti-spasmodic medicine. MB is a specific inhibitor of the enzyme glutathione reductase (GR) and it inhibits haem polymerization within the parasite's food vacuole, preventing haem detoxification [276]. This inhibitory effect of GR is one of the probable reasons for the renewed interest in this substance for malaria therapy [6]. Since high levels of glutathione are usually found in the digestive vacuole of resistant strains, it is thought that one of the mechanisms of resistance is the fact that GSH reduces the level of free haem available for CQ binding. Hence PfCRT mutant strains are less susceptible to CQ. This has led to the theory that a combination of CQ with a glutathione reductase inhibitor might help overcome resistance [6]. However, initial studies of MB in combination with CQ showed that they are antagonistic *in vitro*. The combination artesunate-amodiaquine is nowadays one of the ACTs recommended by WHO for the treatment of malaria. MB-AQ could provide an alternative medicine if resistance developed. In trials in Burkina-Faso to treat uncomplicated falciparum malaria in children, a 95% efficacy at day 28 was obtained with the combination AQ-MB [277]. Methylene blue also has the property of preventing methemoglobinemia, a serious complication that may arise in malarial anaemia [276]. MB is also capable of inhibiting gametocyte development at all stages [278], and the combination AQ-MB, two gametocytocidal drugs, could be a potent agent to prevent transmission of malaria and even lead to its eradication in areas where it is used.

Monotherapies in Phase IIA of development include OZ439, a synthetic peroxide **46**. Its IC_{50} values are comparable to those of artemisinin derivatives presently in clinical use [279]. However, due to the fact that this synthetic molecule has a more stable peroxide bond, which, as it happens with the artemisinins, is the unit responsible for activity, the half-life of OZ439 is much longer, approximately 32 h. Clearance is also reduced and the drug shows a much longer blood *versus* time profile [280].

Also at this stage of development is a novel type of antimalarial **47**, spiroindole NITD609. This synthetic molecule, prepared as a single active enantiomer, is as effective as artesunate. Against *P. falciparum* and *P. vivax* strains from the Thai-Burmese border, it showed $IC_{50s} < 10nM$. It is a blood schizonticide, and it kills both mature trophozoite and immature *P. vivax* ring stages, in contrast to the trophozoite stage-specific activity of chloroquine [281]. Its mechanism of action is different from those of existing antimalarial drugs, suppressing protein synthesis in the parasite. Its pharmacokinetic properties are compatible with once a day oral dosing, it has prophylatic activity, and it is a potent inhibitor of gametocytogenesis, blocking transmission to *P. falciparum* [282].

The fact that it was observed in the past that chloroquine analogues with shortened side-chains are good schizonticides, led to the development of another prospective antimalarial, ferroquine **48** [283], a derivative of chloroquine. In this drug, a ferrocene unit replaces the carbon side-chain of chloroquine. Ferroquine has potent activity against *P. vivax* schizont maturation (IC_{50} = 15 nM) and it is also effective against *P. falciparum* [284]. Its mechanism of action is probably similar to that of chloroquine, involving hematin as the drug target and inhibition of hemozoin formation. Since chloroquine is still the most common first-line treatment for *P. vivax* malaria, ferroquine could provide another alternative [285, 286].

A new semi-synthetic second-generation derivative of artemisinin **20**, artemisone **49**, is also being developed. Artemisone and analogues, with a nitrogen substituent at position 10, were designed to have improved bioavailability and metabolic stability over the first generation artemisinin derivatives [287]. These N,O-acetals cannot be metabolised to dihydroartemisinin, and it was thought that in this way the neurotoxicity associated with artemisinin derivatives could be eliminated. In fact, artemisone has a slightly longer half-life than other artemisinin derivatives ($t_{1/2}$ 2.8 h), better bioavailability [288] and it shows no neurotoxicity [289].

Table 5: Endoperoxide Nomenclature [293]

Nomenclature	Structure	Number of Oxygens	Ring Size
1,2-Dioxolane	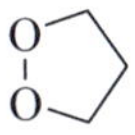	2	5
1,2,4-Trioxolane	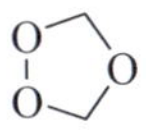	3	5
1,2-Dioxane	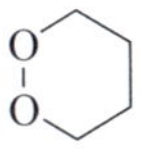	2	6
1,2,4-Trioxane	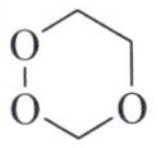	3	6
1,2,4,5-Tetraoxane	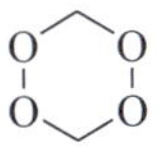	4	6
1,2-Dioxepane	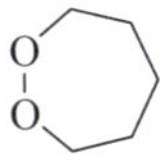	2	7

An antimalarial with an entirely different structure is SAR97276, now named Albitiazolium, a bis-thiazolium compound **50** [263]. This choline analogue inhibits phospholipid metabolism, interfering with plasmodial

Table 6: New Antimalarial Medicines Under Development in the First Quarter of 2012 [266]

Phase of Development	Drug	Active Ingredient and Chemical Class	Properties	Ref.
Waiting registration	A 2.2:1 fixed-dose combination of mefloquine **7** (MQ) and artesunate **23** (AS) [Farmanguinhos/ Drugs for Neglected Diseases Initiative, (DNDi)]	MQ: Quinoline, aryl amino alcohol CAS = 53230-10-7 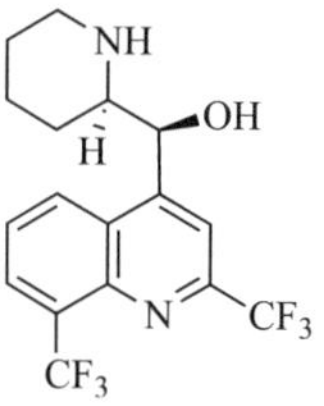 AS: Endoperoxide CAS = 88495-63-0 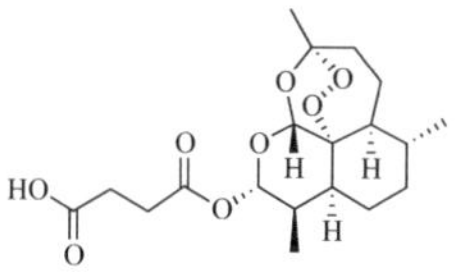 DHA, 21	ACT for the treatment of uncomplicated *P. falciparum* malaria, *P. vivax* malaria, severe malaria. MQ: Synthetic; used as a racemic mixture; it acts as a blood schizonticide effective against erythrocyte stages of *P. falciparum* and *P. vivax*. It inhibits hemozoin formation and hence haem detoxification in the parasite; IC_{50} = 27 nM (*P. falciparum*); $t_{½}$ 2-4 weeks; F (tablet *vs* oral solution) > 85%. AS: Semi-synthetic derivative of artemisinin; blood schizonticide, active on all 4 species of Plasmodium; it has been proposed that it generates fatal free radicals in the lysosomal food vacuole, which damage the parasite, but this may not be the only mechanism of action; IC_{50} = 1.62 nM (*P. falciparum*); $t_{½}$ 1 h; F(oral) = 61%. ACT pharmacokinetics: [8:4 mg kg^{-1}/day MQ:AS for 3 d]: For MQ: C_{max} 2,202 ng mL^{-1}, T_{max} 2.4 d, $AUC_{0-\infty}$ 31,395 d ng mL^{-1}, $t_{½}$ = 10.5 d; PCT = 48 h.	[1, 58, 159, 293-295]
Waiting registration	Artesunate **23** intrarectal (i.r.) [WHO/ The special Programme for Research and Training in Tropical Diseases (TDR)]	AS: Structure as above in this table.	For the treatment of acute malaria. AS is quickly converted in the body to dihydroartemisinin (DHA), the active metabolite, by blood esterases and the hepatic metabolism. Pharmacokinetics of the suppositories (DHA): 10 mg kg^{-1} suppositories: F = 58%, PCT = 20 h; 20 mg kg^{-1} suppositories: F = 23%, PCT = 22 h. For both (mean): C_{max} 4.5 μM, T_{max} 0.2 h, AUC = 4.1 h μmol L^{-1}, $t_{½}$ 0.3 h.	[296-298]

(Table 6) contd…..

Phase of Development	Drug	Active Ingredient and Chemical Class	Properties	Ref.
Phase IIb/III	A fixed-dose combination of azithromycin **35** (AZ) and chloroquine **3** (CQ) (Pfizer)	AZ: macrolide antibiotic, of the azalide class CAS = 83905-01-5 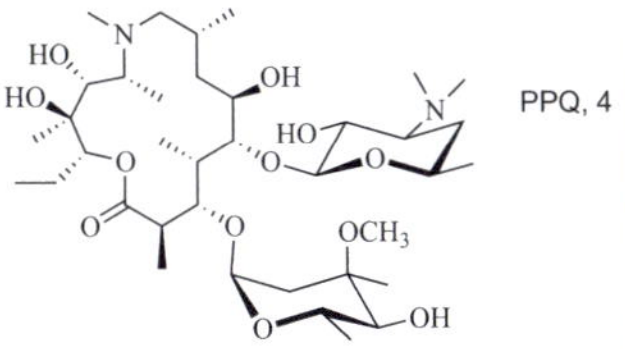 CQ: 4-aminoquinoline CAS = 54-05-7 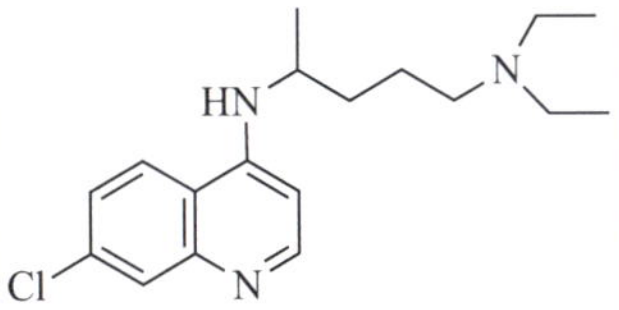 	To be adopted as Intermittent Preventative Treatment in Pregnant Women. The combination is designed to be synergistic against CQ-resistant strains of *P. falciparum*. It may simultaneously have activity against bacterial sexually-transmitted diseases. AZ: Semi-synthetic widely used broad-spectrum antibiotic; it is also an efficient blood schizonticide; it inhibits protein biosynthesis inside the apicoplast; destruction of this plastid prevents the parasite from entering a new cell; IC_{50} (laboratory strains) = 3.0-6.5 μM, IC_{50} (wild isolates) = 29.3 μM (*P. falciparum*); $t_{½}$ 68 h; F = 37%. CQ: Synthetic, highly effective against erythrocytic forms of *P. vivax*, *P. ovale* and *P. malariae*, sensitive strains of *P. falciparum* and gametocytes of *P. vivax;* it is thought to inhibit heme polymerase activity, resulting in accumulation of free heme, toxic to the parasites; IC_{50} = 49.8 ng mL^{-1} (*P. vivax*); IC_{50} = 167 nM (*P. falciparum*); $t_{½}$ 1-2 months F = 89% (as phosphate, in tablets). AZ+CQ: the pharmacokinetics of the two drugs when used alone or in combination are very similar. Together, they are effective against CQ-resistant *P. falciparum in vivo*.	[58, 299-305]

(Table 6) contd.....

Phase of Development	Drug	Active Ingredient and Chemical Class	Properties	Ref.
Phase IIb/III	Tafenoquine **42** (WR-238605) (GlaxoSmith-Kline)	8-aminoquinoline CAS = 106635-81-8 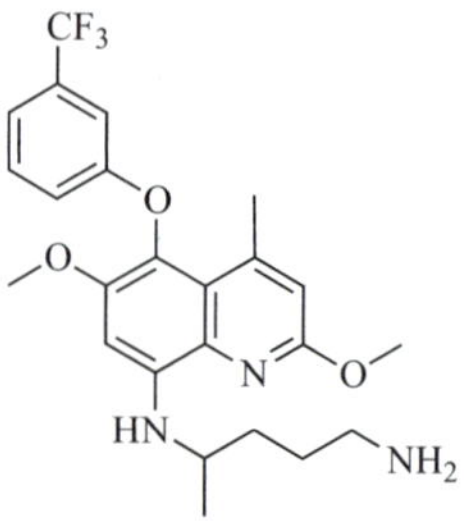	For the treatment of *P. vivax* (relapsing) malaria. Synthetic; active against the dormant liver form of *P. vivax* (the hypnozoites) *in vitro* and in patients. It is thought to act by inhibiting electron transport in the respiratory chain and to inhibit heme polymerization. This is the only molecule in the pipeline with activity against *P. vivax* hypnozoites. IC_{50} = 9.7 μM (wild strains of *P. vivax*); $t_{½}$ 2 weeks. It is also active against all stages of *P. falciparum*: IC_{50} = 4.43 μM (wild strains in Central, West and East Africa); IC_{50} = 0.06-0.3 μM in MDR *P. falciparum* lines.	[6, 53, 306-308]
Phase IIb/III	Pyramax® Paediatric: a 3:1 fixed-dose combination of pyronaridine **39** (PYR) and artesunate **23** (AS) (Shin Poong Pharmaceuticals/ University of Iowa)	PYR: 9-anilinoazaacridine CAS = 74847-35-1 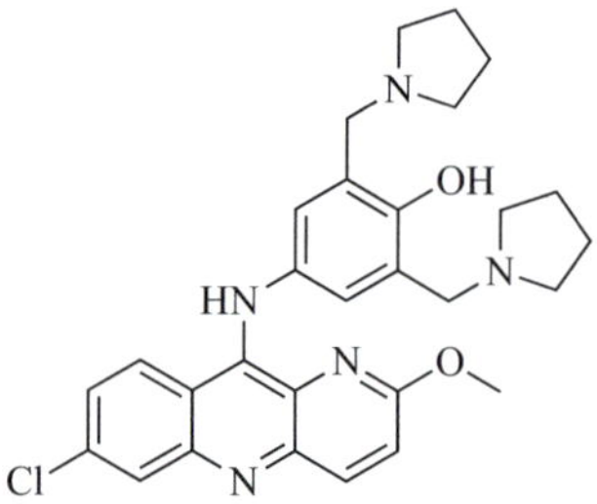 AS: Endoperoxide Structure as above in this table	For uncomplicated *P. falciparum* malaria and for the blood stage of *P. vivax* malaria. A child-friendly granule formulation developed for use in paediatric patients from 3 months. PYR: Synthetic drug that inhibits the formation of β-haematin, preventing the malarial parasite from neutralising haem, thus being toxic to it. IC_{50} = 1.92 nM (*P. falciparum*); IC_{50} = 2.58 (*P. vivax*). AS: Information as above in this table. Pharmacokinetics of the granules (9:3 mg kg^{-1} dose of ACT): PYR: C_{max} 168 ng mL^{-1}, T_{max} 2.4 h, $AUC_{0-\infty}$ 25,325 h ng mL^{-1}, $t_{½}$ = 6.7 d; AS: C_{max} 171 ng mL^{-1}, T_{max} 0.5 h, $AUC_{0-\infty}$ 179 h ng mL^{-1}, $t_{½}$ = 1.2 h; PCT = 8 h.	[58, 293, 309-311]

(Table 6) contd…..

Phase of Development	Drug	Active Ingredient and Chemical Class	Properties	Ref.
Phase IIb/III	Euratesim® Paediatric: a 1:8 fixed-dose combination of dihydroartemi-sinin **21** (DHA) and piperaquine **4** (PPQ) Sigma-Tau Pharmaceuticals Inc./MMV	DHA: Endoperoxide CAS = 71939-50-9 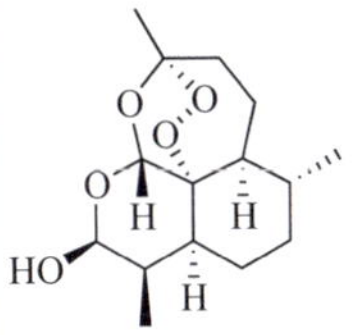 PPQ: 4-aminoquinoline; bisquinolone CAS = 4085-31-8; 85547-56-4 (phosphate) 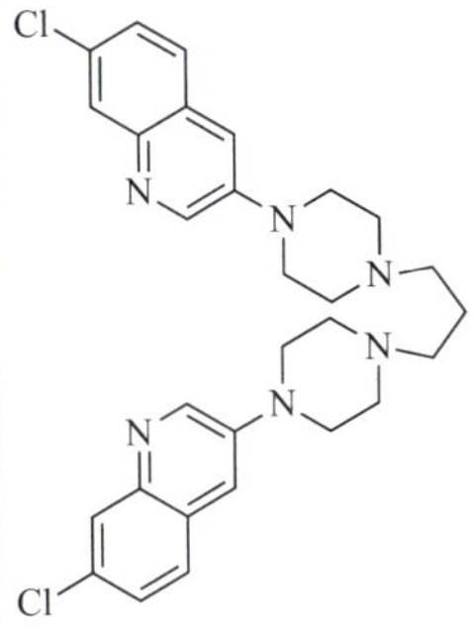	Child-friendly dispersible formulation of the ACT to treat uncomplicated *P. falciparum* malaria in infants and children. The adult formulation is recommended for *P. vivax* too. DHA: Semi-synthetic derivative of artemisinin, potent blood schizonticide; it has been proposed that it generates fatal free radicals in the lysosomal food vacuole, which damage the parasite, but this may not be the only mechanism of action; IC_{50} = 1.22 nM; $t_{½}$ = 0.36 h. PPQ: Synthetic drug; it inhibits the parasite by binding to toxic haem (derived from the patient's haemoglobin) within the malaria parasite, and preventing its detoxification *via* a polymerisation step. IC_{50} = 36-41 nM (field isolates in Africa); $t_{½}$ = 23 days. Pharmokinetics for children (DHA+PPQ tetraphosphate, three daily 2.5:20 mg kg^{-1} doses as tablets): PPQ: $AUC_{0-\infty}$ = 44,556 µg h^{-1} L^{-1}; $t_{½}$ (PPQ) 20 d; $t_{½}$ (DHA) > 1.2 h. PCT (standard dosage of 2.25 mg kg^{-1} and 18 mg kg^{-1} per dose of DHA and PPQ, for uncomplicated malaria) = 2 days.	[6, 312-317]
Phase IIb/III	Synriam®: a 1.5:7.5 fixed-dose combination of arterolane **41** (AR) (OZ277, RBX 11160) and piperaquine **4** (PPQ) (Ranbaxy Laboratories)	AR: Endoperoxide CAS = 664338-39-0 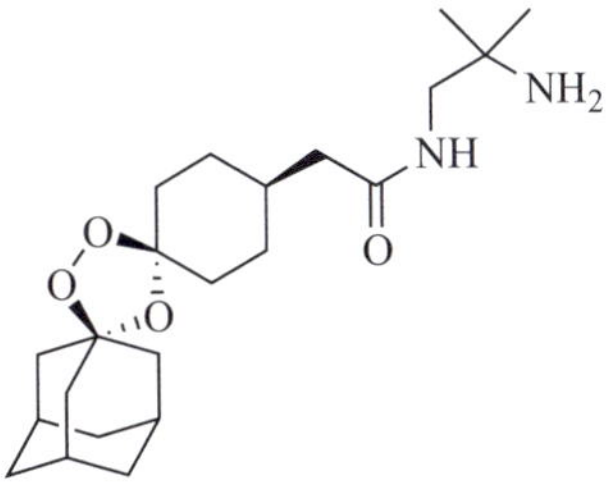 PPQ: aminoquinoline; bis-quinolone, as phosphate Structure as above in this table	For the treatment of uncomplicated *P. falciparum* malaria. AR: synthetic 1,2,4-trioxolane; a blood schizonticide. IC_{50} = 1.5 nM (*P. falciparum*), $t_{½}$ = 0.8-4.2 h. Pharmacokinetics of arterolane (once a day for 7 days, in uncomplicated falciparum malaria): for a 100 mg dose, on day 1, $AUC_{0\rightarrow8}$ = 105 h ng mL^{-1}; for a 200 mg dose, 239 h ng mL^{-1}. Median PCT (both doses) 32 h. PPQ: data as above in this table. Pharmacokinetics (AR:PPQ 150 mg AR maleate and 750 mg PPQ phosphate): PCT = 30 hours;	[318-320]

(Table 6) contd.....

Phase of Development	Drug	Active Ingredient and Chemical Class	Properties	Ref.
Phase IIb/III	Co-trimoxazole (Bactrim): a 1:5 fixed-dose combination of trimethoprim **37** (TMP) and sulphamethoxazole **38** (SMZ) (Institute of Tropical Medicine)	TMP: Diaminopyrimidine CAS = 738-70-5 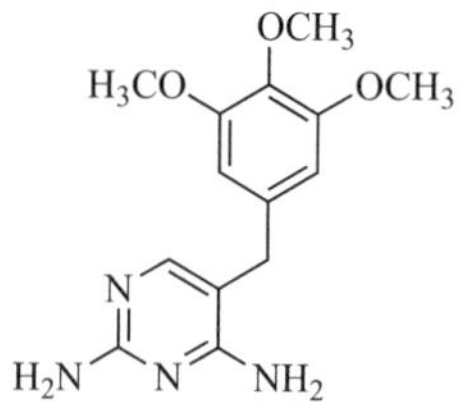 SMZ: Anilinosulphonamide CAS = 723-46-6 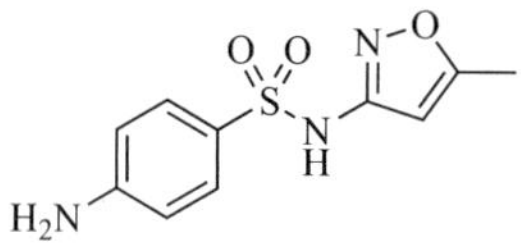	The combination is an antibiotic used to treat various bacterial infections, but also effective in malaria treatment and prophylaxis. It inhibits successive steps in folate synthesis, an essential part of the thymidine synthesis pathway, thus preventing the synthesis of nucleotides necessary for DNA replication. Together they have a synergistic effect. Recommended as part of the treatment for people infected with HIV and with AIDS. TMP: synthetic; it blocks folic acid synthesis in the microorganism by inhibiting dihydrofolate reductase; EC_{50} = 2.5 × 10^{-8} M (*in vitro*); $t_{½}$ 8-11 h ; F (oral): 85-90%. SMZ: Synthetic anilinosulphonamide; it inhibits dihydropteroate synthetase, an enzyme involved further upstream in the thymidine synthesis pathway; EC_{50} = 1.2 × 10^{-7} M (*in vitro*); $t_{½}$ 10 h. Pharmacokinetics of TMP+SMZ [TMP 20 mg kg^{-1}, SMZ 100 mg kg^{-1}, administered orally for 3 days, divided in 3 portions taken every 6 h]: TMP: C_{max} 13.6 μgmL^{-1}, T_{max} 1.9 h, $AUC_{0-\infty}$ 70.9 h mgL^{-1}; $t_{½}$ = 13.6 h; SMZ: C_{max} 372 μg mL^{-1}, T_{max} 2.6 h, $AUC_{0-\infty}$ 2,069 h mg L^{-1}, $t_{½}$ = 14.0 h. PCT (acute uncomplicated malaria) = 2.9 days in adults; 2.6 days in children.	[58, 321-326]

(Table 6) contd…..

Phase of Development	Drug	Active Ingredient and Chemical Class	Properties	Ref.
Phase IIb/III	ARCO^{TM}: a 2.5:1 fixed-dose combination of artemisinin **20** (ART) and naphthoquine **40** (NQ) Kunming Pharmaceutical Corporation (KPC)	ART: Endoperoxide CAS = 63968-64-9 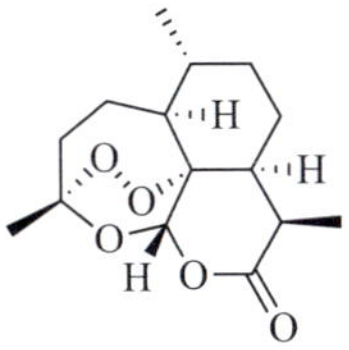 NQ: 4-aminoquinoline CAS = 663215-06-3 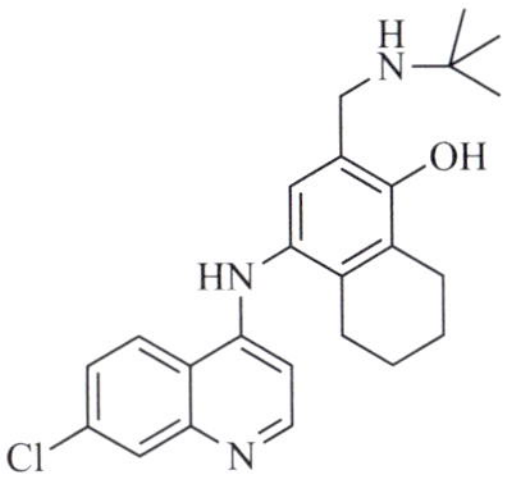	ACT indicated for the treatment of all forms of malaria, including multi-drug resistant malaria. ART: Isolated from the plant *Artemisia annua*. It has been proposed that it generates fatal free radicals in the lysosomal food vacuole, which damage the parasite, but this may not be the only mechanism of action; Fast schizonticidal action. IC_{50} = 12.1 nm-21nM; $t_{½}$ = 1.9-2.61 h. NQ: Synthetic, registered in China in 1993; a *P. falciparum* schizonticide; IC_{50} = 7.0 nM (*P. falciparum*); $t_{½}$ 276 h. Pharmacokinetics (ART+NQ) [single dose 1,000 mg ART/400 mg NQ]: The combination increases $AUC_{(0\rightarrow t)}$ and C_{max} of both components relative to their monotherapies. The increases are: ART: $AUC_{(0\rightarrow t)}$ 71%, C_{max} 49%; NQ: $AUC_{(0\rightarrow t)}$ 135%, C_{max} 104%. With various doses, $t_{½}$ = 255 h; PCT = 21-28 h. ED_{50} (combination) = 8.5 mg kg^{-1}.	[6, 126, 300, 327-332]
Phase IIb/III	Argemone Mexicana (Mali/Geneva)		Mexican poppy or prickly poppy, of the *Papaveraceae* family. A decoction made from extracts of the aerial parts of the plant is used by traditional healers in Mali to cure malaria. IC_{50} = 1.00-5.89 µg mL^{-1} (*P. falciparum* chloroquine-resistant K1 strain)	[270-271]
Phase IIb/III	PR 259 CT1 (DRC/Antwerp)	CAS = 23141-25-5 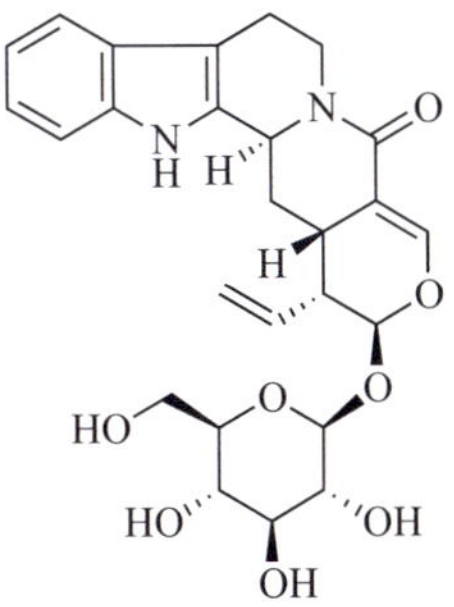	An antimalarial herbal medicinal consisting of a quantified 80% ethanol extract from the stem bark of *Nauclea pobeguinii*, a plant of the Rubiaceae family. It has been shown to display moderate *in vitro* activity against *P. falciparum*; IC_{50} = 32-44 µg mL^{-1}. Strictosamide **43** is the major alkaloid present.	[272]

(Table 6) contd…..

Phase of Development	Drug	Active Ingredient and Chemical Class	Properties	Ref.
Phase IIb/III	ArTiMist: a sublingual formulation of artemether **22** (AM) (Proto Pharma Ltd)	AM: Endoperoxide CAS = 71963-77-4 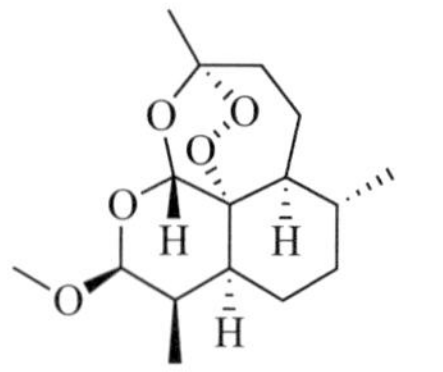	A sublingual spray to treat *P. falciparum* uncomplicated malaria in young children and infants. Also effective for severe malaria. AM is a semi-synthetic derivative of artemisinin. It has properties and a mode of action similar to those of artemisinin, including gametocytocidal activity. IC_{50} = 1.54-16.2 nM (wild isolates). Pharmacokinetics [6× 3 mg kg^{-1} doses of ArTiMist at 0, 8, 24, 36, 48, 60 h]: for AM: C_{max} = 271 ng mL^{-1}, T_{max} = 1.6 h, $AUC_{0-\infty}$ 1,004 h ng mL^{-1}, $t_{½}$ = 4.5 h; for DHA: C_{max} = 106.5 ng mL^{-1}, T_{max} = 1.75 h. F = 2.5 × F (oral artemether). PCT_{90} = 17.6 h.	[6, 53, 333]
Phase IIa	OZ439 Monash Institute of Pharmaceutical Sciences/University of Nebraska Medical Centre/ Swiss Tropical and Public Health Institute (Monash/ UNMC/STI)	Endoperoxide **46** CAS = 1029939-86-3 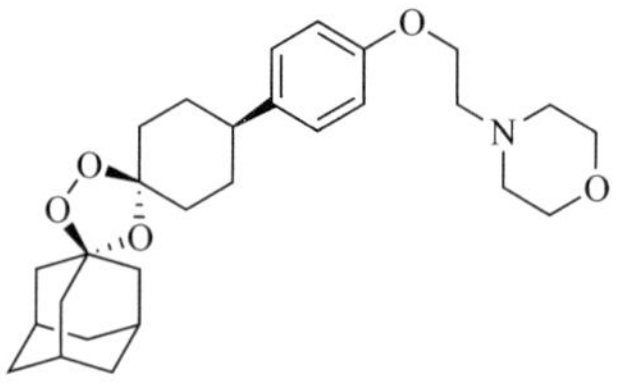	Synthetic peroxide, a 1,2,4-trioxolane, with similar efficacy as artemisinin against both *P. falciparum* and *P. vivax*. It inhibits gametocyte maturation/gamete formation and impact sporogony. It is thought to act by alkylating haem and other molecules and degrading membrane phospholipids. IC_{50} = 1.6-1.9 ng mL^{-1} (*P. falciparum* strains); it has *in vitro* activity against all asexual erythrocytic stages: IC_{50} = 1.9, 3.0, and 2.8 ng mL^{-1} for rings, trophozoites, and schizonts. Pharmacokinetics (single dose, 800 mg): C_{max} 315 ng mL^{-1}, T_{max} 3.0 h, $AUC_{0-\infty}$ 4,690 h ng mL^{-1}, $t_{½}$ = 27.9 h; (single dose, 1,200 mg): C_{max} 701 ng mL^{-1}, T_{max} 3.0 h, $AUC_{0-\infty}$ 9,130 h ng mL^{-1}, $t_{½}$ = 31.6 h; the PK parameters were approximately dose proportional.	[280, 293, 334]

(Table 6) contd…..

Phase of Development	Drug	Active Ingredient and Chemical Class	Properties	Ref.
Phase IIa	NITD609 (Novartis Institute for Tropical Diseases)	Spiroindole **47** CAS = 1193314-23-6 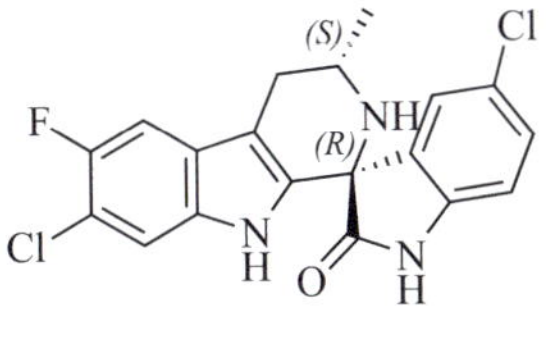	Synthetic molecule; potent against the intraerythrocytic stages of *P. falciparum* and *P. vivax*. It inhibits protein synthesis in *P. falciparum*. It targets both liver and blood stages of the parasite. One of only a handful of molecules capable of completely curing a *P. berghei* model of blood-stage malaria. At a high concentration (≈100 × IC_{50} value), all stages of the parasite (rings, trophozoites, and schizonts) are similarly sensitive. At low concentrations (≈1 or 10 × IC_{50} value), schizonts are the most susceptible. It also inhibits gametocytogenesis. IC_{50} = 0.5-1.4 nM (*P. falciparum* laboratory strains); IC_{50}< 10nM (*P. falciparum* and *P. vivax* blood isolates) Human phase II trials begin in 2012.	[281, 335]
Phase IIa	Ferroquine **48** (Sanofi-Aventis)	4-Aminoquinoline CAS = 185055-67-8 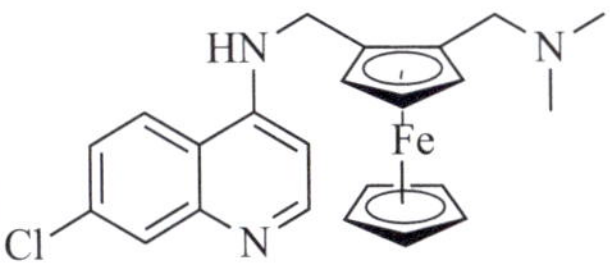	A ferrocenic derivative of chloroquine being developed to treat *P. falciparum* malaria. It may be useful for the treatment of drug-resistant *P. vivax* malaria too. The mechanism of action is probably similar to that of chloroquine, with hematin as the drug target. IC_{50} = 14-42 nM (laboratory strains of *P. falciparum*); IC_{50} = 1-62 nM (field isolates); IC_{50} (*ex vivo P. vivax* schizont maturation) = 15 nM. Pharmacokinetics in asymptomatic carriers of *P. falciparum* infections (400-1200 mg dose): C_{max} = 82-270 ng mL^{-1}, T_{max} = 6.00-5.52 h; (400-1,600 mg dose): AUC = 13,100-49,200 h ng mL^{-1}; $t_{½}$ 16 d.	[6, 336-338]

(Table 6) contd…..

Phase of Development	Drug	Active Ingredient and Chemical Class	Properties	Ref.
Phase IIa	A fixed-dose combination of fosmidomycin **44** (FOS) and piperaquine **4** (PPQ) (Jomaa Pharma GMbH) (and MMV)	FOS: N-Hydroxyformamide phosphonic acid CAS = 185055-67-8 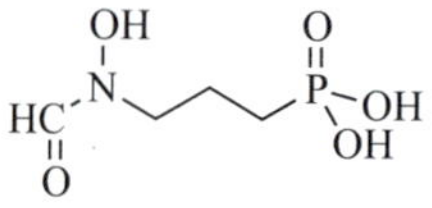 PPQ: structure as above in the table	For the treatment of acute *P. falciparum* malaria. FOS: It was initially developed as an antibacterial agent. In malaria it is an effective blood schizonticide. It acts on *P. falciparum* by inhibiting 1-deoxy-D-xylulose 5-phosphate reductoisomerase, a key enzyme in the non-mevalonate pathway of isoprenoid biosynthesis. It blocks biosynthesis of isoprenoids, essential for cellular functions in *P. falciparum*. The pathway is different in humans, which are therefore not affected. IC_{50} = 400 nM. It is the most potent and rapid acting antibiotic against malaria. Fosmidomycin pharmokinetics [1200 mg dose every 8 h for 7 days]: in patients with acute uncomplicated *P. falciparum* malaria, C_{max} = 4.58 μg mL^{-1}, T_{max} 2 h, $AUC_{0-\infty}$ = 29.7 h μg mL^{-1}, $t_{½}$ 3.4 h; PCT = 44 h. PPQ: as above in the table. Fosmidomycin + PQ: trials will start at the end of 2011 in Thailand.	[6, 274, 339]
Phase IIa	A fixed-dose combination of methylene blue **45** (MB) and amodiaquine **5** (AQ) (University of Heidelberg)	MB: Phenothiazinium derivative CAS = 61-73-4 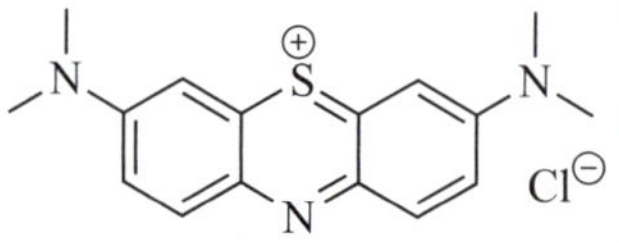 AQ: 4-Aminoquinoline CAS = 86-42-0 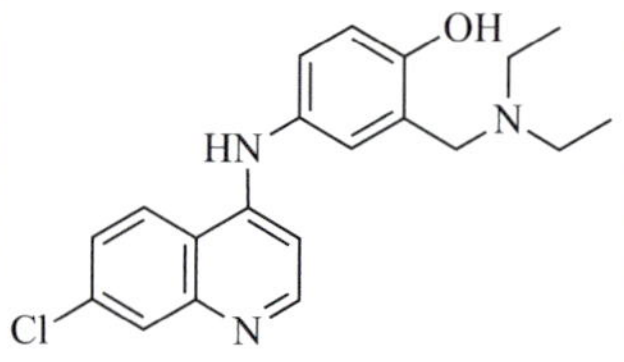	MB was one of the first synthetic drugs used against malaria. Not recommended for this purpose nowadays. The combination is being studied for this purpose. It has a gametocytocidal effect. MB: A gametocytocide; it acts by inhibiting disulfide reductases and heme detoxification. For European Pharmacopoeia-grade MB, Proveblue, mean IC_{50} = 3.62 nM (against 23 *Plasmodium falciparum* strains from several countries). AQ: Aminoquinoline with anti-inflammatory properties. It is indicated for the treatment of acute malaria. The combination: In a study MB-AQ gave adequate clinical and parasitological response after 14 days.	[53, 58, 340]

(Table 6) contd.....

Phase of Development	Drug	Active Ingredient and Chemical Class	Properties	Ref.
Phase IIa	Artemisone **49** (AMS) Hong Kong University of Science and Technology (UHKST)	Endoperoxide CAS = 255730-18-8 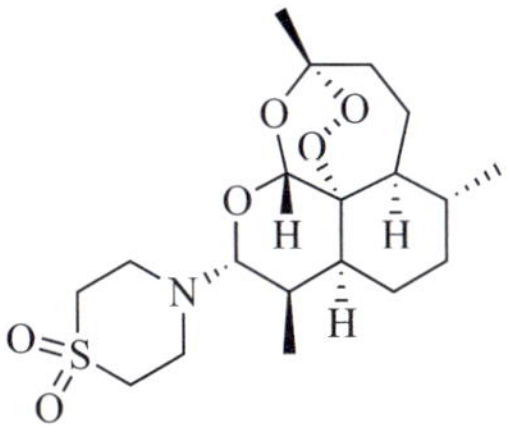	For the treatment of *P. falciparum* malaria. Semi-synthetic derivative of artemisinin, with no neurotoxicity. It is a non-lipophilic drug. The probable drug target is the parasite's Ca^{2+} pump *Pf*ATP6. IC_{50} < 1 nM (*P. falciparum* strains); EC_{50}= 0.14 nM (*P. falciparum* isolates). Pharmacokinetics (single 80 mg oral dose): C_{max} = 140.2 ng mL^{-1}, T_{max} = 0.875 h, AUC = 281.6 h ng mL^{-1}, $t_{½}$ 2.79 h. In a phase IIa trial with patients infected with uncomplicated malaria, after oral AMS (2 mg kg^{-1}/d) for 2 days, MFQ (25 mg kg^{-1}) on day 2: PCT = 26 h.	[287, 341-343]
Phase IIa	Albitiazolium **50** (SAR97276, T3/SAR97276) (Sanofi Aventis)	Bis-thiazolium compound CAS = 321915-72-4 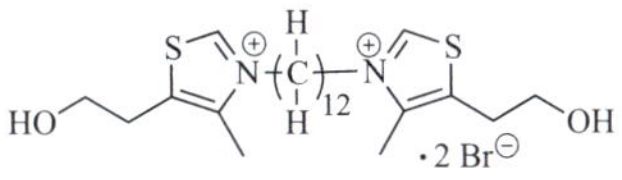	For the treatment of *P. falciparum* malaria. It targets the phospholipid metabolism of *P. falciparum.* *P. falciparum* asexual blood stages: IC_{50} = 3 nM;	[344, 345]

phosphatidylcholine biosynthesis in infected erythrocytes [290, 291]. This potent antimalarial, with an IC_{50} of 3 nM, has low bioavailability because of its two permanent cationic charges, and the development of prodrugs, which overcome this drawback, is the subject of active research [292].

Drugs in Phase I and in a Stage of Preclinical Development (see Table 7)

Two potent new 4-aminoquinolines are now in Phase I of development: GSK369796, N-*tert*-butyl isoquine **51**, structurally analogous to amodiaquine, and AQ13, CQ-analogue **52** with a shorter side-chain. GSK369796 is a fluorinated derivative of amodiaquine, designed to be a cheap antimalarial to overcome CQ-resistance [346]. In addition it was hoped that it would not be hepatotoxic or promote agranulocytosis, two conditions that may arise with prolonged administration of amodiaquine, and have led to some restrictions on its use. It turned out to be more resistant to metabolic cleavage than amodiaquine, and when tested, it did not cause gene mutations or chromosomal damage *in vitro* in a bacterial mutation assay and mouse lymphoma assay or in an *in vivo* mouse micronucleus assay [346].

AQ13 is predicted to have a similar mode of action to chloroquine, but the presence of the shorter side chain might enable the compound to overcome the parasite's resistance mechanism to chloroquine. It is active against multi-drug resistant strains of *P. falciparum* [347]. A Phase I trial has already been carried out with humans [348]. CQ was compared with chloroquine, and no hematologic, hepatic, renal, or other organ toxicity was observed with AQ-13 or with chloroquine at the doses tested. AQ-13 was cleared more rapidly than CQ and QTc prolongation was greater with CQ than AQ-13. There were minimal differences in toxicity between the two compounds and the pharmacokinetics were similar. AQ-13 has a shorter half-life of 14.3 days *versus* 23.3 days for CQ, but a slightly lower bioavailability too: the mean AUC was 140.8 μM for AQ-13 *versus* 241.2 μM for CQ, which implies that a slightly higher dose of AQ-13 may be necessary in treatment. The results indicated that this drug should proceed to further trials to determine its efficiency treating malaria [349].

NPC-1161-B is an 8-aminoquinoline in a phase of preclinical development. It has potent antimalarial action against the blood and tissue stages of *Plasmodium*. This primaquine analogue **53** was prepared originally as a racemic mixture, NPC-1161-C. When the two enantiomers were separated, it was found that the (-)-enantiomer, NPC-1161-B, was several times more active than the (+)-enantiomer in its antiparasitic activity *in vivo* [350]. When the racemic compound was tested in animal models, administered orally in multiple doses at 1 mg kg^{-1} of body weight for 3 days, it gave 100% cure rate and did not show any toxicity at the highest dose tested (64 mg kg^{-1} for 3 days). It also showed promising antimalarial efficacy for radical cure [349]. NPC-1161-B is also active against other protozoa, like the *Leishmania*.

New synthetic endoperoxides are also at these two stages of development [351]: CDRI 97-98, RKA 182 and SAR116242. CDRI, 1,2,4-trioxane **54**, was developed to be used against multidrug-resistant *P. falciparum* and to treat cerebral malaria. When *Anopheles stephenses* mosquitoes were fed on blood from gametocyte carrying *P. cytnomolei* and *P. yoelii* models [352], the oocysts which developed had no infectivity if this trioxane had been previously administered to the hosts, which showed the gametocytocidal activity of CDRI 97-98, and its potential transmission blocking activity.

RKA 182, diaspiro compound **55**, was selected out from a series of 150 novel 1,2,4,5-tetraoxanes during a study on thc antimalarial properties of these molecules [353]. Since it was known that fusion of an adamantane moiety to the 1,2,4-trioxolane system was essential for good antimalarial activity in the ozonide series, this moiety was also incorporated in the new diaspiro peroxide. It was found that the diaspiro compounds were more stable than their 1,2,4-trioxolane or 1,2,4-trioxane counterparts. RKA 182 has superior properties to the semi-synthetic artemisinins in current use [353]. It is water soluble, having solubility greater than 40 mg mL^{-1}, and it has IC_{50s} less than 6 nM against CQ-sensitive and CQ-resistant *P. falciparum* strains. Its half-life is between that of OZ277 and OZ439 [354]. It was also demonstrated that it forms adducts resulting from the formation of covalent bonds between carbon atoms of the haem porphyrin ring and carbon radicals generated from the tetraoxane peroxide ring system [353]. The demonstration that RKA 182 can alkylate haem is in line with what is expected to occur with peroxide-containing antimalarials, on the basis of current knowledge on the mechanism of action of these compounds. Although the exact mechanism of action artemisinin and its derivatives is not entirely clear yet, and more than one target has been suggested (see under The Artemisinins), haem alkylation is thought to be one of the ways in which these and other peroxide antimalarials interact with *Plasmodia* leading to their destruction. As the parasite degrades the host's haemoglobin, toxic free haem is produced which, to eliminate, the parasite converts into the redox-inactive iron (III) polymer, hemozoin. When peroxide drugs interact with iron (II)-haem, short-lived alkoxy radicals are produced, which quickly rearrange to C-centered primary radicals. These carbon radicals can alkylate haem *via* an intramolecular process to produce covalent haem-drug adducts [355], resulting in the accumulation of redox-active haem derivatives, thought to be toxic to the parasite. The ability of synthetic trioxanes or trioxolanes to alkylate haem correlates well with their antimalarial activity [355]. Although RKA contains two peroxide bonds, and scale-up of the chemistry related to its synthesis could be potentially dangerous, a safe method to produce it on industrial kilogram-scale was developed using the Dussault's protocol, in which Re_2O_7 is used as a mild Lewis acid to generate the key tetraoxane ring, without the need for isolation of the required intermediate gem-dihydroperoxide [353].

SAR116242 is a hybrid molecule consisting of a 1,2,4-trioxane moiety and an aminoquinoline moiety, and hence it is named a trioxaquine. It is expected that by having two distinct pharmacophores, molecule **56** will have the activity characteristic of both [356]. In fact SAR116242 is highly active *in vitro* against several sensitive and resistant strains of *P. falciparum* at nanomolar concentrations. This drug was selected from a collection of 120 hybrid molecules. Its dual mode of action was shown: not only was SAR116242 able to inhibit the polymerization of β-hematin as CQ does, but it also promoted haem alkylation *via* the production of free radicals, indicated by the formation of several haem adducts [356]. This drug showed nearly the same transepithelial permeability as chloroquine (P_{tot} between 10 and 20 x 10^{-7} cm s^{-1}), which suggests that oral absorption will be efficient. Tests to show its toxicological profile revealed no mutagenic or clastogenic activity [357]. Once it was demonstrated that the two diastereoisomers have the same *in vitro* activities, subsequent tests were carried out using a mixture of both diastereoisomers. Recent reports indicate, however, that further development of this drug may have been discontinued [354].

A new substance is also being developed for adjunctive therapy, DF-02, or sevuparin sodium **57**. DF-02 is derived from heparin, a naturally occurring polysaccharide, after depolymerization [354]. Heparin is used in medicine, as an anticoagulant, to prevent thrombosis. It has been used in malaria in the past, but its use has been discontinued due to the occurrence of haemostatic side effects such as bleedings. Adjunctive therapy is an additional or secondary therapy given in malaria together with a schizonticide to reduce the effects of malaria. DF-02 has much lower anti-coagulation activity than heparin [358]. In malaria it prevents rosetting, a condition that develops in severe malaria, when *P. falciparum*-parasitized erythrocytes bind to uninfected erythrocytes blocking the flow of blood in the capillaries of the brain and other organs, and hence causing severe complications [359]. DF-02 has been shown to be safe for used in humans [358].

A few nitrogen-containing heterocycles are at these stages of development. The most advanced is GNF156, in Phase I, synthetic imidazolopiperazine **58**. Imidazolopiperazines are novel scaffolds to the antimalarial arsenal [360]. GNF156 resulted from optimization after SAR studies on a series of analogues found to have good antimalarial activity [361]. It is active against the blood, liver and gametocyte stages of Plasmodium but not against the hypnozoites [354].

There are also other piperazine-based antimalarials now a preclinical phase of development, by Actelion Pharmaceuticals. The structures of 14 compounds with general structure **59**, with IC_{50s} of less than 20 nM against P. falciparum have been revealed [362].

There are also two pyrimidine derivatives at this stage of development, DSM265 and P218. DSM265, synthetic triazolopyrimidine **60**, was found to be a *P. falciparum* dihydroorotate dehydrogenase (DHODH) inhibitor, potent against CQ-sensitive and resistant *P. falciparum* strains. The enzyme DHODH catalyzes the rate-limiting step in the pyrimidine biosynthetic pathway (Fig. **10**). Since *P. falciparum* is unable to salvage pyrimidines and must rely on *de novo* biosynthesis for survival, DSM265 leads to parasite death. Human studies are planned for early 2013 [363]. P218 or **61** is a dihydrofolate reductase inhibitor, and hence it prevents folic acid synthesis by the parasite [364].

BCX4945 is another DNA synthesis blocker currently under development. *P. falciparum* is a purine auxotroph. It can't synthesize the purines it requires for synthesis of nucleotides, co-factors, and nucleic acids, but it uses the enzyme purine nucleoside phosphorylase (PNP) to synthesize hypoxanthine. Hypoxanthine is then converted to inosine monophosphate (IMP), a precursor for all the purines, by the action of hypoxanthine-guanine-xanthine phosphoribosyl-transferase (PfHGXPRT). This pyrimidine **62** is a transition state analogue and inhibitor of PNP [365]. When the action of PNP is blocked, the parasites are killed in culture by purine starvation. PNP inhibition is an attractive option, since it is a new target for malaria treatment.

In a screen of approximately 70,000 compounds in the Broad Institute's small molecule library and the ICCB-L compound collection at Harvard Medical

School, Genz-644442, an aminoindole, was selected as a novel lead compound for malaria treatment [366]. Based on its structure, a library of 321 aminoindoles was selected for screening, which led finally to Genz-668764 being selected for further studies in representation of this novel class of antimalarials. Single enantiomer **63** has IC_{50} values in the range 28-65 nM against *P. falciparum in vitro*.

MK4815, aminoalkylphenol **64**, is an inhibitor of the electron transport chain in the mitochondrion, which when administered concentrates in infected erythrocytes. It is active against *P. falciparum* drug-resistant strains in the low nanomolar range, and at present it is in a preclinical stage of development [367]. Tests showed that this antimalarial is most effective against the metabolically active late trophozoite and early schizont stages of the parasite's life cycle. Since it is a small molecule readily synthesized from cheap starting materials, it is an attractive option for an antimalarial.

THE PRESENT DAY PANORAMA, MARKET SHORTCOMINGS AND CONCLUSIONS

When the UN adopted in 2000, as one of its goals for the Millennium, to halt and begin to reverse the incidence of malaria by the year 2015, several initiatives were set in motion to achieve this (see also The Pipeline of Antimalarials in Development). To prevent transmission at community level greater efforts at vector control were adopted. In the African region alone the percentage of indoor residual spraying rose from less than 5% in 2005 to 11% in 2010 and the number of households owing at least one insecticide-treated net (ITN) increased from 3% in 2000 to 53% in 2011 in the sub-Sahara [2]. By 2011, 32 countries in the African region and 78 other countries where malaria is endemic had adopted WHO's recommendation to provide ITNs to persons at risk of malaria and many distributed them free of charge [2]. Sub-Saharan Africa has the greatest burden of malaria, with 90% of the worldwide number of malaria-related deaths occurring in this region. The economic consequences are severe too, and malaria uses up to 2% of the gross domestic product of countries in this region. Since pregnant women and children are the most vulnerable to the disease, besides vector control

Table 7: New Antimalarial Medicines in Phase I or Preclinical Development in the First Quarter of 2012 [266]

Phase of Development	Drug	Active Ingredient and Chemical Class	Properties	Ref.
Phase I	GNF156 (Novartis)	Imidazolopiperazine **58** 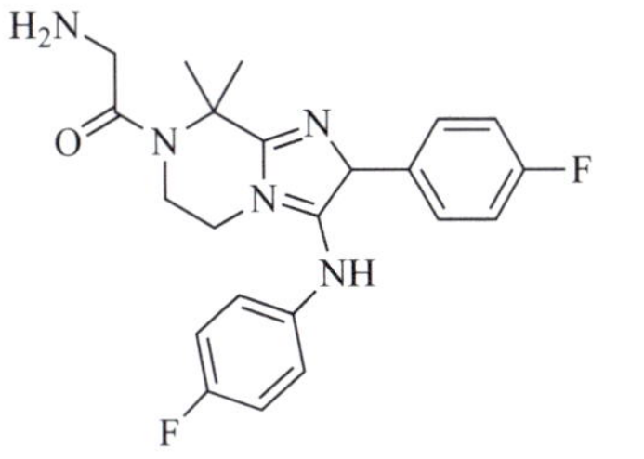	Imidazole-based compound, synthetic. *In vitro* activity: IC_{50} = 6 and 10 nM respectively against W2 and 3D7 *P. falciparum* multidrug resistant strains. Active against the blood, liver and gametocyte stages of *Plasmodium*.	[361, 368]
Phase I	CDRI 97-78 (IPCA Pharmaceuticals Ltd.)	1,2,4-Trioxane **54** 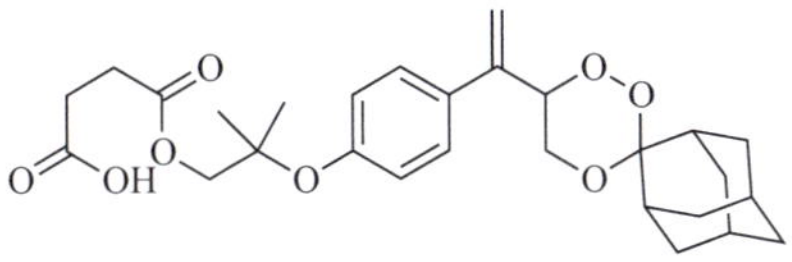	Synthetic. To be used against drug resistant *P. falciparum* and cerebral malaria.	[352]
Phase I	DF02 (Sevuparin sodium) (Dilafor)	Depolymerized heparin **57**	Semi-synthetic; obtained from the glycosaminoglycan heparin. Developed to be used as an adjunct treatment in severe malaria. Mode of action: it prevents rosetting, a complication in malaria, by reducing capillary blocking and releasing blood cells.	[358, 359]
Phase I	N-*Tert*-butyl isoquine (GSK369796) [Liverpool School of Tropical Hygiene/GlaxoSmith-Klyne (GSK)]	4-Aminoquinoline **51** 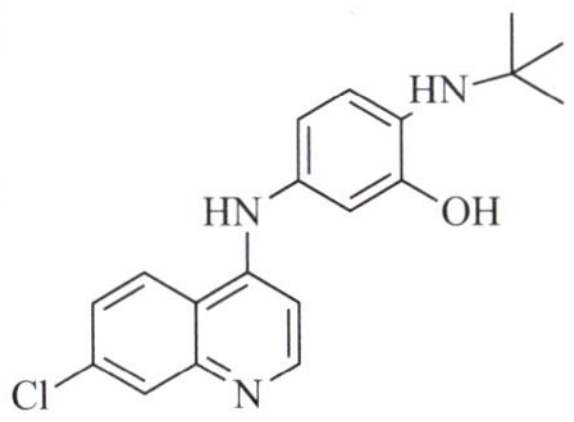	Amodiaquine analogue, synthetic. *In vitro* activity: IC_{50} = 11.2, 12.6 nM (CQ-sensitive 3D7, HB3 *P. falciparum* strains); IC_{50} = 13.2 nM (CQ-resistant K1 *P. falciparum* strain). Mode of action: hemozoin formation is inhibited and hence haem detoxification.	[346]

(Table 7) contd…..

Phase of Development	Drug	Active Ingredient and Chemical Class	Properties	Ref.
Phase I	AQ13 (Immtech Pharmaceuticals, Inc.)	4-Aminoquinoline **52** 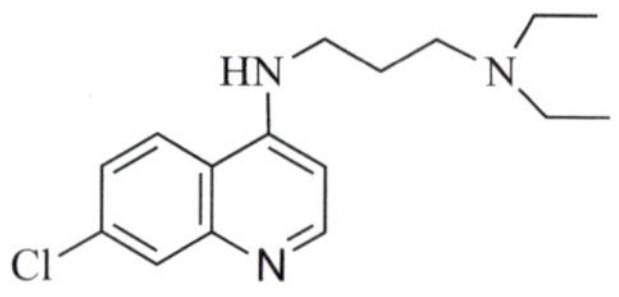	Synthetic, CQ-analogue with a shorter side chain. *In vitro* activity: IC_{50} = 18 nM (drug susceptible NF54 *P. falciparum* strain), 59 nM (K1 CQ-resistant *P. falciparum* strain) Mode of action: hemozoin formation is inhibited and hence haem detoxification.	[347, 348]
Preclinical	DSM265 (UTSW/UW/ Monash)	Triazolopyrimidine **60** 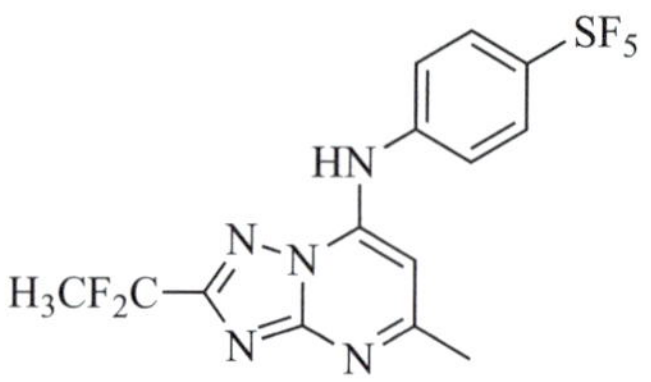	Triazolopyrimidine-based synthetic antimalarial. *In vitro* activity: IC_{50} = 33 nM (*Pf*DHODH), 2.5 μM (*Pb*DHODH), >100 μM (*human* DHODH) and 46 nM (*P. falciparum* CQ-sensitive 3D7 cell) Mode of action: selective inhibitor of the *P. falciparum* enzyme dihydroorotate dehydrogenase (DHODH). It blocks pyrimidine synthesis.	[363]
Preclinical	Genz-668764 (Broad/ Genzyme)	Aminoindole **63** 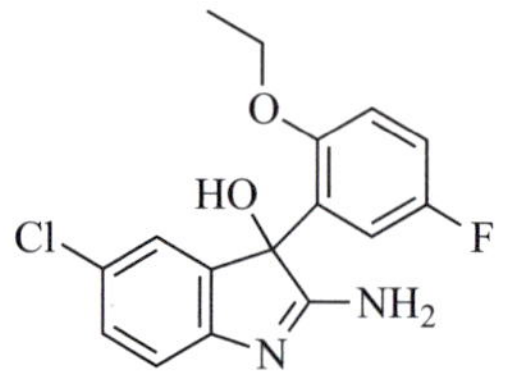	Synthetic indole derivative. *In vitro* activity: IC_{50} = 28-65 nM (*P. falciparum*) A single enantiomer.	[366]
Preclinical	P218 (Biotec/ Monash/ LSHTM)	2,4-Diaminopyrimidine **61** 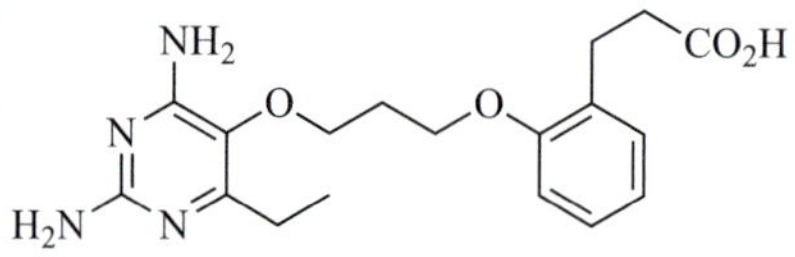	Synthetic. *In vitro* activity: IC_{50} => 0.01 µM (wild type); Mode of action: inhibitor of the dihydrofolate reductase (DHFR) enzyme in *P. falciparum*. It prevents folic acid synthesis.	[364]

(Table 7) contd…..

Phase of Development	Drug	Active Ingredient and Chemical Class	Properties	Ref.
Preclinical	MK4815 (Merck)	Aminoalkylphenol **64** 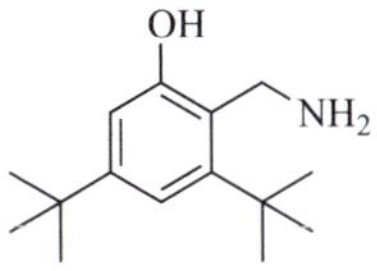	Synthetic. *In vitro* activity: IC_{50} = 0.004-0.030 μg mL^{-1} (a variety of drug-resistant *P. falciparum* isolates) Mode of action: inhibition of haem polymerization is a possibility.	[354, 367]
Preclinical	NPC-1161-B (University of Mississippi)	8-Aminoquinoline **53** 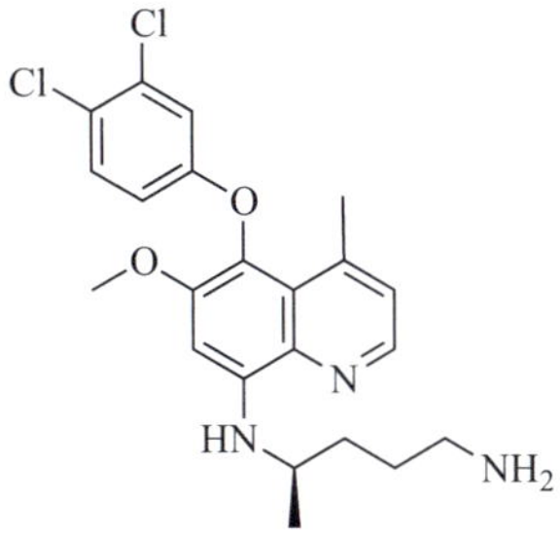	A dichlorophenoxy analogue of primaquine. The (-)-enantiomer shows promising antimalarial efficacy for radical cure and significant activity against the blood stages of *Plasmodium*. *In vitro* activity: IC_{50} = 50-500 nM (*P. falciparum* laboratory strains) It inhibits sporogony	[350]
Preclinical	RKA182 (Liverpool)	1,2,4,5-Tetraoxane **55** CAS = 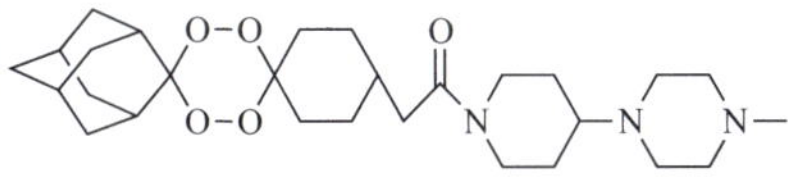	Synthetic endoperoxide. Dispiro-tetraoxane compound with two peroxide moieties. *In vitro* activity: IC_{50} = 1.5-6.0 nM (laboratory strains of *P. falciparum*), 0.87 nM (*P.f.* 3D7 strain) and 1.1 nM (*P.f.* K1 strain). Mode of action: it induces formation of free radicals, which damage the parasite	[353]
Preclinical	Antimalarial (Actelion Pharmaceuticals Ltd)	Piperazine **59** 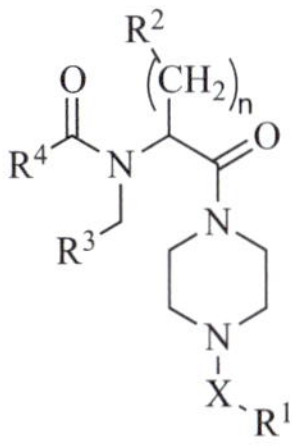	Synthetic. The exact structure of the antimlarial is unknown. Fourteen piperazine derivatives with IC_{50s} < 20 nM (*P. falciparum* K1 strain) have been disclosed.	[354, 362]

(Table 7) contd.....

Phase of Development	Drug	Active Ingredient and Chemical Class	Properties	Ref.
Preclinical	BCX4945 (Byocryst/Albert Einstein College of Medicine)	Deazaguanine **62** 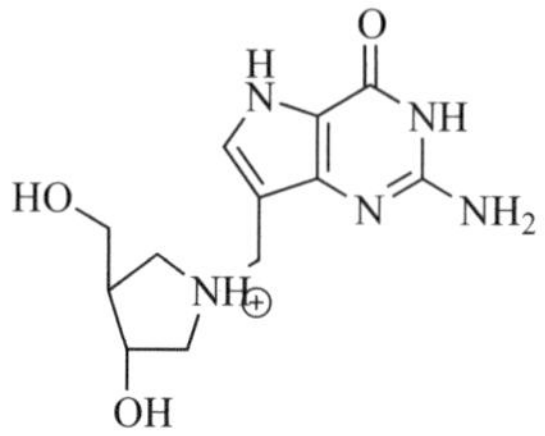	Deazaguanine derivative, an analogue of Immucillin-G. Mode of action: purine nucleoside phosphorylase (PNP) inhibitor. It blocks purine synthesis from hypoxanthine, and hence DNA synthesis.	[365]
Preclinical	SAR116242 (PA1103/ SAR116242) (Palumed)	Trioxaquine **56** CAS = 1096519-66-2 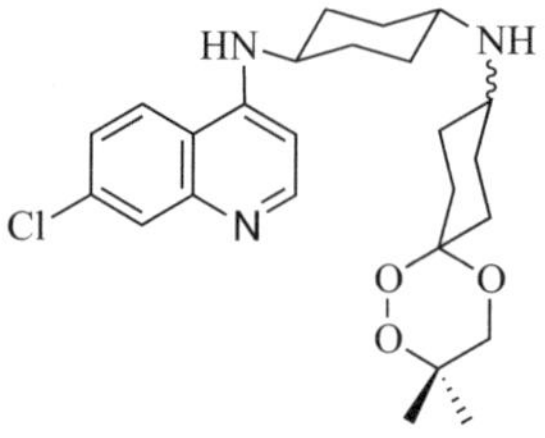	Hybrid combination of a synthetic peroxide, which mimics the 1,2,4-trioxane group of artemisinins and an aminoquinoline. Gametocytocidal. *In vitro* activity: IC_{50} = 7-24 nM (*P. falciparum* laboratory strains) Mode of action: dual, reactive free radicals are formed, which can alkylate haem, and polymerization to β-hematin and detoxification are inhibited.	[53, 357]

programmes, chemoprevention through the adoption of Intermittent Preventive Treatment for pregnant women became part of the national policy in 36 of 45 sub-Saharan African countries by the end of 2011 and also in Papua New Guinea in 2009 [2]. For infants and children the adoption of these measures has been slower to implement. Presently increased vector control and prevention, increased diagnostics and treatment with quality assured antimalarials have led to what appears to be a situation in which the incidence of malaria is in fact retreating [1, 2, 369]. These short-term massive targets will however need a follow-up by long term strategies [370].

The scientific community has also responded to the appeal for increased efforts to fight malaria. A search through the databases of Web of Knowledge (Thompson Corporation), revealed a steep increase in the number of publications on malaria control in later years (Fig. **17**). From 2000 to 2011 the number of publications with the key-words "antimalarial" OR "anti-malarial" OR "anti-malaria drug" has almost tripled. However, the arsenal of antimalarials for prevention and control of the disease is still small. There have been no new classes of antimalarials introduced into clinical practice since 1996 [371]. This situation is due not only to the intrinsic difficulties in discovering and developing new drugs, but also due to low financial resources [372]. Worst of all, many existing drugs may have to be discarded as a result of the fast development of resistance.

Studies involving large sets of compounds have been a very useful recent contribution. In one such study, undertaken at St. Jude Children's Research Hospital, approximately 310,000 compounds were screened for their ability to inhibit growth of *P. falciparum* in asexual blood stages. More than 1,100 were found to inhibit parasite growth by more than 80% at a concentration of 7 μM, and 560 at concentrations lower than 2 μL [372]. A closer look at a selection of 172 of these, with novel structures for antimalarials, revealed that at least 80% seemed to act on targets different from those of the antimalarials used commonly nowadays. The researchers predicted that the targets of many of these new compounds were kinase enzymes of *P. falciparum*, *i.e.,* the enzymes that transfer phosphate from high energy donor molecules like ATP to specific substrates in the phosphorylation process, or that they were targets related to interactions between the pathogen and its host. This being true, they represent new classes of targets for antimalarials. The pharmacokinetics studied also suggested that many of these compounds were suitable for further development. At Novartis, another large compound study involving the in-house library of 12,000 pure compounds, yielded 275 prospective antimalarials, of which 17 were selected for further studies due to their favourable potency and low toxicity [373, 374]. Phenotypic screening like this, which in its simplest variation may employ cell lines and monitor the influence of the drug on a single parameter (the phenotype), like cellular death or the influence on a certain enzyme-catalyzed process, has been used historically as the basis for the discovery of new drugs. These new studies, however, distinguish themselves by the large numbers of samples covered, and they are referred to as Global phenotypic screening. However, the process of determining the relevant target or target molecules subsequently is usually slow and difficult [375]. Phenotypic screening is an alternative to target-based screening, in which the effect of a drug on a purified target protein is observed.

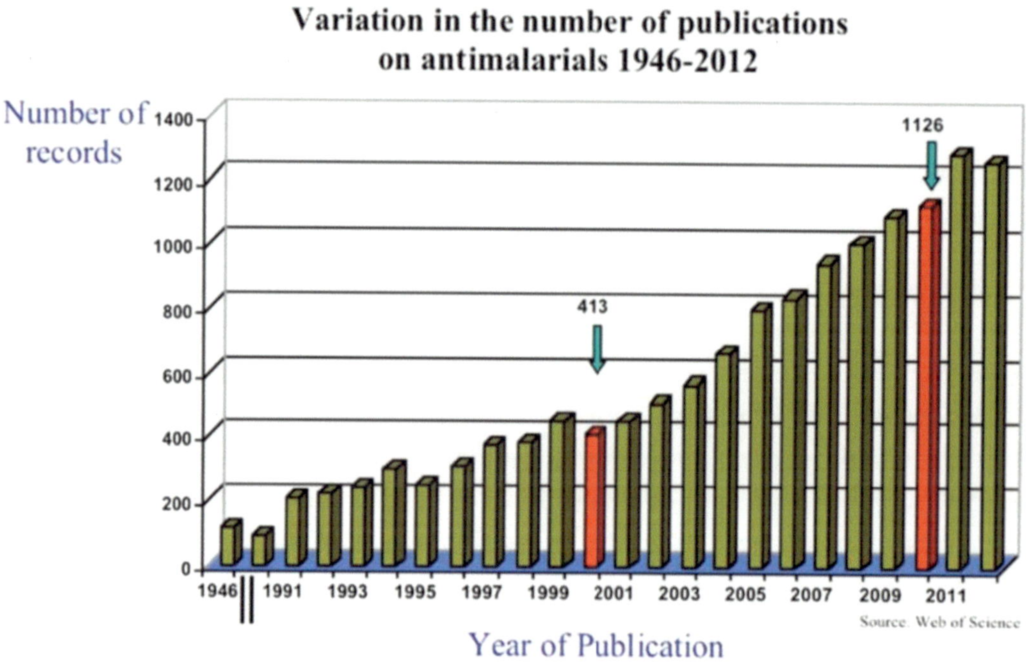

Figure 17: Evolution in the numbers of publications on malaria control since 1990. The number published in 1946 is representative of the number of records found for the previous decades.

In a separate study at GlaxoSmithKline [376], the in-house database was screened for compounds possessing activity against the blood stages of *P. falciparum*. More than 2 million compounds were included in this search. Approximately 13,500 were found to be active in concentrations of up to 2 μM. The data on more than 11,000 of these compounds as well as from the studies described above, was subsequently made available to the general research community at the European Bioinformatics Institute's CHEMI database at https//www.ebi.ac.uk/chemblntd/. The studies described so far did not present the discovery of novel antimalarials, but the information available provides a collection of novel chemical structures, which may be the basis for future research in this area [377]. These databases are nowadays being the subject of several screening studies, in different attempts to prioritize target antimalarials [378, 379].

Genomics is also being used to identify appropriate targets in the parasite. Another area where genome information can be useful, is in the identification of targets that have already been validated for another organism [167]. This has been of importance in the area of drug repositioning [167]. For example, the malaria genome information revealed that bacterial and malaria parasites utilize the same non-mevalonic pathway to synthesize isoprene [380]. Based on this knowledge, the antibiotic fosmidomycin, known to target this pathway, was selected for testing, and not only was its antimalarial activity discovered, but it was also afterwards selected as a prospective antimalarial drug, and it is nowadays undergoing clinical trials (see also under Drugs in Phase IIA).

At present there are no vaccines approved for malaria. Several attempts have been made, but the road to discovery has proven to be difficult. There are at present a few undergoing testing [381]. The most advanced is RTS, S/AS01, which is being developed by PATH, GlaxoSmithKline and the Bill & Melinda Gates Foundation. Large clinical trials are underway in 7 countries in Africa. The final results are expected at the end of 2014 [381].

As mentioned under The Pipeline of Antimalarials Under Development, one aspect of anti-malarial drug development that may help overcome parasite resistance is to have new drug targets. This may be achieved through an increased understanding of the parasite's biology and the mode of action of current antimalarials. Many studies are underway in this area. Table **8** lists possible life cycle processes that appear not to be affected by present-day antimalarials and which could be future targets for antimalarial development [369].

Recent plans at malaria control aim to reduce the parasite's basic reproduction rate [369]. In terms of parasite numbers, there are two critical events in the parasite's life cycle: the transmission of sporozoites from the parasite to the human host and the transmission of gametocytes from the host to the parasite. Only a few dozen to a few hundred parasites are transmitted in these events, compared to the billions which are formed during asexual blood replication. Nevertheless medicines targeting the blood stage are essential because it is during this stage that the disease manifests itself in the host. During a blood meal, 15-123

Table 8: *Plasmodium* Cell Components or Life-Cycle Processes that Could be Future Drug Targets. Until Now, no Antimalarials have been Designed which Aim Specifically at these Targets [369]

Parasite Cell Components or Life-Cycle Processes	Enzyme (Life Stage)	Enzyme Function	Ref.
Cytoplasm	**Serine hydroxymethyl transferase (BS/LS)**	It acts on the pyrimidine biosynthetic pathway; it promotes the conversion of serine and tetrahydrofolate to glycine and methylenetetrahydrofolate.	**[382]**
Endoplasmic reticulum	**Plasmepsin V (BS/LS)**	Enzyme which cleaves the export element (protease recognition sequence) PEXEL;RxLxE/Q/D from parasite proteins which are to be transferred to the erythrocyte.	**[383]**
Food vacuole	**Falcipains (BS)**	Haemoglobin degradation proteases.	**[384]**
	Plasmepsins (BS)	Haemoglobin degradation proteases.	**[384]**
Parasitophorus vacuole (PVM)	**Putative translocon (BS/LS)**	Complex that exports proteins across the Parasitophorus vacuole membrane into the human host cell.	**[385]**
Merozoite invasion	**Rhomboid 4 (BS)**	Merozoites interact with the erythrocytes before invasion *via* parasite ligands, transmembrane adhesins. Romboid 4 releases the adhesins so that the parasite can subsequently enter the cell.	**[386]**
	Subtilisin 2	It is involved in processing and shedding proteins on the merozoite surface during invasion.	**[387]**
Merozoite egress	**DPAP3 (BS/LS)**	*Pf* protease that regulates erythrocyte rupture.	**[388]**
	SERA5 (BS/LS)	Enzyme which mediates PVM and erythrocytic membrane breakdown to allow merozoite invasion.	**[389]**
	Subtilisin 1 (BS/LS)	**Enzyme which mediates PVM and erythrocytic membrane breakdown to allow merozoite invasion.**	**[390]**

sporozoites are deposited under the skin of the host [391]. They move through the dermis until they find a blood vessel, and then migrate to the liver, invading the liver parenchyma cells. Here thousands of merozoites form. Ideally this would be a good point to control the disease, or even the hepatic stage, but these stages are asymptomatic, and hence they are not targets for therapy. The liver stage is appealing for vaccine development, and some of the current research is aimed at this stage of the disease. Later, as a result of gametocytogenesis, a small proportion of parasites are transmitted and reproduce asexually in the middle gut of the mosquito. The numbers are also low: 10-103 [369]. Artemisinin and primaquine are the only antimalarials currently available which kill stage 4 gametocytes, although a few others, which do not kill them, have the effect of rendering them incapable replicating in the mosquito, and hence also allow for transmission control (see under Currently Available Antimalarial Drugs).

Research on *P. vivax* has been slower, because this species is difficult to grow in the laboratory. Even nowadays it is not known how hypnozoite dormancy is induced.

According to a few sources, some of needs for the future of malaria control, besides efficient drugs to replace existing ones in case they fall to resistance [371, 377], are the following [392]:

1. A drug with potential to act at several stages of the parasite's life cycle, which could be taken in one dose.

2. Assays to identify drugs having the capacity to eliminate *P. vivax* hypnozoites from the liver.

3. The development of *P. vivax* and *P. falciparum* culture systems for every stage of the parasite life cycle

4. The implementation and validation of *in vitro* and *in vivo* G6PD deficiency-dependent haemolysis assays.

5. New molecules to block the development of mature gametocytes and hence prevent transmission.

6. To develop and validate high throughput screening assays, to test new drugs against *P. falciparum* and *P. vivax* gametocytes and parasite transmission.

7. An efficacious vaccine.

8. Improved diagnostic tests for malaria.

ACKNOWLEDGEMENTS

The financial support from Fundação para a Ciência e a Tecnologia, Ministério da Educação e Ciência, is gratefully acknowledged.

CONFLICT OF INTEREST

The author confirms that this chapter content has no conflict of interest.

REFERENCES

[1] World Health Organization. World Malaria Report 2011. Geneva, WHO Press, 2011. Available online from: http://www.who.int/malaria/world_malaria_report_2011/en/

[2] World Health Organization. World Malaria Report 2012. Geneva, WHO Press, 2012. Available online from: http://www.who.int/malaria/publications/world_malaria_report_2012/en/

[3] World Health Organization. Guidelines for the Treatment of Malaria: second edition 2010. Geneva, WHO Press, 2010. Available online from: http://www.who.int/malaria/publications/atoz/9789241547925/en/index.html.

[4] Astelbauer F, Walochnik J. Antiprotozoal compounds: state of the art and new developments. International Journal of Antimicrobial Agents 2011; 38(2): 118-24.

[5] Carter R, Mendis KN. Evolutionary and historical aspects of the burden of malaria. Clinical Microbiology Reviews 2002; 15(4): 564-73.

[6] Schlitzer M. Malaria chemotherapeutics, part I: history of antimalarial drug development, currently used therapeutics, and drugs in clinical development. ChemMedChem 2007; 2(7): 944-86.

[7] World Health Organization. Global Report on Antimalarial Drug Efficacy and Drug Resistance: 2000-2010. Geneva, WHO Press, 2010. Available online from: http://whqlibdoc.who.int/publications/2010/9789241500470_eng.pdf.

[8] Solomon AW, Nayagam S, Pasvol G. Recent advances in tropical medicine. Transactions of the Royal Society of Tropical Medicine and Hygiene 2009; 103(7): 647-52.

[9] Kissinger JC, Brunk BP, Crabtree J, *et al.* The Plasmodium genome database. Nature 2002; 419(6906): 490-92.

[10] Achan J, Talisuna AO, Erhart A, *et al.* Quinine, an old anti-malarial drug in a modern world: role in the treatment of malaria. Malaria Journal 2011; 10: 144.

[11] Foley M, Tilley L. Quinoline antimalarials: mechanisms of action and resistance and prospects for new agents. Pharmacology & Therapeutics 1998; 79(1): 55-87.

[12] World Health Organization. Chemotherapy of Malaria. Monograph series No. 27, second edition. Geneva, WHO Press, 1986. Chapter 3. Available online from: http:// whqlibdoc.who.int/monograph/WHO_MONO_27_(2ed)_(chp3).pdf.

[13] Newton PN, Angus BJ, Chierakul W, *et al.* Randomized comparison of artesunate and quinine in the treatment of severe falciparum malaria. Clinical Infectious Diseases 2003; 37(1): 7-16.

[14] Obonyo CO, Juma EA. Clindamycin plus quinine for treating uncomplicated falciparum malaria: a systematic review and meta-analysis. Malaria Journal 2012; 11: 2.

[15] Food and Drug Administration. Center for drug evaluation and research. Qualaquin® (quinine sulfate) capsules. Mutual Pharmaceutical Company, Inc., application number NDA 21-799. Philadelphia. Available from: http://www.fda.gov/downloads/drugs/drugsafety/postmarketdrugsafetyinformationforpatientsandproviders/ucm217721.pdf

[16] Olliaro OL, Yuthavong Y. An overview of chemotherapeutic targets for antimalarial drug discovery. Pharmacology & Therapeutics 1999; 81(2): 91-10.

[17] Mungthin M, Bray PG, Ridley RG, *et al.* Central role of hemoglobin degradation in mechanisms of action of 4-aminoquinolines, quinoline methanols, and phenanthrene methanols. Antimicrobial Agents and Chemotherapy 1998, 42(11): 2973-77.

[18] Olliaro PL, Goldberg DE. The *Plasmodium* digestive vacuole: metabolic headquarters and choice drug target. Parasitology Today 1995; 11(8): 294-97.

[19] Orjih AU. Heme polymerase activity and the stage specificity of antimalarial action of chloroquine. The Journal of Pharmacology and Experimental Therapeutics 1997; 282(1): 108-12.

[20] Giao PT, de Vries PJ. Pharmacokinetic interactions of antimalarial agents. Clinical Pharmacokinetics 2001; 40(5): 343-73.

[21] Soyinka JO, Onyeji CO, Omoruyi SI, *et al.* Pharmacokinetic interactions between ritonavir and quinine in healthy volunteers following concurrent administration. British Journal of Clinical Pharmacology 2010; 69(3): 262-70.

[22] Pukrittayakamee S, Wanwimolruk S, Stepniewska K, *et al.* Quinine pharmacokinetic-pharmacodynamic relationships in uncomplicated falciparum malaria. Antimicrobial Agents and Chemotherapy 2003, 47(11): 3458-63.

[23] Wilby KJ, Ensom MHH. Pharmacokinetics of antimalarials in pregnancy. A systematic review. Clinical Pharmacokinetics 2011; 50(11): 705-23.

[24] Abdelrahim II, Adam I, Elghazali G, *et al.* Pharmacokinetics of quinine and its metabolites in pregnant Sudanese women with uncomplicated Plasmodium falciparum malaria. Journal of Clinical Pharmacology and Therapeutics 2007; 32(1): 15-9.

[25] Jensen M, Mehlhorn H. Seventy-five years of Resochin® in the fight against malaria. Parasitology Research 2009; 105(3): 609-27.

[26] O'Neill PM, Bray PG, Hawley SR, *et al.* 4-Aminoquinolines-past, present, and future: a chemical perspective. Pharmacology & Therapeutics 1998; 77(1): 29-58.

[27] O'Neill PM, Barton VE, Ward SA *et al.* 4-Aminoquinolines: Chloroquine, Amodiaquine and Next-generation Analogues. In: Treatment and Prevention of Malaria: Antimalarial Drug Chemistry, Action and Use, Staines HM, Krishna S (Eds). Basel, Springer, 2012; pp 19-44.

[28] Kaur K, Jain M, Reddy RP, *et al.* Quinolines and structurally related heterocycles as antimalarials. European Journal of Medicinal Chemistry 2010; 45(8): 3245-64.

[29] Castelli F, Tomasoni LR, Matteelli A. Advances in the treatment of malaria. Mediterranean Journal of Hematology and Infectious Diseases 2012; 4(1): e2012064.

[30] Gustafsson LL, Walker O, Alván G, *et al.* Disposition of chloroquine in man after single intravenous and oral doses. British Journal of Clinical Pharmacology 1983; 15(4): 471-79.

[31] Cook JA,, Randinitis EJ, Bramson CR, *et al.* Lack of a pharmacokinetic interaction between azithromycin and chloroquine. American Journal of Tropical Medicine and Hygiene 2006; 74(3): 407-12.

[32] Dunne MW, Singh N, Shukla M, *et al.* A multicenter study of azithromycin, alone and in combination with chloroquine, for the treatment of acute uncomplicated *Plasmodium falciparum* malaria in India. Journal of Infectious Diseases 2005; 191(10): 1582-88.

[33] Lee SJ, McGready R, Fernandez C, *et al.* Chloroquine pharmacokinetics in pregnant and nonpregnant women with vivax malaria. European Journal of Pharmacology 2008; 64(10): 987-92.

[34] Davis TME, Hung T-H, Sim I-K, *et al.* Piperaquine: a resurgent antimalarial drug. Drugs 2005; 65(1): 75-87.

[35] Basco LK, Ringwald P. *In vitro* activities of piperaquine and other 4-aminoquinolines against clinical isolates of *Plasmodium falciparum* in Cameroon. Antimicrobial Agents and Chemotherapy 2003; 47(4): 1391-94.

[37] Tarninga J, Lindegardha N. Quantification of the antimalarial piperaquine in plasma. Transactions of the Royal Society of Tropical Medicine and Hygiene 2008; 102(5): 409-11.

[38] Tarning J, Bergqvist Y, Day NP, *et al.* Characterization of human urinary metabolites of the antimalarial piperaquine. Drug Metabolism and Disposition 2006; 34(12): 2011-19.

[39] Chinh NT, Quang NN, Thanh NX, *et al.* Short report: pharmacokinetics of the antimalarial drug piperaquine in healthy Vietnamese subjects. American Journal of Tropical Medicine and Hygiene 2008; 79(4): 620-23.

[40] Sim I-K, Davis TME, Ilett KF. Effects of a high-fat meal on the relative oral bioavailability of piperaquine. Antimicrobial Agents and Chemotherapy 2005; 49(6): 2407-11.

[41] Olliaro P, Mussano P. Amodiaquine for treating malaria. Cochrane Database of Systematic Reviews 2003, Issue 2. Art. No.: CD000016.

[42] Olliaro P, Nevill C, LeBras J, *et al.* Systematic review of amodiaquine treatment in uncomplicated malaria. The Lancet 1996; 348(9036) 1196-01.

[43] Tagbor HK, Chandramohan D, Greenwood B. The safety of amodiaquine use in pregnant women. Expert Opinion on Drug Safety 2007; 6(6): 631-35.

[44] White NJ, Looareesuwan S, Edwards G, *et al.* Pharmacokinetics of intravenous amodiaquine. British Journal of Clinical Pharmacology 1987; 23(2): 127-35.

[45] Winstanley PA, Simooya O, Kofi-Ekue JM, *et al.* The disposition of amodiaquine in Zambians and Nigerians with malaria. British Journal of Clinical Pharmacology 1990; 29(6): 695-01.

[46] Nair A, Abrahamsson B, Barends DM, *et al.* Commentaries. Biowaiver monographs for immediate-release solid oral dosage forms: primaquine phosphate. Journal of Pharmaceutical Sciences 2012; 101(3): 936-45.

[47] Elderfield RC, Mertel HE, Mitch RT, *et al.* Synthesis of primaquine and certain of its analogs. Journal of the American Chemical Society 1955; 77(18): 4816-19.

[48] Vale N, Moreira R, Gomes P. Primaquine revisited six decades after its discovery. European Journal of Medicinal Chemistry 2009; 44(3): 937-53.

[49] Brueckner RP, Ohart C, Baird JK, *et al.* 8-Aminoquinolines. In: Rosenthal PJ, Ed. Antimalarial Chemotherapy, Mechanism of Action, Resistance and New Directions in Drug Discovery. New Jersey, Humana Press, 2001; pp. 123-51.

[50] Hill DR, Baird JK, Parise ME, *et al.* Primaquine: report from CDC expert meeting on malaria chemoprophylaxis I. American Journal of Tropical Medicine and Hygiene 2006; 75(3): 402-15.

[51] Baird JK, Hoffman SL. Primaquine therapy for malaria. Clinical Infectious Diseases 2004; 39(9): 1336-45.

[52] Tekwani BL, Walker LA. 8-Aminoquinolines: future role as antiprotozoal drugs. Current Opinion in Infectious Diseases 2006; 19(6): 623-31.

[53] Kiszewski AE. Blocking *Plasmodium falciparum* malaria transmission with drugs: the gametocytocidal and sporontocidal properties of current and prospective antimalarials. Pharmaceuticals 2011; 4(1): 44-68.

[54] Mihaly GW, Ward SA, Edwards G, *et al.* Pharmacokinetics of primaquine in man: identification of the carboxylic acid derivative as a major plasma metabolite. British Journal of Clinical Pharmacology 1984; 17(4): 441-46.

[55] Ward SA, Mihaly GW, Edwards G, *et al.* Pharmacokinetics of primaquine in man II. Comparison of acute *vs* chronic dosage in Thai subjects. British Journal of Clinical Pharmacology 1985; 19(6): 751-55.

[56] Schlagenhauf P. Mefloquine for malaria chemoprophylaxis 1992-1998: a review. Journal of Travel Medicine 1999; 6(2): 122-33.

[57] Simpson JA, Watkins ER, Price RN, *et al.* Mefloquine pharmacokinetic-pharmacodynamic models: implications for dosing and resistance. Antimicrobial Agents and Chemotherapy 2000; 44(12): 3414-24.

[58] DrugBank [homepage on the Internet]. Departments of Computing Science & Biological Sciences, University of Alberta and The Metabolomics Innovation Centre. Available from: http://www.drugbank.ca.

[59] Wilby KJ, Ensom MHH. Pharmacokinetics of antimalarials in pregnancy. A systematic review. Clinical Pharmacokinetics 2011; 50(11): 705-23.

[60] Schlagenhauf P, Adamcova M, Regep L, *et al.* The position of mefloquine as a 21st century malaria chemoprophylaxis. Malaria Journal 2010; 9: 357.

[61] Karle JM, Olmeda R, Gerena L, *et al.*: *Plasmodium falciparum*: role of absolute stereochemistry in the antimalarial activity of synthetic amino alcohol antimalarial agents. Experimental Parasitology 1993, 76(4): 345-51.

[62] Gimenez F, Pennie RA, Koren G, *et al.* Stereoselective pharmacokinetics of mefloquine in healthy Caucasians after multiple doses. Journal of Pharmaceutical Sciences 1994; 83(6): 824-27.

[63] Schlagenhauf P. Mefloquine for malaria chemoprophylaxis 1992-1998: a review. Journal of Travel Medicine 1999; 6(2): 122-33.

[64] Bourahla A, Martin C, Gimenez F, *et al.* Stereoselective pharmacokinetics of mefloquine in young children. European Journal of Clinical Pharmacology 1996; 50(3): 241-44.

[65] Fletcher A, Shepherd R. Use of (+)-mefloquine for the treatment of malaria. WO98/39003. 1998.

[66] Brocks DR, Vakily M, Mehvar R. Stereospecific Pharmacokinetics and Pharmacodynamics: Selected Classes of Drugs. In: IK Reddy IK, Mehvar R, Eds. Chirality in Drug Design and Development. New York, Marcel Dekker, 2004; pp 191-80.

[67] Mullié C, Jonet A, Desgrouas C, *et al.* Differences in anti-malarial activity of 4-aminoalcohol quinoline enantiomers and investigation of the presumed underlying mechanism of action. Malaria Journal 2012; 11: 65.

[68] Tansley R, Lotharius J, Priestley A, Fiona *et al.* A randomized, double-blind, placebo-controlled study to investigate the safety, tolerability, and pharmacokinetics of single enantiomer (+)-mefloquine compared with racemic mefloquine in healthy persons. American Journal of Tropical Medicine and Hygiene 2010; 83(6): 1195-01.

[69] J. Karbwang J, Na Bangchang K, Thanavibul A *et al.* Pharmacokinetics of mefloquine alone or in combination with artesunate. Bulletin of the World Health Organization 1994; 72(1): 83-7.

[70] Jiang J-B, Guo X-B, Li G-Q, *et al.* Antimalarial activity of mefloquine and qinghaosu. The Lancet 1982; 320(8293): 285-88.

[71] Pukrittayakamee S Chantra A, Simpson JA *et al.* Therapeutic responses to different antimalarial drugs in vivax malaria. Antimicrobial Agents and Chemotherapy 2000, 44(6):1680-85.

[72] Karbwang J, Na Bangchang K. Clinical pharmacokinetics of halofantrine. Clinical Pharmacokinetics 1994; 27(2): 104-19.

[73] Nothdurft HD, Clemens R, Bock HL *et al.* Halofantrine: a new substance for treatment of multidrug-resistant malaria. Clinical Investigator 1993; 71(1): 69-73.

[74] Halfan label (GlaxoSmithKline). FDA, U.S. Food and Drug Administration. Available at http://www.accessdata.fda.gov/scripts/cder/drugsatfda/index.cfm?fuseaction=Search.Label_ApprovalHistory#apphist.

[75] Wernsdorfer WH, Landgraf B, Kilimali VAEB, *et al.* Activity of benflumetol and its enantiomers in fresh isolates of *Plasmodium falciparum* from East Africa. Acta Tropica 1998; 70(1): 9-15.

[76] Nosten F, White NJ. Artemisinin-based combination treatment of falciparum malaria. American Journal of Tropical Medicine and Hygiene 2007; 77(Suppl 6): 181-92.

[77] The past, present and future of antifolates in the treatment of *Plasmodium falciparum* infection. Nzila A. Journal of Antimicrobial Chemotherapy 2006; 57(6): 1043-54.

[78] Salcedo-Sora J.E., Ward S.A. The folate metabolic network of falciparum malaria. Molecular & Biochemical Parasitology 2013. Available online 15 March 2013.

[79] Metz J. Folic acid metabolism and malaria. Food and Nutrition Bulletin 2007; 28(Suppl 4): S540-49.

[80] Gregson, A, Plowe, CV. Mechanisms of resistance of malaria parasites to antifolates. Pharmacology Reviews 2005; 57(1): 117-45.

[81] World Health Organization. Chemotherapy of Malaria. Monograph series No. 27, second edition. Geneva, WHO Press, 1986. Chapter 2. Available online from: http://whqlibdoc.who.int/monograph/WHO_MONO_27_(2ed)_(chp2).pdf.

[82] Ridley RG. Medical need, scientific opportunity and the drive for antimalarial drugs. Nature 2002; 415(6872): 686-93.

[83] Schapira A, Schwalbach JFL. Evaluation of four therapeutic regimens for falciparum malaria in Mozambique, 1986. Bulletin of the World Health Organization 1988; 66(2): 219-26.

[84] Attlmayr B, Thriemer K, Haque R, *et al.* Untersuchungen zur *in vitro* Arzneimittelresistenz bei Malaria tropica in Bangladesch. Wien Klin Wochenschr 2006; 118(19-20, suppl 3): 58-61.

[85] Basko LK, Ramiliarisoa O, Le Bras J. *In vitro* activity of pyrimethamine, cycloguanil, and other antimalarial drugs against African isolates and clones of *Plasmodium falciparum*. American Journal of Tropical Medicine and Hygiene 1994; 50(2): 193-99.

[86] Charman SA, Arbe-Barnes S, Bathurst IC *et al.* Synthetic ozonide drug candidate OZ439 offers new hope for a single-dose cure of uncomplicated malaria. Proceedings of the National Academy of Sciences of the United States of America 2011; 108(11) 4400-05.

[87] Barnes KI, Little F, Smith PJ, *et al.* Sulfadoxine-pyrimethamine pharmacokinetics in malaria: pediatric dosing implications. Clinical Pharmacology and Therapeutics 2006; 80(6): 582-96.

[88] Sulfalene with pyrimethamine and chloroquine with pyrimethamine in single-dose treatment of Plasmodium falciparum infections. Storey J, Rossi-Espagnet A, Mandel SPH, *et al.* Bulletin of the World Health Organization 1973; 49(3): 275-82.

[89] Baruah I, Talukdar PK, Das SC. The drug sensitivities of *Plasmodium falciparum* in the Sonitpur district, Assam, India. The Southeast Asian Journal of Tropical Medicine and Public Health 2005; 36(3): 587-90.

[90] Winstanley P, Ward S, Snow R, *et al*. Therapy of falciparum malaria in Sub-Saharan Africa: from molecule to policy. Clinical Microbiology Reviews 2004; 17(3): 612-37.

[91] Winstanley P, Mberu EK, Szwandt ISF, *et al*. The *in vitro* activity of novel antifolate drug combinations against *Plasmodium falciparum* and human granulocyte colony-forming units. Antimicrobial Agents and Chemotherapy 1995; 39(4): 948-52.

[92] Zuidema J, Hilbers-Modderman ESM, Merkus FWHM. Clinical pharmacokinetics of dapsone. Clinical Pharmacokinetics 1986; 11(4): 299-15.

[93] Alloueche A, Bailey W, Barton S, *et al*. Comparison of chlorproguanil-dapsone with sulfadoxine-pyrimethamine for the treatment of uncomplicated falciparum malaria in young African children: double-blind randomised controlled trial. The Lancet 2004; 363(9424): 1843-48.

[94] Edstein MD, Rieckmann KH, Veenendaal JR. Multiple-dose pharmacokinetics and *in vitro* antimalarial activity of dapsone plus pyrimethamine (Maloprim®) in man. British Journal of Clinical Pharmacology 1990; 30(2): 259-65.

[95] Edstein MD, Veenendaal JR, Rieckmann KH. Multiple-dose kinetics in healthy volunteers and *in vitro* antimalarial activity of proguanil plus dapsone. Chemotherapy 1990; 36(6): 169-76.

[96] World Health Organization. Review of the safety of chlorproguanil-dapsone in the treatment of uncomplicated falciparum malaria in Africa. Report of a technical consultation. Geneva, WHO Press, 2004.

[97] Mutabingwa T, Nzila A, Mberu E, *et al*. Chlorproguanil-dapsone for treatment of drug-resistant falciparum malaria in Tanzania. The Lancet 2001; 358(9289): 1218-23.

[98] Rollo IM. Antiplasmodial efficacy of 2,4-diaminopyrimidine-sulfonamide combinations, especially against choroquine-resistant malaria. Canadian Medical Association Journal 1975; 112 (13 Spec No): 50-3.

[99] Hitchings GH, Elion GB, Falco EA, *et al*. Antagonists of nucleic acid derivatives: The *lactobacillus casei* model. Journal of Biological Chemistry 1950, 183(1), 1-9.

[100] Yuthavonga Y, Tarnchompooa B, Vilaivanb T *et al*. Malarial dihydrofolate reductase as a paradigm for drug development against a resistance-compromised target. Proceedings of the National Academy of Sciences 2012; 109(42): 16823-28.

[101] Winstanley P, Ward S, Snow R, *et al*. Therapy of falciparum malaria in Sub-Saharan Africa: from molecule to policy. Clinical Microbiology Reviews 2004; 17(3): 612-37.

[102] Marra F, Salzman JR, Ensom MH. Atovaquone-Proguanil for Prophylaxis and Treatment of Malaria. The Annals of Pharmacotherapy 2003; 37(9): 1266-75.

[103] Kain KC. Current status and replies to frequently posed questions on atovaquone plus proguanil (Malarone) for the prevention of malaria. BioDrugs 2003; 17(Suppl 1): 23-8.

[104] Gillotin C, Mamet JP, Veronese L. Lack of a pharmacokinetic interaction between atovaquone and proguanil. European Journal of Clinical Pharmacology 1999; 55(4): 311-15.

[105] Looareesuwan S, Chulay JD, Canfield CJ *et al*. Malarone™ (atovaquone and proguanil hydrochloride): a review of its clinical development for treatment of malaria. American Journal of Tropical Medicine and Hygiene 1999; 60(4): 533-41.

[106] World Health Organization. Guidelines for the Treatment of Malaria. Geneva, WHO Press, 2006. Available online from: http://helid.digicollection.org/en/d/Js13418e/
[107] Bukirwa H, Garner P, Critchley JA. Chlorproguanil-dapsone for treating uncomplicated malaria. Cochrane Database of Systematic Reviews 2004, Issue 4. Art. No.: CD004387.
[108] Fanello CI, Karema C, Avellino P *et al.* High risk of severe anaemia after chlorproguanil-dapsone+artesunate antimalarial treatment in patients with G6PD (A-) deficiency. PLoS ONE 2008; 3: e4031.
[109] Veenendaal R, Edstein MD, Rieckmann KH. Pharmacokinetics of chlorproguanil after a single oral dose of Lapudrine®. Chemotherapy1988; 34(4): 277-83.
[110] Looareesuwan S, Wilairatana P, Chalermarut K, *et al.* Efficacy and safety of atovaquone/proguanil compared with mefloquine for treatment of acute *Plasmodium falciparum* malaria in Thailand. American Journal of Tropical Medicine and Hygiene 1999; 60(4): 526-32.
[111] Bouchaud O, Mühlberger N, Parola P, *et al.* Therapy of uncomplicated falciparum malaria in Europe: MALTHER - a prospective observational multicentre study. Malaria Journal 2012, 11: 212.
[112] Seeber F, Limenitakis J, Soldati-Favre D, *et al.* Apicomplexan mitochondrial metabolism: a story of gains, losses and retentions. Trends in Parasitology 2008; 24(10): 468-78.
[113] Painter HJ, Morrisey JM, Mather MW, *et al.* Specific role of mitochondrial electron transport in blood-stage *Plasmodium falciparum*. Nature 2007; 446 (7131); 88-91.
[114] Baggish AL, Hill DR. Antiparasitic agent atovaquone. Antimicrobial Agents and Chemotherapy 2002, 46(5):1163-73.
[115] Basselin M. Hunt SM, Abdala-Valencia H, *et al.* Ubiquinone synthesis in mitochondrial and microsomal subcellular fractions of *Pneumocystis* spp.: differential sensitivities to atovaquone. Eukaryotic Cell 2005; 4(8): 1483-92.
[116] de Macedo CS, Uhrig ML, Kimura EA, *et al.* Characterization of the isoprenoid chain of coenzyme Q in *Plasmodium falciparum*. FEMS Microbiology Letters 2002; 207 (1) 13-20.
[117] Rodrigues T, Lopes F, Moreira R. Inhibitors of the mitochondrial electron transport chain and *de novo* pyrimidine biosynthesis as antimalarials: the present status. Current Medicinal Chemistry 2010, 17(10), 929-56.
[118] Delves M, Plouffe D, Scheurer C, *et al.* The activities of current antimalarial drugs on the life cycle stages of *Plasmodium*: a comparative study with human and rodent parasites. PLoS Med 2012; 9(2): e1001169.
[119] Fivelman QL, Adagu IS, Warhurst DC. Modified fixed-ratio isobologram method for studying *in vitro* interactions between atovaquone and proguanil or dihydroartemisinin against drug-resistant strains of *Plasmodium falciparum*. Antimicrobial Agents and Chemotherapy 2004; 48(11): 4097-02.
[120] Brockmann A, Price RN, van Vugt M, *et al. Plasmodium falciparum* antimalarial drug susceptibility on the north-western border of Thailand during five years of extensive use of artesunate-mefloquine. Transactions of the Royal Society of Tropical Medicine and Hygiene 2000; 94(5), 537- 44.
[121] Pradines B, Tall A, Ramiandrasoa F, *et al. In vitro* activity of iron-binding compounds against Senegalese isolates of *Plasmodium falciparum*. Journal of Antimicrobial Chemotherapy 2006; 57 (6), 1093-99.

[122] Anderson TJC, Nair S, Qin H, *et al.* Are transporter genes other than the chloroquine resistance locus (*pfcrt*) and multidrug resistance gene (*pfmdr*) associated with antimalarial drug resistance? Antimicrobial Agents and Chemotherapy 2005; 49(6), 2180-88.

[123] Marra F, Salzman JR, Ensom MH. Atovaquone-Proguanil for Prophylaxis and Treatment of Malaria. The Annals of Pharmacotherapy 2003; 37(9): 1266-1275.

[124] Osei-Akoto A, Orton LC, Owusu-Ofori S. Atovaquone-proguanil for treating uncomplicated malaria. Cochrane Database of Systematic Reviews 2005, Issue 4. Art. No.: CD004529.

[125] Miller LH, Su X. Artemisinin: Discovery from the Chinese Herbal Garden. Cell 2011; 146(6), 855-58.

[126] World Health Organization. Nonclinical Overview for Artemisinin Derivatives. Available from: http://apps.who.int/prequal/info_applicants/Guidelines/Nonclinical_Overview_Artemisinin-Derivatives.pdf

[127] Woodrow CJ, Haynes RK, Krishna S. Artemisinins. Postgraduate Medical Journal 2005; 81(952): 71-8.

[128] Chaturvedi D, Goswami A, Saikia PP, *et al.* Artemisinin and its derivatives: a novel class of anti-malarial and anti-cancer agents. Chemical Society Reviews 2010; 39(2): 435-54.

[129] Haynes RK, Krishna S. Artemisinins: activities and actions. Microbes and Infection 2004; 6(14): 339-46.

[130] Kyle DE, Teja-Isavadharm P, Li Q, *et al.* Pharmacokinetics and pharmacodynamics of qinghaosu derivates: how do they impact on the choice of drugs and the dosage regiments? Médecine tropicale 1998; 58(3), 38-44.

[131] Meshnick, SR. Artemisinin: mechanisms of action, resistance and toxicity. International Journal of Parasitology 2002; 32(13): 1655-660.

[132] O'Neill PM, Barton VE, Ward SA. The molecular mechanism of action of artemisinin - The debate continues. Molecules 2010, 15(3), 1705-21.

[133] Krishna S, Uhlemanna A-C, Haynes RK. Artemisinins: mechanisms of action and potential for resistance. Drug Resistance Updates 2004; 7(4-5): 233-44.

[134] Avery MA, Gao F, Chong WKM, *et al.* Structure-activity relationships of the antimalarial agent artemisinin. 1. Synthesis and comparative molecular field analysis of C-9 analogs of artemisinin and 10-deoxoartemisinin. Journal of Medicinal Chemistry 1993; 36 (26): 4264-75.

[135] Ye B., Wu Y-L. Synthesis of carba-analogues of Qinghaosu. Tetrahedron 1989; 45(23), 7287-90.

[136] Ye B., Wu YL, Li GF, *et al.* [Antimalarial activity of deoxoqinghaosu]. Yao Xue Xue Bao 1991; 26(3), 228-30.

[137] Meshnick S. Artemisinin and its Derivatives. In: Rosenthal P, Ed. Antimalarial Chemotherapy:. Mechanisms of Action, Resistance, and New Directions in Drug Discovery. New Jersey, Springer-Science + Business Media LLC, 2001; pp 191-02.

[138] Olliaro P, Haynes R, Meunier B., *et al.* Possible modes of action of the artemisinin-type compounds. Trends in Parasitology 2001; 17(3), 122-26.

[139] Cazelles, J.; Robert, A.; Meunier, B. Alkylation of heme by artemisinin, an antimalarial drug. Comptes Rendus de l'Académie des Sciences - Series IIC - Chemistry 2001, 4(2), 85-89.

[140] Robert A, Benoit-Vical FO, Claparols C, *et al.* The antimalarial drug artemisinin alkylates heme in infected mice. Proceedings of the National Academy of Sciences of the United States of America 2005; 102(38), 13676-80.

[141] Meshnick SR, Thomas A, Ranz A, *et al.* Artemisinin (qinghaosu): the role of intracellular hemin in its mechanism of antimalarial action. Molecular and Biochemical Parasitology 1991; 49(2): 181-89.

[142] Posner GH, Wang D, Cumming JN, *et al.* Further evidence supporting the importance of and the restrictions on a carbon-centered radical for high antimalarial activity of 1,2,4-trioxanes like artemisinin. Journal of Medicinal Chemistry 1995; 38(13), 2273-75.

[143] Jefford CW, Vicente MGH, Jacquier Y, *et al.* The deoxygenation and isomerization of artemisinin and artemether and their relevance to antimalarial action. Helv. Chim. Acta 1996; 79(5): 1475-87.

[144] Wu WM, Wu Y, Wu YL, *et al.* Unified mechanistic framework for the Fe(II)-induced cleavage of qinghaosu and derivatives/analogues. The first spin-trapping evidence for the previously postulated secondary C-4 radical. Journal of the American Chemical Society 1998; 120(14): 3316-25.

[145] Butler AR, Gilbert BC, Hulme P, *et al.* EPR evidence for the involvement of free radicals in the iron-catalysed decomposition of qinghaosu (artemisinin) and some derivatives; antimalarial action of some polycyclic endoperoxides. Free Radical Research. 1998; 28(5): 471-76.

[146] O'Neill PM, Bishop LPD, Searle NL, *et al.* Biomimetic Fe(II)-mediated degradation of arteflene (Ro-42-1611). The first EPR spin-trapping evidence for the previously postulated secondary carbon-centered cyclohexyl radical. Journal of Organic Chemistry 2000; 65(5): 1578-82.

[147] Haynes RK, Chan WC, Lung CM, *et al.* The Fe^{2+}-mediated decomposition, *Pf*ATP6 binding, and antimalarial activities of artemisone and other arteminisins: the unlikehood of C-centered radicals as bioactive intermediates. ChemMedChem 2007; 2(10): 1480-97.

[148] Haynes RK, Vonwiller SC. The behaviour of qinghaosu (artemisinin) in the presence of heme iron(II) and (III). Tetrahedron Letters 1996; 37(2): 253-56.

[149] Olliaro PL, Haynes RK, Meunier B, Yuthavong Y. Possible modes of action of the artemisinin-type compounds. Trends in Parasitology 2001; 17(3): 122-26.

[150] Zhang S, Gerhard G. Heme activates artemisinin more efficiently than hemin, inorganic iron, or hemoglobin. Bioorganic Medicinal Chemistry 2008; 16(16): 7853-61.

[151] Hartwig CL, Rosenthal AS, D'Angelo J, *et al.* Accumulation of artemisinin trioxane derivatives within neutral lipids of *Plasmodium falciparum* malaria parasites is endoperoxide-dependent. Biochemical Pharmacology 2009; 77(3): 322-36.

[152] Ashton M, Gordi T, Hai TN, *et al.* Artemisinin pharmacokinetics in healthy adults after 250, 500 and 1000 mg single oral doses. Biopharmaceutics & Drug Disposition 1998; 19(4): 245-50.

[153] Dien TK, de Vries PJ, Khanh NX, *et al.* Effect of food intake on pharmacokinetics of oral artemisinin in healthy Vietnamese subjects. Antimicrobial Agents and Chemotherapy 1997; 41(5): 1069-72.

[154] Hassan AM, Ashton M, Kihamia CM, *et al.* Multiple dose pharmacokinetics of oral artemisinin and comparison of its efficacy with that of oral artesunate in falciparum malaria patients. Transactions of the Royal Society of Tropical Medicine & Hygiene; 90(1): 61-5.

[155] Newton PN, van Vugt M, Teja-Isavadharm P *et al.* Comparison of oral artesunate and dihydroartemisinin antimalarial bioavailabilities in acute falciparum malaria. Antimicrobial Agents and Chemotherapy 2002; 46(4): 1125-27.

[156] Silamut K, Newton PN, Teja-Isavadharm P, *et al.* Artemether bioavailability after oral or intramuscular administration in uncomplicated falciparum malaria. Antimicrobial Agents and Chemotherapy 2003; 47(12): 3795-98.

[157] Teja-Isavadharm P, Nosten F, Kyle DE, *et al.* Comparative bioavailability of oral, rectal, and intramuscular artemether in healthy subjects: use of simultaneous measurement by high performance liquid chromatography and bioassay. British Journal of Clinical Pharmacology 1996; 42(5): 599-04.

[158] Looareesuwan S, Oosterhuis B, Schilizzi BM, *et al.* Dose-finding & efficacy study for i.m. artemotil (beta-arteether) and comparison with i.m. artemether in acute uncomplicated *P. falciparum* malaria. British Journal of Clinical Pharmacology 2002; 53(5): 492-00.

[159] Batty KT, Thu LT, Davis TM, *et al.* A pharmacokinetic and pharmacodynamic study of intravenous *vs* oral artesunate in uncomplicated falciparum malaria. British Journal of Clinical Pharmacology 1998; 45(2): 123-29.

[160] Newton P, Suputtamongkol Y, Teja-Isavadharm P, *et al.* Antimalarial bioavailability and disposition of artesunate in acute falciparum malaria. Antimicrobial Agents and Chemotherapy 2000; 44(4): 972-77.

[161] Morris CA, Duparc S, Borghini-Fuhrer I, *et al.* Review of the clinical pharmacokinetics of artesunate and its active metabolite dihydroartemisinin following intravenous, intramuscular, oral or rectal administration. Malaria Journal 2011; 10: 263.

[162] Newton P.N., van Vugt M., Teja-Isavadharm P., Comparison of oral artesunate and dihydroartemisinin antimalarial bioavailabilities in acute falciparum malaria. Antimicrobial Agents and Chemotherapy 2002; 46(4): 1125-27.

[163] Binh TQ, Illett KF, Batty KT, *et al.* Oral bioavailability of dihydroartemisinin in Vietnamese volunteers and in patients with falciparum malaria. British Journal of Clinical Pharmacology 2001; 51(6): 541-46.

[164] Rieckman KH. Antibiotics. In: Peters W, Richards WHG, Eds. Antimalarial Drugs II: Handbook of Experimental Pharmacology vol 68/2. Berlin, Springer 1984; pp 443-70.

[165] Fichera ME, Roos DS. A plastid organelle as a drug target in apicomplexan parasites. Nature 1997; 390(6658): 407-409.

[166] Fleige T, Limenitakis J, Soldati-Favre D. Apicoplast: keep it or leave it. Microbes and Infection 2010; 12(4): 253-62.

[167] Pradel G, Schlitzer M. Antibiotics in malaria therapy and their effect on the parasite apicoplast. Current Molecular Medicine 2010; 10(3): 335-49.

[168] Nzila A, Ma Z, Chibale K. Drug repositioning in the treatment of malaria and TB. Future Medicinal Chemistry 2011; 3(11): 1413-26.

[169] Dahl EL, Rosenthal PJ. Multiple antibiotics exert delayed effects against the *Plasmodium falciparum* apicoplast. Antimicrobial Agents and Chemotherapy 2007; 51(10): 3485-90.

[170] Lim L, McFadden GI. The evolution, metabolism and functions of the apicoplast. Philosophical Transactions of the Royal Society B 2010; 365(1541): 749-63.

[171] Noedl H. ABC - antibiotics-based combinations for the treatment of severe malaria? Trends in Parasitology 2009; 25(12): 540-44.

[172] Chopra I, Roberts, M. Tetracycline antibiotics: mode of action, applications, molecular biology, and epidemiology of bacterial resistance. Microbiology and Molecular Biology Reviews 2001; 65(2): 232-60.

[173] Patrick GL. An Introduction to Medicinal Chemistry. Oxford: University Press 2009.

[174] Pradines B, Rogier C, Fusai T, *et al. In vitro* activities of antibiotics against *Plasmodium falciparum* are inhibited by iron. Antimicrobial Agents and Chemotherapy 2001; 45(6): 1746-750.

[175] Griffith KS, Lewis LS, Mali S, *et al.* Treatment of malaria in the United States. A systematic review. The Journal of the American Medical Association 2007; 297(20): 2264-277.

[176] Ekland EH, Schneider J, Fidock DA. Identifying apicoplast-targeting antimalarials using highthroughput compatible approaches. FASEB Journal 2011; 25(10): 3583-93.

[177] Agwuh KN, MacGowan A. Pharmacokinetics and pharmacodynamics of the tetracyclines including glycylcyclines. Journal of Antimicrobial Chemotherapy 2006; 58(2): 256-65.

[178] Welling PG, Koch PA, Lau CC *et al.* Bioavailability of tetracycline and doxycycline in fasted and nonfasted subjects. Antimicrobial Agents and Chemotherapy 1977; 11(3): 462-69.

[179] Karbwang J, Na-Bangchang K, Thanavibul A, *et al.* Comparison of oral artesunate and quinine plus tetracycline in acute uncomplicated falciparum malaria. Bulletin of the World Health Organization 1994; 72(2): 233-238.

[180] Clyde DF, DuPont HL, Hornick RB, *et al.* Antimalarial effects of tetracyclines in man. The Journal of Tropical Medicine and Hygiene 1971; 74(11): 238-42.

[181] Connor BA. Expert recommendations for antimalarial prophylaxis. Journal of Travel Medicine 2001; 8(Suppl 3): S57-S64.

[182] Tan KR, Magill AJ, Parise ME, *et al.* Doxycycline for malaria chemoprophylaxis and treatment: report from the CDC expert meeting on malaria chemoprophylaxis. The American Journal of Tropical Medicine and Hygiene 2011; 84(4): 517-31.

[183] Wiesner J, Henschker D, Hutchinson DB *et al. In vitro* and *in vivo* synergy of fosmidomycin, a novel antimalarial drug, with clindamycin. Antimicrobial Agents and Chemotherapy 2002; 46(9): 2889-94.

[184] Pradines B, Spiegel A, Rogier C, *et al.* Antibiotics for prophylaxis of *Plasmodium faciparum* infections: *in vitro* activity of doxycycline against Senegalese isolates. The American Journal of Tropical Medicine and Hygiene 2000; 62(1): 82-5.

[185] Briolant S, Fusaï T, Rogier C, *et al.* Tetracycline antibiotics in malaria. The Open Tropical Medicine Journal 2008; 1: 31-46.

[186] Nelis HJ, de Leenheer AP. Evidence for metabolic inertness of doxycycline. Journal of Pharmaceutical Sciences 1981; 70(2): 226-28.

[187] Newton PN, Chaulet J-F, Brockman A, *et al.* Pharmacokinetics of oral doxycycline during combination treatment of severe falciparum malaria. Antimicrobial Agents and Chemotherapy 2005; 49(4): 1622-25.

[188] Peragallo MS, Croft AM, Kitchener SJ. Malaria during a multinational military deployment: the comparative experience of the Italian, British and Australian Forces in East Timor. Transactions of the Royal Society of Tropical Medicine & Hygiene 2002; 96(5): 481-82.

[189] Spízek J, Rezanka T. Lincomycin, clindamycin and their applications. Applied Microbiology and Biotechnology 2004; 64(4): 455-64.

[190] Smieja M. Current indications for the use of clindamycin: A critical review. Canadian Journal of Infectious Diseases 1998; 9(1): 22-8.

[191] Clyde, DF, Gilman RH, McCarthy VC. Antimalarial effects of clindamycin in man. The American Journal of Tropical Medicine and Hygiene 1975; 24(2): 369-70.

[192] Lell B, Kremsner PG. Clindamycin as an antimalarial drug: review of clinical trials. Antimicrobial Agents and Chemotherapy 2002; 46(8): 2315-320.

[193] Chow AW, Jewesson PJ. Pharmacokinetics and safety of antimicrobial agents during pregnancy. Reviews of Infectious Diseases 1985; 7(3): 287-13.

[194] Philipson A, Sabath LD, and D. Charles. Erythromycin and clindamycin absorption and elimination in pregnant women. Clinical Pharmacology and Therapeutics 1976; 19(1): 68-77.

[195] Auerbach T, Bashan A, Harms J, *et al.* Antibiotics targeting ribosomes: crystallographic studies. Current Drug Targets. Infectious Disorders 2002; 2(2): 169-86.

[196] Wilson DN, Harms JM, Nierhaus KH, *et al.* Species-specific antibiotic-ribosome interactions: implications for drug development. Biological Chemistry 2005; 386(12): 1239-252.

[197] Dahl EL, Rosenthal PJ. Apicoplast translation, transcription and genome replication: targets for antimalarial antibiotics. Trends in Parasitology 2008; 24(6): 279-84.

[198] Gatfi G, Flaherty J, Bubp J, *et al.* Comparative study of bioavailabilities and pharmacokinetics of clindamycin in healthy volunteers and patients with AIDS. Antimicrobial Agents and Chemotherapy 1993; 37(5): 1137-143.

[199] Obonyo CO, Juma EA. Clindamycin plus quinine for treating uncomplicated falciparum malaria: a systematic review and meta-analysis. Malaria Journal 2012; 11: 2.

[200] Pukrittayakamee S, Chantra A, Vanijanonta S, *et al.* Therapeutic responses to quinine and clindamycin in multidrug-resistant falciparum malaria. Antimicrobial Agents and Chemotherapy 2000; 44(9): 2395-398.

[201] Mutak S. Azalides from azithromycin to new azalide derivatives. Journal of Antibiotics 2007; 60(2): 85-122.

[202] Kobrehel G, Djokic S (PLIVA). Nouveaux derives de l'erythromycine A. Procede pour leur preparation et leur utilisation comme substances antibacteriennes, BE 892 357, July 1, 1982.

[203] Kobrehel G, Radobolja G, Tamburasev Z, *et al.* (PLIVA). 11-Aza-10-deoxo-10-dihydroerythromycin A and derivatives thereof as well as a process for their preparation. Patent US 4328334. 1982.

[204] Dunn CJ, Barradell LB. Azithromycin: a review of its pharmacological properties and use as a 3-day therapy in respiratory tract infection. Drugs 1996; 51(3): 483-05.

[205] Gingras BA, Jensen JB. Antimalarial activity of azithromycin and erythromycin against *Plasmodium berghei*. The American Journal of Tropical Medicine and Hygiene 1993; 49(1): 101-05.

[206] Kuschner RA, Heppner DG, Andersen SL, *et al.* Azithromycin prophylaxis against a chloroquine-resistant strain of *Plasmodium falciparum*. The Lancet 1994; 343(8910): 1396-397.

[207] Anderson SL, Berman J, Kuschner R, *et al.* Prophylaxis of *Plasmodium falciparum* malaria with azithromycin administered to volunteers. Annals of Internal Medicine 1995; 123(10): 771-73.

[208] Nakornchai S, Konthiang P. Activity of azithromycin or erythromycin in combination with antimalarial drugs against multidrug-resistant *Plasmodium falciparum in vitro.* Acta Tropica 2006; 100(3): 185-91.

[209] Ekhland EH, Schneider J, Fidock DA, *et al.* Identifying apicoplast targeting antimalarials using high-throughput compatible approaches. The FASEB Journal 2011; 25(10): 3583-93.

[210] Friesen JO, Silvie ED, Putrianti JC, *et al.* Natural immunization against malaria: Causal prophylaxis with antibiotics. Science Translational Medicine 2010; 2(40): 40-9.

[211] Dahl EL, Rosenthal PJ. Multiple antibiotics exert delayed effects against the *Plasmodium falciparum* apicoplast. Antimicrobial Agents and Chemotherapy 2007; 51(10): 3485-90.

[212] Taylor WR, Richie TL, Fryauff DJ, *et al.* Malaria prophylaxis using azithromycin: a double-blind, placebo-controlled trial in Irian Jaya, Indonesia. Clinical Infectious Diseases 1999; 28(1): 74-81.

[213] Andersen SL, Oloo AJ, Gordon DM, *et al.* Successful double-blinded, randomized, placebo-controlled field trial of azithromycin and doxycycline as prophylaxis for malaria in western Kenya. Clinical Infectious Diseases 1998; 26(1): 146-50.

[214] van Eijk AM, Terlouw DJ. Azithromycin for treating uncomplicated malaria. Cochrane Database of Systematic Reviews 2011, Issue 2. Art. No.: CD006688.

[215] Andersen SL, Ager A, McGreevy P, *et al.* Activity of azithromycin as a blood schizonticide against rodent and human plasmodia *in vivo.* The American Journal of Tropical Medicine and Hygiene 1995; 52(2): 159-61.

[216] Thriemer K, Starzengruber P, Khan WA, *et al.* Azithromycin combination therapy for the treatment of uncomplicated falciparum malaria in Bangladesh: An open-label randomized, controlled clinical trial. The Journal of Infectious Diseases 2010; 392-98.

[217] Sidhu ABS, Sun Q, Nkrumah LJ, *et al. In vitro* efficacy, resistance selection, and structural modeling studies implicate the malarial parasite apicoplast as the target of azithromycin. The Journal of Biological Chemistry 2007; 282(4): 2494-04.

[218] Chico RM, Pittrof R, Greenwood B, *et al.* Azithromycin-chloroquine and the intermittent preventive treatment of malaria in pregnancy. Malaria Journal 2008; 7: 255.

[219] McEvoy GK, Ed. American Hospital Formulary Service - Drug Information 2003. Bethesda, MD: American Society of Health-System Pharmacists, Inc. (Plus Supplements) 2003; pp. 302-04.

[220] Price R, Van Vugt M, Phaipun L, *et al.* Adverse effects in patients with acute falciparum malaria treated with artemisinin derivatives. American Journal of Tropical Medicine and Hygiene 1999; 60(4): 547-55.

[221] Ahmed MU, Islam MS, Shohag H, *et al.* Comparative pharmacokinetic and bioequivalence study of azithromycin 500 mg tablet in healthy Bangladeshi volunteers. International Journal of Clinical Pharmacology and Therapeutics 2012; 50(6): 452-58.

[222] Sinclair D, Zani B, Donegan S, Olliaro P, Garner P. Artemisinin-based combination therapy for treating uncomplicated malaria. Cochrane Database of Systematic Reviews 2009, Issue 3. Art. No.: CD007483.

[223] Castelli F, Tomasoni LR, Matteelli A. Advances in the treatment of malaria. Mediterranean Journal of Hematology and Infectious Diseases 2012; 4(1): e2012064.

[224] Ibezim EC, Odo U. Current trends in malarial chemotherapy. African Journal of Biotechnology 2008; 7(4): 349-56.

[225] Phyo AP, Nkhoma S, Stepniewska K, *et al.* Emergence of artemisinin-resistant malaria on the western border of Thailand: a longitudinal study. Lancet 2012; 379(9830): 1960-66.

[226] World Health Organization. Update on artemisinin resistance - April 2012. Available from: http://www.who.int/malaria/publications/atoz/arupdate042012.pdf

[227] Nosten F, White NJ. Artemisinin-based combination treatment of falciparum malaria. American Journal of Tropical Medicine and Hygiene 2007; 77(Suppl 6): 181-92.

[228] Jamsen KM, Duffull SB, Tarning J, *et al.* Optimal designs for population pharmacokinetic studies of oral artesunate in patients with uncomplicated falciparum malaria. Malaria Journal 2011; 10: 181.

[229] Faye B, Ndiaye J-L, Ndiaye D *et al.* Efficacy and tolerability of four antimalarial combinations in the treatment of uncomplicated *Plasmodium falciparum* malaria in Senegal. Malaria Journal 2007; 6: 80.

[230] Orrell C, Little F, Smith P, *et al.* Pharmacokinetics and tolerability of artesunate and amodiaquine alone and in combination in healthy volunteers. European Journal of Clinical Pharmacology 2008; 64(7): 683-90.

[231] Faye B, Ndiaye J-L, Ndiaye D *et al.* Efficacy and tolerability of four antimalarial combinations in the treatment of uncomplicated *Plasmodium falciparum* malaria in Senegal. Malaria Journal 2007; 6: 80.

[232] Krudsood S, Looareesuwan S, Tangpukdee N, *et al.* New fixed-dose artesunate-mefloquine formulation against multidrug-resistant *Plasmodium falciparum* in adults: a comparative phase iib safety and pharmacokinetic study with standard-dose nonfixed artesunate plus mefloquine. Antimicrobial Agents and Chemotherapy 2010; 54(9): 3730-37.

[233] Martinelli A, Moreira R, Cravo PVL. Malaria combination therapies: advantages and shortcomings. Mini-Reviews in Medicinal Chemistry 2008; 8(3): 201-12.

[234] Guthmanna J-P, Ampuerob J, Fortes F, *et al.* Antimalarial efficacy of chloroquine, amodiaquine, sulfadoxine-pyrimethamine, and the combinations of amodiaquine + artesunate and sulfadoxine-pyrimethamine + artesunate in Huambo and Bié provinces, central Angola. Transactions of the Royal Society of Tropical Medicine and Hygiene 2005; 99(7): 485-492.

[235] Dondorp AM, Nosten F, Yi P, *et al.* Artemisinin resistance in *Plasmodium falciparum* malaria. The New England Journal of Medicine 2009; 361(5): 455-67.

[236] Karbwang J, Na Bangchang K, Thanavibul A, *et al.* Pharmacokinetics of mefloquine alone or in combination with artesunate. Bulletin of the World Health Organization 1994; 72(1): 83-87.

[237] Minzi OMS, Gupta A, Haule AF, *et al.* Lack of impact of artesunate on the disposition kinetics of sulfadoxine/pyrimethamine when the two drugs are concomitantly administered. European Journal of Clinical Pharmacology 2007; 63(5): 457-62.

[238] Ibrahium AM, Kheir MM, Osman ME *et al.* Efficacies of artesunate plus either sulfadoxine-pyrimethamine or amodiaquine, for the treatment of uncomplicated *Plasmodium falciparum* malaria in eastern Sudan. Annals of Tropical Medicine and Parasitology 2007; 101(1): 15-21.

[239] Ashley EA, Stepniewska K, Lindegårdh, *et al.* How much fat is necessary to optimize lumefantrine oral bioavailability? Tropical Medicine and International Health 2007; 12(2): 195-00.

[240] Colussi D, Parisot C, Legay F *et al.* Binding of artemether and lumefantrine to plasma proteins and erythrocytes. European Journal of Pharmaceutical Sciences 1999; 9(1): 9-16.

[241] Lefèvre G, Looareesuwan S, Treeprasertsuk S, *et al.* A clinical and pharmacokinetic trial of six doses of artemether-lumefantrine for multidrug-resistant *Plasmodium falciparum*

malaria in Thailand. American Journal of Tropical Medicine and Hygiene 2001; 64 (5,6): 247-56.

[242] Ezzet F, van Vugt M, Nosten F, *et al.* Pharmacokinetics and pharmacodynamics of lumefantrine (benflumetol) in acute falciparum malaria. Antimicrobial Agents and Chemotherapy 2000; 44(3): 697-04.

[243] van Agtmael MA, Cheng-Qi S, Qing JX, *et al.* Multiple dose pharmacokinetics of artemether in Chinese patients with uncomplicated falciparum malaria. International Journal of Antimicrobial Agents 1999; 12(2): 151-58.

[244] White NJ, van Vugt M, Ezzet F. Clinical pharmacokinetics and pharmacodynamics of artemether-lumefantrine. Clinical Pharmacokinetics 1999; 37(2): 105-25.

[245] Omari AAA, Gamble CL, Garner P. Artemether-lumefantrine for treating uncomplicated falciparum malaria. Cochrane Database of Systematic Reviews 2003, Issue 2. Art. No.: CD003125.

[246] Wong RPM, Salman S, Ilett KF, *et al.* Desbutyl-lumefantrine is a metabolite of lumefantrine with potent *in vitro* antimalarial activity that may influence artemether-lumefantrine treatment outcome. Antimicrobial Agents and Chemotherapy 2011; 55(3): 1194-98.

[247] Na-Bangchang K, Krudsood S, Silachamroon U, *et al.*The pharmacokinetics of oral dihydroartemisinin and artesunate in healthy Thai volunteers. Southeast Asian Journal of Tropical Medicine and Public Health 2004; 35(3): 575-82.

[248] Liu C, Zhang R, Hong X, *et al.* Pharmacokinetics of piperaquine after single and multiple oral administrations in healthy volunteers. Yakugaku Zasshi 2007; 127(10): 1709-14.

[249] Hong X, Liu C-H, Huang X-T, *et al.* Pharmacokinetics of dihydroartemisinin in Artekin tablets for single and repeated dosing in Chinese healthy volunteers. Biopharmaceutics & Drug Disposition 2008; 29(4): 237-44.

[250] Chinh NT, Quang NN, Thanh NX, *et al.* Pharmacokinetics and bioequivalence evaluation of two fixed-dose tablet formulations of dihydroartemisinin and piperaquine in Vietnamese subjects. Antimicrobial Agents and Chemotherapy 2009; 53(2): 828-31.

[251] Nguyen DVH, Van Hoang D, Nguyen QP, *et al.* Pharmacokinetics and *ex vivo* pharmacodynamic antimalarial activity of dihydroartemisinin-piperaquine in patients with uncomplicated falciparum malaria in Vietnam. Antimicrobial Agents and Chemotherapy 2009; 53(8): 3534-37.

[252] Binh TQ, Ilett KF, Batty KT, *et al.* Oral bioavailability of dihydroartemisinin in Vietnamese volunteers and in patients with falciparum malaria. British Journal of Clinical Pharmacology, 51(6), 541-46.

[253] Wilairatana P, Krudsood S, Sombat T, *et al.* The future outlook of antimalarial drugs and recent work on the treatment of malaria. Archives of Medical Research 2002; 3(4): 416-21.

[254] White NJ. Assessment of the pharmacodynamic properties of antimalarial drugs *in vivo*. Antimicrobial Agents and Chemotherapy 1997; 41(7):1413-22.

[255] Barnes KI, Watkins WM, White NJ. Antimalarial dosing regimens and drug resistance. Trends in Parasitology 2008; 24(3): 127-34.

[256] Antimalarial drug resistance, N. J. White, The Journal of Clinical Investigation 2004; 113(8): 1084-92.

[257] Talisuna AO, Bloland P and D'Alessandro U. History, dynamics, and public health importance of malaria parasite resistance. Clinical Microbiology Reviews 2004; 17(1): 235-54.

[258] Woodrow CJ, Krishna S. Antimalarial drugs: recent advances in molecular determinants of resistance and their clinical significance. Cellular and Molecular Life Sciences 2006; 63(14): 1586-96.

[259] Kano S, Kimura M. Trends in malaria cases in Japan. Acta Tropica 2004; 89(3) 271-78.

[260] Olliaro PL, Yuthavong Y. An overview of chemotherapeutic targets for antimalarial drug discovery, Pharmacology & Therapeutics 1999; 81(2): 91-10.

[261] Rosenthal PJ. Antimalarial drug discovery: old and new approaches. The Journal of Experimental Biology 2003; 206(Pt 21), 3735-44.

[262] Padmanaban G, Nagaraj VA, Rangarajan PN. Drugs and drug targets against malaria. Current Science 2007; 92(11): 1545-55.

[263] Medicines for Malaria Venture. MMV at a Glance, July 2012. Available from http://www.mmv.org/sites/default/files/uploads/docs/publications/at%20a%20glance.pdf

[264] BIO Ventures for Global Health (BVGH). Global Health Landscape, a Report. 2010. Available from: http://www.bvgh.org/Biopharmaceutical-Solutions/Data-Center/BVGH-Reports.aspx

[265] UNITAID, World Health Organization. HIV, tuberculosis and malaria medicines landscape. Progress report on emerging issues and potential opportunities to improve access. WHO, Geneva, 2012. Available from: http://www.accesstomedicineindex.org/sites/www.accesstomedicineindex.org/files/unitaid_hiv_tuberculosis_and_malaria_medicines_landscape_2012.pdf

[266] Medicines for Malaria Venture. The Global Malaria Portfolio, 1Q 2012. 2012. Available from: http://www.mmv.org/research-development/science-portfolio

[267] Suvarna V. Phase IV of Drug Development. Perspectives in Clinical Research 2010; 1(2): 57-60.

[268] Khalil IF, Rønn AM, Alifrangis M, *et al.* Response of *Plasmodium falciparum* to cotrimoxazole therapy: relationship with plasma drug concentrations and dihydrofolate reductase and dihydropteroate synthase genotypes. American Journal of Tropical Medicine and Hygiene 2005; 73(1): 174-77.

[269] Valecha N, Looareesuwan S, Martensson A, *et al.* Arterolane, a new synthetic trioxolane for treatment of uncomplicated *Plasmodium falciparum* malaria: a phase II, multicenter, randomized, dose-finding clinical trial. Clinical Infectious Diseases 2010; 51(6): 684-91.

[270] Diallo D, Graz B, Falquet J, *et al.* Malaria treatment in remote areas of Mali: use of modern and traditional medicines, patient outcome. Transactions of the Royal Society of Tropical Medicine and Hygiene 2006; 100(6): 515-20.

[271] Graz B, Willcox ML, Diakite C, *et al.* Argemone mexicana decoction *versus* artesunate-amodiaquine for the management of malaria in Mali: policy and public-health implications. Transactions of the Royal Society of Tropical Medicine and Hygiene 2010; 104(1): 33-41.

[272] Mesia K, Cimanga K, Tona L, *et al.* Assessment of the short-term safety and tolerability of a quantified 80% ethanol extract from the stem bark of *Nauclea pobeguinii* (PR 259 CT1) in healthy volunteers: A clinical phase I study. Planta Medica 2011; 77(2): 111-16.

[273] Wiesner J, Henschker D, Hutchinson DB, *et al. In vitro* and *in vivo* synergy of fosmidomycin, a novel antimalarial drug, with clindamycin. Antimicrobial Agents and Chemotherapy 2002; 46(9): 2889-94.

[274] Lell B, Ruangweerayut R, Wiesner J, *et al.* Fosmidomycin, a novel chemotherapeutic agent for malaria, Antimicrobial Agents and Chemotherapy 2003; 47(2): 735-38.

[275] Gutteridge W, Hutchinson D, New drug combinations for the treatment of malaria. EP 2404601A1. 2012.

[276] Zoungrana A, Coulibaly B, Sié A, *et al.* Safety and efficacy of methylene blue combined with artesunate or amodiaquine for uncomplicated falciparum malaria: a randomized controlled trial from Burkina Faso. Plos One 2008; 3(2): e1630.

[277] Coulibaly B, Zoungrana A, Mockenhaupt FP, *et al.* Strong gametocytocidal effect of methylene blue-based combination therapy against falciparum malaria: a randomised controlled trial. PLOS One 2009; 4(5): e5318.

[278] Adjalleya SH, Johnston GL, Li T, *et al.* Quantitative assessment of *Plasmodium falciparum* sexual development reveals potent transmission-blocking activity by methylene blue. Proceedings of the National Academy of Sciences of the United States of America 2011; 108 (47): E1214-23.

[279] Snyder C, Chollet J, Santo-Tomas J, *et al. In vitro* and *in vivo* interaction of synthetic peroxide RBx11160 (OZ277) with piperaquine in *Plasmodium* models. Experimental Parasitology 2007; 115 (3) 296-00.

[280] Charmana SA, Arbe-Barnesb S, Bathurstc IC, *et al.* Synthetic ozonide drug candidate OZ439 offers new hope for a single-dose cure of uncomplicated malaria. Proceedings of the National Academy of Sciences of the United States of America 2011; 108(11): 4400-05.

[281] Rottmann M, McNamara C, Yeung BKS, *et al.* Spiroindolones, a potent compound class for the treatment of malaria. Science 2010; 329(5996): 1175-80.

[282] van Pelt-Koops JC, Pett HE, Graumans W, *et al.* The spiroindolone drug candidate NITD609 potently inhibits gametocytogenesis and blocks *Plasmodium falciparum* transmission to *Anopheles* mosquito vector. Antimicrobial Agents and Chemotherapy 2012; 56(7): 3544-48.

[283] Biot C, Daher W, Ndiaye CM, *et al.* Probing the role of the covalent linkage of ferrocene into a chloroquine template. Journal of Medicinal Chemistry 2006; 49(15): 4707-14.

[284] Leimanis ML, Jaidee A, Sriprawat K, *et al. Plasmodium vivax* susceptibility to ferroquine. Antimicrobial Agents and Chemotherapy 2010; 54(5): 2228-30.

[285] Biot C, Nosten F, Fraisse L, *et al.* The antimalarial ferroquine: from bench to clinic. Parasite 2011; 18(3), 207-14.

[286] Biot C. Ferroquine: A new weapon in the fight against malaria. Current Medicinal Chemistry - Anti-Infective Agents 2004; 3(2): 135-47.

[287] Haynes RK, Fugmann B, Stetter J, *et al.* Artemisone - a highly active antimalarial drug of the artemisinin class. Angewandte Chemie International Edition 2006; 45(13): 2082-88.

[288] Pooley S, Fatih FA, Krishna S., *et al.* Artemisone uptake in *Plasmodium falciparum*-infected erythrocytes. Antimicrobial Agents and Chemotherapy 2011; 55(2): 550-56.

[289] Schmuck G, Temerowski M, Haynes RK, *et al.* Identification of non-neurotoxic artemisinin derivatives *in vivo* and *in vitro*. In: Research Advances in Antimicrobial Agents and Chemotherapy, vol 5. Kerala, Global Research Network, Hkust Scholarly Publications, 2003; pp. 35-47.

[290] Peyrottes S, Caldarelli S, Wein S, *et al.* Choline analogues in malaria chemotherapy. Current Pharmaceutical Design 2012; 18(24): 3454-66.

[291] Calas M, Ancelin ML, Cordina G, *et al.* Antimalarial activity of compounds interfering with *Plasmodium falciparum* phospholipid metabolism: comparison between mono- and bisquaternary ammonium salts. Journal of Medicinal Chemistry 2000; 43(3): 505-16.

[292] Caldarelli SA, El Fangour S, Wein S, *et al.* New bis-thiazolium analogues as potential antimalarial agents: design, synthesis, and biological evaluation. Journal of Medicinal Chemistry 2013; 56(2): 496-09.

[293] Burrows JN, Chibale K, Wells TNC. The state of the art in anti-malarial drug discovery and development. Current Topics in Medicinal Chemistry 2011; 11(10): 1226-54.

[294] Ashley EA, Stepniewska K, Lindegårdh N, *et al.* Population pharmacokinetic assessment of a new regimen of mefloquine used in combination treatment of uncomplicated falciparum malaria. Antimicrobial Agents and Chemotherapy 2006; 50(7): 2281-85.

[295] Finaurini S, Basilico N, Corbett Y, *et al.* Dihydroartemisinin inhibits the human erythroid cell differentiation by altering the cell cycle. Toxicology 2012; 300(1-2): 57-66.

[296] Krishna S, Planche T, Agbenyega T, *et al.* Bioavailability and preliminary clinical efficacy of intrarectal artesunate in Ghanian children with moderate malaria. Antimicrobial Agents and Chemotherapy 2001; 45(2): 509-16.

[297] Advisory Committee; FDA Division of Anti-Infective Drug Products. Briefing document on artesunate rectal capsules. 2010. Available from: http://www.fda.gov/downloads/AdvisoryCommittees/CommitteesMeetingMaterials/Drugs/Anti-InfectiveDrugsAdvisoryCommittee/UCM2099 23.pdf

[298] Krishna S, Planche T, Agbenyega T, *et al.* Bioavailability and preliminary clinical efficacy of intrarectal artesunate in Ghanian children with moderate malaria. Antimicrobial Agents and Chemotherapy 2001; 45(2): 509-16.

[299] Department of Health and Human Services, United States Food and Drug Administration Center for Drug Evaluation and Research: Anti-infective Drugs Advisory Committee. Paper mill reporting 301 495-5831: Artesunate. 2010.

[300] Wong RPM, Lautu D, Tavul L, *et al. In vitro* sensitivity of *Plasmodium falciparum* to conventional and novel antimalarial drugs in Papua New Guinea. Tropical Medicine & International Health 2010; 15(3): 342-49.

[301] Chico RM, Pittrof R, Greenwood B, *et al.* Azithromycin-chloroquine and the intermittent preventive treatment of malaria in pregnancy. Malaria Journal 2008; 7: 255.

[302] Noedl H, Wernsdorfer WH, Krudsood S, *et al.* Antimalarial activity of azithromycin, artemisinin and dihydroartemisinin in fresh isolates of *Plasmodium falciparum* in Thailand. Acta Tropica 2001; 80 (1): 39-44.

[303] PubChem. Chloroquine - Compound Summary (CID 2719). Available from: http://pubchem.ncbi.nlm.nih.gov/summary/summary.cgi?cid=2719&loc=ec_rcs

[304] Cook JA, Randinitis EJ, Bramson CR, *et al.* Lack of a pharmacokinetic interaction between azithromycin and chloroquine. American Journal of Tropical Medicine and Hygiene 2006; 74(3): 407-12.

[305] Gingras BA, Jensen JB. Activity of azithromycin (CP-62,993) and erythromycin against chloroquine-sensitive and chloroquine-resistant strains of *Plasmodium falciparum in vitro*. American Journal of Tropical Medicine and Hygiene 1992; 47(3): 378-82.

[306] Nasveld P, Kitchener S. Treatment of acute vivax malaria with tafenoquine. Transactions of the Royal Society of Tropical Medicine and Hygiene 2005; 99(1): 2-5.

[307] Russell BM, Udomsangpetch R, Rieckmann KH, *et al.* Simple *in vitro* assay for determining the sensitivity of *Plasmodium vivax* isolates from flesh human blood to antimalarials in areas where *P. vivax* is endemic. Antimicrobial Agents and Chemotherapy 2003; 47(1): 170-73.

[308] Pradines B, Mamfoumbi MM, Tall A, *et al*. *In vitro* activity of tafenoquine against asexual blood stages of *Plasmodium falciparum* isolates from Gabon, Senegal, and Djibouti. Antimicrobial Agents and Chemotherapy 2006; 50(9): 3225-26.
[309] Gamage SA, Tepsiri N, Wilairat P, *et al*. Synthesis and *in vitro* evaluation of 9-anilino-3,6-diaminoacridines active against a multidrug-resistant strain of the malaria parasite *Plasmodium falciparum*. Journal of Medicinal Chemistry 1994; 37(10): 1486-94.
[310] Price RN, Marfurt J, Chalfein F, *et al*. *In vitro* activity of pyronaridine against multidrug-resistant *Plasmodium falciparum* and *Plasmodium vivax*. Antimicrobial Agents and Chemotherapy 2010; 54(12): 5146-50.
[311] Ramharter M, Kurth F, Schreier AC, *et al*. Fixed-dose pyronaridine-artesunate combination for treatment of uncomplicated *Falciparum malaria* in pediatric patients in Gabon. Journal of Infectious Diseases 2008; 198(6): 911-19.
[312] Stepniewska K, White NJ. Pharmokinetic determinants of the window of selection for antimalarial drug resistance. Antimicrobial Agents and Chemotherapy 2008; 52(5): 1589-96.
[313] European Medicines Agency. Eurartesim Assessement report. 2011. Available from: http://www.ema.europa.eu/docs/en_GB/document_library/EPAR_Public_assessment_report/human/001199/WC500118116.pdf
[314] Tarning J, Ashley EA, Lindegardh N, *et al*. Population pharmacokinetics of piperaquine after two different treatment regimens with dihydroartemisinin-piperaquine in patients with *Plasmodium falciparum* malaria in Thailand. Antimicrobial Agents and Chemotherapy 2008; 52(3): 1052-61.
[315] Salman S, Page-Sharp M, Batty KT, *et al*. A pharmacokinetic comparison of two piperaquine-containing artemisinin combination therapies in Papua New Guinean children with uncomplicated malaria. Antimicrobial Agents and Chemotherapy 2012; 56(6): 3288-97.
[316] Irish Pharmaceutical Healthcare Association Ltd. Eurartesim. Available from: http://www-medicines.ie./medicine/15397/SPC/Eurartesim+320+mg+40+mg+film+coated+tablets/medicines.ie
[317] Bassat Q, Mulenga M, Tinto H, *et al*. Dihydroartemisinin-piperaquine and artemether-lumefantrine for treating uncomplicated malaria in African children: a randomised, non-inferiority trial. Plos One 2009; 4(11): e7871.
[318] Uhlemann AC, Wittlin S, Matile H, *et al*. Mechanism of antimalarial action of the synthetic trioxolane RBX11160 (OZ277). Antimicrobial Agents and Chemotherapy 2007; 51(2): 667-72.
[319] Valecha N, Looareesuwan S, Martensson A., *et al*. Arterolane, a new synthetic trioxolane for treatment of uncomplicated *Plasmodium falciparum* malaria: a phase II, multicenter, randomized, dose-finding clinical trial. Clinical Infectious Diseases 2010; 51(6): 684-91.
[320] Valecha N, Krudsood S, Tangpukdee N, *et al*. Arterolane maleate and piperaquine phosphate combination for the treatment of uncomplicated *Plasmodium falciparum* malaria: a comparative, multicentre randomized clinical trial. Clinical Infectious Diseases 2012; 55(5): 663-71.
[321] Gasasira AF, Kamya MR, Ochong EO, *et al*. Effect of trimethoprim-sulphamethoxazole on the risk of malaria in HIV-infected Ugandan children living in an area of widespread antifolate resistance. Malaria Journal 2010; 9: 177.

[322] Daramola OO, Alonso PL, O'Dempsey TJD *et al*. Sensitivity of *Plasmodium falciparum* in The Gambia to co-trimoxazole. Transactions of the Royal Society of Tropical Medicine and Hygiene 1991, 85(3): 345-48.
[323] National Library of Medicine. National Center for Biotechnology Information: PubChem. Trimethoprim-Sulfamethoxazole Combination - Compound Summary (CID 358641). Available from: http://pubchem.ncbi.nlm.nih.gov/summary/summary.cgi?cid=358641&loc=ec_rcs
[324] Stevens RC, Laizure SC, Williams CL, *et al*. Pharmacokinetics and adverse effects of 20-mg/kg/day trimethoprim and 100-mg/kg/day sulfamethoxazole in healthy adult subjects. Antimicrobial Agents and Chemotherapy 1991; 35(9):1884-90.
[325] Khalil IF, Rønn AM, Alifrangis M, *et al*. Response of *Plasmodium falciparum* to cotrimoxazole therapy: relationship with plasma drug concentrations and dihydrofolate reductase and dihydropteroate synthase genotypes. American Journal of Tropical Medicine and Hygiene 2005; 73(1): 174-77.
[326] Fehintola, FA, Adedeji, AA, Tambo E *et al*. Cotrimoxazole in the treatment of acute uncomplicated falciparum malaria in Nigerian children: a controlled clinical trial. Clinical Drug Investigation 2004; 24(3): 149-55.
[327] Wang J-Y, Cao W-C, Shan C-Q, *et al*. Naphthoquine phosphate and its combination with artemisinin. Acta Tropica 2004; 89(3): 375-81.
[328] Hombhanje FW, Qingyun Huang Q. Artemisinin-naphthoquine combination ARCO®): An overview of the progress. Pharmaceuticals 2010; 3(12): 3581-93.
[329] Nigerian-German Chemical PLC. Arco. Available from: http://www.ngcplc.com/arco/arco.html
[330] Medhi B, Patyar S, Rao RS, *et al*. Pharmacokinetic and toxicological profile of artemisinin compounds: an update. Pharmacology 2009; 84(6): 323-32.
[331] Qu, HY, Gao HZ, Hao GT, *et al*. Single-dose safety, pharmacokinetics, and food effects studies of compound naphthoquine phosphate tablets in healthy volunteers. Journal of Clinical Pharmacology 2010; 50(11): 1310-18.
[332] Tjitra E, Armedy R, Hasugian AR, Siswantoro H, *et al*. Efficacy and safety of artemisinin-naphthoquine *versus* dihydroartemisinin-piperaquine in adult patients with uncomplicated malaria: a multi-centre study in Indonesia. Malaria Journal 2012; 11: 153.
[333] Rulisa S, Bendel D, Booles C. Pharmokinetics of artmether sublingual spray. Abstract number A1-050/48, 50th Interscience Conference on Antimicrobial Agents Chemotherapy, Boston MA, USA 2010; Available from: http://www.eastlandmedical.com.au/investors/announcements_news_media_releases/combined_announcements
[334] Van Pelt-Koops JC, Pett HE, Graumans W, *et al*. The spiroindolone drug candidate NITD609 potently inhibits gametocytogenesis and blocks *Plasmodium falciparum* transmission to *Anopheles* mosquito vector. Antimicrobial Agents and Chemotherapy 2012; 56(7): 3544-48.
[335] Moehrle JJ, Duparc S, Siethoff C, *et al*. First-in-man safety and pharmacokinetics of synthetic ozonide OZ439 demonstrates an improved exposure profile relative to other peroxide antimalarials. British Journal of Clinical Pharmacology 2013; 75(2): 535-48.
[336] Mombo-Ngoma G, Supan C, Dal-Bianco MP, *et al*. Phase I randomized dose-ascending placebo-controlled trials of ferroquine - a candidate anti-malarial drug - in adults with asymptomatic *Plasmodium falciparum* infection. Malaria Journal 2011; 10: 53.
[337] Mombo-Ngoma G, Supan C, Dal-Bianco MP, *et al*. Pharmacokinetics of ferroquine, a novel 4-aminoquinoline, in asymptomatic carriers of *Plasmodium falciparum* infections. Antimicrobial Agents and Chemotherapy 2012; 56(6): 3165-73.

[338] Leimanis ML, Jaidee A, Sriprawat K, *et al. Plasmodium vivax* susceptibility to ferroquine. Antimicrobial Agents and Chemotherapy 2010; 54(5): 2228-30.

[339] Na-Bangchang K, Ruengweerayut R, Karbwang J, *et al.* Pharmacokinetics and pharmacodynamics of fosmidomycin monotherapy and combination therapy with clindamycin in the treatment of multidrug resistant falciparum malaria. Malaria Journal 2007; 6: 70.

[340] Pascual A, Henry M, Briolant S, *et al. In vitro* activity of proveblue (methylene blue) on *Plasmodium falciparum* strains resistant to standard antimalarial drugs. Antimicrobial Agents and Chemotherapy 2011; 55(5): 2472-74.

[341] Haynes R, Fugmann B, Stetter J, *et al.* Artemisone - a highly active antimalarial drug of the artemisinin class. Angewandte Chemie International Edition 2006; 45(13): 2082-88.

[342] Ramharter M, Burkhardt D, Nemeth J, *et al.* Short report: *in vitro* activity of artemisone compared with artesunate against *Plasmodium falciparum.* American Journal of Tropical Medicine and Hygiene 2006; 75(4): 637-39.

[343] Nagelschmitz J, Voith B, Wensing G, *et al.* First assessment in humans of the safety, tolerability, pharmacokinetics, and *ex vivo* pharmacodynamic antimalarial activity of the new artemisinin derivative artemisone. Antimicrobial Agents and Chemotherapy 2008; 52(9): 3085-91.

[344] Wein S, Maynadier M, Van Ba CT, *et al.* Reliability of antimalarial sensitivity tests depends on drug mechanisms of action. Journal of Clinical Microbiology 2010; 48(5): 1651-60.

[345] Vial, HJ, Wein S, Farenc C, *et al.* Prodrugs of bisthiazolium salts are orally potent antimalarials. Proceedings of the National Academy of Sciences of the United States of America 2004; 101(43): 15458-63.

[346] O'Neill PM, Park BK, Shone AE, *et al.* Candidate selection and preclinical evaluation of *N-tert*-butyl isoquine (GSK369796), an affordable and effective 4-aminoquinoline antimalarial for the 21st century. Journal of Medicinal Chemistry 2009; 52(5), 1408-15.

[347] Ridley RG, Hofheinz W, Matile H, *et al.* 4-Aminoquinoline analogs of chloroquine with shortened side chains retain activity against chloroquine-resistant *Plasmodium falciparum.* Antimicrobial Agents and Chemotherapy 1996; 40(8): 1846-54.

[348] Mzayek F, Deng H, Mather FJ, *et al.* Randomized dose-ranging controlled trial of AQ-13, a candidate antimalarial, and chloroquine in healthy volunteers. PLoS Clinical Trials 2007; 2(1): DOI: 10.1371/journal.pctr.0020006.

[349] Tekwani BL, Walker LA. 8-Aminoquinolines: future role as antiprotozoal drugs. Current Opinion in Infectious Diseases 2006; 19(6): 623-31.

[350] Ager AL, Bartlett MS, Yardley V, *et al.* Antiparasitic activities and toxicities of individual enantiomers of the 8-aminoquinoline 8-[(4-amino-1-methylbutyl)amino]-6-methoxy-4-methyl-5-[3,4-dichlorophenoxy]quinoline succinate. Antimicrobial Agents and Chemotherapy 2008; 52(6): 2130-37.

[351] Zhang Y-K, Ge M, Plattner JJ. Recent progress in the synthesis of antimalarial agents. Organic Preparations and Procedures International 2012; 44(4): 340-74.

[352] Singh C, Puri SK. Substituted 1,2,4-trioxanes as antimalarial agents and a process of producing the substituted 1,2,4-trioxanes. US 6316493. 2001.

[353] O'Neill PM, Amewu RK, Nixon GL, *et al.* Identification of a 1,2,4,5-tetraoxane antimalarial drug-development candidate (RKA 182) with superior properties to the

semisynthetic artemisinins. Angewandte Chemie International Edition 2010; 49(33): 5693-97.

[354] Anthony MP, Burrows JN, Duparc S, *et al.* The global pipeline of new medicines for the control and elimination of malaria. Malaria Journal 2012, 11: 316

[355] Meunier B, Robert A. Heme as trigger and target for trioxane-containing antimalarial drugs. Accounts of Chemical Research 2010; 43 (11): 1444-51.

[356] Meunier B. Hybrid molecules with a dual mode of action: dream or reality? Accounts of Chemical Research 2008; 41(1): 69-77.

[357] Coslédan F, Fraisseb L, Pellet A. Selection of a trioxaquine as an antimalarial drug candidate. Proceedings of the National Academy of Sciences of the United States of America 2008; 105(45): 17579-84.

[358] Kalatova D, Bordacova J, Mikolasova P, *et al.* Safety, tolerability, pharmacokinetics and pharmacodynamics of sevuparin, a new depolymerised heparin to treat severe malaria. Talk or poster A1-060[a]. Emerging problems in public health, nursing and social work in tropical regions 2010. SEUC Pribram, Czech Republic.

[359] Leitgeb AM, Blomqvist K, Cho-Ngwa F, *et al.* Low anticoagulant heparin disrupts *Plasmodium falciparum* rosettes in fresh clinical isolates. American Journal of Tropical Medicine and Hygiene 2011; 84(3): 390-96.

[360] Meister S, Plouffe DM, Kuhen KL, *et al.* Imaging of *Plasmodium* liver stages to drive next-generation antimalarial drug discovery. Science 2011; 334(6061): 1372-77.

[361] Nagle A, Wu T, Kuhen K, *et al.* Imidazolopiperazines: lead optimization of the second-generation. Journal of Medicinal Chemistry 2012; 55(9), 4244-73.

[362] Binkert C, Boss C, Corminboeuf O, *et al.* Piperazine derivatives as antimalarial agents. WO2007046075A1. 2006. Chem. Abstr. 2007; 146: 462506, Also EP1940814A1. 2008.

[363] Coteron JM, Marco M, Esquivias J, *et al.* Structure-guided lead optimization of triazolopyrimidine-ring substituents identifies potent *Plasmodium falciparum* dihydroorotate dehydrogenase inhibitors with clinical candidate potential. Journal of Medicinal Chemistry 2011; 54(15), 5540-61.

[364] Chairman S. Antimalarial compounds with flexible side-chains. US20090099220A1. 2009.

[365] Cassera MB, Hazleton KZ, Merino EF, *et al.* (2011) *Plasmodium falciparum* parasites are killed by a transition state analogue of purine nucleoside phosphorylase in a primate animal model. PLoS ONE 6(11): e26916. doi:10.1371/journal.pone.0026916.

[366] Barker RH Jr, Urgaonkar S, Mazitschek R, *et al.* Aminoindoles, a novel scaffold with potent activity against *Plasmodium falciparum*. Antimicrobial Agents and Chemotherapy 2011; 55(6): 2612-22.

[367] Powles MA, Allocco J, Yeung L, *et al.* MK-4815, a potential new oral agent for treatment of malaria. Antimicrobial Agents and Chemotherapy 2012; 56(5): 2414-19.

[368] Chatterjee AK, Nagle A, Wu T, *et al.* Fused imidazoles and compositions comprising them for the treatment of parasitic diseases, such as *e.g.,* malaria. WO2011006143. 2011. Chem. Abstr. 2011; 154: 158494.

[369] Kappe SHI, Vaughan AM, Boddey JA, *et al.* That was then but this is now: malaria research in the time of an eradication agenda. Science 2010; 328(5980): 862-66.

[370] Feachem R, Sabat O. A new global malaria eradication strategy. The Lancet 2008; 371(9624): 1633-35.

[371] Fidock DA. Drug discovery: Priming the antimalarial pipeline. Nature 2010; 465 (7296): 297-298.

[372] Guiguemde WA, Shelat AA, Bouck D, *et al.* Chemical genetics of *Plasmodium falciparum*. Nature 2010; 465(7296): 311-15.

[373] Ekland EH, Fidock DA. *In vitro* evaluations of antimalarial drugs and their relevance to clinical outcomes. International Journal of Parasitology 2008; 38(7): 743-47.

[374] Plouffe D, Brinker A, McNamara C, *et al. In silico* activity profiling reveals the mechanism of action of antimalarials discovered in a high throughput screen. Proceedings of the National Academy of Sciences of the United states of America 2008; 105(26): 9059-64.

[375] Kotz J. Phenotypic screening, take two. Science-Business Exchange 2012; 5(15): doi:10.1038/scibx.2012.380.

[376] Gamo F-J, Sanz LM, Vidal J, *et al.* Thousands of chemical starting points for antimalarial lead identification. Nature 2010; 465(7296): 305-10.

[377] Guiguemde WA, Shelat AA, Garcia-Bustos JF, *et al.* Global phenotypic screening for antimalarials. Chemistry & Biology 2012; 19(1): 116-29.

[378] Calderón F, Barros D, Bueno JM *et al.* An invitation to open innovation in malaria drug discovery: 47 quality starting points from TCAMS. ACS Medicinal Chemistry Letters 2011; 2 (10): 741-46.

[379] Waver M, Bajorath J. Extracting SAR information from a large collection of anti-malarial screening hits by NSG-SPT analysis. ACS Medicinal Chemistry Letters 2011; 2(3): 201-06.

[380] Jomaa H, Wiesner J, Sanderbrand S, *et al.* Inhibitors of the nonmevalonate pathway of isoprenoid biosynthesis as antimalarial drugs. Science 1999; 285(5433): 1573-76.

[381] World Health Organization. Malaria Fact sheet 94. Geneva, WHO Press, 2011. Available online from: http://www.who.int/mediacentre/factsheets/fs094/en/.

[382] Pornthanakasem W, Kongkasuriyachai D, Uthaipibull C, *et al.* Plasmodium serine hydroxymethyltransferase: indispensability and display of distinct localization. Malaria Journal 2012, 11: 387.

[383] Boddey JA, Carvalho TG, Hodder AN, *et al.* Role of Plasmepsin V in Export of Diverse Protein Families from the Plasmodium falciparum Exportome. Traffic 2013; 14(5): 532-50.

[384] Moura PA, Dame JB, Fidock DA. Role of *Plasmodium falciparum* digestive vacuole plasmepsins in the specificity and antimalarial mode of action of cysteine and aspartic protease inhibitors. Antimicrobial Agents and Chemotherapy 2009; 53(12): 4968-78.

[385] Bullen HE, Charnaud SC, Kalanon M, *et al.* Biosynthesis, localization, and macromolecular arrangement of the *Plasmodium falciparum* translocon of exported proteins (PTEX). The Journal of Biological Chemistry 2011; 287(11): 7871-84.

[386] Baker RP, Wijetilaka R, Urban S. Two plasmodium rhomboid proteases preferentially cleave different adhesins implicated in all invasive stages of malaria. PLoS Pathogens 2006; 2(10): e113.

[387] Barale J-C, Blisnick T, Fujioka H, *et al. Plasmodium falciparum* subtilisin-like protease 2, a merozoite candidate for the merozoite surface protein 1-42 maturase. Proceedings of the National Academy of Sciences of the United States of America 1999; 96(11): 6445-50.

[388] Arastu-Kapur S, Ponder EL, Fonović UP, *et al.* Identification of proteases that regulate erythrocyte rupture by the malaria parasite Plasmodium falciparum. Nature Chemical Biology 2008; 4(3): 203-13.

[389] Alam A, Chauhan VS. Inhibitory potential of prodomain of *Plasmodium falciparum* protease serine repeat antigen 5 for asexual blood stages of parasite. PLoS ONE 2012; 7(1): e30452.

[390] Withers-Martinez C, Suarez C, Fulle S, *et al. Plasmodium* subtilisin-like protease 1 (SUB1): insights into the active-site structure, specificity and function of a pan-malaria drug target. International Journal of Parasitology 2012; 42(6): 597-12.

[391] Prudêncio M, Rodriguez A, Mota MM. The silent path to thousands of merozoites: the *Plasmodium* liver stage. Nature Reviews. Microbiology 2006; 4(11): 849-56.

[392] Delves M, Plouffe D, Scheurer C, *et al.* The activities of current antimalarial drugs on the life cycle stages of *Plasmodium*. A comparative study with human and rodent parasites. PloS Medicine 2012; 2: e1001169.

INDEX

A

Atta-ur-Rahman / M. Iqbal Choudhary (Eds)

B

C

D

E

F

G

H

I

J

K

L

M

N

Q

R

S

X

Made in the USA
Las Vegas, NV
03 November 2026

57424628R00250